Ultrasound of
Superficial Structures

Commissioning Editor: Geoff Nuttall
Copy Editors: Heather Russell, Ruth Swan
Indexer: Nina Boyd
Design Direction: Sarah Cape
Cover design: Keith Kail
Project Manager: Mark Sanderson
Sales Promotion Executive: Caroline Boyd

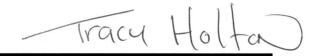

Ultrasound of Superficial Structures
High frequencies, Doppler and interventional procedures

Edited by

Luigi Solbiati MD
Department of Radiology, General Hospital,
Busto Arsizio (VA), Italy

Giorgio Rizzatto MD
Department of Radiology, General Hospital,
Gorizia, Italy

Foreword by
J. William Charboneau MD
Department of Radiology, Mayo Clinic,
Rochester, Minnesota, USA

CHURCHILL LIVINGSTONE
EDINBURGH HONG KONG LONDON MADRID MELBOURNE NEW YORK
AND TOKYO 1995

CHURCHILL LIVINGSTONE
An imprint of Harcourt Brace and Company Limited

© Harcourt Brace and Company Limited 1999

◢◗ is a registered trademark of Harcourt Brace and
Company Limited

First published 1995
Reprinted 1995
Reprinted 1999

ISBN 0 443 05131 3

British Library Cataloguing in Publication Data
A catalogue record for this book is available from the British
Library.

Library of Congress Cataloging in Publication Data
A catalog record for this book is available from the Library of
Congress.

Note
Medical knowledge is constantly changing. As new
information becomes available, changes in treatment,
procedures, equipment and the use of drugs become
necessary. The editors/authors/contributors and the
publishers have, as far as it is possible, taken care to ensure
that the information given in this text is accurate and up-to-
date. However, readers are strongly advised to confirm that
the information, especially with regard to drug usage,
complies with the latest legislation and standards of practice.

The
publisher's
policy is to use
**paper manufactured
from sustainable forests**

Printed in Hong Kong
CTPS/03

Contents

v

Contributors

Michela Abbona MD
Department of Radiology, General Hospital, Gorizia, Italy

Ivo Bergamo Andreis MD
Department of Radiology, University Hospital, Verona, Italy

Giuseppe Balconi MD
Department of Radiology, San Raffaele Hospital, Milan, Italy

Silvia Baldassarre MD
Institute of Radiology, University Hospital Torrette, Ancona, Italy

Enrico Ballarati MD
Department of Radiology, General Hospital, Busto Arsizio (VA), Italy

Jean-Noel Bruneton MD
Department of Radiology, Centre Hospitalier Universitaire Pasteur, Faculté de Médecine, Nice, France

Francesco Candiani MD
Institute of Radiology, University Hospital, Padua, Italy

Angelina Cavallo MD
Department of Radiology, San Paolo Hospital, Savona, Italy

Roberta Chersevani MD
Department of Radiology, General Hospital, Gorizia, Italy

Luca Crespi MD
Department of Radiology, General Hospital, Busto Arsizio (VA), Italy

Luigi De Pra MD
Department of Radiology, General Hospital, Legnano, (MI), Italy

Lorenzo E. Derchi MD
Institute of Radiology, University Hospital, Genoa, Italy

Giulio Di Candio MD
Institute of General and Experimental Surgery, University Hospital, Pisa, Italy

Carlo Fugazzola MD
Department of Radiology, University Hospital, Verona, Italy

Anne Geoffray MD
Department of Radiology, Hôpital Lenval, Nice, France

Gianmarco Giuseppetti MD
Institute of Radiology, University Hospital, Torrette, Ancona, Italy

Barry B. Goldberg MD
Division of Diagnostic Ultrasound, Department of Radiology, Thomas Jefferson University Hospital and Medical College, Philadelphia, Pennsylvania, USA

Tiziana Ierace MD
Department of Radiology, General Hospital, Busto Arsizio (VA), Italy

W. R. Lees FRCR
Department of Radiology, The Middlesex Hospital, London, UK

Ji-Bin Liu MD
Division of Diagnostic Ultrasound, Department of Radiology, Thomas Jefferson University Hospital and Medical College, Philadelphia, Pennsylvania, USA

Tito Livraghi MD
Department of Radiology, General Hospital, Vimercate (MI), Italy

Masatoshi Makuuchi MD PhD
First Department of Surgery, Shinsyu University, Nagano; Professor and Chairman, Second Department of Surgery, University of Tokyo, Tokyo, Japan

Carlo Martinoli MD
Institute of Radiology, University Hospital, Genoa, Italy

Glauco Mininel MD
Department of Radiology, General Hospital, Gorizia, Italy

S. Miyagawa MD
First Department of Surgery, Shinsyu University, Nagano, Japan

Giuseppe Monetti MD
Institute of Sports Medicine, University of Bologna, Bologna, Italy

Franco Mosca MD
Institute of General and Experimental Surgery, University Hospital, Pisa, Italy

Anna Maria Offidani MD
Institute of Dermatology, General Hospital, Umberto I, Ancona, Italy

Uday Patel FRCR
Department of Radiology, The Middlesex Hospital, London, UK

Andrea Pietrabissa MD
Institute of General and Experimental Surgery, University Hospital, Pisa, Italy

Giorgio Rizzatto MD
Department of Radiology, General Hospital, Gorizia, Italy

Leopoldo Rubaltelli MD
Institute of Radiology, University Hospital, Padua, Italy

Giovanni P. Serafini MD
Department of Radiology, San Paolo Hospital, Savona, Italy

Luigi Solbiati MD
Department of Radiology, General Hospital, Busto Arsizio (VA), Italy

E. Tohno MD
Institute of Clinical Medicine, University of Tsukuba, Japan

H. Tsunoda-Shimizu MD
Institute of Clinical Medicine, University of Tsukuba, Japan

E. Ueno MD
Institute of Clinical Medicine, University of Tsukuba, Japan

Foreword

One of the most significant advances in medical imaging in the last 15 years is high-frequency sonography. It is remarkable not only because of its clear display of morphologic detail, but also because of the wide variety of organs and structures which can be imaged. This book is devoted to an increasingly important segment of ultrasound imaging – the superficial structures also called 'small parts'.

This textbook reflects current concepts of examination technique and high-frequency sonographic diagnosis. It also reviews the newer interventional applications of needle biopsy and tumor ablation. These authors are among the few in the world who have broad expertise in these new frontiers of ultrasound-guided therapy. The editors, Dr Solbiati and Dr Rizzatto, are widely recognized for their talents as clinicians, researchers and educators. The 37 authors have combined their unparalleled experience with a review of the great body of published material on high-frequency sonography, and have distilled it into a concise, readable reference text. Experienced physicians and beginning students are fortunate to have this comprehensive state-of-the-art information accessible in a single source.

J.W.C.

Preface

The study of superficial structures is one of the fastest-growing fields in the application of ultrasound. The spatial resolution of both high-frequency B-mode and colour Doppler ultrasound has improved in the past few years to such an extent that sonographic images are increasingly comparable with anatomic and pathologic specimens, a feature frequently demonstrated in this volume.

Furthermore, high-frequency ultrasound can now be used to guide interventional procedures applied to superficial structures, either for diagnostic or for therapeutic purposes, with great precision.

In this book, it is our aim to provide the most up-to-date information available on all of these applications of high-frequency ultrasound. To help us achieve this aim, we are indebted for their contributions to some internationally recognized experts in the field: Professor Barry Goldberg, President of the World Federation of the Societies for Ultrasound in Medicine and Biology, Dr Jean-Noel Brune-

ton, Dr W. R. Lees, Dr Masatoshi Makuuchi and Dr E. Ueno.

We are also very grateful to our friend Dr William Charboneau for his encouragement and for his suggestions regarding the draft contents list.

The opportunity of collaborating with Esaote Biomedica, an Italian manufacturer involved in the development of high-frequency ultrasound equipment, was extremely beneficial in the book's initial stages. We would also like to thank all of the manufacturers who allowed us to use their instruments to generate the images shown here: Acuson, ATL, Diasonics, Esaote and Toshiba.

Finally, we would like to express our sincere thanks to our families for their continuing support, and to Enrico Caccia for the computer editing of many of the illustrations.

Busto Arsizio and   L.S.
Gorizia, 1995   G.R.

Abbreviations

AFTN	autonomously functioning thyroid nodule	MIBI	methoxyisobutyl-isonitrile
AI	acceleration index	MRI	magnetic resonance imaging
ANDI	aberrations of normal development and involution	MTI	moving target indicator
		PDS	penile Doppler study
AV	arteriovenous	PECAM	platelet/endothelial cell adhesion molecules
BBC	benign breast changes	PEI (T)	percutaneous ethanol injection (treatment)
BMD	bone mineral density	PHPT	primary hyperparathyroidism
BUA	broad-band ultrasound attenuation	PI	pulsatility index
CFM	color-flow mapping	PRF	pulse repetition frequency
CT	computerized tomography	PSC	pancreatic pseudocyst
CVI	colour velocity imaging	PTH	parathyroid hormone
DTPA	diethylene-triaminepentaacetic acid	RI	resistance index
DXA	dual energy X-ray absorptiometry	RIA	radioimmunoassay
FGF	fibroblast growth factor	SE	spin echo
FNAB	fine-needle aspiration biopsy	SHPT	secondary hyperparathyroidism
FT$_3$	free triiodothyronine	SOS	speed of sound
FT$_4$	free thyroxine	TAF	tumor angiogenic factors
HAD	human adjuvant disease	TG	thyroglobulin
HPT	hyperparathyroidism	TGF	transforming growth factor
ICP	intracavernosal pressure/intracranial pressure	TSH	thyroid stimulating hormone
IOUS	intraoperative ultrasonography	US	ultrasound
MEN	multiple endocrine neoplasia	VEGF	vascular endothelial growth factor

1

Instrumentation

G. Rizzatto

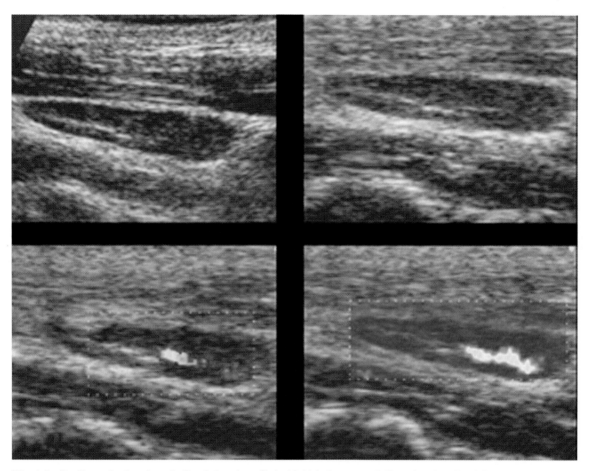

Fig. 1.1 Small reactive lymph node (9 × 2.5 mm) studied with high-frequency dedicated probes. Top left: 13 MHz, small parts; top right: 10 MHz, linear array; bottom left: 10 MHz linear array and 7 MHz color Doppler; bottom right: power Doppler.

ULTRASOUND

Correct ultrasound examination of the superficial structures requires appropriate equipment. Nowadays, instruments are available that make use of high-frequency transducers, sophisticated focusing and computing facilities; the same instrument may allow high quality B-mode imaging and sensitive Doppler analysis (Fig. 1.1).

High-frequency real-time hand-held specific transducers ranging from at least 7.5 MHz up to 15 MHz and more, and focused in the near field, may allow enough resolution to discern very subtle differences of acoustic impedance among soft tissues.[1] High-frequency probes can enhance both *spatial* (axial and lateral) and *contrast resolution*. They provide better definition of normal as well as pathologic features and thus increase the diagnostic potential and clinical precision of this technique (Fig. 1.2).

The location of these superficial structures also makes it possible to increase the frequency of the Doppler signal that is used both for spectrum analysis and color flow mapping; as a result, the *resolution of vascular structures* may also increase.

Spatial resolution

In ultrasonic images, the spatial resolution varies within every image and among the three directions defined by the scan plane.[2–4]

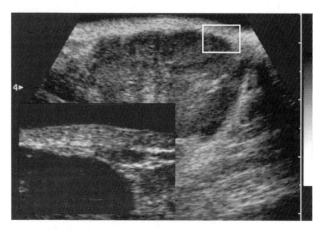

Fig. 1.2 Phyllodes tumor of the breast. The 'pushing' type border is clearly defined by the 20 MHz small-parts probe (bottom left).

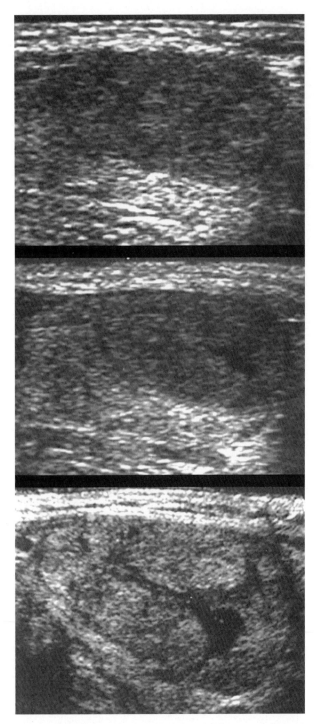

Table 1.1 Wavelength of ultrasound for different frequencies

Frequency (MHz)	Wavelength (mm)
2.5	0.616
3.5	0.440
5.0	0.308
7.5	0.205
10	0.154
13	0.118
15	0.102
20	0.090

with the frequency of the transducer. For a constant number of cycles, as the frequency is increased, the shortened wavelength decreases the spatial pulse length and improves the axial resolution (Fig. 1.3). On the other hand, ultrasound waves of higher frequencies will be absorbed more rapidly. The higher the frequency, the lower is the penetration. The high-frequency ultrasound waves require a more powerful impulse to achieve a useful level of acoustic energy in the deeper tissues. In order to overcome this limitation many probes use new composite ceramics with a wider bandwidth; they improve axial resolution up to the limits set by the wavelength (Table 1.1), without exposing

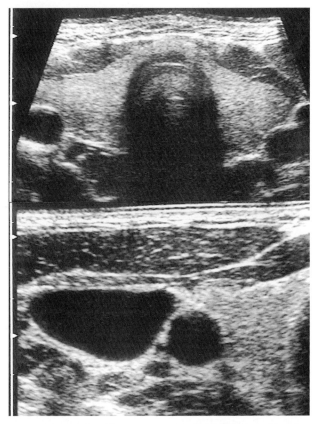

Fig. 1.3 Hyperplastic nodule of the thyroid, with cystic changes. The thin peripheral halo, suggestive of a benign lesion, is better defined with the highest frequency. Top: 7.5 MHz, conventional linear array; middle: 10 MHz, broad-band linear array; bottom: 13 MHz, broad-band annular array with liquid path.

Axial resolution may be defined as the minimum separation of two targets in tissue in a direction parallel to the beam that results in a display of two distinct structures. The main factor that determines axial resolution is the length of the ultrasound pulse, which is closely correlated

Fig. 1.4 Normal thyroid: transverse scan. A 7.5 MHz broad-band annular array with liquid path allows good resolution and large field of view. Also shown in zoom mode.

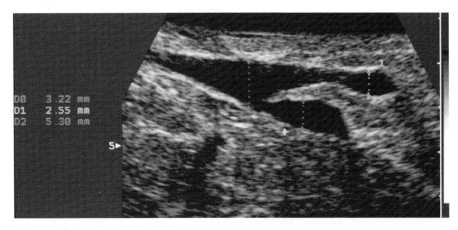

Fig. 1.5 Ectasia of the mammary ducts studied with a 13 MHz broad-band annular array with liquid path; the resolution of the system means that the caliper output must be precise enough to measure the small size of the displayed images.

the tissue to too high a peak of acoustic intensity. These broad-band ceramics allow a range of operating frequencies in a single transducer and in linear arrays. Compared with a narrow band transducer they are easier to match electronically with the other components of the ultrasonic system. This allows the receiver to be tuned to variable frequencies to maximize the sensitivity at various depths. Resolution is improved and, at the same time, there is sufficient penetration. Consequently, there is no need for very high receiver gain for the deeper echoes, and the signal-to-noise ratio and contrast resolution are preserved (Figs 1.4, 1.5). Broad-band technology is also useful for

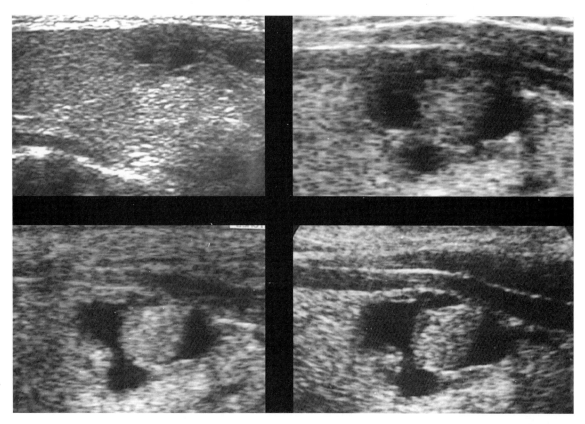

Fig. 1.6 Cystic papillary carcinoma of the thyroid presenting as a mixed lesion. The increasing resolution allows better evaluation of the solid internal projection; the absence of invasion of the strap muscles is defined only with the 13 MHz small-parts probe. Top left: 5 MHz conventional linear array; top right: 7.5 MHz broad-band linear array; bottom left: 10 MHz broad-band linear array; bottom right: 13 MHz broad-band annular array with liquid path.

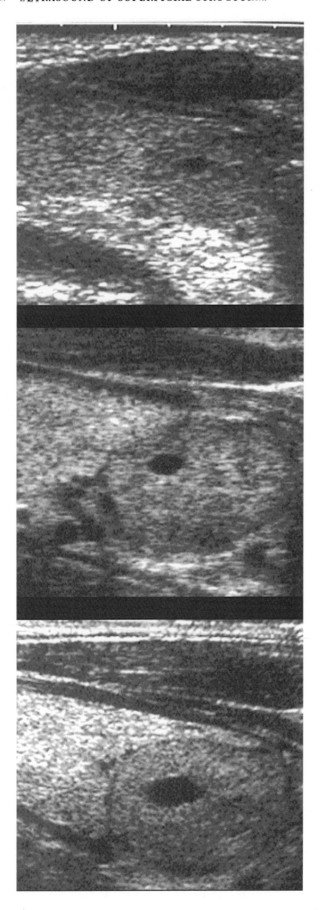

systems offering both Doppler analysis and B-mode imaging: the low-frequency component optimizes flow evaluation, while the higher-frequency component allows an adequate study of morphology and structure through gray-scale imaging.

Lateral resolution describes the ability to resolve two objects next to each other that are perpendicular to the beam axis. In general, it is inferior to, or at best comparable with, the axial resolution. The principal determinant is the width of the ultrasound beam; consequently, the lateral resolution increases with thin beams and is maximum in the focal zone of the ultrasonic beam. Narrower beams are obtained with the use of higher-frequency transducers (Fig. 1.6). Given a narrow beam width, the lateral resolution is proportional to the ultrasound lines which define the image.

Lateral resolution is the major limiting factor in the quality of diagnostic ultrasound images. Artifacts originating outside the focal zone are important: they may lead to an incorrect diagnosis, because of important changes in the structural pattern shown in the image.

The depth of the area of interest is a primary consideration when selecting the optimum transducer. Transducers with high frequencies and wide diameters maintain a narrow beam width to greater depths.

A weakly focused 5 or 7.5 MHz transducer shows very poor resolution in the near and far fields (Fig. 1.7). To reduce the artifacts of the near field, the distance between the transducer and the skin surface must be increased. This can be achieved with the use of an external stand-off pad, which optimizes the position of the focal zone of the beam within the tissue and improves the quality of the final images (Fig. 1.8). Nevertheless, this also brings disadvantages, in that probe handling is less convenient, and palpation and any interventional procedures cannot be carried out while scanning. A better way to reduce the artifacts in the near field is by use of the higher frequencies and the more advanced technology of liquid-path dedicated probes. In these probes, the transducer has been moved inside the probe and there is a fluid path between the transducer and the skin surface (Fig. 1.9). Such probes incorporate oscillating annular arrays or single crystal transducers with wide diameters and higher frequencies. These produce high-intensity and correctly focused beams, which achieve very homogeneous resolution. There may be minimal limitations due to the mechanical movement, but probe handling is comfortable, and the transducer frequency may be increased up to 15 MHz and more. An increase in frequency results in a deeper near field and a less diverging far field; as a result, the region of best lateral

Fig. 1.7   Large hyperplastic nodule of the thyroid (52 × 28 mm). Comparison between two conventional linear-array probes (top: 5 MHz; middle: 7.5 MHz) and a 7.5 MHz small-parts dedicated probe (broadband 12-ring annular array) with liquid path.

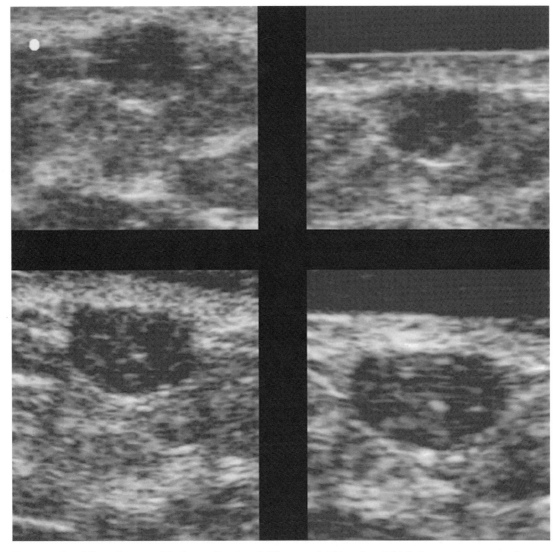

Fig. 1.8   Small fibroadenoma of the breast (9 × 4 mm). The superficial location of this lesion requires the use of a stand-off pad. The synthetic material does not alter the acoustic beam and allows good evaluation of the superficial tissues. Only with the higher frequency is it possible to appreciate the type of border and the small calcifications inside the lesion. Top: 7.5 MHz linear array; bottom: 10 MHz linear array, images obtained with the stand-off pad on the right.

resolution is extended. In practice, deep structures may not be visualized because the reflected waves are too weak to be detected; a broad-band transducer will overcome this problem, by producing multiple frequencies that tend to make the near field more uniform, while the lower frequencies are better able to penetrate to greater depths and to permit the gain settings to be reduced. The wide diameter of these transducers produces beams of higher intensity and narrower width that help penetration into the tissues. The depth reached is dependent on the specific liquids used in the fluid path inside the probe. A different liquid is used for each frequency, chosen to have minimal effect on penetration and to suppress artifacts within the fluid path. Palpation is straightforward while scanning with liquid-path probes and there are no limitations to inter-

ventional procedures whatsoever. An increase in line density and a wide proximal field of view, as well as optimal resolution, are achieved.

Lateral resolution and sensitivity can be improved by selective focusing of the ultrasonic beams (Figs 1.10, 1.11). Single-element transducers can be produced with specifically curved shapes (internal focusing method). Annular array transducers have a central element surrounded by concentric rings of additional elements. Each element is pulsed in such a fashion that external electronic focusing can achieve a narrow beam width at all depths along the beam axis; dynamic focusing in reception is also possible. Linear array transducers may require more complex focusing owing to the large number of elements sometimes involved and their very thin size (Fig. 1.12). Until recently,

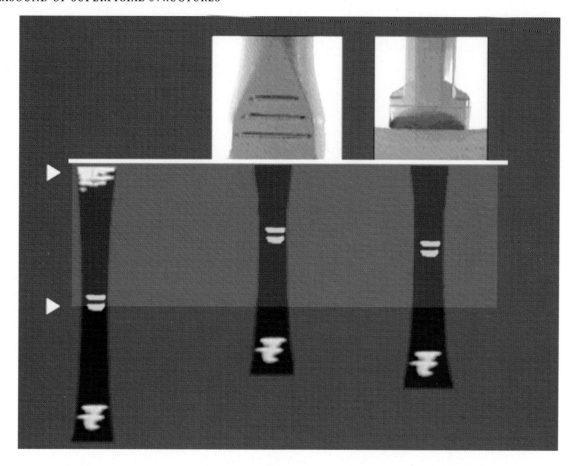

Fig. 1.9   Different ways of putting the area of interest within the focal zone of the probe: using a stand-off pad (top right) or having a liquid path inside the probe. Both methods allow the targets to be resolved.

the transmit focus remained fixed at either one or only a few locations, while the receive focus was continuously or dynamically altered with depth. However, recent substantial advances in computing facilities have enabled several transmit and receive focal zones to be provided throughout the field of view, while still maintaining adequate frame rates. With the aid of such powerful focusing configurations, some 10 MHz linear arrays are now producing high-quality diagnostic images; however, owing to the low efficiency of the small elements, these images are still of lower definition than those obtained with liquid-path transducers.

Contrast resolution

Contrast resolution is defined as the ability to discriminate the differences of acoustic impedance among tissues. It is affected by echo amplitude and tissue attenuation. If the echoes arising from a particular tissue are weak, it will be impossible to detect them without increasing the receiver gain and, therefore, the noise. All techniques that increase the signal-to-noise ratio will enhance spatial resolution and beam penetration, and increase contrast (Figs 1.13, 1.14).

Contrast enhancement is also a particularly powerful processing technique of the digitized image.[4] Changing the gray-scale maps will cause pixels that have similar values over a narrow range to be displayed with different degrees of brightness. Correct selection of gray-scale mapping requires understanding of the quality of the investigated tissues and large digital memories; dedicated gray-scale assignment must be available as a preprocessing function.

Vascular resolution

Vascular resolution describes sensitivity for detection of very low Doppler signal intensities and Doppler frequency shifts. In color-flow mapping (CFM) systems (where flow information is superimposed as colors on a gray-scale image) it is a measure of the system's ability to recognize the presence of flow. Although the advantage of the directional resolution and of the quantitative analysis on Doppler spectrum is extremely useful, determination of whether flow is present or not is the simplest and most useful clinical application of Doppler.[2]

According to the principles of blood and ultrasound interaction, the intensity of the Doppler signal is related to

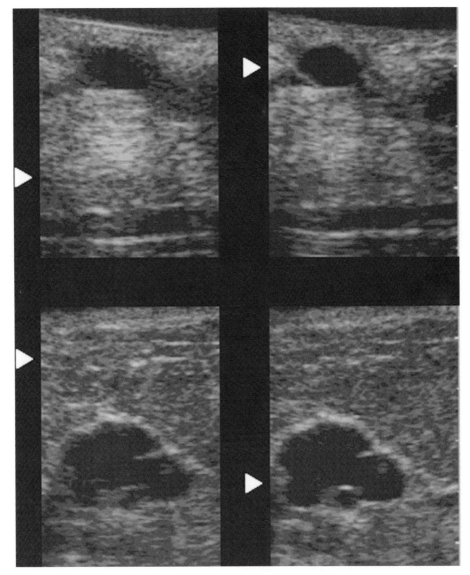

Fig. 1.10 Selective beam focusing (white arrow) is responsible for dramatic changes in the quality of the ultrasound image. Incorrect focusing impairs morphology, echo structure and acoustic enhancement or shadowing.

the number of erythrocytes within the sensitive region of the Doppler beam; as a result, vascular resolution is limited by the lower number of scatterers in small vessels. At the same time the more slowly moving blood in the small vessels acts as the main limiting factor in the current sensitivity to low Doppler frequency shifts.

Another factor that determines Doppler performance is that the intensity of the scattered wave is proportional to the fourth power of frequency; as a consequence, doubling the frequency will result in an echo from the blood that is 16 times stronger.[2] At present, the ability to localize low flow in superficial structures has increased without significant cost to spatial resolution and frame rate. New broad-band linear array probes permit the imaging of rela-

tively deep-seated areas of interest (up to 4–6 cm) with peak frequencies ranging from 7.5 to 13 MHz; at the same time these probes use frequencies of 4.5–7 MHz to optimize the Doppler analysis of the lower flow rate (Fig. 1.15).

The final quality of a CFM image is chiefly dependent on the selection of the highest ultrasonic frequency that can be employed at the depth of the structure of interest; correct beam focusing avoids exaggerated attenuation and increases the efficiency of scattering at higher frequencies, thus giving a more precise morphological picture (Fig. 1.16). Different color palettes act like tailored windows to enhance flows of different velocity and turbulence, or to minimize artifacts (Fig. 1.17).[5]

At superficial locations the angle of incidence and there-

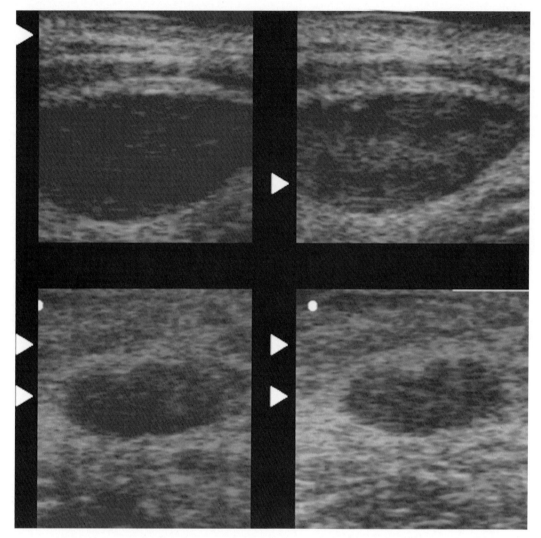

Fig. 1.11 Effect of beam focusing (arrows) and frequency on the amplitude of the returning echoes, without changing the receiver gain, in two different cases of breast fibroadenoma. Top: 13 MHz annular array with liquid path; bottom: 7.5–10 MHz broad-band, linear array used at 10 (left) and 7.5 MHz (right).

fore the beam steering do not influence the detection of low flow in small structures. In contrast, sensitivity increases when the cut-off value of the moving target indicator (MTI) filter (a complex system designed to minimize the artifacts due to the movements originating from heart, thorax, vessel wall and ultrasound probe) and the pulse repetition frequency (PRF) are reduced.[5] However, too low a value of the MTI filter or the PRF lead to major CFM artifacts. This occurs because most color Doppler instruments indicate local flow by encoding in color an estimate of all the mean frequency shifts present at a particular position. Random noise has a random frequency shift and, therefore, noise can look like flow (Fig. 1.18). Aliasing is an other problem that occurs with the frequency detection technique, especially where a low PRF is required,[5,6] for example where the machine has been set up to measure slow flow. Aliasing can make vessels look discontinuous

and impairs the morphologic analysis of vascular distribution; this is already limited by the reduced sensitivity of Doppler instruments to flows that are perpendicular to the sound field.

Instead of measuring Doppler frequency shifts, the technique of color velocity imaging (CVI) measures flow velocity directly by using time-domain processing.[7] CVI tracks individual clusters of blood cells, using ultrasound to measure the distance and the time traveled. CVI maintains high frame rate and low PRF, and improves the detection of low-velocity blood flow.

Recently many manufacturers have developed another technique that encodes the amplitude of the returning Doppler signal in color; this technique is termed Power Doppler, Ultrasound Angio, Color Doppler Energy or Color Intensity Doppler, by different manufacturers. It does not provide information about the speed or direction

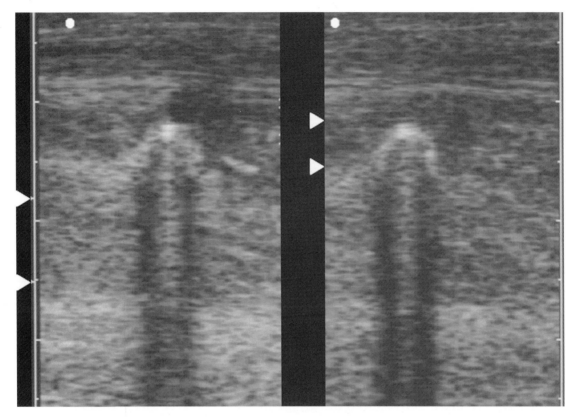

Fig. 1.12 External fixation of tibial fracture: section thickness artifact, due to incorrect focusing, distorts the image returning from a fixation pin. Section thickness represents the observer's window; it is a section with a thickness equivalent to the width of the beam that produced the image. Echoes located from tissues positioned near the edges of the beam are represented as if they are arranged on the central axis of the beam, causing a superimposition effect. Correct focusing (arrows) reduces the beam thickness and minimizes the characteristic blurred edges of round structures.

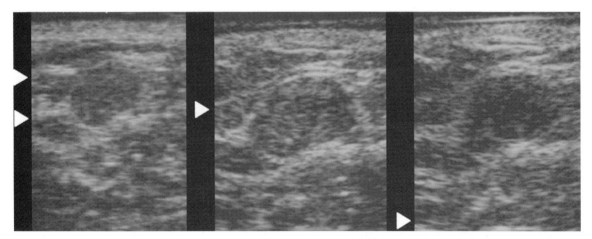

Fig. 1.13 Effect of frequency and beam focusing (arrows) on contrast resolution. A small breast fibroadenoma (7 × 3 mm) is well defined by the 10 MHz broad-band linear array (left). The 13 MHz broad-band annular array with liquid path resolves texture and morphology to a greater extent (middle); nevertheless, with incorrect focusing there is no benefit (right).

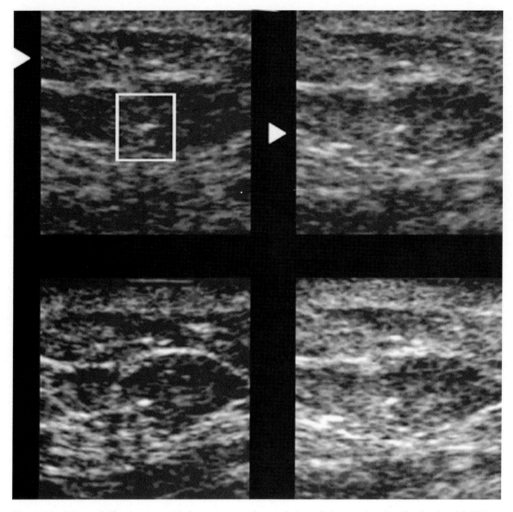

Fig. 1.14   Microcalcifications, outside homogeneous hypoechoic nodules, can be visualized only with high-frequency transducers. Focusing (top right) and digital processing methods (bottom) enhance contrast resolution and increase their visibility.

of flow; with some instruments, power Doppler may be extremely motion sensitive, requiring slow probe movement and low respiration, a limitation that is more crucial in the abdominal scans. On the other hand, power Doppler has many advantages:[6] it eliminates aliasing, is three to five times more sensitive than the mean frequency shift, and does not lose sensitivity with an increasingly perpendicular angle of incidence.

The frequency information in the echo signal is ignored. Hence, the vascular image is angle and direction independent; the display changes with increasing attenuation and with the local density of the red blood cells. If the angle of the insonification is changed, the mean Doppler shift of these blood cells will change, but not the power. Even when flow is almost at right angles to the beam, although the power is reduced, it is not completely zero, as would be the case with estimation of mean frequency, where the negative and positive shifts of energy tend to cancel each other out. In power Doppler the positive as well as the negative

components are summed, giving rise to strong signals; hence, vessels are rendered as continuous structures, significantly increasing diagnostic capability (Fig. 1.19). In addition, power Doppler is inherently more sensitive than color flow mapping; this means that it will always visualize smaller vessels at greater depths than will the equivalent color Doppler image. The amplitude of the signal does not depend on velocity and is therefore not pulsatile; as a result the frame-to-frame averaging techniques are used more effectively to enhance the signal–noise ratio. The amplitude of the signal is always greater than that of noise; thus each signal is assigned a color that differs from that of noise and can be differentiated clearly even at the weakest intensities (Fig. 1.20).

INTERVENTIONAL

Guided percutaneous needle maneuvers have emerged as one of the most important advances in the characterization

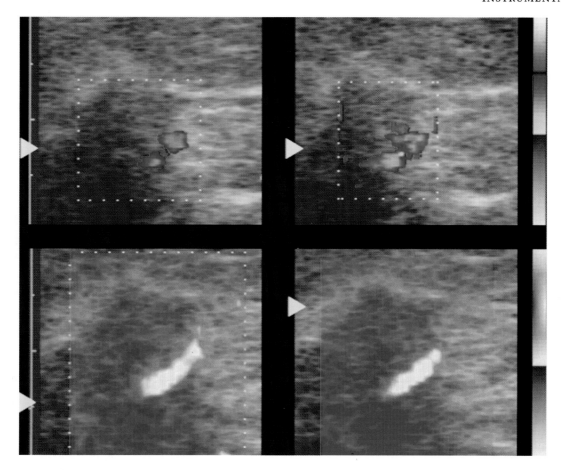

Fig. 1.15 Breast carcinoma evaluated with a 7.5 MHz broad-band linear array. Vascular resolution increases using higher Doppler frequencies and correct beam focusing, or encoding the amplitude of the returning Doppler signal. (Top left: 4.7 MHz Doppler; top right: 7 MHz Doppler; bottom left: 4.7 MHz, power Doppler, with correct focusing and noise due to overamplified signal; bottom right: 4.7 MHz, power Doppler, with reduction of the signal intensity due to incorrect focusing).

of most lesions.[8] Owing to improvements in instrumentation and biopsy techniques, any interventional approach to very small, deeply located alterations can be easily achieved.

Ultrasound as a guidance method

For optimum results it is essential to use high-frequency (7.5–10 MHz) linear arrays or small-parts probes; the focusing of their beams allows good contrast and spatial resolution, and guarantees better visibility of the lesion and of the needle tip.

Different techniques are available for ultrasound (US)-guided needle insertion. Some intraoperative probes have a central biopsy hole, enabling very precise *perpendicular* needle insertion. It is possible to use very short needles, but tip visibility is limited and the needle depth must be marked before the procedure.[9] Most biopsies involve *vertical* or *lateral* insertion (Fig. 1.21).[10] For *vertical* insertion the lesion is displayed approximately at the midline of the

scan plane and the needle is then inserted lateral to the midpoint of the probe. The needle is not seen until the tip has reached the scan plane; this technique requires experience, therefore, and cannot be used for the biopsy of small lesions adjacent to vital structures. For *lateral* insertion, the lesion is displayed close to the lateral margin of the scan plane. The needle is then placed close to the corresponding end of the probe and inserted along the scan plane. The distance involved is greater than with a vertical insertion, but the entire distal portion of the needle is seen as soon as it approaches the lesion within the scan plane.

Both these maneuvers can be performed freehand; no special probes are required and great flexibility is provided. The only problem is in acquiring experience in adjusting the needle's degree of obliquity depending on the depth of the lesion. The freehand technique allows slight adjustments during the course of the biopsy, thus compensating for deviations from the correct path and for movement of the patient.[8] Its major advantages include fanlike sampling, unrestricted site of entry and tilt of the needle.[10] Con-

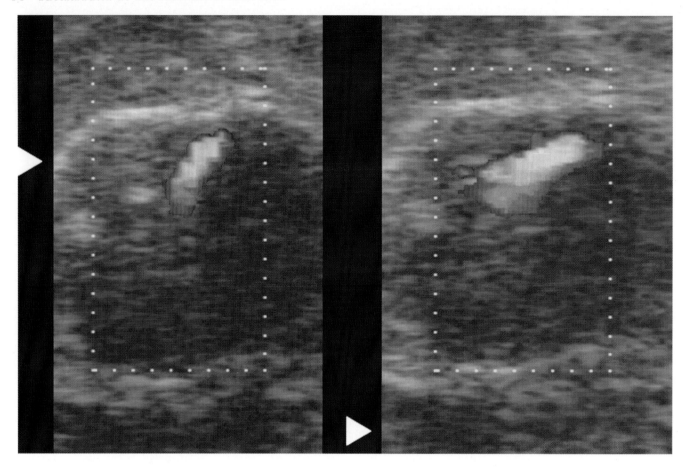

Fig. 1.16   With high-amplitude Doppler signals, incorrect focusing reduces color spatial resolution, imaging artifactual lumens (right).

versely, needle guides that are fitted to the side of the probe restrict the possibility to perform a fanlike sampling in multiple directions or to reposition a deviating needle. In addition, they require longer needles and cannot be used to biopsy very superficial lesions (Fig. 1.22). The major advantage of using the needle guides is the suppression of all uncertainty regarding the needle track.[10] This may be important in case of small lesions adjacent to vital structures, especially when therapeutic procedures have been planned. Precise localization of the needle during the biopsy shortens the procedure and reassures the examiner. The needle is poorly or not visualized mainly because of its misalignment; in addition, if an organ or a lesion are relatively hyperechoic, it is usually difficult to visualize the echogenic tip in this background. Needle visibility has been increased by modifying the needle design. The distal portions of some needles are roughened to increase sound reflection; a special needle stylet with a transponder sensor at its tip, electronically displays a bright echo (Biosponder, Advanced Technology Laboratories, Bellevue, Washington, USA); an external mechanical exciter creates minimal vibrations of the needle shaft and the needle appears as a stripe of color in color Doppler mode

(Colormark, EchoCath, Princeton, New Jersey, USA). Color Doppler information is essential to avoid puncturing or hypervascular areas (Fig. 1.23) and to control the result of US guided therapeutic injections.

Materials

Biopsies

Fine needles, ranging from 20 to 25 gauge, are used to perform *fine-needle aspiration biopsy* (FNAB). The size of the needle depends mostly on the cytologist's choice; 20 or 22-gauge hypodermic needles, 4 cm (1.5 inch) in length, are used routinely. A 10 cm (4 inch), Chiba or Franseen type needle may be necessary for deeply located lesions or for insertions with guided devices. A 10 or 20 ml syringe provides adequate vacuum of aspirate. Syringe handling guns have been designed for easy, comfortable, one-handed aspiration; an alternative is to connect an external tube to the syringe and have the aspiration performed by an assistant.[10] Sampling of solid masses is usually performed with to-and-fro and rotating movements to dissociate the tissue and load the distal lumen of the needle while suction

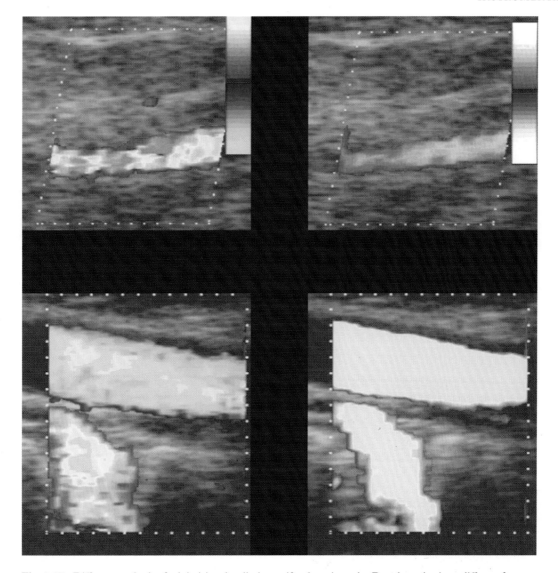

Fig. 1.17 Different methods of minimizing the aliasing artifact by using color Doppler: selecting a different frequency range, which brings about a different color palette (top right), or encoding the amplitude of the returning signals (power Doppler) (bottom right).

is applied. For 'hard' solid lesions it is better to avoid aspiration during the sampling procedure. In this technique, capillarity drives the dissociated tissue fragments and cells into the needle; a short suction is performed only at the end of the procedure. This technique reduces the percentage of inadequate smears and allows an increase of the sampled volume. *Large-core needle biopsy* requires large-bore Tru-Cut needles. These needles can be used with spring-driven automatic devices (Fig. 1.24). The needle tip is placed near the margin of the lesion; the firing of the device will trigger the spring mechanism, propelling the stylet and the cutting cannula forward (12–24 mm) for a core biopsy sample. The Tru-Cut needles range from 14 to 20 gauge and yield large tissue cores that can be read by any pathologist. However, local anesthesia and skin incision

may be required; in addition, there is an increased risk of local hemorrhage. The subsequent fibrosis may induce alterations and increase the equivocal reports in follow-up examinations. Because of the instantaneous advancement of the needle, it is difficult to monitor the procedure. For this reason, Tru-Cut biopsies must always be performed with the oblique needle insertion technique and are less safe for sampling small lesions adjacent to vital structures.

Aspiration

Fluid collections are usually easily aspirated with 20 gauge needles and 20–50 ml syringes. Inspissated cysts, hematomas and abscesses require large-bore needles (14 to 18 gauge), with Teflon cannula. Some drainage procedures

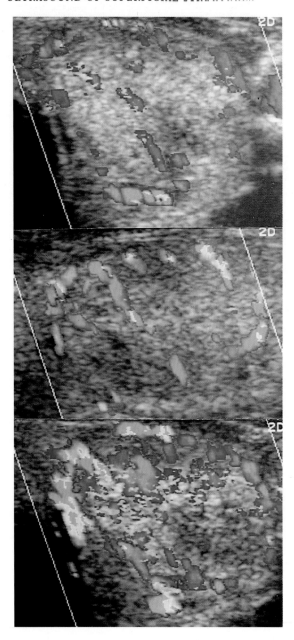

Fig. 1.18 Thyroid adenoma with vascular capsule and transnodular vessels. Too high PRF values (top) reduce the visibility of the vessels, while too low values result in diffuse noise (bottom).

require percutaneous placement of appropriate pigtail catheters.

Therapeutic injection

Various therapeutic percutaneous procedures are currently performed. Most of them are performed with the same needles that are used for the aspiration procedure (antibiotic injection after abscess drainage, ethanol injection after cyst aspiration) or with 18–22 gauge spinal needles (injection of ethanolamine oleate for spermatocele sclerotherapy).

Therapeutic procedures in the neck usually require needles 9 cm in length; this length is needed because all therapeutic interventions are carried out with direct ultrasound guidance, using lateral biopsy devices and high-frequency probes. Percutaneous ethanol injection treatment (PEIT) of solid masses (e.g. thyroid autonomous nodules and parathyroid tumors) can be performed either with the type of spinal needles used for cysts or (a more recent development) with 8 cm long 21 gauge needles with a closed conical tip and three sideholes (Fig. 1.25). With spinal needles the injections of sterile 95% ethanol can be precisely guided into small targets or into small areas of the tumors left unperfused by multihole needles. With the multihole needles, large volumes of tissue can be perfused in single sessions (Fig. 1.26); furthermore the reflux of ethanol in the blood vessels is more uncommon, as well as the posterior extravasation of ethanol that may cause, for example, damage to the laryngeal recurrent nerve in the treatment of neck pathologies.

Color Doppler is more and more widely employed in PEIT, chiefly in order to assess either the immediate effect of ethanol (sudden reduction of perfusion) or, on the follow-up, the presence of hypervascular areas requiring further treatment.

Localization

Different methods of localization of non-palpable lesions have been developed. A small amount of a solution of carbon particles can be injected after proper placement of the needle under US guidance. Continuous injection while the needle is withdrawn allows surgical identification of the needle track for some months. This technique is inexpensive and safe; however, it does not allow radiographic confirmation unless a contrast agent is added. As preoperative localization is used mostly in breast diagnosis, the most popular design consists of a radiopaque hook wire loaded into 20 or 22 gauge needles that allow secure placement of the open hook within the lesion or adjacent to it (Fig. 1.27). The same technique can be used for non palpable lesions in other areas. In some cases a lesion is not seen equally well on radiograms and sonograms. Although more expensive, various adjustable devices allow the wire or the needle to be moved if they are incorrectly placed.

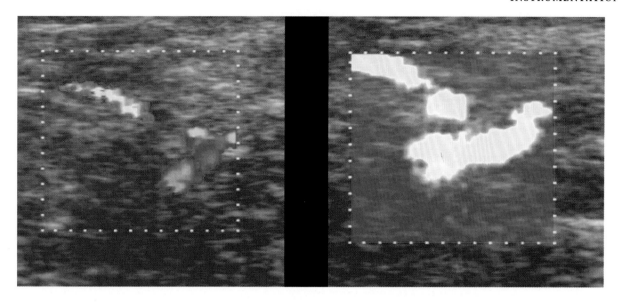

Fig. 1.19 Intramammary vessels visualized with a 10–13 MHz linear array with a 7 MHz Doppler. With power Doppler (right), vessels kept their anatomical continuity.

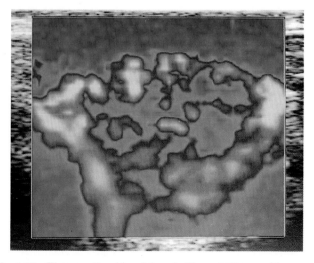

Fig. 1.20 The same thyroid nodule as in Figure 1.18 seen with power Doppler; this technique allows better evaluation of vascular morphology.

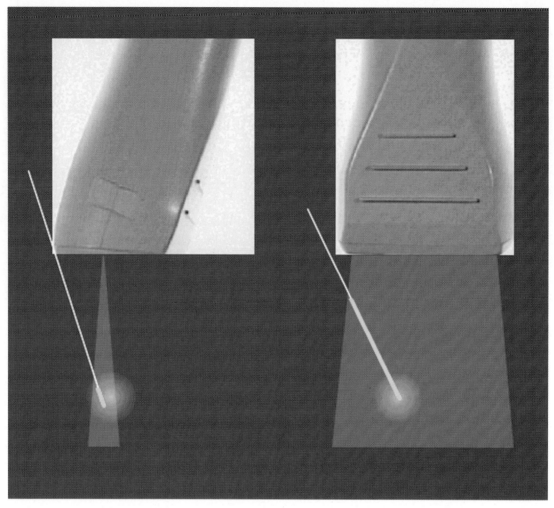

Fig. 1.21 Vertical and lateral approaches during US-guided interventional maneuvers. The bold yellow line, representing the needle portion visualized on the US display, is longer in the lateral approach (right)

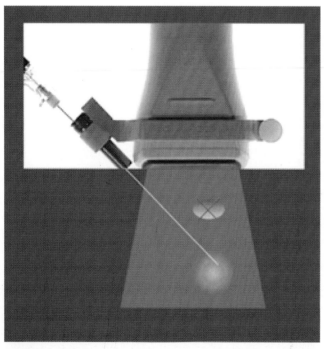

Fig. 1.22 Small-parts probe with lateral adaptor. The system is useful for deep lesions but does not allow adequate puncturing of superficial non-palpable lesions.

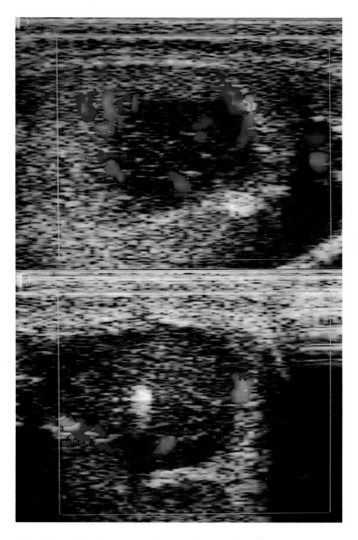

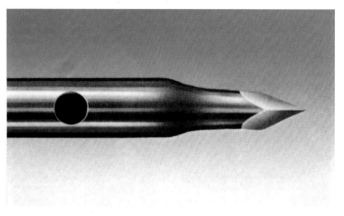

Fig. 1.25 PEIT needle with closed conical tip and three sideholes (21 gauge PEIT needle, Hakko, Tokyo, Japan).

Fig. 1.23 Color Doppler used as a guide to avoid puncturing of the vascular rim of a hypoechoic testicular nodule. The bright echo with ring-down artifacts is clearly seen using vertical insertion (bottom).

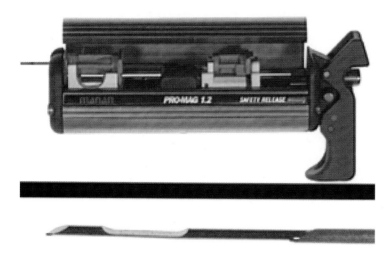

Fig. 1.24 Spring-driven automatic device for Tru-Cut needles. After releasing the safety catch and depressing the firing button, the stylet moves forward and the surrounding tissue prolapses into the sampling notch (bottom).

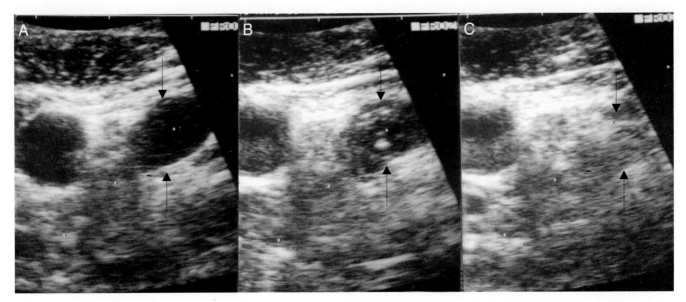

Fig. 1.26 PEIT of 10 mm parathyroid hyperplasia (arrows). After centering the lesion (**A**), a multihole needle (arrowhead) is inserted (**B**) and complete perfusion of the target is obtained (**C**).

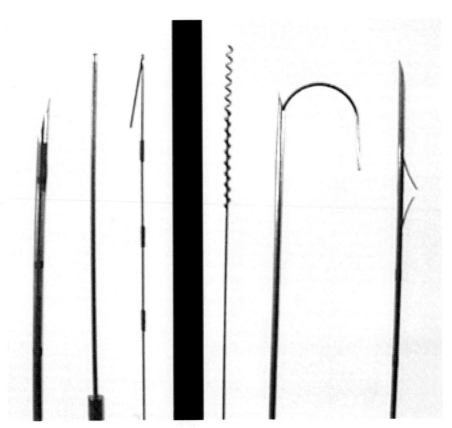

Fig. 1.27 Different localization needles. On the left the Kopan's non repositionable needle (localization needle, steering sheath and spring-hookwire positioning mark). On the right various repositionable needles: from left the Homer's, Helixx and Hawkins needles.

REFERENCES

1. Rizzatto G, Chersevani R, Solbiati L 1993 High-resolution ultrasound assists in breast diagnosis. Diagn Imag Int 5: 42–45
2. Burns P N 1991 Principles of US. In: Rifkin M D, Charboneau J W, Laing F C (eds) Ultrasound 1991. RSNA, Oak Brook, pp 33–55
3. Fish P 1990 Physics and instrumentation of diagnostic medical ultrasound. John Wiley, Chichester
4. Hykes D L, Hedrick W R, Starchman D E 1992 Ultrasound physics and instrumentation, 2nd edn. Mosby Year Book, St Louis
5. Miyajima Y 1993 Ultrasound color Doppler imaging: current technology and future prospects. Med Rev 44: 47–56
6. Rubin J M, Adler R S 1993 Power Doppler expands standard color capability. Diagn Imag Int 12: 66–69
7. Tegeler C H, Kremkau F W, Hitchings L P 1991 Color velocity imaging: introduction to a new ultrasound technology. Neuroimag 1: 85–90
8. Charboneau J W 1991 US-guided biopsy. In: Mueller P R, van Sonnenberg E, Becker G J (eds) Interventional radiology. RSNA, Oak Brook, pp 9–16
9. Rizzatto G, Solbiati L, Croce F, Derchi L E 1987 Aspiration biopsy of superficial lesions: ultrasonic guidance with a linear array probe. AJR 148: 623–625
10. Fornage B D, Coan J D, David C L 1992 Ultrasound-guided needle biopsy of the breast and other interventional procedures. Radiol Clin North Am 1: 167–185

2

Ultrasound contrast agent evaluation of superficial masses

B. B. Goldberg   J.-B. Liu

DEVELOPMENT OF ULTRASOUND CONTRAST AGENTS

The concept of using ultrasound contrast agents was first introduced in the late 1960s by Gramiak and Shah while performing echocardiography during cardiac catheterization.[1] They injected a solution (saline or indocyanine green) through a catheter into the great vessels and heart, which resulted in multiple reflections being recorded from within the vessels or chambers. Using this method they were able effectively to demonstrate a variety of cardiovascular structures. Others who followed used it to demonstrate a variety of vessels and even to confirm that ultrasound could visualize the common bile duct.[1-5] Over the years many investigators have utilized ultrasound contrast agents in the evaluation of cardiac abnormalities, including ventricular shunts and retrograde flows.[6,7] It has been shown that any solution not left standing for any length of time contains microbubbles of gas. In fact, if the solution is agitated the quantity of microbubbles increases. One of the problems, however, is that after a relatively short distance these microbubbles go back into solution or are removed as they pass through the lungs.

As a result of this early work many researchers, at both universities and companies throughout the world, have tried to produce ultrasound contrast agents that can be injected into a peripheral vein and circulate throughout the body. It was only toward the end of the 1980s that such a possibility became practical. One of the first successful agents was an albumen product containing microbubbles of gas (Albunex®, Molecular Biosystems Inc, San Diego, California, USA) that has been produced by sonification. These albumen particles, on average, are small enough to pass through the capillary system and can be used to visualize not only the right side of the heart but also the left.[8] In animal models this agent showed significant B-mode image enhancement in both chambers of the heart as well as significant enhancement of the Doppler signals in vessels elsewhere in the body.[9-11] Increased visualization of the parenchyma using B-mode imaging could not be demonstrated.

In animal experiments a VX2 tumor grown in the ear of a rabbit was used to evaluate the effectiveness of Albunex in visualizing superficial tumors. Without Albunex, minimal Doppler signals could be demonstrated in the small normal vessels but were not clearly seen in the tumor vessels. However, a small amount of the albumen-containing microbubble agent, injected into a peripheral vein of the rabbit, circulated throughout the body, resulting in significantly improved visualization of both the normal as well as the tumor vessels. This method shows promise for evaluation of blood flow in other superficial structures.

Another agent, consisting of galactose in which microbubbles of gas are trapped within the crevices (Echovist®, Schering AG, Berlin, Germany), has become the first commercially approved agent in Europe for visualization of the right side of the heart.[12-15] However, more recently an agent modified in terms of size, in which the galactose-trapped microbubbles of gas are coated with a thin layer of a fatty acid, has resulted in a stabilized product (Levovist®, Schering AG) that is small enough to recirculate throughout the body. Work in animals and subsequently in humans has shown recirculation times in excess of 3–5 minutes. This product significantly enhances Doppler signals, both color and spectral, in both normal and abnormal vessels as well as in the chambers of the heart.[16-18] No significant gray-scale enhancement of tissues could be demonstrated although there was visualization of this agent within slower-moving blood as in the portal vein and vena cava.

Animal studies

The galactose-based product (Levovist) has been tested in a variety of animal models in both normal and abnormal vessels, such as in naturally occurring tumors in the liver of the woodchuck. Significant enhancement of both tumor and adjacent normal vessels could be clearly documented (Fig. 2.1A,B). In an effort to demonstrate the effectiveness of contrast enhancement in more superficial structures, experiments were carried out imaging the eye of the dog. Pre-injection studies delineated the ophthalmic artery and vein using both pulsed and color Doppler. No significant flow could be demonstrated in the region of the retina or anterior chamber of the eye. After the injection of a small quantity of this ultrasound contrast material into a peripheral vein, there was significant enhancement of the ophthalmic artery as well as visualization of vessels in the retina and the anterior chamber of the eye (Fig. 2.2A, B). Using spectral analysis for pre- and postevaluation of the ophthalmic artery and vein showed a dramatic enhancement of the intensity of the Doppler signals after contrast was injected. The enhancement in the ophthalmic vein clearly demonstrated that this agent was small enough to pass through the capillary system.[19]

Human evaluation programs

As a result of these initial animal experiments, research was carried out in humans to evaluate the effectiveness of this ultrasound contrast agent in enhancing both normal and tumor vessels throughout the body. Medical centers in Europe, Asia and the United States participated in these human evaluation programs. In our facility we evaluated both normal and abnormal vessels throughout the body and examined the effectiveness of Levovist in enhancing Doppler signals, both color and spectral. In general, there was improvement in the intensity of the visualized vessels, as well as the demonstration of vessels not seen before injection of the agent.

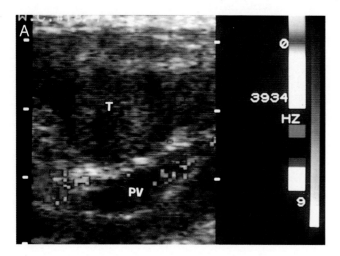

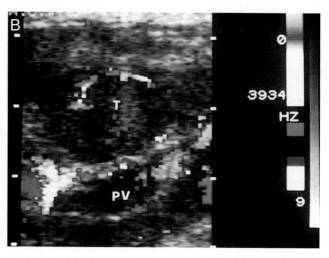

Fig. 2.1   Color Doppler signal enhancement is seen within a woodchuck hepatocellular tumor (T) before (**A**) and after (**B**) a peripheral intravenous injection of 1.0 ml Levovist. Note the appearance of tumor vessels within the poorly defined solid mass. PV: portal vein. Reproduced from ref. 19, with permission.

Dose response

The reflectivity of ultrasound contrast agents is significantly greater than that of red blood cells and, thus, a smaller quantity of this material is needed for significant improvement in the signal-to-noise ratio. It was seen to be effective in the visualization of small vessels, such as are found in tumors, as well as in visualizing vessels deeper in the body. Experimental work in measuring dose response carried out with Doppler cuffs placed around the aorta and celiac artery in a rabbit model, as well as in a superficially located tumor in the liver of the woodchuck, showed increased Doppler signal enhancement with increasing amounts of contrast. The dose–response curves showed that as increasing quantities of the agent were injected there was sig-

nificant enhancement in the Doppler signals, with changes of up to 24 dB in normal vessels and almost 14 dB in tumor vessels (Figs 2.3, 2.4). In humans, contrast effects were seen with doses of 10 ml of Levovist injected into a peripheral vein. As previously noted, the circulation time of this ultrasound agent was in excess of 3–5 minutes.

EVALUATION IN SUPERFICIAL MASSES

Although masses were studied throughout the body, particular attention was directed to evaluation of the contrast agent in breast and other superficial masses. As seen elsewhere in the body there was significant enhancement in the Doppler signals, both color and pulsed, after the injection of Levovist into a peripheral vein. It was possible, in

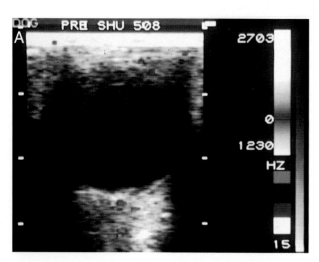

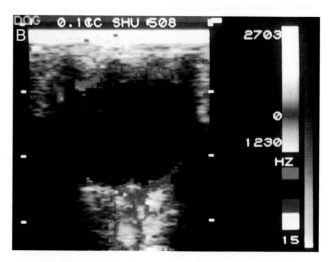

Fig. 2.2   Color Doppler images of the dog eye before (**A**) and after (**B**) a peripheral intravenous injection of 0.1 ml Levovist. Vessels in both the retina and the anterior portion of the eye are rendered visible by the contrast agent. Reproduced from ref. 19, with permission.

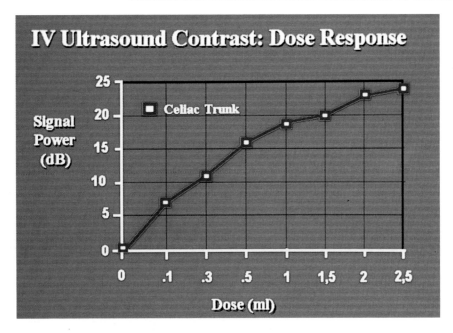

Fig. 2.3   Doppler spectrum measurements obtained from the celiac artery with increasing intravenous doses (0.1–2.5 ml) of contrast agent demonstrate progressive increase in the signal intensity (up to 24 dB).

some cases, to see tumor vessels before the injection of contrast but, even in these cases, after injection of the agent there was a significant increase in the number of vessels seen and in the intensity of the signal arising from the vessels previously imaged (Fig. 2.5). This enhancement of the color Doppler signals often made it easier to obtain spectral Doppler signals. The potential to record the rate of ultrasound contrast agent uptake and outflow within breast masses has been reported.[20] This approach has been used in magnetic resonance imaging (MRI) with gadolinium to differentiate benign from malignant breast masses.[21,22] The possibility therefore exists that these ultrasound contrast agents could prove useful for the evaluation of other superficial masses.

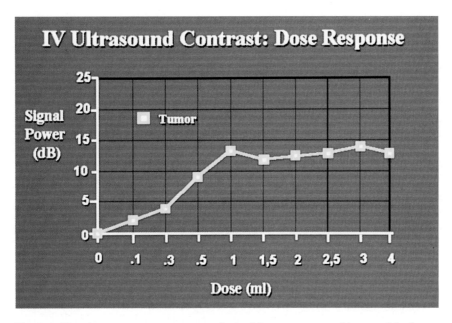

Fig. 2.4   Doppler spectrum measurements obtained from a tumor vessel in a woodchuck hepatocellular tumor with increasing intravenous doses (0.1–4 ml) of contrast agent demonstrate progressive increase in the signal intensity (up to 14 dB).

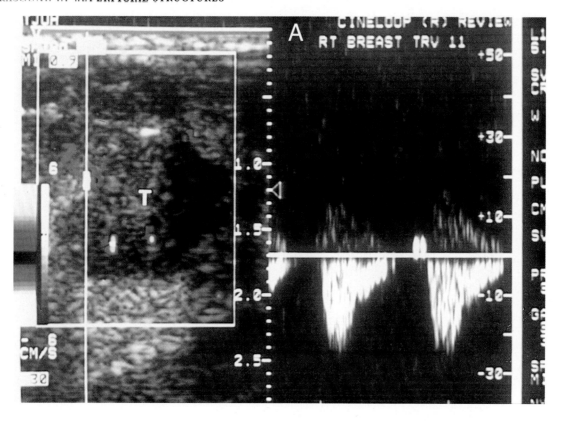

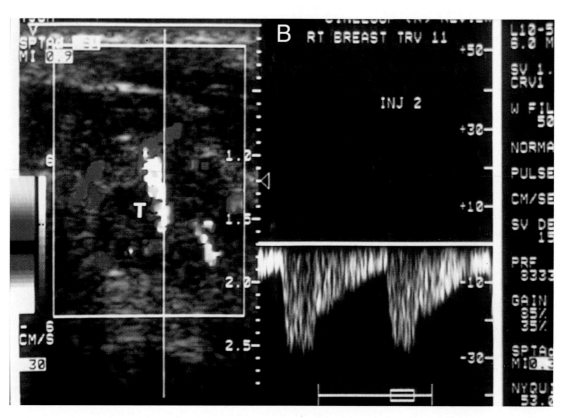

Fig. 2.5 In a patient with a breast tumor, a peripheral intravenous injection of Levovist demonstrated color and spectrum Doppler tumor vessel enhancement. **A** Before contrast injection; **B** after contrast injection.

FUTURE DEVELOPMENTS

Several ultrasound contrast agents are already undergoing evaluation in humans and many more agents are under development. Some agents, such as a form of a perfluorochemical (Echogen[R], Sonus Pharmaceuticals, Costa Mesa, California, USA), which is a liquid emulsion at room temperature and which turns to a gas at body temperature, shows promise in animal and preliminary human studies in being able not only to increase the Doppler signals but also to enhance gray-scale visualization of the parenchyma of the kidney and liver. No research has yet been carried out using this agent for the evaluation of superficial masses. Ultrasound contrast agents appear to hold great promise for provision of additional useful information in the evaluation of a wide variety of abnormalities.

REFERENCES

1. Gramiak R, Shah P M 1968 Echocardiography of the aortic root. Invest Radiol 3: 356–366
2. Feigenbaum H, Stone J, Lee D et al 1970 Identification of ultrasound echoes from the left ventricle by use of intracardiac injections of indocine green. Circulation 41: 615–621
3. Kerber R E, Kioschos J M, Lauer R M 1974 Use of an ultrasonic contrast method in the diagnosis of valvular regurgitation and intracardiac shunts. Am J Cardiol 34: 722–727
4. Goldberg B B 1971 Ultrasonic measurement of the aortic arch, right pulmonary artery, and left atrium. Radiology 101(2): 383–390
5. Goldberg B B 1976 Ultrasonic cholangiography, gray-scale B-scan evaluation of the common bile duct. Radiology 118: 401–404
6. Sahn D J, Valdez-Cruz L M 1984 Ultrasonic contrast studies for the detection of cardiac shunts. J Am Coll Cardiol 3: 978–985
7. Reid C L, Kawanishi D T, McKay C R et al 1983 Accuracy of evaluation of the presence and severity of aortic and mitral regurgitation by contrast 2-dimensional echocardiography. Am J Cardiol 52: 519–524
8. Feinstein S R, Cheirif J, Ten Cate F J et al 1990 Safety and efficacy of a new transpulmonary ultrasound agent: initial multicenter clinical results. J Am Coll Cardiol 16: 316–324
9. Hilpert P L, Mattrey R F, Mitten R M, Peterson T 1989 IV injection of air-filled human Albumin Microspheres to enhance arterial Doppler signal: a preliminary study in rabbits. AJR 153: 613–616
10. Goldberg B, Hilpert P, Burns P et al 1990 Hepatic tumors: signal enhancement of Doppler US after intravenous injection of a contrast agent. Radiology 177: 713–717
11. Keller M, Glasheen W, Kaul S 1989 Albunex: a safe and effective commercially produced agent for myocardial contrast echocardiography. J Am Soc Echocardiol 2: 48–52
12. Becher H, Schlief R, Lüderitz B 1989 Improved sensitivity of color Doppler by SHU 454. Am J Cardiol 64: 374
13. Smith M D, Kwan O I, Reiser H J, DeMaria A N 1984 Superior intensity and reproducibility of SHU 454, a new right heart contrast agent. J Am Coll Cardiol 3: 992–998
14. Fritzsch T H, Hilmann J, Mutzel W, Lange L 1986 Right-heart echocontrast in the anaesthetized dog after i.v. administration of a new standardized sonographic contrast agent (I). Arzneimittelforschung 36: 1030–1033
15. Lange L, Fritzsch T H, Hilmann J, Kubowicz G, Mutzel W 1986 Right-heart echocontrast in the anaesthetized dog after i.v. administration of a new standardized sonographic contrast agent (II). Arzneimittelforschung 36: 1034–1036
16. Smith M D, Elion J L, McClure R R et al 1989 Left heart opacification with peripheral venous injection of a new saccharide echo contrast agent in dogs. J Am Coll Cardiol 13: 1622–1628
17. Fritzsch T, Hilmann J, Kampfe M, Muller N, Schoobel C, Siegert J 1990 SHU 508, a transpulmonary echocontrast agent: initial experience. Invest Radiol 25: 160–161
18. Schlief R, Staks T, Mahler M, Rufer M, Fritzsch T, Seifert W 1990 Successful opacification of the left heart chambers on echocardiographic examination after intravenous injection of a new saccharide-based contrast agent. Echocardiography 7: 1–4
19. Goldberg B B, Liu J B, Burns P N, Merton D A, Forsberg F 1993 Galactose-based intravenous sonographic contrast agent: experimental studies. J Ultrasound Med 12: 463–470
20. Kedar R P, Cosgrove D O, McCready V R, Bamber J C 1993 Microbubble Doppler angiography of breast masses: dynamic and morphologic features (abstract). Radiology 189(P): 154
21. Stack J P, Redmond O M, Codd M B et al 1990 Breast disease: tissue characterization with Gd-DTPA enhancement profiles. Radiology 174: 491–494
22. Beck R, Heywang S H, Schlegel A et al 1990 KST der mamma mit GD-DTPA-Erfahrungen von 600 Fallen. Zentralbl Radiol 141: 3–4: 215

3

Morphology and structure related to pathology

G. Rizzatto   L. Solbiati

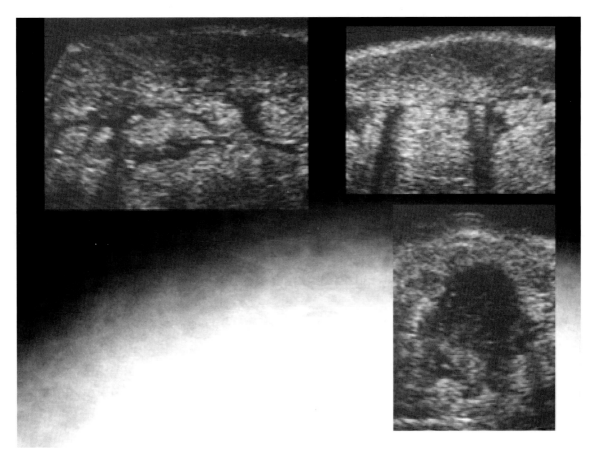

Fig. 3.1 Hyperechoic edema of breast soft tissues following carcinomatosis of the dermal lymphatics. Skin thickening and dilated lymphatics (top); small nodule of undifferentiated carcinoma (bottom right); typically dense mammographic pattern (bottom).

High-frequency transducers can be employed in small-parts sonography. The resolution is the greatest achievable in ultrasound studies; as a result, a good correlation between pathologic and imaging patterns can be obtained. This is particularly true for focal abnormalities; diffuse processes give a less specific sonographic pattern.

DIFFUSE ABNORMALITIES

Diffuse abnormalities (such as thyroiditis, orchitis, testicular atrophy or inflammatory carcinoma of the breast) are usually characterized by variations in size and by diffuse alterations in the echo texture. Enlargement is more typical of acute or progressive diseases, whereas reduction in size is usually related to chronic or atrophic processes. Variably echogenic patterns may be caused by edema, hypervascularity, fibrosis, neoplastic or inflammatory infiltration, necrosis, hemorrhage and infarction. The same pathologic process may exhibit an increase or decrease of signal intensity in different organs or tissues. It is widely accepted that this phenomenon is probably attributable to the number and size of the acoustic interfaces and their relationship

with the macrostructure of the organ. In inflammatory carcinoma of the breast the infiltration of dermal lymphatics by cancer cells causes capillary congestion, edema and a highly echogenic thickening of soft tissues (Fig. 3.1).

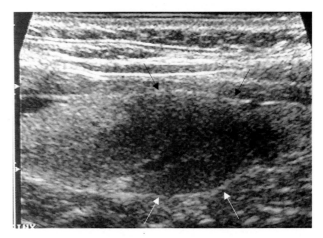

Fig. 3.2 Subacute thyroiditis of the caudal portion of the thyroid lobe (arrows). Inflammatory edema and lymphocytic infiltration markedly reduce the echogenicity of the thyroid parenchyma.

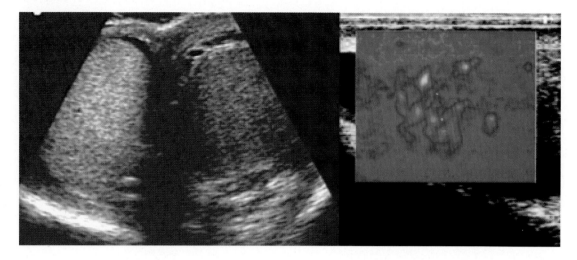

Fig. 3.3 Acute inflammation of the left testis. The typical decrease in echogenicity is mainly related to the increased vascularity, as shown by color Doppler.

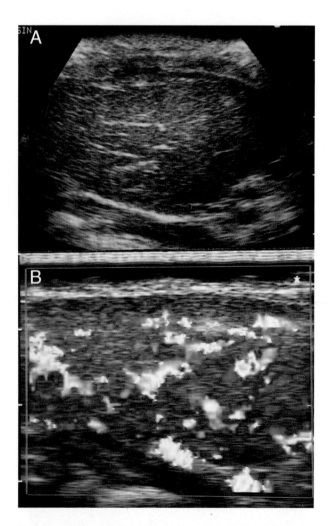

Fig. 3.4 Hypertrophic Hashimoto thyroiditis. Diffusely hypoechoic pattern (A) with hypervascularity (B). Most vessels are located in the hyperechogenic septa (visible in A) which may represent either fibrous strands or vessel walls.

In subacute thyroiditis, parenchymal inflammatory edema causes a marked decrease in glandular echogenicity (Fig. 3.2). Most acute inflammatory diseases cause diffuse hypoechogenicity; color Doppler has shown that this pattern is related more to increased vascularization than to edema (Fig. 3.3). In chronic abnormalities hyperechogenic lines may represent either fibrous strands or the walls of thin vessels (Fig. 3.4).

FOCAL ABNORMALITIES

The nature and type of growth of focal abnormalities are described in terms of the following parameters:

- morphology and type of borders
- relationship with nearby structures
- internal echogenicity and sound through-transmission
- vascularity.

The morphological pattern allows an initial assessment of the type of growth – expansive or infiltrating. Where the longitudinal diameter, parallel to the skin, is greatest, the pathology is usually benign, as in most breast fibroadenomas[1], enlarged reactive lymph nodes[2] or soft tissue lipomas, for example. A greater anteroposterior diameter, perpendicular to the skin, is more often found in malignant growths. The shape of metastatic nodes changes from oval to rounded. The greatest diameter of most infiltrating breast carcinomas is perpendicular to the skin.

The second parameter to be considered is the type of border. An expansive growth shows regular, well-defined borders that simply push into the nearby tissues, causing compression but no distortion. There may be a true anatomic capsule (Fig. 3.5), or the compressed tissues may form a pseudocapsule (Fig. 3.6). An infiltrating growth has irregular, ill-defined borders, that invade and alter the surrounding tissues.

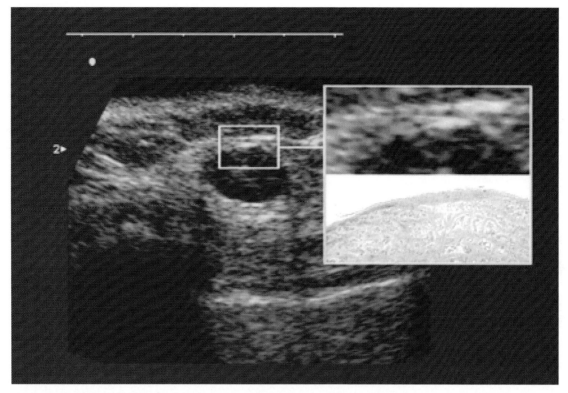

Fig. 3.5 The regular, 'pushing' type border (not infiltrating, but compressing and displacing the surrounding tissues) of a small fibroadenoma of the breast correlates well with the histologic encapsulated margin.

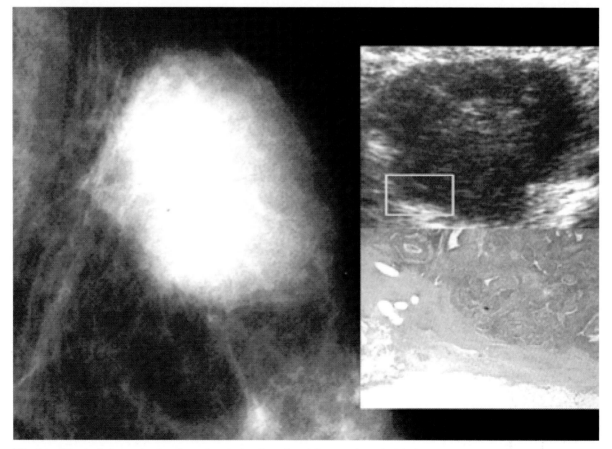

Fig. 3.6 Histological examination shows that the borders of medullary carcinoma of the breast are always of the 'pushing' type. At the periphery of the tumor, the host tissues react by producing a prominent lymphoplasmacytic infiltrate.

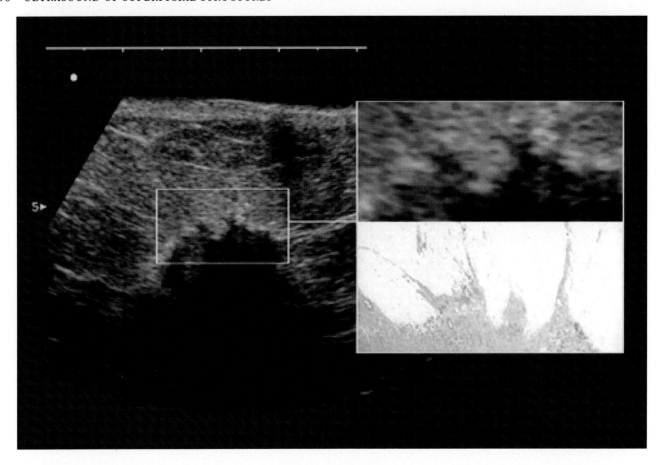

Fig. 3.7 Invasive carcinoma of the breast exhibits mostly 'infiltrating' borders. The tumoral strands, radiating through the surrounding parenchyma into the fat, are responsible for the notorious stellate configuration. The large amount of stroma within the tumor gives rise to a marked acoustic shadow.

The real-time ultrasound examination reveals compressibility and a degree of mobility, under pressure from the probe, in any lesion that does not adhere firmly to the surrounding structures. The type of border correlates to the interface between a focal abnormality and its surroundings, and explains the relationship of an abnormality with nearby structures. Some examples of different interfaces are the echogenic rim of desmoplasia in breast infiltrating carcinomas, the different types of hypoechogenic halos in thyroid nodules, and the loss of the hyperechogenic central band of the lymph sinus in invaded superficial nodes. Normal breast tissue reacts to neoplastic infiltration with desmoplasia, which represents the production of connective tissue around the tumour. The sonographic pattern is a fairly thick, echogenic and irregularly shaped band surrounding the tumor (Fig. 3.7). The hypoechoic halo of thyroid nodules is due to peripheral vessels, edema and/or necrosis of nearby tissues and the capsule, when present. Slowly growing thyroid nodules, benign in most cases, usually have a thin and regular peripheral halo, due either to a capsule (adenomas) or to perilesional vessels (nodular goiters; Fig. 3.8). Rapidly growing nodules, with a thick and irregular halo, are more often malignant; in such cases

the capsule is destroyed with resultant edema and prevalent peripheral necrosis (Fig. 3.9).

Sonography can also demonstrate the extension of an abnormality outside the borders of an organ. Examples are the invasion of nerves[2] (Fig. 3.10), of fat and soft tissues (Fig. 3.11), of mammary ducts[3] (Fig. 3.12) and of blood vessels.[4]

Internal echogenicity is not merely an oversimplified differentiation between a solid and liquid focal abnormality. A homogeneous or an inhomogeneous echo pattern correlates with macrostructure. The elements that build up the macrostructure not only determine its homogeneity, but also the behaviour of sound transmission and the vascular pattern that is seen (Figs 3.13, 3.14). Nevertheless there is no general rule that clearly differentiates between a benign or malignant sonographic pattern. An exception to this is the demonstration of microcalcifications suggesting malignancy. Ultrasound screening for breast microcalcifications should never be attempted; they are readily detected with mammography, and magnification permits correct morphological analysis. Sonography is very insensitive to calcifications that are interspersed in breast parenchyma, whereas even very small microcalcifications –

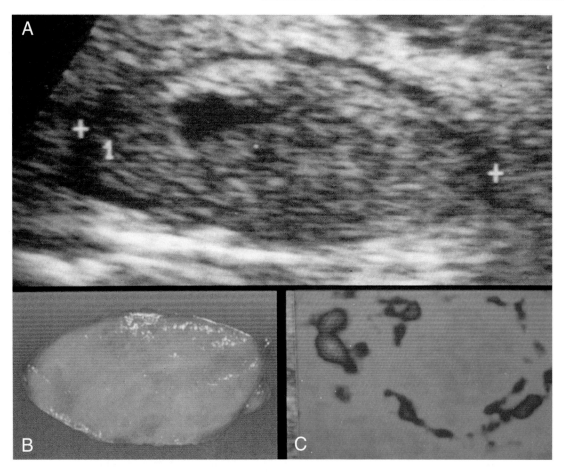

Fig. 3.8 Nodular goiter. The thin hypoechoic peripheral halo (A) consists of perilesional vessels, as power Doppler (C) clearly shows. In the surgical specimen (B) these vessels are collapsed and appear as a thin, regular border.

about $110\,\mu$m in diameter – can be shown inside hypoechoic nodules.[5]

The use of high-frequency dedicated probes improves ultrasound sensitivity.[3] Such probes can detect microcalcifications as small as $50\,\mu$m in diameter, which are almost exclusively found in thyroid malignancies, such as papillary and medullary cancers.[2] Sonography is the only imaging modality that allows these microcalcifications to be demonstrated in vivo: they are displayed as hyperechoic dots, with or without posterior shadowing (Fig. 3.15), or as 'microshadows' with no visible dots. The same pattern is characteristic of node metastatic involvement (Fig. 3.16).

Degree and type of vascularity and their correlation with structure are discussed in Chapter 4.

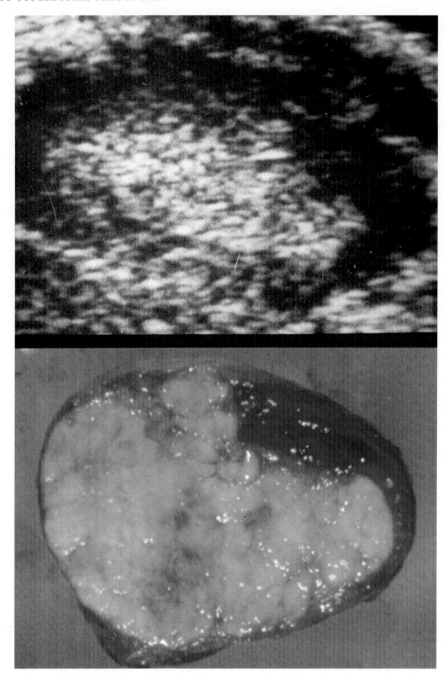

Fig. 3.9   Follicular carcinoma of the thyroid gland. The large, irregular peripheral halo is due to necrosis and hemorrhage of the surrounding tissues compressed by the rapidly growing tumor, as is demonstrated in the surgical specimen.

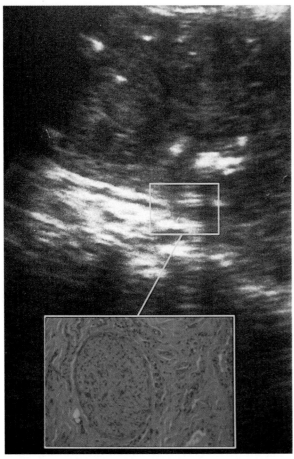

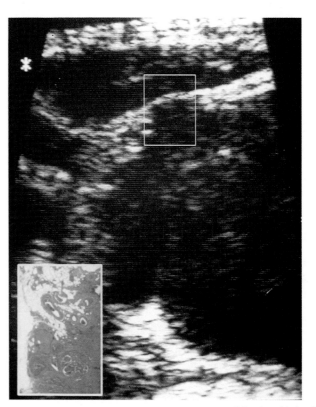

Fig. 3.11 Large, lobulated invasive follicular carcinoma of the thyroid gland. The invasion of perithyroideal fibrous and fatty tissues by the tumor is confirmed histologically.

Fig. 3.10 Undifferentiated carcinoma of the thyroid gland, studied with a 5 MHz probe because of its large size. The mass encases the laryngeal recurrent nerve, which is represented as a thin hypoechoic line posterior to the thyroid lobe. Histological examination reveals an oval nerve branch embedded in the neoplastic tissue.

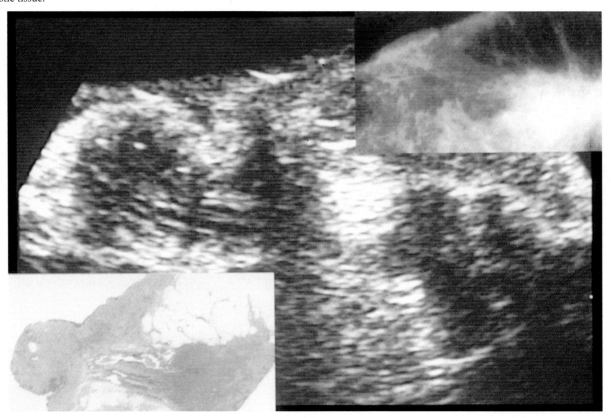

Fig. 3.12 Cancer spreading within the mammary ducts causes segmentary ductal dilatation. The ducts connecting the tumor to the nipple are typically hypoechoic, stretched and rigid.

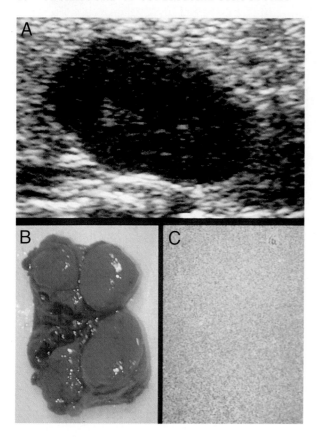

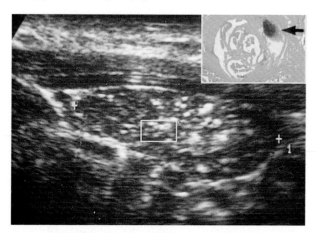

Fig. 3.13 The typical homogeneously hypoechoic pattern of parathyroid tumors (A) is closely related to the homogeneity of the specimen (B) and of the histological section (C), which consists of small, closely packed and regularly spaced cells.

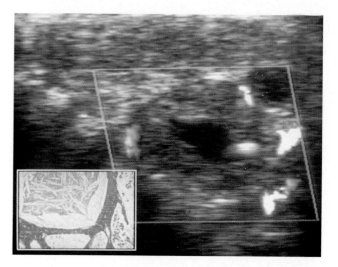

Fig. 3.14 Parathyroid hyperplasia with unusually inhomogeneous and avascular pattern due to anechoic necrotic changes, confirmed by histological examination.

Fig. 3.15 Scan (13 MHz) of papillary carcinoma involving the whole thyroid lobe. The tumor is characterized by many scattered hyperechoic dots which histologically correspond to the tiny (30–50 μm) calcific psammoma bodies (arrow) representing one of the hallmarks of papillary carcinoma.

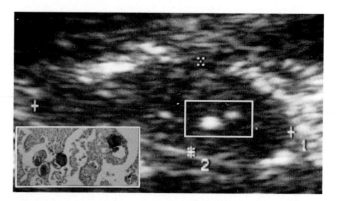

Fig. 3.16 Lymph node of the deep jugular chain with metastasis from papillary cancer of the thyroid gland. Few microcalcifications due to calcific psammoma bodies are detected.

REFERENCES

1. Fornage B, Lorigan J, Andry E 1989 Fibroadenoma of the breast: sonographic appearance. Radiology 172: 671–675
2. Solbiati L, Cioffi F, Ballarati E 1992 Ultrasonography of the neck. Radiol Clin North Am 30: 941–954
3. Rizzatto G, Chersevani R, Solbiati L 1993 High-resolution ultrasound assists in breast diagnosis. Diagn Imag Int 5: 42–45
4. Gritzmann N, Grasl MC, Helmer M et al 1990 Invasion of the carotid artery and jugular vein by lymph node metastases: detection with sonography. AJR 154: 411–414
5. Kasumi F 1988 Identification of microcalcification in breast cancers by ultrasound. Ultrasound Med Biol 14: 175–182

4

Spectral and color Doppler signals related to pathology

E. Ueno   E. Tohno

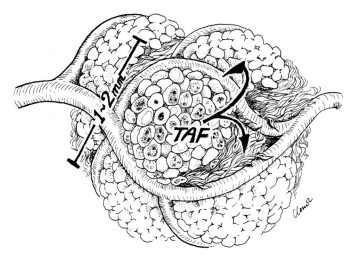

Fig. 4.1 Most tumors will never grow to more than 1–2 mm in diameter. Angiogenetic factors cause neovascularization and fibrosis.

Tumor neovascularization is a process that is similar in all organs apart from features specific to some pathological processes. In this chapter particular reference is made to the breast because of the good correlation between imaging and pathology in that organ.

TUMOR NEOVASCULARIZATION

Without the ability to recruit new blood vessels or to enter and leave the bloodstream, most tumors would never attain more than 1–2 mm in diameter.[1] There is a strong correlation between vacularization and tumor growth. Neovascularization is due to tumor angiogenetic factors (TAF) secreted by cancer cells[2] (Fig. 4.1).

Many angiogenetic factors have been investigated, including fibroblast growth factor (FGF), vascular endothelial growth factor (VEGF) and transforming growth factor α (TGF-α). FGF is the representative TAF and is classified into seven factors. One of these, the basic FGF, with paracrine activities, is rapidly secreted from fibrosarcomas, after their transformation from fibromas; as a result, tumor growth and neovascularization are markedly accelerated.[3] This phenomenon probably occurs with other malignant tumors also.

Tumor neovascularization is initiated from a starting vessel, at the level of a terminal arteriole. The new vessel anastomoses with host capillaries, resulting in a rich network of tumor vessels.[4] With neoplastic growth, the blood pressure in the starting vessel (normally 30–40 cmH$_2$O) increases to 120–130 cmH$_2$O, while the already existing postcapillaries become deformed and dilated, causing a decrease in blood pressure.[5] Reduction in blood capillary pressure is likely to disturb capillary exchange. Neovascularization occurs in particular at the periphery of the tumor, while low-pressure capillaries inside the tumor are reduced or occluded, producing central necrosis. Thus, the degree of vascularization differs in different parts of the tumor, being high at the periphery and low in the center.

Tumoral cell invasion is due to destruction of the basement membrane. This process is possible because cancer cells attach themselves to the laminin (a glycoprotein of the basement membrane) by means of their laminin receptors and secrete type IV collagenase that destroys the basement membrane. On the other hand, arteries are not invaded by this process: tumor angiogenetic factors affect the fibrous tissues, causing encasement of the arteries, which become tortuous and may be obstructed (Fig. 4.2).

As well as differences in degree of vascularization, angiographic studies have demonstrated different vascular patterns in the center and the periphery of tumors.[6,7] In the center there are numerous abnormal, chaotically arranged vessels that represent abnormally proliferated capillaries. These capillaries are dilated, with an irregular diameter

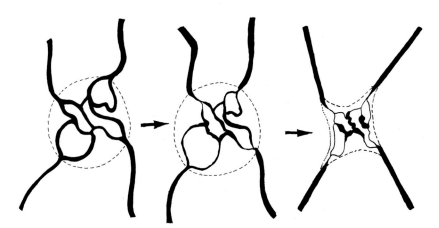

Fig. 4.2 TAF affect the fibroblasts, causing stenosis and obstruction of arteries and producing desmoplasia, with convergence of surrounding tissues. The center of the tumor becomes necrotic, in spite of neovascularization, and displays a chaotic vascular network.

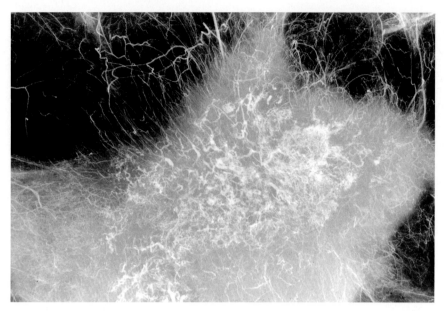

Fig. 4.3 Specimen angiography shows vessels at the periphery of tumor and interruption of some main feeding arteries. Dilated vessels form a chaotic network in the center of the tumor.

that varies from 50 to 500 μm. Blood flow is stagnant because of the low pressure and low resistance in the center of the tumour and the concurrent high degree of resistance of the drainage veins (Fig. 4.3). At present the slow flow in these veins cannot be detected with color flow imaging. At the periphery of a malignant tumor, arteries enter more or less at a right angle, together with the accompanying veins. The feeding arteries are encased and obstructed. Angi-

ography reveals early venous drainage, which means that there are arteriovenous (AV) shunts at the periphery. The existence of these AV shunts has also been demonstrated by the higher oxygen concentration in the drainage vein than in the normal tissue, despite the high metabolic rate of the tumor.[6] The presence of arteries on the tumoral surface is typical of expanding tumors, such as fibro-adenomas.

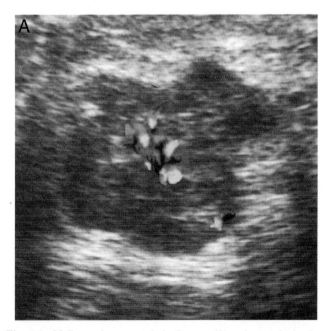

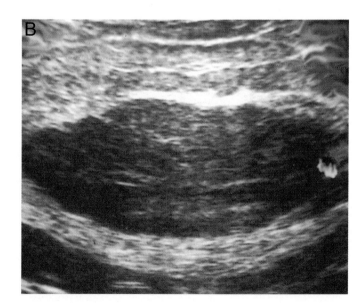

Fig. 4.4 Malignant hypervascularized tumor (A) and avascular benign mass (B).

Table 4.1 Percentage of cases of malignant (n = 125) or benign (n = 103) breast tumor in which no vessel (0), a single vessel (+) or multiple vessels (+ + +) were detected by ultrasound

Tumor size (mm)	Malignant (0)	(+)	(+ + +)	Benign (0)	(+)	(+ + +)
<10	72.7	18.2	9.1	86.4	13.6	0
10–20	21.8	28.2	50.0	56.8	31.8	11.4
20–40	18.6	15.2	66.2	46.6	20.0	33.4
>40	13.1	8.6	78.3	28.5	14.3	57.2

Table 4.2 Percentage distribution of morphological and color tone features in color Doppler maps from vessels in malignant and benign breast tumors

Color Doppler findings	Tumor Benign	Malignant
Feeding artery	(n = 28)	(n = 24)
Irregular	14.3	75.0
Regular	78.6	20.8
Unclassified	7.1	4.2
Color tone	(n = 23)	(n = 23)
Mosaic	43.5	78.3
Monotone	56.5	17.4
Unclassified	–	4.3

MORPHOLOGICAL ASSESSMENT BY COLOR DOPPLER

Tumoral vascularization is usually evaluated qualitatively.

Previously, it was thought that masses with visible vessels were malignant, and that non-vascularized masses were benign (Fig. 4.4).[8–10] However, improved detection of low-flow signals has allowed demonstration of vessels in benign tumors also, mostly in fibroadenomas. As a consequence, there has been confusion in the diagnosis of tumors that has been based only on the visibility of vessels. Study of the vascularization of breast tumors has shown that there are more vessels in carcinomas; when comparing vascularity in tumors of the same size, however, the difference between carcinomas and fibroadenomas is not so marked (Table 4.1); the reduced vascularization of fibroadenomas can be influenced by tumor size. Technical developments probably will not affect the percentage of hypervascular tumors recorded, but will undoubtedly bring about an increase in the number of hypovascular compared with avascular type documented.

The morphology of the vessels is also informative. As previously stated, the feeding artery enters a malignant tumor more or less at a right angle, whereas an artery associated with an expansive growth, such as a fibroadenoma, runs along the surface of the tumor (Fig. 4.5). The demonstration of a penetrating artery and its encasement in the tumoral tissues permits the diagnosis of cancer (Fig. 4.6). Some feeding arteries become the tumor vessels themselves, whereas others pass through the mass.

Vessels inside the tumor are irregular and tortuous, compressed by the surrounding tumoral tissues. The color map from these vessels appears as a 'mosaic' because of frequent velocity changes and vessel tortuosity. Conversely, fibro-

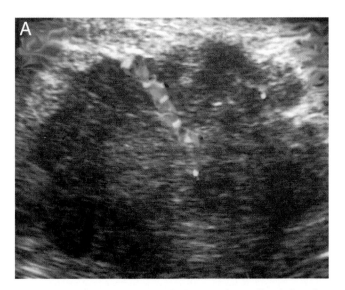
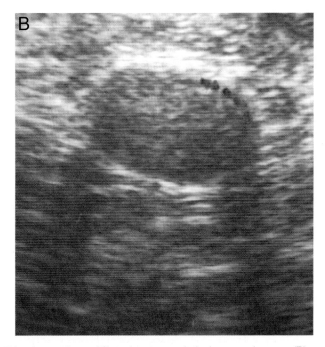

Fig. 4.5   In malignant tumors the feeding arteries go directly into the tumor (A), whereas those of fibroadenomas encircle the expansive mass (B).

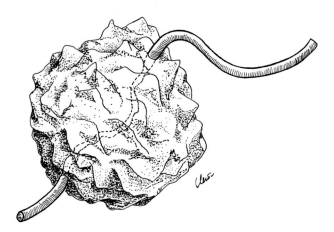

Fig. 4.6   Encased artery penetrating a malignant tumor.

adenomas have one or more surrounding, peripheral arteries, which show fairly regular and 'monotone' features (Fig. 4.7). In fibroadenomas even the intratumoral vessels may appear monotone. Because aliasing affects the color map, special care must be given to equipment settings (see Ch. 1). In our patients, feeding vessels of malignant tumors were tortuous in 75% of cases and mosaic in 78.3%. In benign tumors these values were 14.3% and 43.5% respectively (Table 4.2).

Both an early venous opacification on the angiogram, as well as a pulsating Doppler spectrum related to the drainage vein, suggests the existence of AV shunts. Color Doppler cannot demonstrate blood pooling in the center of the tumor, which can be seen on the specimen angiogram.

PATHOLOGIC CORRELATIONS

The appearance of invasive ductal carcinoma depends on the amount of fibrous stroma and on the growth pattern. Hence, we can distinguish stellate or scirrhous carcinomas and circumscribed carcinomas. Stellate carcinomas with variable distal sound attenuation are hypovascular; their arteries are encased and compressed by the surrounding tissue; blood flow in the center of the tumor is poor. Conversely, circumscribed carcinomas, such as invasive ductal carcinomas with a papillotubular or solid tubular pattern, and medullary hypercellular carcinomas, show distal sound enhancement and vacularization. Their arteries do not collapse and they produce Doppler signals[11] (Fig. 4.8).

A correlation has been established between vascularization and prognosis. In breast cancer, an abundance of microvessels in the tumor indicates a great degree of axillary lymph node involvement and a poor prognosis.[12,13] Stellate carcinoma is highly fibrotic, is hypovascular on angiography and gives few, if any, Doppler signals; nevertheless, microangiographic studies[7] show many vessels at the periphery of the tumor (Fig. 4.9) and this carcinoma has a poor prognosis. Weak Doppler signals are probably due to beam attenuation and vessel interruption, as well as to reduced Doppler sensitivity; nevertheless, vascularization can be demonstrated with monoclonal antibodies to platelet/endothelial cell adhesion molecules (PECAM) or factor VIII-related antigen. There is still a poor correlation between microvessel density as evaluated by immunohistochemical methods and that indicated by

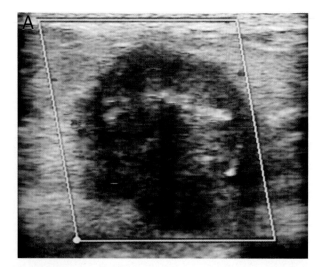

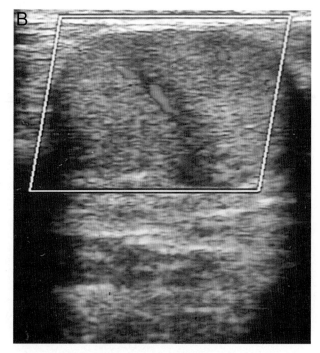

Fig. 4.7   Irregular arteries in a malignant tumor showing a 'mosaic' color Doppler pattern (A); regular vessels with a 'monotone' pattern in a fibroadenoma (B).

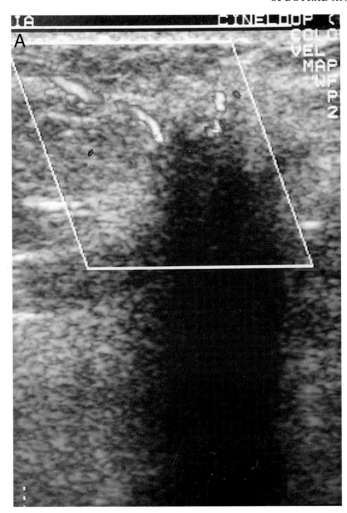

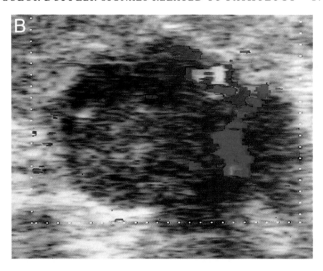

Fig. 4.8 Stellate carcinomas, which are highly fibrotic, cause distal sound attenuation and are hypovascular (A). Non-attenuating carcinoma, with posterior enhancement, is rich in malignant cells and vascularization: circumscribed ductal carcinoma (B).

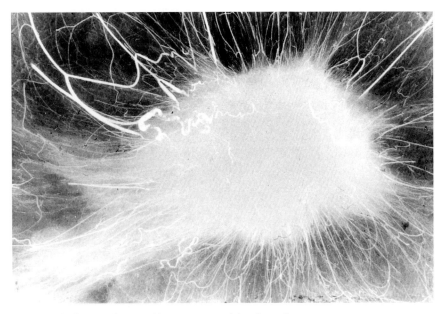

Fig. 4.9 Stellate carcinoma with numerous peripheral vessels.

Doppler flow assessment; this discrepancy is probably due to the inadequate sensitivity of current technology, as discussed in Chapter 1.

FUNCTIONAL ASSESSMENT BY SPECTRAL ANALYSIS

Pulsed Doppler can measure blood flow velocity. The Pulsatility Index (PI), Resistance Index (RI) and Acceleration Index (AI) can be calculated from maximum velocity (V_{max}), mean velocity (V_{mean}), minimum velocity (V_{min}) and the time between V_{max} and V_{min} (t), as follows:

$$PI = (V_{max} - V_{min})/V_{mean}$$

$$RI = (V_{max} - V_{min})/V_{max}$$
$$AI = (V_{max} - V_{min})/(t \times V_{max})$$

These indices are more reliable than velocity, which is angle dependent. The correct evaluation of blood flow velocities requires angle compensation; thus if the incident angle is more than 70 degrees, velocity is not a reliable parameter. High resistance indices are reported for malignant tumors, but with a low specificity. The acceleration index has been considered important recently. Breast cancer shows a high acceleration index and a cut-off value of 15.5/s has been reported.[14] Benign lesions have an acceleration index less than 15.5/s, whereas malignant lesions have a higher value, with a sensitivity for breast cancer of 77.8% and a specificity of 78.8%.

REFERENCES

1. Blood C H, Zetter B R 1990 Tumour interaction with the vasculature: angiogenesis and tumour metastasis. Biochim Biophys Acta 1032: 89–118
2. Folkman J, Merler E, Abernathy C 1970 Isolation of a tumor factor responsible for neovascularization. J Exp Med 133: 275–288
3. Kandel J, Bossy-Wetzel E, Radavanyi F et al 1991 Neovascularization is associated with a switch to the export of FGF in the multistep development of fibrosarcoma. Cell 66: 1095
4. Hori K, Suzuki M, Abe I, Saito S, Sato H 1981 New technique for measurement of microvasculature pressure in normal and tumour vessels of rats. Invasion Metastasis 1: 248–260
5. Hori K, Suzuki M, Saito S, Tanda S 1990 Development of the angioarchitecture and microcirculatory characteristics in rat tumor. Jpn J Cancer Chemother 17: 554–563
6. Bierman H R, Kelly K H, Singer G 1952 Studies on the blood supply of tumors in man. IV. The increased oxygen content of venous blood draining neoplasms. J Natl Cancer Inst 12: 701–707
7. Maeda M 1977 Angiography of breast using the Lo-Dose Mammography system (Dupont). Nippon Acta Radiol 37: 1101–1108
8. Cosgrove D O, Bamber J C, Davey J B, McKinna J A, Sinnett H D 1990 Color Doppler signals from breast tumors. Radiology 176: 175–180
9. Ueno E, Tsunoda-Shimizu H, Nakamura N et al 1991 Colour Doppler imaging for the diagnosis of solid masses. In: Topics in Breast Ultrasound. Shinohara, Tokyo, pp 58–62
10. Hamada M, Konishi Y, Shimada K et al 1992 Color Doppler echography of breast diseases: detection rate of color flow signals and significance of color Doppler echography in breast diseases. Jpn J Med Ultrason 19: 329–336
11. Tsunoda-Shimizu H, Ueno E, Hirano M, Nakamura N, Imamura A, Itai Y 1991 Correlation of color Doppler imaging with B mode pattern in diagnosis of breast carcinoma. Jpn Soc Ultrasound Med Proc 18: 353–354
12. Horak E R, Leek R, Klenk N et al 1992 Angiogenesis, assessed by platelet/endothelial cell adhesion molecule antibodies, as indicator of node metastases and survival in breast cancer. Lancet 340: 1120–1124
13. Toi M, Kashitani J, Tominga T 1993 Tumor angiogenesis is an independent prognostic indicator in primary breast carcinoma. Int J Cancer 55: 371–374
14. Konishi Y, Hamada M, Simada K et al 1992 Value of Doppler spectral analysis of the intratumoral waveform in the breast diseases. Jpn Soc Ultrasound Med Proc 62: 490–491

5

Thyroid gland

L. Solbiati   T. Livraghi   E. Ballarati   T. Ierace
L. Crespi

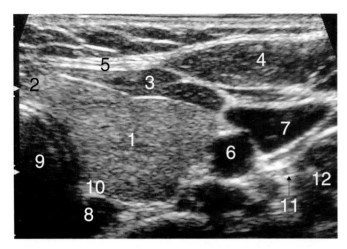

Fig. 5.1 Transverse scan of the left thyroid compartment. 1: left thyroid lobe; 2: thyroid isthmus; 3: prethyroid muscles; 4: sternocleidomastoid muscle; 5: anterior cervical fascia; 6: carotid artery; 7: deep jugular vein; 8: esophagus; 9: trachea; 10: tracheo-esophageal groove (with minor neurovascular bundle); 11: vagus nerve; 12: anterior scalene muscle.

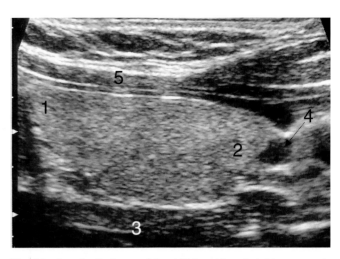

Fig. 5.2 Longitudinal scan of thyroid lobe with typical thin upper pole (1) and rounded lower pole (2). 3: longus colli muscle; 4: lower thyroid vein; 5: prethyroid muscles.

ANATOMY

The thyroid gland lies in the antero-inferior aspect of the neck (infrahyoid compartment), in a space outlined by muscles, fascias, the larynx, trachea and esophagus and also including blood vessels, nerves and the parathyroid glands.

With regard to the muscles and aponeuroses of the neck, numerous structures can be discerned at high ultrasound frequencies (7.5–13 MHz). Immediately below the subcutaneous plane is a thin (1–2 mm) hypoechoic line corresponding to the platysma. Anterior to it is a thin hyperechoic line representing the superficial cervical apo-

neurosis and dorsal to it are the three principal infrahyoid prethyroid muscles (sternocleidomastoid, sternohyoid and omohyoid). Lateral to them is the largest muscular structure of the neck, the sternocleidomastoid muscle (Fig. 5.1). Anteriorly, the prethyroid muscles taper off to end, along the midline, in the fibrous median raphe together with aponeurotic and ligamentous formations. This raphe is not of much importance sonographically and the same applies to the more lateral cervical aponeurosis and to the perithyroid sheath that envelops the thyroid and the neurovascular bundle of the neck. An important ultrasound landmark is the longus colli muscle, which lies dorsal to the medial wall of the thyroid lobes in close contact with

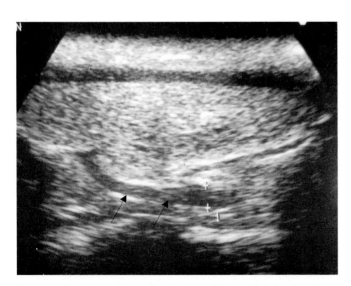

Fig. 5.3 Longitudinal scan. Arrow: normal (2 mm) inferior thyroid artery in its longitudinal course behind the thyroid lobe.

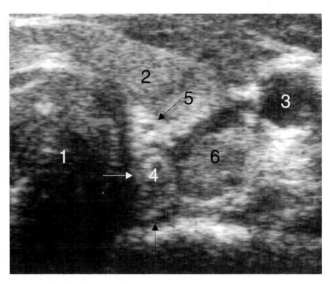

Fig. 5.4 Transverse scan of the left thyroid compartment. 1: trachea; 2: thyroid lobe; 3: carotid artery; 4: esophagus; 5: recurrent laryngeal nerve; 6: parathyroid tumor.

the prevertebral planes (Fig. 5.2). Lateral to these planes, especially in thin patients, the anterior scalene muscle can be discerned behind the outermost portion of the thyroid lobes and the great muscles of the neck (see Fig. 5.1).

The principal vessels of the infrahyoid compartment are the thyroid arteries and veins. There are two thyroid arteries on each side, superior and inferior; rarely, a third is present on the midline, the arteria ima. The mean diameter of these arteries is about 1–2 mm. The superior thyroid artery arises from the external carotid artery and descends towards the homolateral thyroid lobe, dividing at the upper pole of the lobe into two branches, anterior and posterior. The latter is visible on the ultrasound scan. The inferior thyroid artery arises from the thyrocervical trunk and appears on the scans starting at the point at which it crosses the common carotid artery posteriorly at right angles. In its subsequent upward course the artery describes a 90 degree curve and lies longitudinally, at the level of the posteromedial angle of the thyroid lobes (Fig. 5.3), in the tracheo-esophageal space, in close contact with the recurrent laryngeal nerve (Fig. 5.4). Normally, with pulsed Doppler, thyroid arteries have peak systolic velocities of 20–40 cm/s (the highest values of all the vessels supplying superficial organs) with diastolic velocities of 10–15 cm/s. In goiters, but mostly in thyroid diseases with hyperfunction, arteries increase their size and peak systolic values can even attain 70–90 cm/s (Fig. 5.5). The thyroid veins

originate from the perithyroid venous network and join to form three groups (upper, middle and lower) and drain into the homolateral jugular vein. The largest vessel is the lower vein, which occasionally can attain 7–8 mm at its largest diameter (Fig. 5.6).

Of the nerves in the infrahyoid compartment, the only one of importance for ultrasound implications is the recurrent laryngeal nerve. Originating from the vagus, it runs initially behind the subclavian artery (on the right) and the aortic arch (on the left), describing a loop around these vessels, to take an upward course, running in the angle between the trachea, esophagus and thyroid lobe (see Fig. 5.4). In this segment it images on the longitudinal scans as a thin hypoechoic line, circumscribed anteriorly and posteriorly by thin hyperechoic lines between the thyroid lobe and the longus colli muscle on the right (Fig. 5.7) and between thyroid lobe and esophagus on the left. In this portion of its course the nerve lies in close contact with the posterior wall of the thyroid lobe and with the anatomical sites of the inferior parathyroids situated in front of it. This anatomical arrangement explains the frequent involvement of the nerve in the course of space-occupying diseases of the thyroid (Fig. 5.8) or parathyroid glands and the possibility of functional deficits of the laryngeal apparatus.

The thyroid gland is made up of two lobes, connected medially by the isthmus, which has a transverse course. From 10 to 40% of normal subjects have a third thyroid

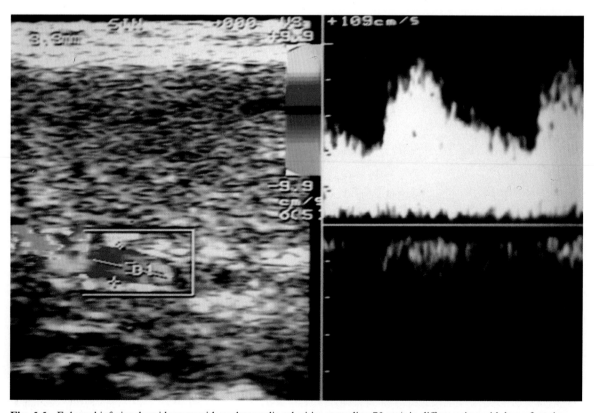

Fig. 5.5   Enlarged inferior thyroid artery with peak stystolic velocities exceeding 70 cm/s in diffuse goiter with hyperfunction.

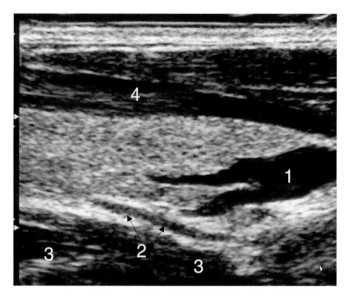

Fig. 5.6 Longitudinal scan. 1: large lower thyroid vein (8 mm); 2: inferior thyroid artery; 3: longus colli muscle; 4: prethyroid muscles.

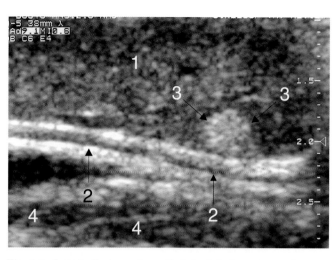

Fig. 5.7 Longitudinal scan (magnified view). 1: thyroid parenchyma; 2: recurrent laryngeal nerve; 3: tiny (4 mm) fibrotic area of thyroid lobe; 4: longus colli muscle.

lobe (pyramidal) arising from the isthmus and running upwards along the same longitudinal axis as the thyroid lobes and lying in front of the thyroid cartilage[1] (Fig. 5.9). It can be imaged in the young but it undergoes progressive atrophy in adulthood.

The morphology, size and even site of the thyroid lobes with reference to the laryngeal and tracheal structures behind them vary widely in normal subjects, depending particularly on body built. The lateral lobes examined in sagittal planes are roughly pear-shaped with the tip at the cranial end and a rounded base (see Fig. 5.2). In longilineal individuals the pear shape is slimmer and longer; in brachymorphic (brevilineal) types it is more globose. Conse-

quently, the normal dimensions of the lobes vary widely between individuals. In the newborn the lobes are normally between 18 and 20 mm long with an anteroposterior diameter of 8–9 mm. At 1 year of age the mean length is 25 mm and the anteroposterior diameter 12–15 mm.[2] In adults the mean length is in the range of 40–60 mm and the mean anteroposterior diameter 13–18 mm. The mean thickness of the isthmus is 4–6 mm.[3]

At present, sonography is the most accurate method by which to calculate thyroid volume: this is particularly important in clinical situations such as the diagnosis of goiter, the calculation of the dose of ^{131}I to be administered in thyrotoxicosis, or assessment of the response to sup-

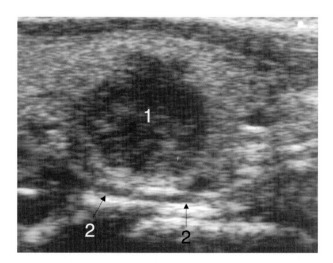

Fig. 5.8 15 mm papillary cancer (1) in close proximity with the laryngeal recurrent nerve (2), displaced posteriorly, but not infiltrated by the tumor.

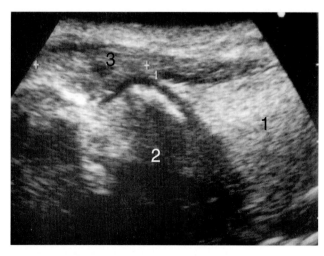

Fig. 5.9 Longitudinal scan of the upper pole (1) of thyroid gland. 2: thyroid cartilage; 3: pyramidal lobe.

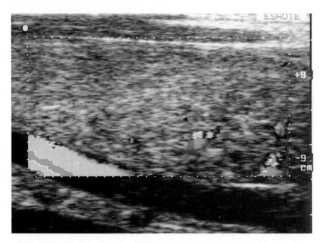

Fig. 5.10   Normal thyroid gland with few blood flow signals, mostly localized at the poles.

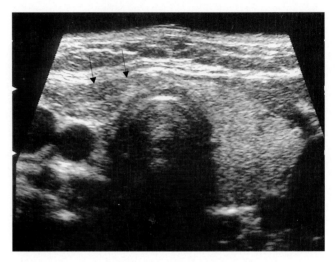

Fig. 5.11   Severe congenital hypoplasia of the right lobe (arrow) of the thyroid gland.

pression treatments.[4] Compared with sonographic measurements, physical examination is incorrect in 32–39% of cases.[5]

Thyroid volume can be calculated with linear parameters or, more precisely, with mathematical formulae. Among the linear parameters, the anteroposterior diameter is now regarded as the most important, as it is relatively independent of possible dimensional asymmetries (especially longitudinal) between the two lobes. It is measured by placing the transducer parallel to the longest axis of the thyroid lobe, with slight lateromedial obliquity. A longitudinal diameter of more than 2 cm is grounds for suspicion of thyroid enlargement; when this diameter is 2.5 cm, the thyroid is definitely enlarged.

The most precise method of calculating thyroid volume is an integration of formulae of serial areas obtained from US contiguous scans.[6] In neonates, thyroid volume ranges from 0.40 to 1.40 ml, increasing by approximately 1.0–1.3 ml for each 10 kg of weight, up to a normal volume in adults of 10–11 ± 3–4 ml.[7] Thyroid volume is related to some physiological conditions, being greater in men than in women and increasing with the patient's age and body surface area. Furthermore, it is generally larger in regions with iodine deficiency and in patients with acute hepatitis and chronic renal failure, and it is smaller in chronic hepatitis.[4,8]

The echo texture of the thyroid parenchyma is fine, homogeneous, more echogenic than that of the contiguous muscular structures, and interrupted at the periphery (and especially at the poles) by the arterial and venous vessels. In normal conditions, blood flow signals detectable with color Doppler are few, mainly localized at the poles and in thin intraparenchymal septa (Fig. 5.10). The thin hyperechoic line that bounds the parenchyma (the capsule) is clearly identifiable on the US scans (see Fig. 5.2) and may present extensive foci of calcification, mostly in cases of

uremia or in disorders of calcium metabolism.

The homogeneous ultrasound pattern of the thyroid parenchyma is often interrupted, especially in the elderly, by small (5–6 mm) clear-cut echo-free spaces corresponding to accumulation of colloid, of no pathological significance. Less frequently there may be calcified spots and patches of fibrotic tissue (see Fig. 5.7) within the parenchyma; both of these are expressions of tissue aging and are of no pathological importance.[3]

CONGENITAL PATHOLOGY

Congenital diseases of the thyroid include agenesia or hemi-agenesia, total or partial hypoplasia and ectopia.

In agenesia or hypoplasia, the chief symptoms are those of hypothyroidism, which is earlier and more severe in agenesia and in total hypoplasia. Ultrasound scans easily demonstrate these malformations and their extent (Fig. 5.11). In hemiagenesis the compensatory hypertrophy of the contralateral lobe is evident.[2,3]

There are many forms of thyroid ectopia – lingual, sublingual, paralaryngeal, intratracheal, infrasternal.[1] Lingual ectopia is the one most easily discerned by ultrasound: the ectopic thyroid appears as a roundish or ovoid structure with sharply defined contours, highly vascularized and homogeneous in texture and with the same levels of echogenicity as the normal parenchyma.[9] The mean diameter of these thyroids does not as a rule exceed 20–25 mm; when the glands are larger, they may undergo the same colloid-cystic colliquative degeneration as thyroids in the typical site (Fig. 5.12).

High-frequency ultrasound is at present the first-line imaging procedure in the study of congenital hypothyroidism, as it permits accurate measurement of the thyroid lobes, as stated earlier, and differentiation between hypothyroidism secondary to agenesia or hypoplasia, or goitrous in nature (with enlargement of the thyroid gland), or hypothyroidism with a thyroid gland normal or below borderline in size, usually accompanied by the clinical findings of hyperthyrotropinemia.[10]

ACQUIRED PATHOLOGY

Acquired diseases of the thyroid include numerous pathologies that are not easy to classify. The first distinction is between functional and histological diseases: the former include hypothyroidism and hyperthyroidism. Hypothyroidism may be due to congenital anomalies (described above), diseases of the pituitary gland or hypothalamus, autoimmune thyroiditis, iodine excess, incorrect treatment with antithyroid drugs, or it may occur following surgery

or radioiodine ablation. Hyperthyroidism is mostly caused by Graves' disease, toxic multinodular goiter, autonomous nodule (Plummer's disease), inappropriate thyroid-stimulating hormone (TSH) secretion, drug administration, or thyroiditis [both of autoimmune etiology (Hashitoxicosis) and as a result of early follicular disruption]. In this chapter, however, thyroid pathologies will be described according to the histological classification, which is better suited to the peculiarities of an imaging modality such as ultrasound.

The histological features of thyroid diseases are not always clearly distinguishable and the terminology to be used in defining them is not always unequivocal. The current complete classification of the principal acquired diseases of the thyroid is given in Table 5.1.

From the imaging point of view, the first line of demarcation is between diseases with nodules, single or multiple, and diffuse diseases without evidence of nodules. Even here, there are frequent variants due to the association of one or more nodular lesions with a diffuse structural

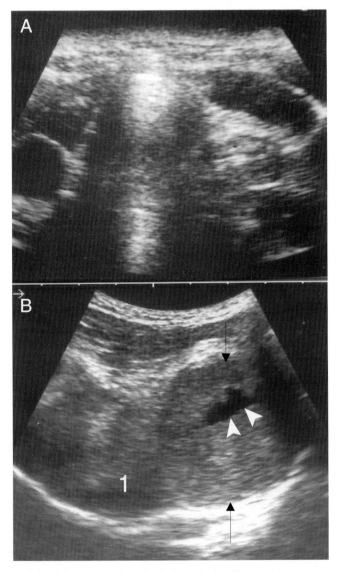

Fig. 5.12 Lingual ectopia of the thyroid gland. **A** The thyroid compartment is completely empty. **B** The rounded lingual thyroid gland (arrow), with small fluid changes (arrowhead) is close to the base of the tongue (1).

Table 5.1 Classification of acquired diseases of the thyroid

Hyperplasia	Diffuse	
	Nodular	Uninodular Multinodular
Adenoma	Follicular	Trabecular (embryonal) Tubular Microfollicular (fetal) Normofollicular (simple) Macrofollicular (colloid) Oxyphilic (Hurthle cells)
	Non-follicular	
Malignant tumors	Carcinomas of the follicular epithelium	Differentiated (follicular, papillary) Poorly differentiated (with tall, oxyphilic columnar cells, follicular and papillary carcinomas) Undifferentiated (with large cells, spindle cells, sarcomas)
	Medullary carcinomas Lymphomas	
Thyroiditis	Acute/Subacute	Acute suppurative Subacute (De Quervain's) Silent (painless) Post-partum
	Chronic	Lymphocytic (Hashimoto's and variants) Riedel's Tuberculous Parasitic

change, or of a lesion that usually is single (adenoma, carcinoma) with pre-existing multiple nodules.

Nodular disease is much more common than diffuse disease, affecting up to 8–10% of the adult population, with a clear prevalence of females and with incidence varying with such factors as geographical area, or exposure to ionizing radiation.[11] Unsuspected thyroid nodules have been detected incidentally in up to 13–40% of patients undergoing carotid or parathyroid ultrasound examinations.[12,13]

Other features peculiar to thyroid nodules are the definite prevalence of benign diseases (some 90% of the total) and the high incidence of small (diameters under 10–15 mm) clinically occult nodules.[14]

The aims of an ultrasound examination are identification of masses as intra- or extrathyroidal, the detection of thyroid nodules (in these applications high-frequency ultrasound is the most accurate imaging modality) and, possibly, characterization of nodules, differentiating 'benign' (or non-surgical) lesions (merely followed up) from those that are questionable or malignant (to be biopsied).[4]

Hyperplasia and goiter

Thyroid hyperplasia is the commonest pathological condition of the gland (80–85% of the total), occurring in up to 5% of any population.[15] It has several causes, including iodine deficiency (endemic), disorders of hormonogenesis (hereditary familial forms), poor utilization of iodine as a result of drugs or goiter-inducing foods.

When hyperplasia leads to an overall increase in the volume of the thyroid, it is correct to use the term 'goiter'. The sex ratio is 3:1 in favour of females and the peak age group is between 35 and 50 years.

The histological presentation of hyperplasia varies but the starting point is always diffuse cellular hyperplasia of the thyroid acini. In children and in cases of recent onset this feature remains constant and may extend to the whole gland (diffuse hyperplasia) until it reaches the point of an overall increase in volume (diffuse goiter). In adults and in case of longer standing, micronodules develop and reproduce in clusters the structure of thyroid follicles and vesicles containing colloid substance, enveloped in a non-vascularized eosinophilic mass. Progression of the disease is marked by the formation of macronodules, which may contain a homogeneous solid structure but which often undergo colliquative degeneration with the accumulation of serous fluid (false cysts), colloid substance or blood (hemorrhagic 'cysts'). Nodular hyperplasias (uni- or multinodular) or nodular goiters are formed in this way. According to the type of fluid within the areas of degeneration they are termed cystic, colloid–cystic or hemorrhagic hyperplasia or goiters. The hemorrhagic type is much swifter in onset than the others, owing to the rapid formation of intralesional hemorrhages. Cystic hyperplasia (or cystic goiter) is the only cystic disease of the thyroid, true cysts (with secretory epithelium) being practically non-existent in this gland.

The ultimate stage of hyperplasia or goiter in the degenerative variants is calcification, which may present in two ways – coarse calcifications throughout the thyroid parenchyma and shell-shaped calcifications that surround nodules and clusters of nodules.[4,16,17]

Functionally, too, hyperplasia and goiter may present extremely variable characteristics. In diffuse disease, function may be normal or increased (Graves' or Basedow's disease); in nodular disease, function may be decreased (rarely), normal, or increased (toxic nodules). These functional differences have important repercussions on the radionuclide scans (not covered here) and also on the ultrasound patterns.

In diffuse hyperplasia and goiter, sonography shows not only increased volume, but also rounding of the poles of the gland (Fig. 5.13); in long-standing goiters a somewhat coarse and patchy structure without nodular lesions develops. In diffuse goiters, the blood vessels feeding and draining the thyroid gland are found to be increased in number and size, which is due solely to the increased volume of the parenchyma. Spectrum analysis does not usually highlight increases in flow velocities.

In hyperplasia accompanied by hyperfunction (Graves' disease) the gland contours are lobulated and the size is increased, with usually prompt response to effective medical treatment: size reduction is a useful indicator of therapeutic success.[18] The echo texture may be less homogeneous than in diffuse goiter, mainly because of the presence of numerous large intraparenchymal vessels (Fig. 5.14). Furthermore, especially in young patients, the parenchyma may be diffusely hypoechoic, owing either to the extensive lymphocyte infiltration or to the predominantly cellular content of the parenchyma, which is almost devoid of colloid substance.[19]

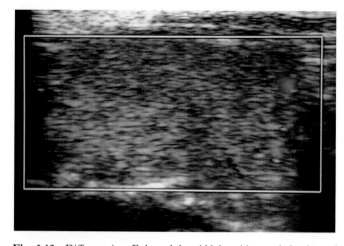

Fig. 5.13 Diffuse goiter. Enlarged thyroid lobe with rounded poles and sparse, scattered flow signals.

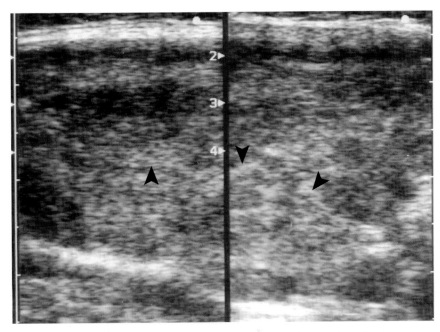

Fig. 5.14 Graves' disease. Coarse echo texture with thin fibrotic septa (arrowhead).

Color flow Doppler and spectrum analysis confirm the hypervascular pattern that Ralls termed the 'thyroid inferno'[20] (Fig. 5.15): the intrathyroid arteries present turbulent blood flow with AV shunts and the highest peak systolic velocities found in thyroid diseases (50–120 cm/s) (Fig. 5.16), owing to a flow rate usually exceeding 70 ml/min.[21]

There are at present no demonstrations of correlation among degree of thyroid hyperfunction as assessed by laboratory parameters, extent of hypervascularization and flow velocity values. It is, however, known that in the course of treatment the vascular pattern revealed by color flow Doppler tends to regress as the functional data normalize.

The ultrasound pattern of nodular hyperplasia (or nodular goiter) varies widely, according to the number of colliquative areas and their extent (or size). The most typical hyperplastic nodule is isoechoic to the normal thyroid tissue, consisting of echoes of the same size, arranged regularly: the only feature that permits its identification in normal thyroid tissue is the fine hypoechoic peripheral halo of uniform thickness (Fig. 5.17). Histologically, these nodules do not have a fibrous capsule and their outlines are represented by the walls of the clusters of follicular structures and by supplying the periphery blood vessels (always collapsed on histological specimens) (see Fig. 5.17). In vivo, on the other hand, thin peripheral vessels (Fig. 5.18) and mild edema of perinodular normal tissue seem to be responsible for the thin halo. As the volume gradually increases, the nodule may assume a hyperechogenic structure, due to the macrofollicular structure, with interfaces between cells and colloid substance[4,19] (Fig. 5.19). This echo texture, found in 20–25% of nodular goiters, is highly suggestive, if not pathognomonic, of a benign lesion.

In 5–7% of cases, solid nodular goiters may also appear hypoechoic, owing to the prevailing cellular content: this structural feature, unlike those previously described, may erroneously suggest surgical disease (adenoma, carcinoma) on ultrasound examination. Only the color Doppler demonstration of poor, exclusively perinodular vascularization (Fig. 5.20A) and/or posterior acoustic enhancement suggesting a 'sponge-like' colloid content (Fig. 5.20B) can allow a confident diagnosis of a benign nature.

Irrespective of their structure, hyperplasia and nodular goiter usually have regular margins;[14,22,23] they show no signs of invasion of adjacent anatomical structures. Color

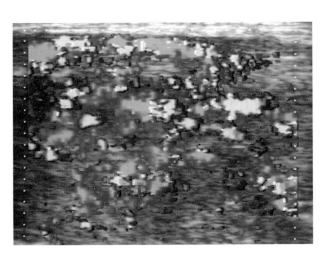

Fig. 5.15 Graves' disease: markedly hypervascular pattern ('thyroid inferno').

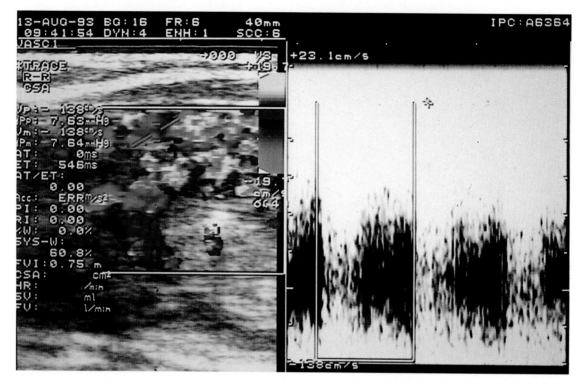

Fig. 5.16 Graves' disease. Spectral analysis shows turbulent flow with extremely high peak stystolic velocities.

Doppler shows a complete absence of flow signals in 10–15% of cases (type I pattern, according to Lagalla),[24] or exclusively perinodular arterial-flow signals (type II), with no intranodular component (see Fig. 5.18). Systolic peak flow velocities range between 15 and 40 cm/s and diastolic velocities are 5–20 cm/s.[4,17,25–27]

When a hyperplastic nodule becomes hyperfunctional (autonomous or toxic nodule), perinodular blood vessels increase in size and thickness; in 40–50% of cases the color flow pattern changes to type III (intranodular flow with multiple vascular poles, associated with perinodular signals) (Fig. 5.21) and the systolic flow velocities often exceed 30–40 cm/s, with diastolic velocities of 15 cm/s or higher.[25–27] In about 25% of cases, hyperplastic disease may have a partly (mixed pattern) or wholly fluid content, owing to extensive colloid–cystic or hemorrhagic changes (Fig. 5.22). Completely anechoic nodules are benign in 100% of cases, in our experience. These collections may be completely echo free or contain fine mobile echoes, or even show a typical fluid–fluid level varying with the patient's position (upright or supine): both aspects may be attributable to the echogenicity of the colloid substance or to the hemorrhagic content[14,23] (Fig. 5.23). The walls of the areas of colliquation may be regular or present tiny hyperechoic papillae (2–3 mm) that represent the starting point of intranodular colliquation. Multiple concamerations due to septa, sometimes thickened but always devoid of blood flow signals, are often found (Fig. 5.24): this complete absence of vascularity is important for differentiation from

cystic-papillary carcinoma.[16,25]

Lastly, nodular goiters often show scattered coarse calcifications or, more significantly, shell-like or 'egg-shell' calcifications[4,14,23] at the periphery; these are sometimes very thin, sometimes thickened so that their acoustic shadow masks the content of the nodule. Peripheral calcifications are rarely detected (2–4% of cases), but are considered the only single finding diagnostic of a benign condition[4] (Fig. 5.25). Hyperplastic (or goitrous) disease of the thyroid is multinodular in 70–80% of cases; this fact, combined with the long-held view that a solitary nodule with low uptake has a 15–25% probability of malignancy whereas a hypofunctioning nodule in a multinodular gland is malignant in less than 1% of cases[28] has led to reliance on the high sensitivity of ultrasound in the search for small nodules alongside the principal one, in order to rule out the possibility of malignancy. In fact, recent studies have shown the following:

- 70% of nodules considered solitary on scintigraphy or physical examination are actually multiple when assessed with high-frequency ultrasound[23,29]
- thyroid neoplasms are found in over 30% of cases in multinodular thyroid[30]
- papillary carcinoma is multinodular in 20% of cases in non-occult form.

Thus multinodularity is not synonymous with a benign condition and, in multinodular thyroids, sonography should be performed in conjunction with the clinical and

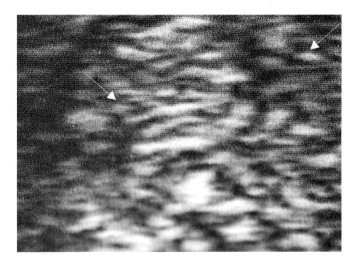

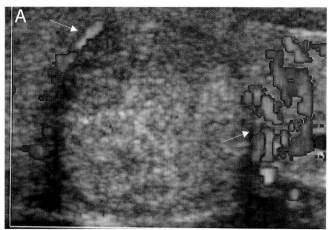

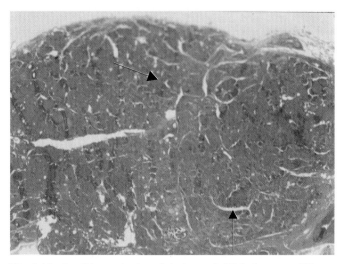

Fig. 5.17 Small hyperplastic nodule (arrows). High-frequency US depicts a very thin peripheral halo which corresponds histologically to the demarcation of the surrounding thyroid tissue, since the nodule is not outlined by fibrous capsule.

Fig. 5.18 Nodular goiters. Both color Doppler (**A**) and power Doppler (**B**) feature only perinodular (type II) flow signals (arrows).

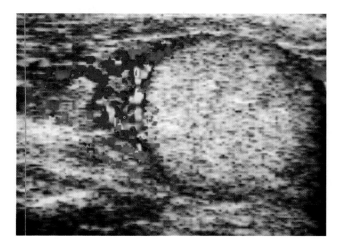

Fig. 5.19 Typical hyperechoic nodular goiter with perinodular (type II) flow signals.

perhaps radionuclide data, analyzing the structural and, if possible, vascular characteristics of every nodule. The fundamental aim of ultrasound examination is to identify one or more suspect lesions within a multinodular gland and to direct percutaneous needle aspiration biopsy for cytology at these targets, thereby reducing the number of biopsies and increasing the chances of positive findings (Fig. 5.26).

In large goiters, high-frequency sonography cannot be employed, owing to the depth of the field of view and, moreover, because the possible mediastinal extension cannot be assessed: in these circumstances computerized tomography (CT) studies are mandatory (Fig. 5.27).

Adenomas

Thyroid adenomas are histologically distinguishable into follicular (micro-, normo- and macrofollicular) and non-

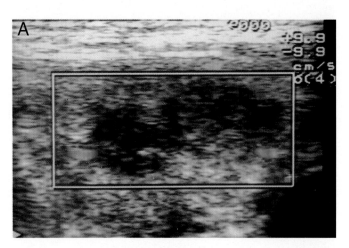

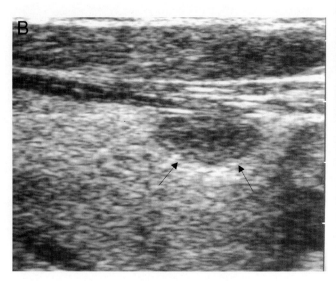

Fig. 5.20 Nodular goiters with hypoechoic structure. Hypovascularity (**A**) and acoustic distal enhancement (**B**) (arrow) suggesting colloid content are helpful for the sonographic diagnosis.

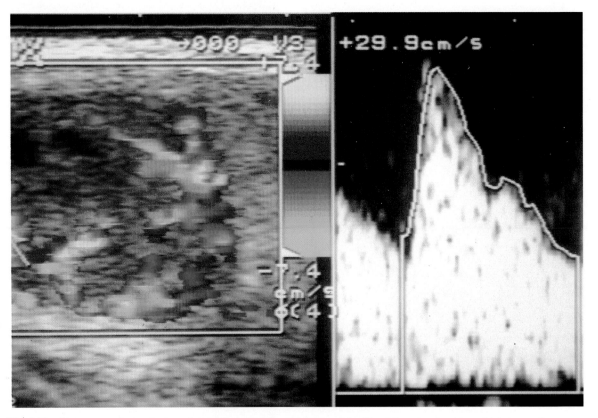

Fig. 5.21 Autonomous hyperplastic nodule with perinodular and intranodular blood flow signals with multiple internal vascular poles. Peak systolic velocities are in the normal range.

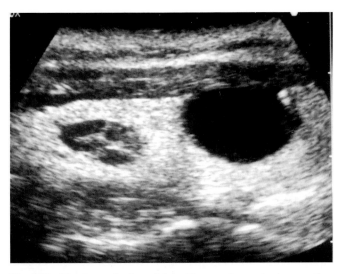

Fig. 5.22 Two hyperplastic nodules with extensive cystic changes: the smaller is partly septated.

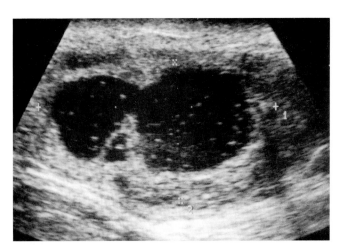

Fig. 5.23 Cystic cavity in nodular goiter: hyperechoic mobile spots in the fluid are due to hemorrhagic changes ('hemorrhagic cyst').

follicular (trabecular and fetal adenoma, papillary cysto-adenoma, Hurthle-cell adenoma). All are focal glandular proliferations outlined by a fibrous capsule (see Fig. 5.28); in the capsule most of the blood supply of the lesion is localized, with several vascular branches directed to the center of the nodule. Adenomas are much less common than hyperplastic–goitrous lesions, representing only 5–10% of all nodular diseases of the thyroid.[4] They mostly affect adult women (7:1) often being functional but very occasionally (1–2% of cases) hyperfunctional. Adenomas are commonly solitary, but they may develop within multinodular goiters. Follicular adenomas, which are found more frequently than the non-follicular variety, have cytological features indistinguishable from those of follicular carcinomas: the only distinguishing features are vascular and capsular invasiveness, which can be detected only by histological examination (see Fig. 5.32B). A cytological diagnosis of a follicular lesion therefore, as a rule, implies surgical removal. Unlike hyperplasias and nodular goiters, adenomas fall within the purview of surgical pathology.

There are no sonographic elements characteristic of thyroid adenomas. In some 50% of cases follicular adenomas are isoechoic (reproducing the normal follicular

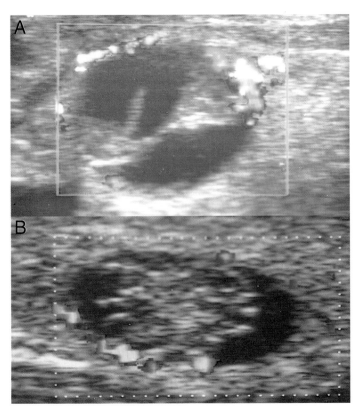

Fig. 5.24 Two nodular goiters with mixed echo texture: the solid component is very thin in **A** and thick in **B**. No flow signals are detected within the solid projections.

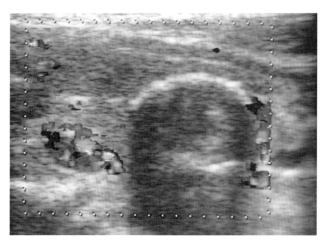

Fig. 5.25 Nodular hyperplasia with 'egg-shell' calcification and few peripheral flow signals.

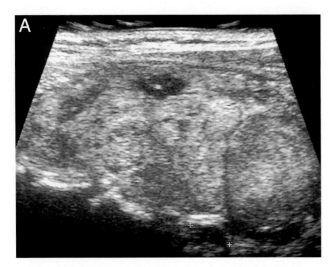

Fig. 5.26 Multinodular goiters. **A** Many nodules with the same structure (iso-hyperechoic) suggesting a benign nature are present. No further diagnostic assessments are performed. **B** Longitudinal scans of two hypoechoic nodules in the same patient, studied with power Doppler. The lesion (**Bi**) shows only perinodular flow (histology: nodular goiter) whereas in the mass (**Bii**) mainly intranodular flow signals are found (histology: papillary carcinoma).

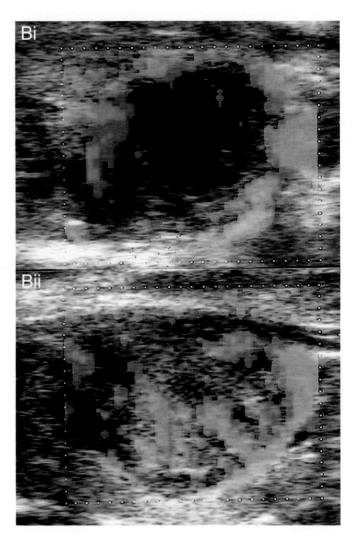

pattern of the thyroid gland), although hyperechoic mixed and, very rarely, hypoechoic patterns are possible. Non-follicular adenomas are mostly hypoechoic, although hyperechoic and mixed patterns are possible. Most adenomas show a thick peripheral halo, corresponding to the histological capsule, to the edema of the surrounding normal parenchyma (in rapidly growing nodules), or, more often, to the blood supply mainly localized along the capsule. In fact, 80–90% of adenomas show predominantly

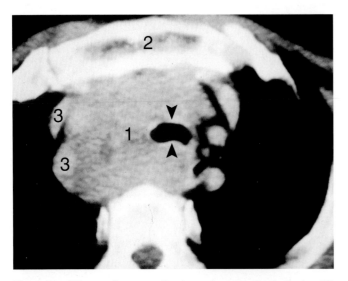

Fig. 5.27 CT scan of upper mediastinum. Large mediastinal goiter (1) which develops behind the sternum (2), displaces the blood vessels (3) and envelops the trachea (arrowhead).

perinodular blood flow signals with possible central branches (type III), whereas only 10–20% have intranodular flow signals only[24–27] (Figs 5.28–5.30). All thyroid adenomas may undergo colliquation and calcification but far less frequently than in hyperplasia and goiter. The solid portions of partly cystic adenomas, unlike those of goiters, show intense flow signals (Fig. 5.31). The systolic peak flow velocities do not differ from those measured in nodular goiters.[27]

When thyroid adenomas, especially the follicular variety, break out of the hormonal regulation mechanism and become autonomous (toxic adenomas or Plummer's disease), with increased uptake of radionuclide and inhibited function of the remaining thyroid tissue, then the echo texture does not reveal any distinguishing characteristics; with color Doppler accentuation of the type III vascular pattern may be detected, together with an increase of peak systolic velocity.[24–27] These findings are helpful in the sonographic follow-up of the autonomous nodules treated percutaneously with ethanol injections (see below). However, the most important contribution of ultrasound

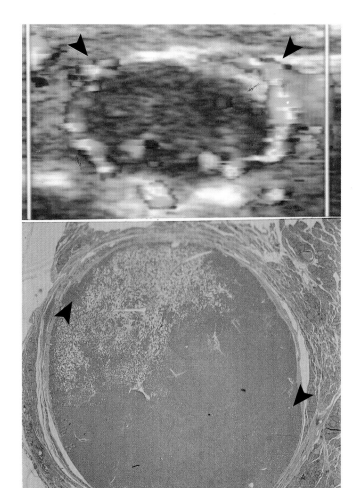

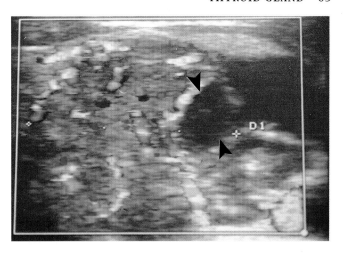

Fig. 5.29 Large follicular adenoma with small cystic changes (arrowhead). Many intranodular blood vessels with regular arrangement and course are visible, originating from pericapsular vessels.

Fig. 5.28 Follicular adenoma. Color Doppler shows mostly perinodular flow (arrowheads), at the level of the peripheral halo which corresponds histologically to a thick fibrous capsule (arrowheads). Blood vessels are not visible in the histological specimen because of their collapse. (Courtesy of Dr C. Ravetto, Second Department of Pathology, Busto Arsizio Hospital, Italy.)

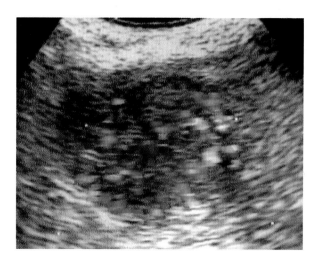

Fig. 5.30 Hypervascular toxic adenoma with exclusively intranodular vascular arrangement.

in toxic adenoma is the information it provides regarding the extranodular thyroid tissue, if present – its extent, morphology and structure in the affected and in the opposite lobe. This tissue cannot be studied by radioisotope scans unless a TSH stimulation test is performed.

Malignant tumors

Tumors of the follicular epithelium

The follicular epithelium of the thyroid may give rise to several histological forms of malignancies – slow-growing well-differentiated tumors (papillary and follicular

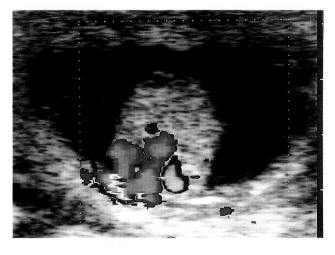

Fig. 5.31 Oncocytic adenoma with mixed echo texture. In the solid projection large blood vessels are visible.

carcinoma), poorly differentiated tumors with intermediate prognosis, and highly malignant undifferentiated (formerly termed anaplastic) tumors (Table 1). Follicular carcinoma accounts for about 5% of thyroid carcinomas, but its incidence is higher in areas of endemic goiter, since it develops in most cases from pre-existing adenoma. It is more frequent in females and in the sixth decade of life. There are two variants differing greatly in histology and course – 'minimally invasive' and 'frankly invasive'.[31] In the former (encapsulated follicular carcinoma), only invasion of the blood vessels of the tumor capsule (see Fig. 5.32B) and, in some cases, of the pericapsular thyroid parenchyma, permits differentiation from thyroid adenoma. With regard to the histological outlines, most follicular carcinomas have a fibrous peripheral capsule, which is not present in some frankly invasive forms. In the frankly invasive variant the diagnostic criteria are invasion of the vessels and invasion of the adjacent thyroid (see Fig. 3.11). In both variants follicular carcinoma has a distinct propensity to spread by way of the blood, with secondary deposits most frequently in bone, lung, brain and liver, especially in the frankly

invasive variant. Lymph node metastases in the neck are practically unknown. The minimally invasive variant rarely metastasizes (8–10% of cases) and is the cause of death in about 20% of cases. The frankly invasive variant metastasizes in about 50% of cases.

The prognosis is worse in the elderly, in males and in cases with marked extrathyroid growth. Only in minimally invasive tumors, in subjects under 50 years of age and in tumors having a diameter under 5 cm should non-radical surgery be contemplated (hemithyroidectomy).[31]

Follicular carcinoma is the most difficult thyroid malignancy to detect and diagnose by ultrasound. In fact, it is associated with nodular goiter in over 60–70% of cases, especially in areas of endemic goiter, and there are few conventional ultrasound signs that can be helpful in the differentiation of follicular carcinoma from nodular goiter: such signs are irregular and multilobate margins, large peripheral halo of uneven thickness, or signs of invasion of the perithyroid anatomical structures, especially muscles (rarely found in this disease). As for the peripheral halo, it is mostly due to the rich vascular supply of the capsular

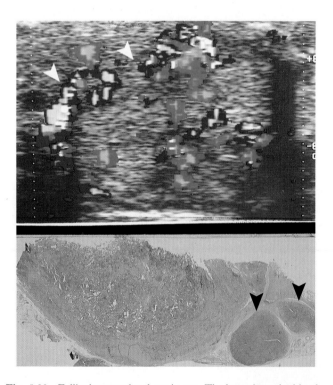

Fig. 5.32 Follicular capsulated carcinoma. The large, irregular blood vessels demonstrated by color Doppler at the periphery of the lesion (arrowhead) correspond histologically to the dilated capsular vessels which enclose neoplastic thrombi (arrowhead). Intranodular large vessels with uneven distribution are also present. (Histological specimen: courtesy of Dr C. Ravetto.)

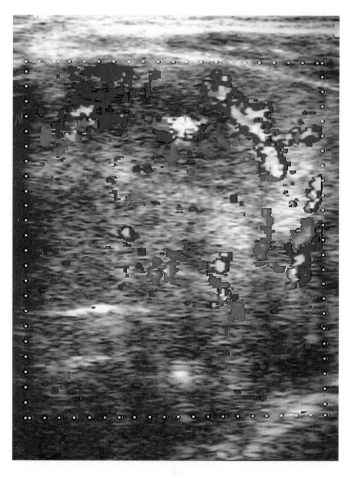

Fig. 5.33 Partial view of large follicular invasive carcinoma. Only intranodular blood vessels are assessable, with chaotic distribution and uneven size. Some vessels show high flow velocities probably attributable to AV shunts.

structure: because of the collapse of blood vessels in specimens, the sonographic halo and capsule with blood supply can be compared only when tumor thrombi maintain the enlarged status of the vessels in histological specimens (Fig. 5.32). The ultrasound texture is isoechoic to the surrounding thyroid parenchyma in over 60% of cases (Fig. 5.33) and hypoechoic in the remaining 40%. Follicular carcinoma lacks two cardinal ultrasound signs of malignancy – microcalcifications and cervical lymph node metastases.

Color Doppler is somewhat more informative. Like other thyroid malignancies, with the sole exception of undifferentiated tumors, follicular carcinoma presents a type III vascular pattern in over 90% of cases,[24,25,32] with mostly intranodular arterial vessels, chaotically disposed, with tortuous course and uneven diameter (mainly in invasive forms) (see Fig. 5.33). Although these ultrasound features do not justify a definite suspicion of malignancy, they do identify (especially in lesions located in multinodular goiters) the most suspect nodule and act as a guide for percutaneous needle aspiration biopsy. Ultrasound is far less important than radioisotope scan and X-rays in the follow-up of follicular carcinoma, because recurrences in the thyroidectomy cavity and in the laterocervical lymph node chains are very infrequent.

Papillary carcinoma accounts for more than 80% of thyroid carcinomas. It affects females more than males and has its peak incidence between 30 and 50 years of age. It is often due to exposure to ionizing radiation and is often associated with an iodine-rich diet. Papillary carcinoma has some peculiar cytological features, such as 'frosted glass' nuclei, cytoplasmic inclusions in the nucleus and indentations of the nuclear membrane;[31] microcalcifications are very frequent, owing to the deposition of calcium salts in the psammoma bodies,[33] present both in the primary tumor and, with the same high frequency, in the cervical lymph node metastases and in post-surgical recurrences. Most papillary carcinomas have a fibrous capsule (see Fig. 5.38).

Papillary carcinoma has three typical biological characteristics:

- frequent multifocality, owing to lymphatic spread within the thyroid (Fig. 5.34)
- spread almost exclusively in the neck, especially to the laterocervical and recurrent lymph nodes (over 50% of cases)
- low degree of aggressiveness, owing to the extremely slow growth.[31]

Even the presence of lymph node metastases does not worsen the prognosis. Distant metastases are very rare (2–3% of cases); as a rule they are to the lung.

Factors that adversely affect the prognosis, apart from certain genetic characteristics, are female patient, aged over 50 years, tumor diameter over 3 cm, and extrathyroid extension of the tumor. Lesions confined to the thyroid, without lymph node metastases, and with a diameter less than 3 cm can be treated by simple hemithyroidectomy.[34]

A variant of papillary carcinoma is the 'microcarcinoma', a non-encapsulated sclerosing tumor usually under 1 cm in diameter and situated under the capsule. Being highly lymphophilic, this tumor manifests in 80% of cases in large metastases to the laterocervical lymph nodes, without clinical signs of the primary tumor. The prognosis is very good, since distant metastases are extremely uncommon. The surgical procedure currently recommended is hemithyroidectomy with removal of the affected lymph nodes only.[35]

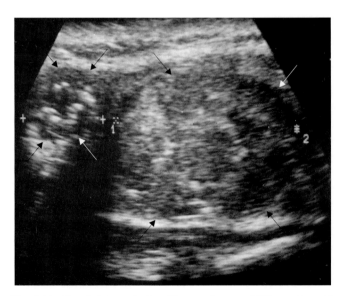

Fig. 5.34 Two foci (arrow) of papillary carcinoma of different size, with disseminated microcalcifications, are visualized in the same thyroid lobe.

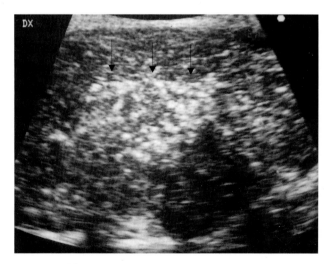

Fig. 5.35 Diffuse sclerosing papillary carcinoma in a child. The whole thyroid lobe is involved; an extensive cluster of microcalcifications is visible in the central portion (arrow).

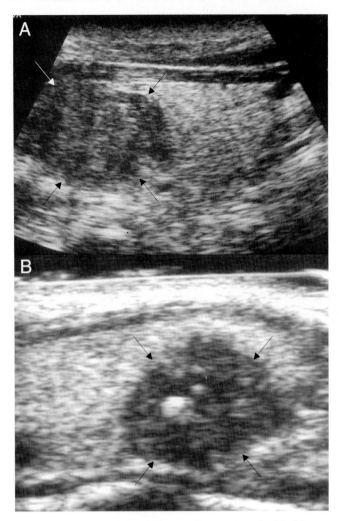

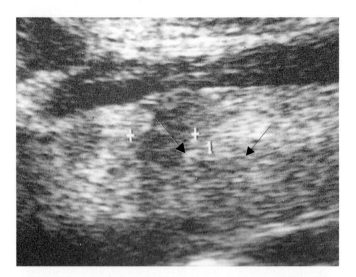

Fig. 5.36 Two hypoechoic papillary carcinomas (arrow) with different types of margins. **A** Invasive carcinoma with irregular margins. **B** Encapsulated cancer with well-defined outlines.

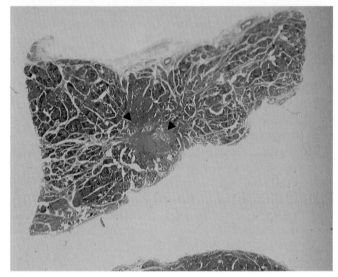

Fig. 5.37 6 mm papillary microcarcinoma (arrow) with corresponding histological representation. Histological specimen also shows structural changes consistent with early chronic thyroiditis. (Courtesy of Dr C. Ravetto.)

In children a diffuse sclerosing variant is possible (Fig. 5.35), with very frequent metastases to the lung.[31]

The ultrasound pattern of papillary carcinoma has more characteristic (even though not pathognomonic) features than follicular carcinoma. In about 90% of cases the structure is hypoechoic (Fig. 5.36), owing to the closely packed cell content with sparse colloid substance; in the remainder it is mixed or, more rarely, isoechoic. Hyperechoic and anechoic ultrasound patterns are extremely uncommon.[14,23] Irregular and ill-defined margins are frequently seen in invasive forms (see Fig. 5.36A) and in microcarcinomas (Fig. 5.37); regular margins and hypoechoic peripheral haloes are frequently encountered in capsulated carcinomas (Figs 5.36B, 5.38). Microcalcifications are, on the other hand, a very important diagnostic feature:[14,16,22,36]

they are found in 85–90% of papillary carcinomas, are attributable to calcification of the psammoma bodies and each measure about 1 mm. They may appear as hyperechoic spots with or without acoustic shadows or as simple fine acoustic shadows (Figs 5.39, 3.15). Microcalcifications are a highly specific sign of malignancy (papillary or medullary cancers), being detected in only 5% of nodular goiters and in 3–4% of adenomas.

Signs of invasion of the contiguous anatomical structures are rare in papillary cancers, given their low invasiveness. When they are present, they may consist of infiltration of the neck musculature, especially the prethyroid muscles, and of the recurrent laryngeal nerve. In the case of infiltration of the neck muscles, imaged only at frequencies of at least 10 MHz, the key diagnostic feature is fixation of

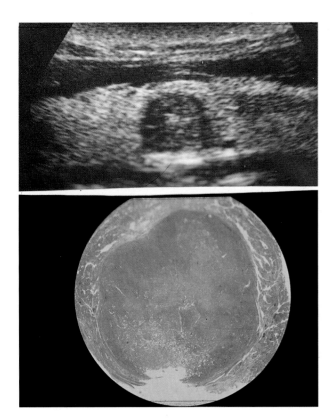

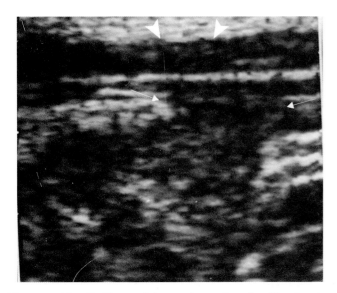

Fig. 5.38 12 mm papillary carcinoma with corresponding histological specimen. The thick peripheral halo corresponds to the thickened fibrous capsule. (Courtesy of Dr C. Ravetto.).

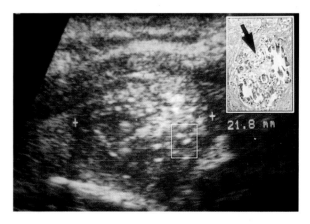

Fig. 5.39 Papillary carcinoma with disseminated microcalcifications, due to calcified psammoma bodies.

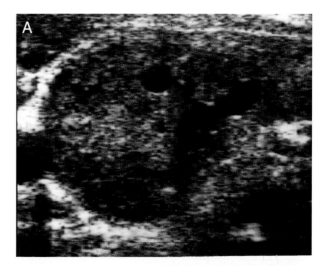

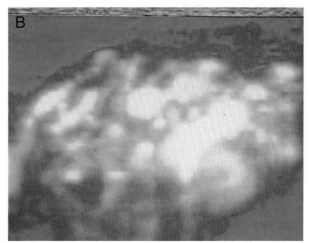

Fig. 5.40 Magnified image of the anterior portion of papillary invasive carcinoma. A solid anterior projection of the tumor (arrow) infiltrates the prethyroid muscles (arrowhead). Real-time observation during bending of the neck confirms the anatomic invasion.

Fig. 5.41 Papillary carcinoma (**A**). Power Doppler (**B**) shows extremely abundant flow signals which fill the whole tumor. (Courtesy of J. W. Charboneau, Department of Radiology, Mayo Clinic, Rochester, USA.)

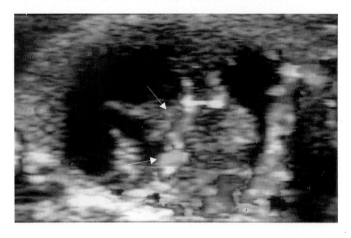

Fig. 5.42 Cystic papillary carcinoma. Presence of arterial blood supply (arrow) in the solid projection.

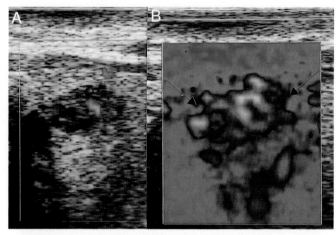

Fig. 5.44 Color Doppler (**A**) and power Doppler (**B**) (arrow) images of papillary microcarcinoma, which shows intense blood flow signals.

the muscles to the thyroid nodule, demonstrated during bending of the neck and swallowing (Fig. 5.40). Invasion of the recurrent laryngeal nerve, preceded by clinical evidence of paralysis of a vocal cord, occurs in tumors with dorsal development (even if small), which tend to be invasive: ultrasound diagnosis is established by demonstrating encasement of the nerve within the neoplastic nodule.[16]

In over 90% of papillary carcinomas, color Doppler shows hypervascular, type III patterns, with even more abundant and widespread flow signals, mostly in forms with low invasiveness and on using power Doppler (Fig. 5.41). This characteristic is very useful in identifying a papillary carcinoma embedded in a multinodular goiter. Spectral analysis yields the same non-specific results as most nodular lesions of the thyroid gland. The distinguishing sonographic characteristics of papillary carcinoma are cystic papillary lesions, microcarcinomas and cervical lymph node metastases.

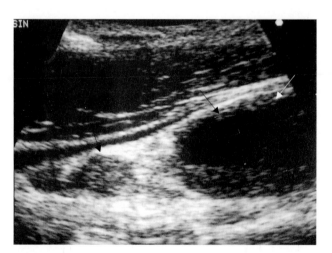

Fig. 5.43 Two metastatic laterocervical adenopathies (arrow) from papillary carcinoma. The larger node has complete cystic changes.

Cystic–papillary carcinoma appears on the ultrasound scan as a mixed nodule with a mainly fluid component but with one or more solid, irregularly marginated projections in the lumen. The solid component may contain microcalcifications and characteristically presents a central arterial blood supply with possible ramifications (Fig. 5.42). Microcalcifications and this particular vascular pattern never appear in the solid components (often consisting of cell debris or fibrous septa) of mixed nodular goiters (see Fig. 5.24). Cystic–papillary carcinomas often give rise to laterocervical lymph node metastases with partially or totally colliquated structure (Fig. 5.43).

Papillary microcarcinoma, usually revealed by the presence of laterocervical lymph node metastases, can be imaged by high-frequency ultrasound in 70–80% of cases. Rarely, it may present as a small hyperechoic patch (like fibrosis) under the capsule, accompanied by thickening and retraction of the capsule. This pattern is very hard to interpret. Much more characteristic and far more frequent is a minute hypoechoic nodule (usually under 6–7 mm in diameter) with a blurred irregular outline (see Fig. 5.37), with no visible microcalcifications, but often with intense vascular signals within and around the lesion (Fig. 5.44).

Laterocervical metastases from microcarcinoma do not differ in site or structure from those generally caused by all papillary carcinomas. The very frequent lymph node metastases from papillary carcinoma have two distinctly prevalent sites: the lower half of the deep jugular chain (Fig. 5.45) and the recurrent chain (Fig. 5.46). The latter, lying dorsal and caudal to the inferior pole of the thyroid lobe, is often difficult to study by ultrasound, especially in patients with a short neck, because of the overlying manubrium sterni. Each individual recurrent lymph node must be carefully distinguished from pathological parathyroid glands, the morphology and structure of which are almost identical. Lymph node metastases from papillary

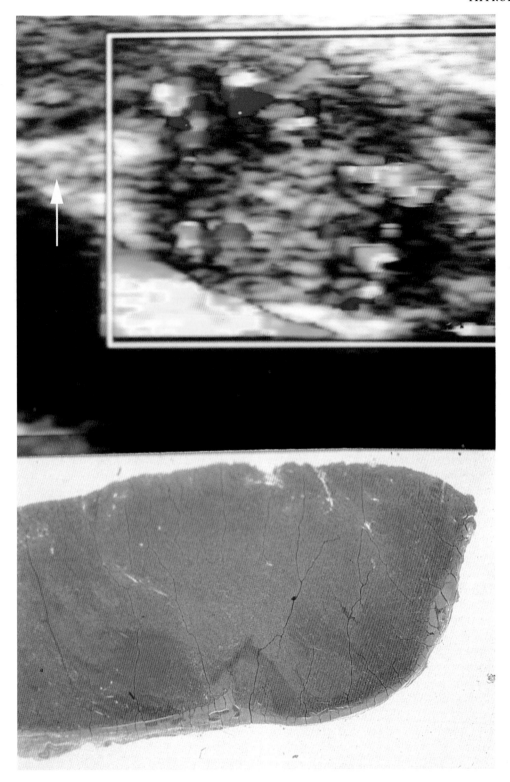

Fig. 5.45 Metastatic lymph node of the deep jugular chain from papillary carcinoma, with corresponding histological specimen. Intense blood flow signals with irregular course and uneven distribution are visible in the lymph node. Arrow: jugular vein. (Courtesy of Dr C. Ravetto.)

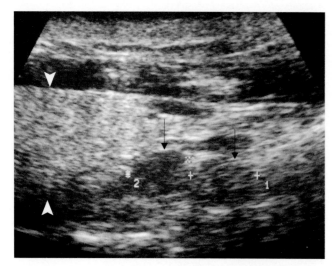

Fig. 5.46 Two metastatic lymph nodes (arrow) of the recurrent chain from papillary thyroid cancer. Arrowhead: lower pole of the thyroid lobe.

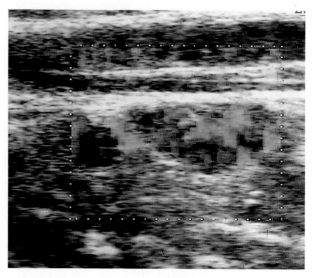

Fig. 5.47 Two recurrences of papillary carcinoma in the thyroid compartment. Power Doppler shows hypervascularity.

carcinoma have the same sonographic characteristics as any malignant superficial lymph node (see Ch. 14). In addition, in 80–90% of cases they present the same micro-calcifications as the primary tumor (see Fig. 3.16). Not infrequently the metastases are completely cystic, with thin regular walls (see Fig. 5.43): the only other tumor that often gives rise to cystic nodal metastases in the neck is carcinoma of the rhinopharynx. When sonography reveals extensive nodal metastatic deposits in the neck, contrast-enhanced CT of the upper mediastinum has to be performed preoperatively in order to assess possible involvement of mediastinal lymph nodes.

Ultrasound has an essential role in the follow-up of papillary carcinoma, especially in radionuclide-negative cases. Recurrences may develop at the same site as the primary tumor – the thyroidectomy cavity, deep jugular lymph node chain and recurrent chain. Recurrences usually appear as nodules hypoechoic to normal thyroid tissue, with or without microcalcifications, with irregular margins, intense flow signals and sometimes with signs of infiltration of the muscular, nervous and vascular structures (Fig. 5.47). These signs combined usually allow differentiation from residual islands of normal thyroid tissue or post-surgical scar tissue. In questionable cases MRI can provide the differential diagnosis.[37] Even so, cytological study of the material supplied by ultrasound-guided aspiration biopsy is the key examination.[38]

It has to be remembered, however, that the essential procedure in the follow-up of differentiated thyroid tumors is the serum assay of thyroglobulin, especially if the examination is done in the absence of hormone replacement therapy. Another essential examination is total body radionuclide scanning with ^{131}I, usually performed 1 month following total thyroidectomy: it reveals any areas of iodine uptake, where they lie anatomically and how much iodine has been taken up.[39]

Poorly differentiated thyroid carcinomas have several histological patterns (Table 1), identified relatively recently. These tumors are mostly papillary or follicular carcinomas that do not follow the preferential route of spread by the lymphatics or blood vessels, but have a strong tendency to local invasion (of muscles or nerves, for example) and to invasion of the vascular structures.[31] The ultrasound pattern of these tumors is much the same as that of differentiated varieties, except that they are very inclined to invade locally, like undifferentiated tumors.

Undifferentiated carcinomas arising from the follicular epithelium of the thyroid gland represent, outside areas where goiter is endemic, about 5% of all thyroid tumors and occur to by far the greatest extent in females and the elderly. They include the histological forms formerly called small cell and spindle cell anaplastic cancers and represent the final state of dedifferentiation of follicular or papillary carcinomas. Patients exhibit a sudden rapid worsening of a pre-existing disease (differentiated carcinoma or generic goiter): the biological evolution is marked by local aggression with lymphatic and blood spread, with a mean survival usually of less than a year.[31]

These tumors cannot usually be examined by high-frequency ultrasound because of their large size and high acoustic absorption. They appear as hypoechoic masses with very irregular, multilobate margins and with calcifications, which may be coarse or 'egg-shell' shaped. Definite signs of invasion of the anatomical structures of the neck are detected in most cases and represent the outstanding sonographic findings[40,41] (Figs 3.10 and 5.48). The infiltration of the walls of the great vessels of the neck may be caused by the primary tumor or by its nodal

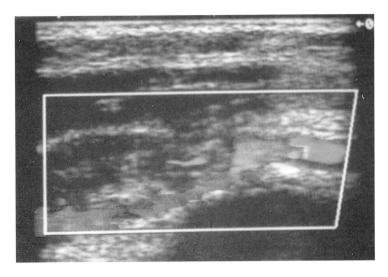

Fig. 5.48 Neoplastic infiltration of the deep jugular vein by undifferentiated carcinoma of the thyroid gland.

metastases:[42,43] this occurrence may also be seen, although rarely, in highly aggressive forms of papillary or follicular cancers. Conversely, the diagnostic findings provided by color Doppler are very poor in undifferentiated carcinomas, probably because of their large necrotic component: only single arterial or venous vessels of large diameter, with tortuous course, are commonly visualized.

Pathognomonic of undifferentiated carcinoma is invasion of the trachea, esophagus, retroesophageal spaces and even, cranially, of the laryngeal cartilages. These signs, not imaged by ultrasound, are clearly assessed by CT (Fig. 5.49). Indeed, currently the main indications for CT in thyroid pathology are the preoperative staging of undifferentiated carcinomas as well as the investigation of large goiters developing into the mediastinum. Sonography may provide more information than CT only in the assessment of the extent of invasion of the large neck vessels and of encasement of the nervous structures.

Medullary tumors

Medullary carcinoma of the thyroid is a relatively uncommon tumor, representing some 10% of all thyroid tumors. It arises from the parafollicular cells (or C cells), which produce calcitonin; this substance is the biochemical marker of medullary carcinoma. In 20% of cases the disease is familial, a component of the multiple endocrine neoplasia syndrome (MEN Chong type II).[44]

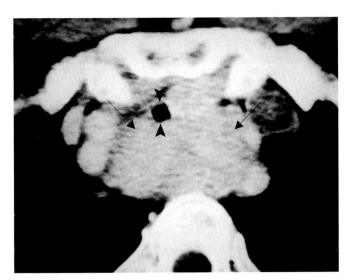

Fig. 5.49 CT scan of the upper mediastinum. Large undifferentiated carcinoma of the thyroid gland (arrow) which invades the mediastinal spaces and causes a malignant encasement of the trachea (arrowhead).

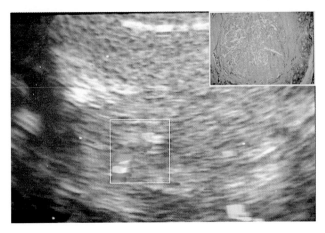

Fig. 5.50 7 mm focus of medullary carcinoma (box with histological specimen) in patient with familial multiple endocrine neoplasms (MEN). Hypervascularity is detectable.

Medullary carcinoma has a more aggressive biological behavior and a poorer prognosis than differentiated carcinomas: it does not take up radioiodine and does not respond to chemotherapy or to radiotherapy. Surgery remains the treatment of choice, both at the initial stage and on recurrence.

On sonography, medullary carcinoma appears mostly hypoechoic or, very occasionally, isoechoic, with irregular outlines and often bounded by a hypoechoic halo of uneven thickness, consisting mainly of arterial and venous vessels. The main feature of the vascular pattern is, however, the intranodular component (type III pattern), exactly like that of differentiated tumors of the follicular epithelium and detectable also in small foci of medullary cancer (Fig. 5.50). The most characteristic sonographic sign comes from microcalcifications (Fig. 5.51), detectable in 80–90% of medullary carcinomas,[45] both in the primary tumor and in nodal metastatic deposits. They are even larger and more numerous than in papillary carcinomas[4,46] and are due to calcified nests of amyloid substance.

Spread to the lymph nodes of the recurrent chain and of the superior mediastinum is reportedly more frequent than in papillary carcinomas: preoperatively, therefore, CT examination of the upper mediastinum is mandatory in all cases in which sonography detects nodal metastatic spread in the neck.

Recurrences of medullary carcinoma in the neck have the same patterns as those described above for papillary carcinoma, but sonography is even more important than in papillary cancers because radiosotope scans with ^{131}I do not yield diagnostic results, owing to the tissue characteristics of this malignancy. Elevation of serum levels of calcitonin is a useful sign of neoplastic recurrence.

Thyroid lymphomas

Thyroid lymphomas account for 4% of all malignancies of the thyroid gland. They are nearly always non-Hodgkin lymphomas, which principally affect women and the aged. The typical sign is a rapidly growing lump, which may cause symptoms of obstruction, such as dyspnea and dysphagia.[47] In 70–80% of cases lymphoma arises on pre-existing chronic thyroiditis with subclinical or overt hypothyroidism. Prognosis depends on the stage of the disease and on its early diagnosis, 5-year survival ranging from 89% in initial cases to 5% in disseminated disease.

The ultrasound scan shows a markedly hypoechoic mass, often large, with multilobate margins and large, anechoic, necrotic areas. Multiple, small hypoechoic foci disseminated in thyroid parenchyma may also occur (Fig. 5.52). The vascular pattern seen on color Doppler is usually not very remarkable, comparable to that of undifferentiated carcinomas; the signs of cervical invasion, in later stages, may also be identical. However, in most occurrences, the peritumoral thyroid tissue is normal in undifferentiated cancers, whereas it features signs of chronic thyroiditis in cases of lymphomas.[48,49] Cytological examination of the percutaneous needle aspiration biopsy material still remains, however, the key procedure in the diagnosis of thyroid lymphoma, even though the differentiation from thyroiditis can occasionally be very difficult. The most accurate imaging method by which to stage thyroid lymphomas is currently CT.

Concluding remarks

The role of ultrasound in the diagnosis of thyroid nodules has steadily gained in importance, especially since the introduction of high-frequency transducers. In the early days sonography was used merely for differentiating lesions with a fluid content from solid nodules; now, a more confident differentiation among the varying histological forms can be achieved in most cases.

Characteristics strongly suggestive of a benign lesion are now anechoic or hyperechoic texture, regular margins, a thin and regular perilesional halo, the presence of large

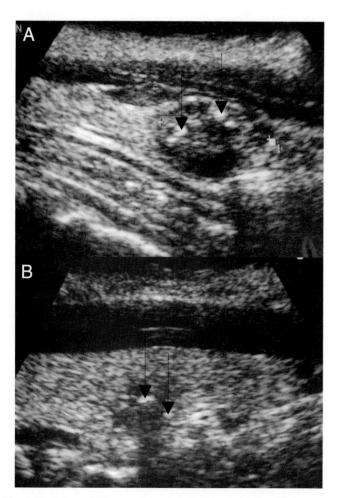

Fig. 5.51 Microcalcifications (arrow) detected by high-frequency ultrasound in medium-size (**A**) and small (**B**) medullary carcinomas.

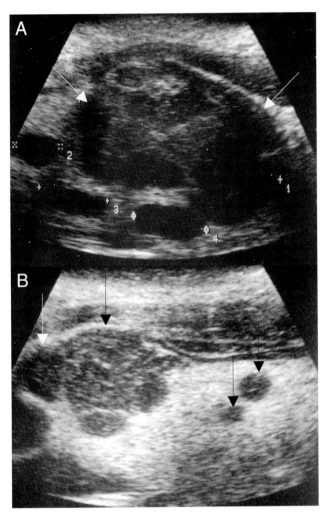

Fig. 5.52 Primary lymphomas (arrow) of the thyroid gland: large, single mass (**A**) and multiple, small foci (**B**).

cystic changes and perilesional flow signals with little or no intranodular component. By contrast, ultrasound signs of malignancy are hypoechogenicity, microcalcifications, irregular margins, thick and irregular peripheral halo, presence of intranodular flow signals in the absence of clinical and radionuclide evidence of hyperfunction. Sure findings of malignancy, present in only a minority of cases, are infiltration or invasion of the perithyroid structures. Grouping these signs, an accuracy of 75% in predicting cancers with US has been reported,[4] while, according to our experience based on more than 300 cases with histological confirmation, this accuracy increases to approximately 80% and even to 85% if differentiation between 'non-surgical' (goiters) and 'surgical' (adenomas and carcinomas) lesions is sought.

Multinodularity is no guarantee of benign disease: every single nodule must be examined for its characteristics; only if multiple lesions all present the same benign structural findings is a diagnosis of goiter or multinodular hyperplasia

justified. The problem raised by the great sensitivity of high-frequency ultrasound is the very common detection of non-palpable nodules in patients examined for non-thyroid disease. These findings must be carefully assessed in order to avoid overdiagnosis of diseases of scant clinical importance. Only nodules exceeding 8–10 mm in diameter now seem worthy of further investigation (especially fine-needle aspiration biopsy), except in very specific situations such as a history of exposure to ionizing radiation or a family history of thyroid malignancies.

A further point to note is that the thyroid carcinoma with the highest incidence, papillary carcinoma, usually develops extremely slowly – so slowly as often to be an incidental post-mortem finding in patients dying of other diseases.[14,50]

Thyroiditis

Thyroiditis includes acute/subacute and chronic diseases (Table 5.1). Acute/subacute forms are of four main types: acute suppurative, subacute (De Quervain's), painless, and post-partum thyroiditis. Acute suppurative thyroiditis caused by pyogenic agents is almost a curiosity in the antibiotic era and therefore is not included in this chapter.

Subacute thyroiditis

Subacute granulomatous (or De Quervain's) thyroiditis is a self-limiting viral disease, usually preceded by infection of the upper airways with prodromal muscular pains and weakness. The clinical findings are fever, and enlargement of all or part of the thyroid gland with increased consistency and pain on palpation. In the initial stages transient hyperthyroidism has been reported (attributable to massive follicular rupture) as well as signs of inflammation. Subsequently, moderate and transient hypothyroidism may occur, related to slowly progressive functional normalization. In the majority of cases subacute thyroiditis responds well to medical therapy, with complete recovery of thyroid function within a few weeks.

Histologically, the disease is marked by interstitial edema and cellular exudation with destruction of follicular cells and consequent release of colloid substance and thyroid hormones.

Although subacute thyroiditis is easily diagnosed clinically, sonographic findings are pathognomonic.[51,52] In the initial stages the affected segments of the thyroid (mostly subcapsular regions) appear enlarged and present ill-defined, irregular margins and markedly hypoechoic structure with high absorption of the acoustic beam (Fig. 5.53A). With color Doppler vascularization appears normal or, more commonly, reduced, owing to the diffuse edema of the gland. As the disease evolves, recovery of the normal thyroid structure may take a pseudonodular form (Fig. 5.53B), usually starting from the central portion of

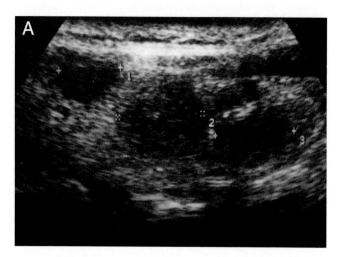

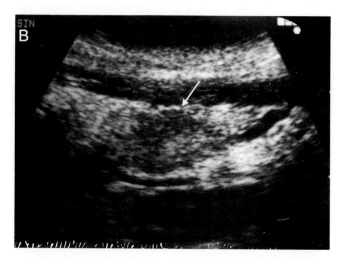

Fig. 5.53 **A** Multiple hypoechoic foci of subacute thyroiditis with severe enlargement of the lobe. **B** Following therapy the gland size is normalized and only one small residual area of inflammation is present in the central portion (arrow).

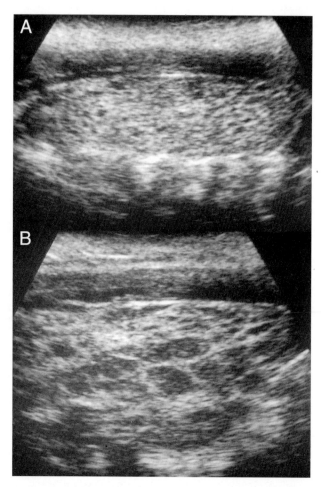

Fig. 5.54 Painless thyroiditis. **A** Mild form with tiny hypoechoic foci representing lymphocytic aggregates. **B** More severe form with larger hypoechoic nodules.

the previously altered area; recovery may involve the various pathologic foci asynchronously. Prognosis is worse when the hypoechoic areas increase in size on follow-up examination, requiring further medical treatment. The main roles of sonography in subacute thyroiditis are, therefore, to assess the evolution of the disease and the timing of medical therapy and to detect early possible recurrences.

Painless (silent or subacute lymphocytic) thyroiditis has the typical histological pattern of chronic autoimmune thyroiditis (lymphocytic infiltration and fibrosis), but the clinical findings resemble those of acute diseases. Moderate hyperthyroidism with thyroid enlargement usually occur in the early phases, followed by hypothyroidism of variable entity and always slowly remitting.

Sonography shows typically small hypoechoic foci (representing lymphocytic aggregates) disseminated throughout the thyroid parenchyma (Fig. 5.54). No signs of hypervascularity are usually detected by color Doppler and the thyroid may be slightly enlarged.

Post-partum thyroiditis, mostly occurring 2–4 months following delivery, often in patients with pre-existing thyroiditis, has the same clinical, histologic and sonographic patterns of silent thyroiditis, but the progression to hypothyroidism is more frequent.

Chronic thyroiditis

The chronic forms of thyroiditis include autoimmune lymphocytic thyroiditis (Hashimoto's and other variants), Riedel's fibrous thyroiditis (to date of extremely rare occurrence and not included in this chapter), tuberculous thyroiditis, and forms related to radiotherapy and iodine treatment. Further differentiations of chronic or Hash-

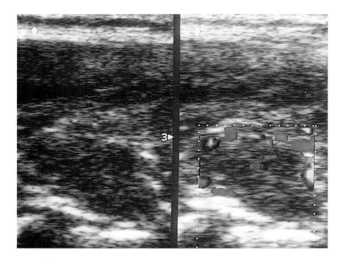

Fig. 5.55 Focal nodular chronic thyroiditis with few peripheral blood flow signals.

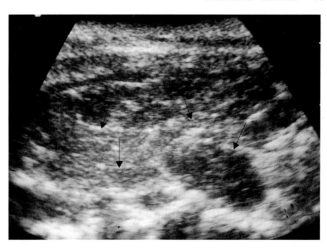

Fig. 5.56 Chronic thyroiditis. The lobe is enlarged, with large hypoechoic areas and fibrous septa (arrow) ('pseudolobulated' appearance).

imoto's thyroiditis include classic, fibrous, juvenile, trophic and other variants.[53,54]

Chronic autoimmune thyroiditis is more frequent in females (9:1) and in patients with other autoimmune pathologies. Thyrotoxicosis may be the initial clinical presentation, related to excessive hormonal release stimulated by antibodies (Hashitoxicosis); following this phase, hypothyroidism slowly develops, together with the progression of histological changes, consisting of lymphocytic infiltration together with atrophy of the parenchymal cells and fibrosis.

These changes can be easily assessed by high-frequency sonography. When the early presentation is focal nodular thyroiditis, the sonographic pattern (hypoechoic nodules with irregular margins and almost complete absence of flow signals) poses problems of differential diagnosis from other nodular diseases of the thyroid, either benign or malignant (Fig. 5.55). Diffuse forms may initially present with the same 'micronodular' sonographic pattern described in painless thyroiditis (see above), with increase in size of the gland.[55] Progressively, together with irreversible hypothyroidism, the typical appearance of chronic hypertrophic thyroiditis develops – increase in size, multilobate margins and ill-defined hypoechoic areas of varying dimensions (attributable to lymphocytic conglomerates) separated by hyperechoic, fibrotic septa ('pseudolobulated' appearance)[4] (Fig. 5.56). At this stage the color Doppler findings are very characteristic, showing marked hypervascularity, chiefly arterial, within the parenchyma and especially inside the hyperechoic septa[4,56] (Fig. 5.57). This pattern does not differ significantly from the 'thyroid inferno' described in Graves' disease. Recent studies[56] have demonstrated that in chronic thyroiditis hypervascularity

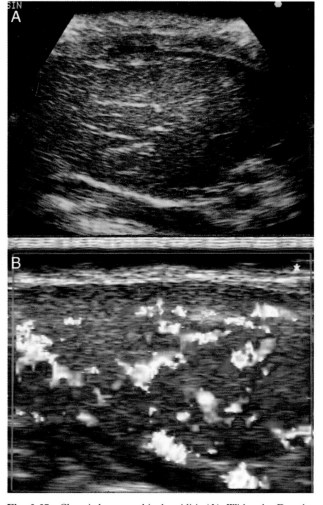

Fig. 5.57 Chronic hypertrophic thyroiditis (**A**). With color Doppler (**B**) hypervascularity is seen, mostly involving the hyperechoic septa.

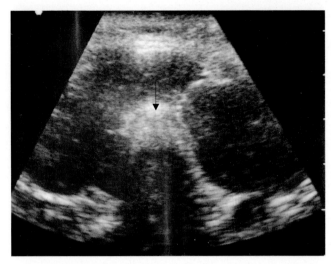

Fig. 5.58 Chronic thyroiditis with marked enlargement and diffusely hypoechoic structure. Arrow: trachea.

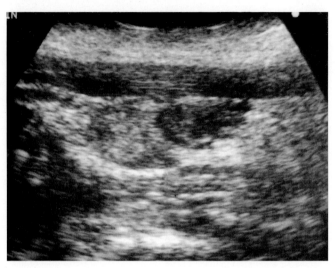

Fig. 5.59 End-stage atrophic thyroiditis, 2 cm in maximum longitudinal diameter.

occurs when hypothyroidism develops: this is likely to be attributable to the hypertrophic action of TSH. Indeed, when TSH progressively falls to normal values (either spontaneously or during successful medical treatment) the color flow signals gradually revert to the normal pattern.[56] In the final stage of chronic hypertrophic thyroiditis the gland is enlarged and diffusely hypo- to anechoic, with rounded outlines (Fig. 5.58).

In a few cases (10–15%)[4,53] cervical lymph nodes are present: for the most part they show the typical pattern of hyperplastic/reactive nodes (see Ch. 14), but if their appearance is questionable further diagnostic assessments (cytology initially) must be conducted in order to evaluate possible thyroid lymphoma.

The end stage of chronic thyroiditis is the atrophic form: the gland is small, with ill-defined margins and heterogeneous texture due to the progressive increase of fibrosis (Fig. 5.59). Blood flow signals are completely absent.

A fairly unusual, though not exceptional, finding is the coexistence of thyroid nodules, benign or malignant, with chronic lymphocytic thyroiditis. In this situation the diffuse, firm consistency of the thyroid parenchyma may hinder clinical recognition of the nodule; hence, sonographic and cytologic (if indicated by ultrasound) assessments are needed. In these cases aspiration biopsy must be performed under direct ultrasound guidance, as the target cannot be detected by palpation.[57]

INTERVENTIONAL PROCEDURES

Interventional US-guided procedures of the thyroid gland include the following:

- fine-needle aspiration biopsy (FNAB)
- ethanol injection of cystic lesions
- ethanol injection of autonomously functioning nodules.

Fine-needle aspiration biopsy

Aspiration biopsies of palpable thyroid lesions are commonly performed by a freehand technique, using short (3–3.5 cm) 22–23 G needles. When the target is not palpable (because of its small size, deep site or lack of identification in multinodular pathologies), ultrasound guidance is mandatory and is commonly performed using longer (9 cm) needles and lateral needle adaptors of high-frequency probes, allowing an oblique approach to the target (Fig. 5.60). One or two rapid needle passages are performed for each target.

The aspirated material can be examined by the routine staining methods, by immunocytochemistry or even as a paraffin microinclusion.[58] Fluid aspirated from cystic lesions is always centrifuged and cellular debris examined in the search for possible cystic papillary cancers.

The choice of the nodules to be punctured is made chiefly on the basis of radioisotope and/or sonographic findings. Because of the increasing rate of detection of small unpredicted nodules of no clinical and biological significance, targets less than 7–8 mm in diameter should be aspirated only in specific circumstances, as follows:

- patients with cervical nodal metastases (cytologically assessed) from undetectable thyroid carcinoma, before scheduling thyroidectomy
- patients with a doubtful nodule in the lobe remaining following contralateral hemithyroidectomy with occasional detection of small neoplastic focus, before planning re-intervention for total thyroidectomy[38]

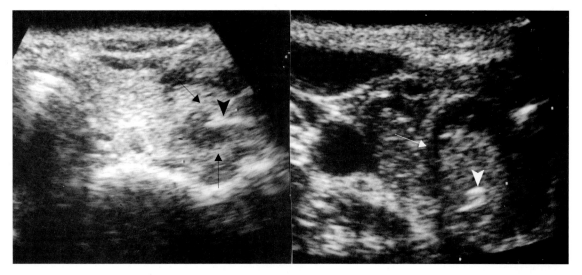

Fig. 5.60 US-guided aspiration biopsies of small hypoechoic nodule (arrow) (**A**) and of larger lesion with mixed echo texture (arrow) (**B**). Arrowhead: tip of the needle.

- nodules of questionable sonographic appearance in patients with a familial history of MEN.

Aspiration biopsy can be employed for the assessment of all nodular lesions of doubtful nature, as well as for the differentiation of chronic thyroiditis from lymphomatous deposits and of malignant recurrences from post-surgical scars or inflammatory tissue. At present, in centers with enough experience, the diagnostic accuracy of FNAB is very high, with rates of sensitivity of approximately 85% and specificity of 99%.[58–60] Particularly high is the identification of 'surgical' pathologies and, among these, of papillary, undifferentiated and medullary carcinomas, owing to the increasing use of immunocytochemistry. Diagnostic problems are currently the differentiation of thyroiditis from low-grade lymphoma and, in particular, of follicular adenoma from follicular carcinoma, because of the impossibility of assessing by cytologic methods the signs of capsular and vascular invasion, which are the only clues for differential diagnosis.

Ethanol injection of cystic lesions

The management of cystic thyroid nodules relies primarily on FNAB in order to rule out malignancy: simple aspiration may result in permanent shrinkage of the lesion in reported rates ranging from 20 to 94% of cases.[61]

In order to avoid recurrence, intranodular injection of several sclerosing agents (including sodium tetradecyl sulfate, tetracycline and monocycline) has been attempted over the past 20 years. Nowadays ethanol is the preferred intracystic sclerosing agent, as for liver malignancies, thyroid autonomous nodules and parathyroid tumors, for example. Where simple aspiration has been unsuccessful

the cyst fluid is completely aspirated with fine needles and a volume of sterile 95% ethanol varying from 30% to 60% (according to different experiences) of that of the aspirated fluid is injected under US guidance.[62,63] This ethanol can be either withdrawn within 1 or 2 days, or left permanently in situ. In large cystic cavities this procedure can be repeated once or twice at variable intervals.

Ethanol injection is usually well tolerated, the only discomfort being transient local pain or a burning sensation. The success rates (total disappearance or drastic reduction in volume) of this treatment range from 70 to 90%,[62,63] without any change in thyroid function (Fig. 5.61). Currently ethanol injection can be considered the percutaneous treatment of choice for cystic lesions of the thyroid gland.

Percutaneous ethanol injection of autonomously functioning thyroid nodules

Introduction

Autonomously functioning thyroid nodule (AFTN) is a portion of the gland that functions independent of the production of TSH. The original work by Plummer[64] on nodular hyperthyroidism described a solitary hyperfunctioning adenoma; today, the term Plummer's disease is more commonly used to describe a toxic multinodular goiter. When AFTN produces thyroid hormones in excess, TSH secretion becomes suppressed and the extranodular tissue becomes quiescent.

On radionuclide scans, AFTN appears 'hot', in contrast to the low or absent extranodular uptake, in relation to the amount of thyroid hormones produced. Scintigraphic differentiation between an autonomous adenoma and a solitary autonomous portion of multinodular goiter is

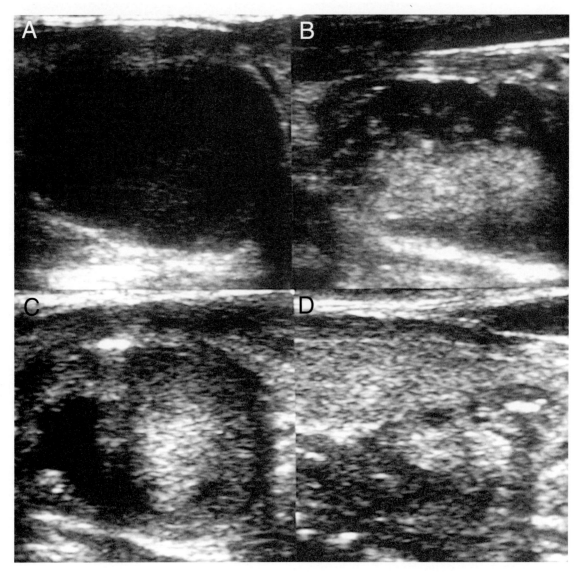

Fig. 5.61   Percutaneous ethanol injection of cystic lesion (**A**) of the thyroid gland. From **B** to **D** the complete disappearance of the cystic cavity is clearly demonstrated.

difficult; the problem is solved by sonography, because the coexistence of other nodules is diagnostic of multinodular goiter whereas the absence of such nodules is diagnostic of adenoma.

Depending on the amount of thyroid hormones secreted, the patient may be toxic or non-toxic. The degree of hyperthyroidism is usually proportional to the volume of the nodule. AFTN can, therefore, cause a range of functional abnormalities, from euthyroidism (compensated AFTN) to subclinical hyperthyroidism (pretoxic AFTN) and clinical hyperthyroidism (toxic AFTN).

The toxic effects of ethanol injected into the solid tissues are attributable to its diffusion into the cells and to its distribution in high concentration into the local vascular supply. The diffusion causes direct damage, due to cell dehydration followed by immediate coagulation necrosis and subsequent fibrotic changes; the vascular distribution causes an indirect damage, due to dehydration of the endothelium and blood cells and aggregation of the latter, followed by thrombus formation and subsequent tissue ischemia.

With regard to solid lesions, PEI was proposed in 1985 for treating hyperplastic parathyroid glands in secondary hyperparathyroidism,[65] in 1986 for treating hepatic neoplasms[66] and in 1987 for treating parathyroid adenomas.[67] In 1990 PEI was proposed for treatment of AFTN.[5] Since then, further experience with this procedure has been acquired by various authors.[68–75]

Technique

Equipment. A 7.5 MHz probe with a guide device is convenient for the US study of the lesions and for guiding the needle within them. Sterile 95% ethyl alcohol is used. Initially, we used a 22 gauge spinal needle (Becton-Dickinson, Rutherford, New Jersey) to inject the alcohol; more recently we have been using a 21 gauge needle with a closed conical tip and three terminal sideholes (PEI needle, Hakko, Tokyo, Japan). The latter permits the injection of a larger volume of ethanol, thereby reducing the total number of sessions required, enabling a greater volume of tissue to be treated and minimizing the risk of laryngeal nerve damage because of the lateral diffusion; however, it is more expensive than the needle previously used.

Procedure. Treatment is given in the outpatient department. After local skin preparation with iodized alcohol, which also is used as the contact medium, ethanol is injected without local anesthesia or sedation, under direct real-time control. The perfused area is clearly seen as a patch of hyperechogenicity (Fig. 5.62). The ethanol is injected slowly and its diffusion checked in real time. The injection is stopped and repeated when diffusion is not clearly visible. As long as the ethanol is seen to disappear rapidly, washed out by the abundant blood supply, the injection is continued until ethanol begins to remain in the lesion.

In nodules located near the posterior region of the gland (i.e. near the recurrent laryngeal nerve), care is taken to avoid ethanol spillage in that direction; in particular, when the needle tip passes beyond the nodule boundaries, the needle is completely retracted and re-inserted at another site, because partial retraction can be followed by ethanol spillage along the needle tract. This problem is avoided when the multihole needle is used.

The procedure is completed in 10–15 min. The injection site is chosen before each session to ensure perfusion of areas considered not to have been treated previously. To facilitate this goal, every session may be recorded on videotape or by simple diagrams. The treatment ends when the nodule is considered to have been completely perfused. PEI usually takes place twice a week for a total of four to eight sessions. The amount of ethanol ranges from 1 to 8 ml per session, given by one to three injections, according to the type of needle, ethanol distribution, patient tolerance and lesion size. At the end of treatment the total volume administered is about one-and-a-half times or double that of the nodule.

Measures of therapeutic efficacy. Before PEI, scintiscan and sonography are conducted and the thyroid hormone profile is evaluated. ^{99m}Tc scintigraphy is routinely used, because when TSH is suppressed the nodule is definitely hyperfunctional. Sonographic examination studies the suppressed tissue and measures the nodule volume, calculated by the ellipsoid formula $(A \times B \times C \times 0.52)/1000$, where A, B and C are the three orthogonal diameters. When color Doppler is available, this is used to map the nodule. Serum levels of free thyroxine (FT_4) and free triiodothyronine (FT_3) are measured by specific radioimmunoassay; TSH is evaluated by means of an ultrasensitive immunoradiometric method. These examinations are repeated 3 months after the final PEI. When TSH remains undetectable, a second cycle of PEI can take place. Thyroid hormone profile evaluation is repeated every 6 months.

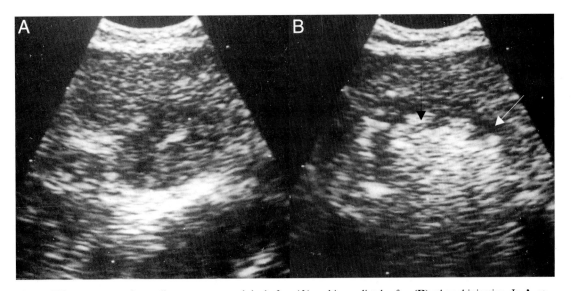

Fig. 5.62 US appearance of a small autonomous nodule, before (**A**) and immediately after (**B**) ethanol injection. In **A**, at the center of the nodule the needle tip is visible as a small hyperechoic spot. In **B** the area perfused by alcohol is clearly hyperechoic (arrow).

Side effects

PEI is generally well tolerated. The most common side effect is a transient burning sensation or moderate pain at the injection site, which can radiate to the mandibular or retroauricular regions; slow withdrawal of the needle and use of the multihole needle reduce this side effect. In a minority of cases, patients complain of local hematoma, slight dysphonia or headache. In some patients with larger nodules, when the amount of necrosis is high, fever lasting 2–3 days may develop after the initial treatment.

Moderate aggravation of symptoms of thyrotoxicosis has sometimes been reported after the initial sessions, but this has not required therapy. Only one case of thyrotoxic crisis has been reported; according to Papini et al[74], methimazole or β-blockers are appropriate for severely thyrotoxic patients.

The only important complication reported is transient damage of the recurrent laryngeal nerve, which occurred in 1–4% of cases.[69–75] Full recovery from vocal cord paresis occurred in all patients, within 1–3 months. Nerve damage is probably induced chemically or by compression; the full recovery is probably due to the fact that, in these cases, in contrast to surgical accidents, there is no anatomic nerve interruption. The multihole needle appears to preclude this occurrence.

Results

During PEI, particularly after the initial injections, some acute changes occur: the serum thyroglobulin level doubles immediately and remains higher than the baseline during the first 24 h; the FT_3 and, more markedly, the FT_4 values show a moderate increase during the first 24 h. At the 3-month assessment, three types of response are obtained, as follows:

1. There is remission of clinical signs, reduction of thyroid hormone levels to within normal range if initially elevated, normalization of TSH concentration, and appear-

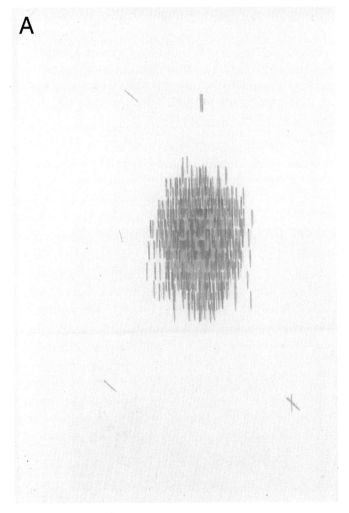

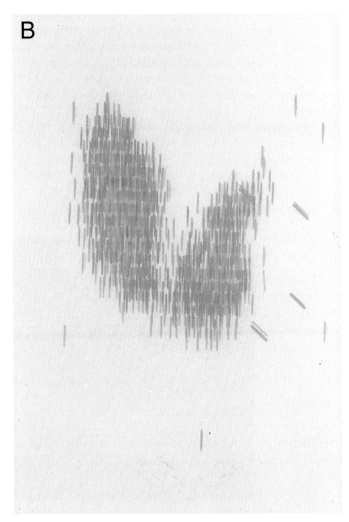

Fig. 5.63 Thyroid scintiscan showing a hot nodule before PEI (**A**) and reactivation of extranodular normal tissue with nodule no longer visible after therapy (**B**).

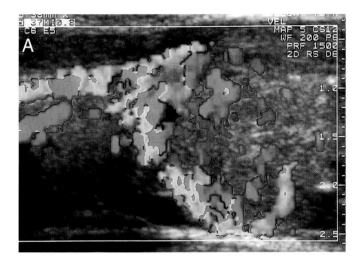

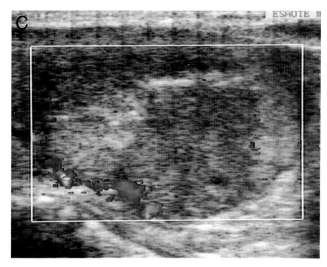

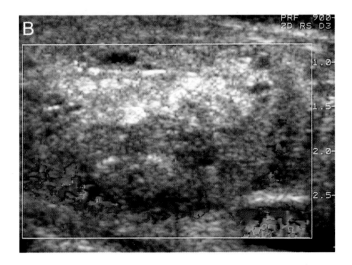

Fig. 5.64 Color Doppler scans showing an autonomous nodule clearly hypervascularized before PEI (**A**) and totally hypovascular immediately after therapy (**B**) and 6 months after therapy (**C**).

ance of extranodular tissue at scintigraphy with the nodule no longer visible, or 'cold' (Fig. 5.63). Color Doppler examination shows complete disappearance of intranodular hypervascularization (Fig. 5.64).

2. There is remission of clinical signs, reduction of thyroid hormone levels to within normal range, detectable-to-normal TSH concentration, and reactivation of extranodular tissue at scintigraphy, but the nodule (or parts of it) is still visible (Fig. 5.65). Color Doppler examination shows the persistence of some areas of intranodular activity.

3. There is remission of clinical signs and reduction of thyroid hormone levels to within normal range, with TSH levels still undetectable, extranodular tissue still suppressed and radionuclide uptake by the nodule only, although in general the nodule is markedly smaller. In these cases the intranodular vascular activity remains clearly detectable in some portions of the nodule.

In the latter types of response, especially in the third one,

a second cycle of PEI is usually conducted. In these patients color Doppler can be useful for guiding the needle into the undamaged areas that are still hypervascular.

In a total of 246 patients reported by different authors,[69–75] the first type of response was obtained in 61–85% of cases. However, recovery from disease, i.e. the first and the second type of response, was obtained in, on average, 86% of cases. The efficacy of response was inversely proportional to the nodule volume:[75] in smaller nodules (<10 ml) the first type of response was achieved in all patients; in medium-sized nodules (11–40 ml) the first and the second types of response were achieved in 95% of patients and in larger nodules (>40 ml) this response was achieved in only 37% of cases.

Marked nodule shrinkage, by about 75%, was observed in all patients, usually accompanied by a reduction in echogenicity (Fig. 5.66). No permanent increase in antithyroid antibodies was observed. No recurrence of disease and no case of hypothyroidism occurred after follow-up for 4 years.[75]

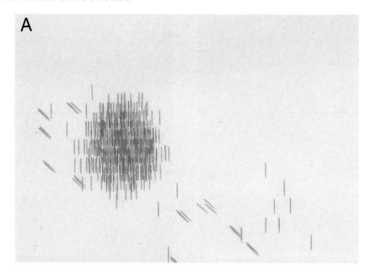

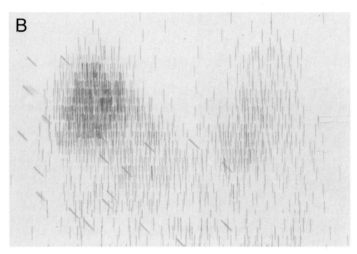

Fig. 5.65 Thyroid scintiscan showing a hot nodule before PEI (**A**) and partial reactivation of extranodular normal tissue with nodule still partially functioning (**B**).

Conclusions

The established methods for the treatment of AFTN are radioiodine and surgery. Radioiodine is followed by hypothyroidism in up to 36% of cases, although a more realistic estimate ranges from 5 to 15% of cases.[76-83] In the patients rendered euthyroid, post-treatment scintigraphy showed compensation in 10–50% of cases, a proportion similar to that observed in patients treated by PEI.[73,80,84] Recent evidence[85] suggests that radioiodine may increase the risk of, and mortality from, gastric cancer. Surgery presents a small risk of permanent damage to vocal cord function and to the parathyroid glands and a mean rate of hypothyroidism of 11%.[76,80,83,86,87] PEI has a high therapeutic efficacy in small and medium-sized nodules, is not followed by hypothyroidism and did not present permanent side effects.

On the strength of these data, the choice of treatment in patients with AFTN depends on various factors, such as patient age, nodule size and number, and the presence or absence of thyrotoxicosis. The indications for therapy may be summarized as follows:

- Surgery for locally symptomatic large nodules and for toxic multinodular goiter in younger patients.
- Radioiodine for bigger single nodules and toxic multinodular goiter in elderly patients.
- PEI for small and medium-sized single nodules, and for patients reluctant to undergo the other types of therapy or not responding to radioiodine. PEI is also proposed as the first option for patients with non-toxic AFTN, for which the choice of aggressive or conservative management is still a question of debate.

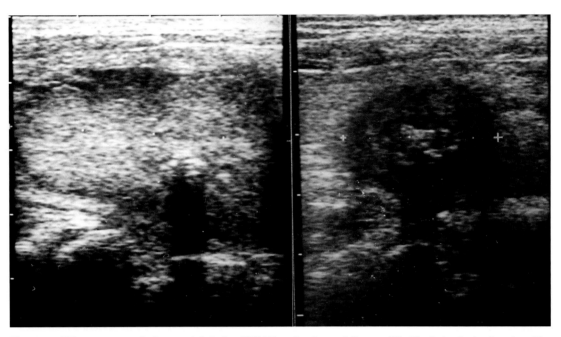

Fig. 5.66 US appearance of a 3 cm nodule before PEI (**A**) and at 2-year follow-up (**B**). The lesion is clearly reduced in volume and decreased in echogenicity.

REFERENCES

1. Rogers W M 1978 Anomalous development of the thyroid. In: Werner S C, Ingbar S H (eds) The thyroid. Harper & Row, New York, pp 416–420
2. Tomá P, Guastalla P P, Carini C, Lucigrai G 1992 Collo. In: Fariello G, Perale R, Perri G, Tomá P (eds) Ecografia pediatrica. Ambrosiana, Milan, pp 139–162
3. Solbiati L, Croce F, Rizzatto G 1992 Tiroide e paratiroidi. In: Rizzatto G, Solbiati L (eds) Anatomia ecografica. Quadri normali, varianti e limiti con il patologico. Masson, Milan, pp 35–45
4. Kerr L 1994 High-resolution thyroid ultrasound: the value of color Doppler. Ultrasound Q 12: 21–43
5. Jarlov A E, Hegedus L, Gjorup T, Hansen J E M 1991 Accuracy of the clinical assessment of thyroid size. Dan Med Bull 38: 87–89
6. Yokoyama N, Nagayama Y, Kakezono F et al 1986 Determination of the volume of the thyroid gland by a high resolutional ultrasonic scanner. J Nucl Med 27: 1475–1479
7. Chanoine J P, Toppet V, Lagasse R, Spehl M, Delange F 1991 Determination of thyroid volume by ultrasound from the neonatal period to late adolescence. Eur J Pediatr 150: 395–399
8. Hegedus L 1986 Thyroid gland volume and thyroid function during and after acute hepatitis infection. Metabolism 35: 495–498
9. Miller J H 1985 Lingual thyroid gland: sonographic appearance. Radiology 156: 83–84
10. Ueda D, Mitamura R, Suzuki N, Yano K, Okuno A 1992 Sonographic imaging of the thyroid gland in congenital hypothyroidism. Pediatr Radiol 22: 102–105
11. Rojeski M T, Gharib H 1985 Nodular thyroid disease: evaluation and management. N Engl J Med 313: 428–436
12. Carrol B A 1982 Asymptomatic thyroid nodules: incidental sonographic detection. AJR 133: 499–501
13. Reading C C, Charboneau J W, James E M et al 1982 High-resolution parathyroid sonography. AJR 139: 539–546
14. James E M, Charboneau J W, Hay I D 1991 The thyroid. In: Rumack C M, Wilson S R, Charboneau J W (eds) Diagnostic ultrasound. Mosby, St Louis, pp 507–523
15. Hennman G 1979 Non toxic goiter. J Clin Metab 8: 167
16. Solbiati L, Cioffi V, Ballarati E 1992 Ultrasonography of the neck. Radiol Clin North Am 30: 941–954
17. Solbiati L, Croce F, Derchi L E 1993 The neck. In: Cosgrove D, Meire H, Dewbury K (eds) Abdominal and general ultrasound. Vol II. Churchill Livingstone, Edinburgh, pp 659–694
18. Sakane S 1990 The prognostic application of thyroid volume determination in patients with Graves' disease. Folia Endocrinol 66: 543–556
19. Muller H W, Schroder S, Schneider C, Seifert G 1985 Sonographic tissue characterisation in thyroid gland diagnosis. Klin Wochenschr 63: 706–710
20. Ralls P W, Mayekawa D S, Lee K P et al 1988 Color-flow Doppler sonography in Graves' disease: 'Thyroid Inferno'. AJR 150: 781–784
21. Hodgson K J, Lazarus J H, Wheeler M H et al 1988 Duplex scan-derived thyroid blood flow in euthyroid and hyperthyroid patients. World J Surg 12: 470–475
22. Brkljacic B, Cuk V, Tomic-Brzac H, Bence-Zigman Z, Delic-Brkljacic D, Drinkovic I 1994 Ultrasonic evaluation of benign and malignant nodules in echographically multinodular thyroids. JCU 22: 71–76
23. Solbiati L, Volterrani L, Rizzatto G et al 1985 The thyroid gland with low uptake lesions: evaluation by ultrasound. Radiology 155: 187–191
24. Lagalla R, Caruso G, Midiri M, Cardinale A E 1992 Echo-Doppler-couleur et pathologie thyroidienne. J Echograph Med Ultrasons 13: 44–47
25. Solbiati L, Ballarati E, Cioffi V 1991 Contribution of color-flow mapping to the differential diagnosis of thyroid nodules. Radiology 181 P: 177
26. Fobbe F, Finke R, Reichenstein E, Schleusener H et al 1989 Appearance of thyroid diseases using colour-coded duplex sonography. Eur J Radiol 2: 29–31
27. Lagalla R, Caruso G, Cardinale A E 1993 Analisi flussimetrica nella patologia tiroidea: ipotesi di integrazione con lo studio qualitativo con color-Doppler. Radiol Med 85: 29–34
28. Brown C L 1981 Pathology of the cold nodule. Clin Endocrinol Metab 10: 235–245
29. Brander A, Viikinkoski P, Nickels J, Kivisaari L 1989 Thyroid gland: US screening in middle-aged women with no previous thyroid disease. Radiology 173: 507–510
30. Hay I D 1990 Papillary thyroid carcinoma. Endocrinol Metab Clin North Am 19: 545–576

31. Pilotti S, Pierotti M A 1992 Classificazione istologica e caratterizzazione molecolare dei tumori dell'epitelio follicolare della tiroide. Argomenti Oncol 13: 365–380

32. Fukunari N, Kawauchi A, Nagakuar H et al 1990 Clinical experience of the color flow mapping in thyroid tumours. Jpn Soc Ultrasound Med Proc 1990: p 429

33. Holtz S, Powers W E 1958 Calcification in papillary carcinoma of the thyroid. Radiology 80: 997–999

34. McConahey W H, Hay I D, Woolner J B et al 1986 Papillary thyroid cancer treated at the Mayo Clinic, 1946 through 1970: initial manifestations, pathologic findings, therapy and outcome. Mayo Clin Proc 61: 978–996

35. Hubert J P, Kiernan P D, Beahrs O H et al 1980 Occult papillary carcinoma of the thyroid. Arch Surg 115: 394–400

36. Solbiati L, Ballarati E, Cioffi V et al 1990 Microcalcifications: a clue in the diagnosis of thyroid malignancies. Radiology 177 (P): 140

37. Auffermann W, Clark O H, Thurnher S, Galante M, Higgins C B 1988 Recurrent thyroid carcinoma: characteristics on MR images. Radiology 168: 753–757

38. Sutton R T, Reading C C, Charboneau J W et al 1988 Ultrasound-guided biopsy of neck masses in postoperative management of patients with thyroid cancer. Radiology 168: 769–772

39. Buraggi G L, Castellani M R, Resnik M 1992 La medicina nucleare nella diagnosi e terapia dei tumori differenziati della tiroide. Argomenti Oncol 13: 393–400

40. Bittman O, Bruneton J N, Fenart D et al 1992 Imagerie des cancers anaplasiques de la thyroïde. J Radiol 73: 35–38

41. Hatabu H, Kasagi K, Yamamoto K et al 1992 Undifferentiated carcinoma of the thyroid gland: sonographic findings. Clin Radiol 45: 307–310

42. Gooding G A W, Langman A W, Dillon W P, Kaplan M J 1989 Malignant carotid artery invasion: sonographic detection. Radiology 171: 435–438

43. Gritzmann N, Grasl M C, Helmer M, Steiner E 1990 Invasion of the carotid artery and jugular vein by lymph node metastases: detection with sonography. AJR 154: 411–414

44. Chong G C, Beahrs O H, Sizemore G W, Woolner L B 1975 Medullary carcinoma of the thyroid gland. Cancer 35: 695–704

45. Gorman B, Charboneau J W, James E M et al 1987 Medullary thyroid carcinoma: role of high-resolution US. Radiology 162: 147–150

46. Schwerk W B, Grun R, Wahl R 1985 Ultrasound diagnosis of c-cell carcinoma of the thyroid. Cancer 55: 624–630

47. Hamburger J I, Miller J M, Kini S R 1983 Lymphoma of the thyroid. Ann Intern Med 99: 685–693

48. Kasagi K, Hatabu H, Tokuda Y et al 1991 Lymphoproliferative disorders of the thyroid gland: radiological appearances. Br J Radiol 64: 569–575

49. Takashima S, Morimoto S, Ikezoe J et al 1989 Primary thyroid lymphoma: comparison of CT and US assessment. Radiology 171: 439–443

50. Mortensen J D, Woolner L B, Bennett W A 1955 Gross and microscopic findings in clinically normal thyroid glands. J Clin Endocrinol Metab 15: 1270–1280

51. Adams H, Jones N C 1990 Ultrasound appearances of De Quervain's thyroiditis. Clin Radiol 42: 217–218

52. Birchall I W J, Chow C C, Metreweli C 1990 Ultrasound appearances of De Quervain's thyroiditis. Clin Radiol 41: 57–59

53. Gutekunst R, Hafermann R, Mansky W, Scriba T 1989 Ultrasonography related to clinical and laboratory findings in lymphocytic thyroiditis. Acta Endocrinol 121: 129–135

54. Holmes H B, Kreutner A, O'Brien P H 1977 Hashimoto's thyroiditis and its relationship to other thyroid diseases. Surg Gynecol Obstet 144: 887–890

55. Sostre S, Reyes M M 1991 Sonographic diagnosis and grading of Hashimoto's thyroiditis. J Endocrinol Invest 14: 115–121

56. Lagalla R, Caruso G, Benza I, Novara V, Calliada F 1993 Echo-color Doppler in the study of hypothyroidism in the adult. (in Italian) Radiol Med 86: 281–283

57. Takashima S, Matsuzuka F, Nagareda T, Tomiyama N, Kozuka T 1992 Thyroid nodules associated with Hashimoto's thyroiditis: assessment with US. Radiology 185: 125–130

58. Lowhagen T 1983 Cytological diagnosis of thyroid disease. Ann Chir Gynaecol 72: 90–98

59. Ravetto C, Colombo L, Assi A 1992 La biopsia per aspirazione con ago sottile dei tumori tiroidei. Argomenti Oncol 13: 387–391

60. Rosen I B, Azadian A, Walfish P G, Salem S, Lansdown E, Bedard Y C 1993 Ultrasound-guided fine-needle aspiration biopsy in the management of thyroid disease. Am J Surg 166: 346–353

61. Miller J M, Hamburger J I, Taylor C I 1981 Is needle aspiration of the cystic thyroid nodule effective and safe treatment? In: Hamburger J I, Miller J M (eds) Controversies in clinical thyroidology. Springer-Verlag, New York

62. Ferrari C, Paracchi A, Macchi R M et al 1994 Treatment of cystic thyroid nodules by percutaneous ethanol injection under ultrasound guidance. Eur J Ultrasound (in press)

63. Yasuda K, Ozaki O, Sugino K et al 1992 Treatment of cystic lesions of the thyroid by ethanol instillation. World J Surg 16: 958–961

64. Plummer H S 1913 Clinical and pathological relationships of simple and exophthalmic goiter. Trans Assoc Am Physicians 28: 588–595

65. Solbiati L, Giangrande A, De Pra L, Bellotti E, Cantù P, Ravetto C 1985 Percutaneous ethanol injection of parathyroid tumors under US guidance: treatment for secondary hyperparathyroidism. Radiology 155: 607–610

66. Livraghi T, Festi D, Monti F, Salmi A, Vettori C 1986 US-guided percutaneous alcohol injection of small hepatic and abdominal tumors. Radiology 161: 309–312

67. Karstrup B S, Holm H H, Torp-Pedersen S, Hegedus L 1987 Ultrasonically guided percutaneous inactivation of parathyroid tumors. Br J Radiol 60: 667–670

68. Livraghi T, Paracchi A, Ferrari C et al 1990 Treatment of autonomous thyroid nodules with percutaneous ethanol injection: preliminary results. Radiology 175: 827–829

69. Goletti O, Monzani F, Caraccio N et al 1992 Percutaneous ethanol injection treatment of autonomously functioning single thyroid nodules: optimization of treatment and short term outcome. World J Surg 16: 784–790

70. Martino E, Murtas M L, Loviselli A et al 1992 Percutaneous intranodular ethanol injection for treatment of autonomously functioning thyroid nodules. Surgery 112: 1161–1165

71. Monzani F, Goletti O, Caraccio N et al 1992 Percutaneous ethanol injection treatment of autonomous thyroid adenoma: hormonal and clinical evaluation. Clin Endocrinol 36: 491–497

72. Paracchi A, Ferrari C, Livraghi T et al 1992 Percutaneous intranodular ethanol injection: a new treatment for autonomous thyroid adenoma. J Endocrinol Invest 15: 353–362

73. Mazzeo S, Toni M G, De Gaudio C et al 1993 Percutaneous injection of ethanol to treat autonomous thyroid nodule. AJR 161: 871–876

74. Papini E, Panunzi C, Pacella C M et al 1993 Percutaneous ultrasound-guided ethanol injection: new treatment of toxic autonomously functioning thyroid nodules. J Clin Endocrinol Metab 76: 411–416

75. Livraghi T, Paracchi A, Ferrari C, Reschini E, Macchi R M, Bonifacino A 1994 Treatment of autonomous thyroid nodules with percutaneous ethanol injection: 4-year experience. Radiology, in press

76. Horst W, Rosler H, Schneider C, Labhart A 1967 306 cases of toxic adenoma: clinical aspects, finding in radioiodine diagnostics, radiochromatography and histology; results of 131-I and surgical treatment. J Nucl Med 8: 515–528

77. Goldstein R, Hart I R 1983 Follow-up of solitary autonomous thyroid nodules treated with 131-I. N Engl J Med 309: 1473–1476

78. Ross D S, Ridgway E C, Daniels G H 1984 Successful treatment of solitary toxic thyroid nodules with relatively low-dose iodine-131, with low prevalence of hypothyroidism. Ann Intern Med 101: 488–490

79. Hegedus L, Veiergang D, Karstrup S, Molholm Hansen J 1986 Compensated 131-I therapy of solitary autonomous thyroid nodules: effect on thyroid size and early hypothyroidism. Acta Endocrinol (Copenh) 113: 226–232

80. Kinser J A, Roesler H, Furrer T, Grutter D, Zimmermann H 1989 Nonimmunogenic hyperthyroidism: cumulative hypothyroidism incidence after radioiodine and surgical treatment. J Nucl Med 30: 1960–1965

81. Huysmans D A, Corstens F H, Kloppenborg P W 1991 Long-term

follow-up in toxic solitary autonomous thyroid nodules treated with radioactive iodine. J Nucl Med 32: 27–30

82. Berglund J, Christensen S B, Dymlig J F, Halengren B 1991 The incidence of recurrence and hypothyroidism following treatment with antithyroid drugs, surgery or radioiodine in all patients with thyrotoxicosis in Malmo during the period 1970–1974. J Intern Med 229: 435–442

83. O'Brien T, Gharib H, Suman V J, Van Heerden J A 1992 Treatment of toxic solitary thyroid nodules: surgery versus radioactive iodine. Surgery 112: 1166–1170

84. Molnar G D, Wilber R D, Lee R E, Woolner L B, Keating F R 1965 On the hyperfunctioning solitary thyroid nodule. Mayo Clin Proc 40: 665–684

85. Holm L E, Hall P, Wiklund K et al 1991 Cancer risk after iodine-131 therapy for hyperthyroidism. J Natl Cancer Inst 83: 1072–1077

86. Eyre-Brook I A, Talbot C H 1982 The treatment of autonomous functioning thyroid nodules. Br J Surg 69: 577–579

87. Bransom C J, Talbot C H, Henry L, Elemenoglou J 1979 Solitary toxic adenoma of the thyroid gland. Br J Surg 66: 590–595

6

Parathyroid glands

C. Fugazzola   I. Bergamo Andreis   L. Solbiati

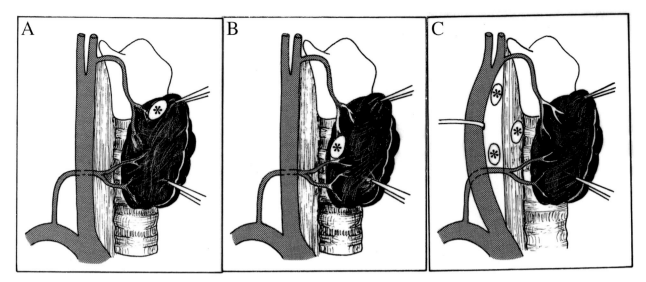

Fig. 6.1 Possible locations of upper parathyroid glands (⋆): behind the upper pole (**A**) or the middle third (**B**) of the thyroid lobe, or ectopic sites (**C**) (retropharyngeal, retrotracheal and retro-esophageal).

ANATOMY

The parathyroid glands are, in most cases, four glands located posterior to the thyroid lobes; their mean size is 5 × 3 × 1 mm, with weight ranging between 10 and 75 mg.[1] Their variable location and number has, however, to be borne in mind, depending on anomalies of embryologic development.

Location

The superior parathyroid glands arise from the fourth branchial pouch along with the lateral lobes of the thyroid gland. Their migration in the fetal period is minimal; in most cases they remain in close association with the posterior portion of either the upper or middle third of the thyroid lobes.[2] Only in about 1% of cases are they ectopically placed (retropharyngeal, retrotracheal, retroesophageal locations) (Fig. 6.1).[1,3]

Conversely, the inferior parathyroid glands arise from the third branchial pouch along with the thymus, with which they descend during the fetal period towards the mediastinum: the variable location of these glands is associated with their migration,[2] only about 60% of cases being located close to the lower thyroid pole;[1,3] in 26–39% of cases they are found within either the thyrothymic ligament or the tongue of the thymus; much more rare (2%) is a location within the intramediastinal thymus. There are, moreover, undescended parathyroid glands (usually associated with thymic remnants) located in the superior latero-cervical region close to the carotid bifurcation and lowest

glands, along the course of the common carotid artery (2%) (Fig. 6.2).[1]

These remarks apply to normal glands; in pathologic conditions the percentage of superior glands with an unusual location increases up to 10%[4,5]; this is due to the fact that the glands, when enlarged, can change their usual position while migrating (owing to the effect of gravity) along the posterior aspect of the esophagus down into the posterior superior mediastinum.[6,7]

The percentage of pathologic inferior glands with an unusual location is not very different from that of the normal glands; nevertheless, some inferior glands may also migrate, usually within the anterior mediastinum (the glands are therefore extrathymic instead of intrathymic in location);[8] the detection of pathologic glands within either the middle mediastinum[9] or even the pericardium[10] is exceedingly rare.

The fairly rare intrathyroidal location (subcapsular or intraparenchymal) has also to be remembered; however, only the intraparenchymal glands are considered to be ectopic, this being exceptional for normal glands (0.2%),[3] slightly less so for pathologic glands (2–5%).[6] Theoretically, these glands should pertain to the superior parathyroid glands; however, intrathyroidal adenomas quite often originate from the inferior glands.[6]

Number

In 85% of cases there are four parathyroid glands; in 3% of cases only three glands are to be found; in about 10–

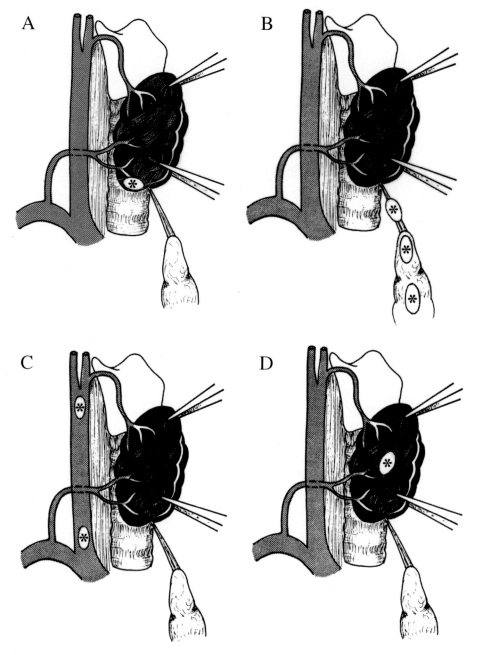

Fig. 6.2 Possible locations of lower parathyroid glands (*): behind the lower thyroid pole (**A**), within the thyrothymic ligament or the thymic tongue (**B**), along the carotid artery (undescended) (**C**) and intrathyroidal (**D**).

13% of cases there are up to 11 supernumerary glands;[3] however, most often a fifth gland is present, usually with a thymic location.[3]

PATHOLOGY

Primary hyperparathyroidism

The pathologic background of primary hyperpara-thyroidism (HPT) [the diagnosis of which is mainly based on laboratory data such as the presence of hypercalcemia and increased serum parathyroid hormone (PTH) levels] is in most cases due to adenomas (80–85%), hyperplasias being rarer (15–20%) and carcinomas very rare (0.5–4%).[2]

Adenomas

An adenoma is usually a single lesion (Fig. 6.3), double adenomas being fairly rare (2–5%).[8] Adenomas are com-posed of chief cells in over 90% of cases; in 5–10% of cases

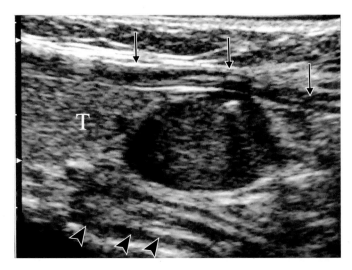

Fig. 6.3 Longitudinal scan. Typical hypoechoic parathyroid adenoma in primary HPT, oval in shape and located between prethyroidal muscles, anteriorly (arrow) and esophagus (arrowhead) posteriorly. T: lower pole of the thyroid lobe.

they consist of oncocytes (or oxyphil cells).[8] Their size is very variable: a microadenoma is slightly larger than a normal gland (6–8 mm), 80–100 mg in weight; the mean size of an adenoma is about 15 mm, the mean weight about 1 g.[8] The volume of the adenoma is often closely related to the biochemical hyperfunctional levels,[11] with the exception of large adenomas with wide areas of necrotic or hemorrhagic degeneration.[8] Cysts have also to be considered in this section; they represent two different types of lesions:

1. *Cystic adenomas.* These contain residual adenomatous tissue within either the cystic cavity or the wall. This sometimes detectable macroscopically, sometimes only at histologic evaluation. Cystic adenomas are always associated with signs of hyperfunction.[8]
2. *True cysts.* These usually develop within the inferior glands close to the lower thyroid pole; they have a fluid content with high PTH levels. The wall is made up of fibrous tissue of variable thickness with islets of parathyroid tissue; unlike cystic adenomas, true cysts are usually non-functional.[12]

The very rare *lipoadenomas* should also be mentioned, being characterized by an epithelial (adenomatous) and a connective tissue (lipomatous) component. These tumors, which present specific sonographic and CT features, are also responsible for HPT.[13]

Hyperplasia

Hyperplasia – usually chief cell hyperplasia – always affects all the parathyroid glands, although in an asymmetric way: on macroscopic examination, only two or three glands may show an increase in volume.[8,14]

Adenoma and hyperplasia are often superimposed, both macroscopically and histologically. With pathologic glands, the easiest way to differentiate adenoma from hyperplasia is to examine a second parathyroid: if this is histologically normal, the first gland assessed is adenomatous.[2]

Carcinoma

Carcinoma presents as a fairly large mass (average diameter 3.5 cm) of firm consistency, with peripheral fibrotic reaction and often adherent to contiguous anatomic structures.[15,16] The histologic differential diagnosis from adenoma is often difficult, especially on frozen sections, being based on few characteristics.[17,18]

The 5-year survival rate is rarely more than 50%; recurrence may be local or distant (25–30% of cases); in 20% of cases distant metastases are already present at the first diagnosis.[16,19,20]

Secondary hyperparathyroidism

Secondary HPT is usually associated with chronic renal failure; hypocalcemia – induced by hyperphosphoremia and deficit of gastrointestinal calcium absorption (due to lack of renal vitamin D activation) – induces hyperplasia (diffuse or nodular) of all glands (Fig. 6.4), consisting mainly of chief cells; the degree of hyperplasia is variable, with a weight range (of the four glands) between 250 mg and 10 g: the mean value is about 2–3 g.[8] However, as in primary HPT, the increase in volume of the gland is often asymmetric.[8]

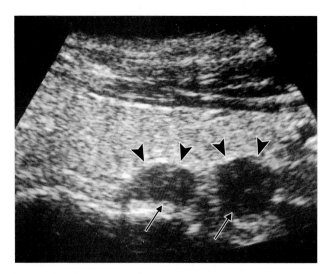

Fig. 6.4 Longitudinal scan. Two contiguous, 1 cm, parathyroid hyperplasias (arrow) in secondary HPT. Both glands show anterior hyperechoic capsule (arrowhead).

Persistent or recurrent hyperparathyroidism

Persistent HPT is a condition characterized by the persistence of hypercalcemia after surgery, whereas recurrent HPT refers to the reappearance of hypercalcemia after a period of normal calcemia lasting from 6 months to 1 year.[21,22] The main causes are due to adenomas not detected at surgery (usually a second adenoma or a tumor in an unusual location) and misdiagnosed primary hyperplasia.[23,24] Much rarer is the recurrence of carcinoma (wrongly diagnosed, at the time of the first surgical intervention, as adenoma). Ever more exceptional is the presence of fragments of hyperfunctional glands (parathyromatosis) left in situ during surgery or reimplanted within the operative field[22,25]; these multiple hyperfunctional nodules scattered through the neck and mediastinum may be due sometimes to the spontaneous spread of parathyroid tissue during ontogenesis (Fig.6.5).[26] There is also the possibility (after total parathyroidectomy) of hyperfunction of glandular fragments autotransplanted into muscular pockets of the forearm or within the sternocleidomastoid muscle.[27]

SONOGRAPHY

Examination technique

The sonographic (US) study is performed with hyperextension of the neck, achieved by placing a pad under the patient's shoulders.

The optimal frequencies for the study of the parathyroid glands are those above 7.5 MHz in medium-sized necks, the best results are achieved with small-parts probes with built-in water path, ranging between 10 and 13 MHz in frequency. In obese patients, with short necks or associated multinodular goiters, one has often to resort to probes of lower frequency (5–7.5 MHz), since the usually retrothyroidal location of the parathyroid glands requires the penetration of the US beam deeper than 3–4 cm from the skin surface.[28]

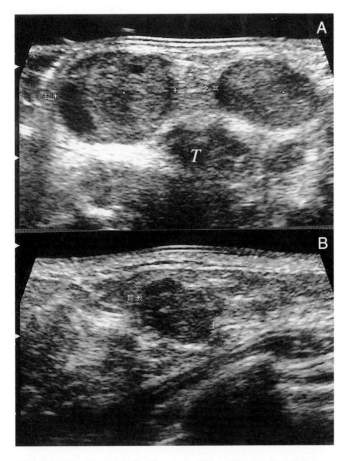

Fig. 6.5 Parathyromatosis. Transverse (**A**) and longitudinal (**B**) scans of the lower neck showing multiple hypoechoic solid nodules (calipers) disseminated in soft tissues. The patient with secondary HPT had undergone two previous surgical explorations with removal of five parathyroid hyperplasias. T: trachea.

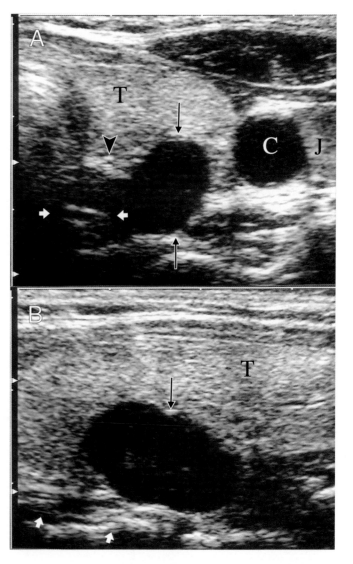

Fig. 6.6 Transverse (**A**) and longitudinal (**B**) scans of parathyroid hyperplasia (arrow) in typical location. White arrows: esophagus; arrowhead: lesser neurovascular bundle; T: thyroid lobe; C: carotid artery; J: jugular vein.

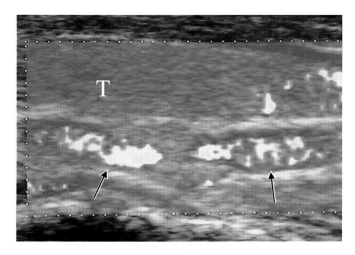

Fig. 6.7 Longitudinal scan obtained with power Doppler. Two hypervascular tubular parathyroid hyperplasias (arrow) lie behind the thyroid lobe (T).

The performance of the US scans (usually longitudinal and axial) requires the identification of a few topographic landmarks that are useful for locating the parathyroid glands: these are the posteromedial angle of the thyroid lobe, the longus colli muscle and the lesser neurovascular bundle (inferior thyroid artery and recurrent laryngeal nerve) (Fig. 6.6). The examination includes not only the thyroid region, but also the neck areas above and below, in order to include those glands that have an unusual location.[28,29]

The search for parathyroid glands with a paratracheal and paraesophageal location is very difficult; it is necessary to angle the probe lateromedially, with rotation of the patient's head to the opposite side.[30] To search for glands within the cervical thymus it is convenient to perform scans while the patient is swallowing, in order to move the thymic tissue upwards into the field of view.[31]

Currently, the use of color Doppler is mandatory in questionable cases, mainly when differentiation from thyroid nodules is needed. Either the conventional frequency-shift based color Doppler or, preferably, the new power (or energy) Doppler can be employed, with 7.5–10 MHz probes and settings for slow-flow analysis.

Features

B-mode sonography

Normal parathyroid glands cannot be demonstrated, even with high-frequency probes (10–13 MHz); this is probably due to their small size but is attributable mainly to their echo structure, which is indistinguishable from that of the thyroid gland.[28]

Adenomas, hyperplasias and carcinomas have similar patterns of morphology and echo structure. Glands with a retrothyroidal location are typically oval, with longitudinal main axis (see Figs 6.3 and 6.6B), since the parathyroid glands develop within longitudinally oriented tissue planes;[32] rounded glands are not infrequent, both for small and large lesions (see Fig. 6.4). Glands with a different shape, however, may be observed: some are tubular (with marked predominance of the longitudinal axis) (Fig. 6.7), some leaf-like (less than 2 mm thick) (Fig. 6.8); sometimes the increase in volume is asymmetric (the cranial or caudal extremity can be more bulbous, thus bringing about a triangular, teardrop-like, or bilobate shape) (Fig. 6.9).[32–34]

Pathologic glands, no matter what their histologic type, are homogeneously hypoechoic compared with the thyroidal parenchyma: this is due to the regular hypercellularity of the lesions, with few acoustic interfaces[30] (see Fig. 3.13). A second structural characteristic (which is fairly frequent in normally sited glands) is a hyperechoic band separating the pathologic parathyroid gland from the

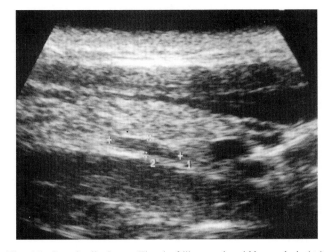

Fig. 6.8 Longitudinal scan. Tiny, leaf-like parathyroid hyperplasia (+), 8 × 2 mm in size.

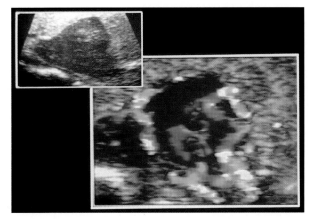

Fig. 6.9 Parathyroid adenoma with triangular shape. B-mode and color Doppler representation. Intranodular blood vessels with fairly regular course.

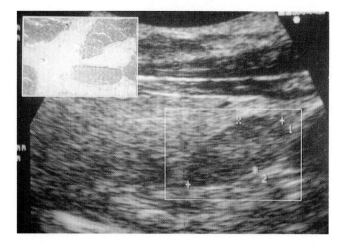

Fig. 6.10 Parathyroid adenoma (yellow box) nearly isoechoic with the thyroid parenchyma. This echo pattern is due to an abundant fibrotic component (see histological specimen).

thyroidal tissue, likely due to the facing capsular leaves of two adjacent glands (see Fig. 6.4).[28]

In 15–20% of cases there are variations in echo structure, for some of which histopathologic correlations can be suggested:

- glands nearly isoechoic with the thyroid gland (Fig. 6.10) from which they may be separated by a thin hypoechoic halo[33]
- glands with inhomogeneous echo structure,[34] characterized by hyperechoic areas interspersed with hypoechoic areas, owing to microcystic degeneration or fibrosis
- glands of mixed echo structure,[33] partly solid, partly anechoic, related to necrotic or hemorrhagic degeneration (Fig. 6.11)
- glands with cystic features[35] (cystic adenomas or parathyroid cysts) (Fig. 6.12)

- glands with calcifications:[34] calcifications are very rare in adenomas, more frequent in carcinomas[36] and hyperplasias of secondary HPT (the latter, possibly in relation to the slow growth of these lesions).[28]

Finally, it should be remembered that the rare lipoadenomas, should the fatty component be predominant, present as hyperechoic masses.[37]

To summarize, although there are usually no features enabling differentiation between adenomas, hyperplasias and carcinomas, the detection of several enlarged parathyroid glands in the same patient is suggestive of hyperplasia.[34] Carcinomas may have irregular and lobulated margins and an inhomogeneous structure with cystic spaces (Fig. 6.13). However, these features are not useful for the differential diagnosis, being detectable also in larger adenomas;[38] the only conclusive sign of malignancy, although rare, is the extensive invasion of adjacent anatomic structures (such as the thyroid, vessels or muscles);[38,39] the invasion of adjacent structures is nevertheless often visible only on microscopic examination and thus is not detectable by US.[38]

Color Doppler sonography

Pathologic parathyroid glands, whatever their histologic type, on color Doppler sonography present a hypervascular pattern which is typical in about 90% of cases:[40] this comprises fairly marked intraparenchymal vascularization (relative to the gland volume), which is mainly arterial, with a fairly straight course (Figs 6.9, 6.14). No perinodular flow is usually detected, apart from that at the hilum, which is usually in the caudal part of the inferior glands and in the cranial part of the superior glands.[28]

With power (or intensity or energy) Doppler both large and small (parenchymal perfusion) intraglandular vessels

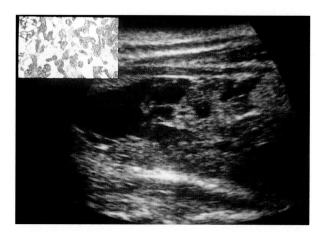

Fig. 6.11 Large (4 cm) parathyroid adenoma with mixed structure, due to necrotic and hemorrhagic changes (see specimen).

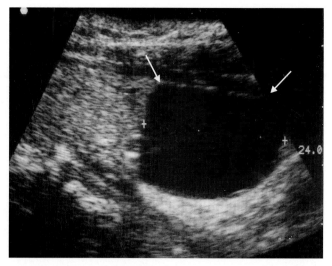

Fig. 6.12 Cystic adenoma (arrow) of the lower parathyroid gland.

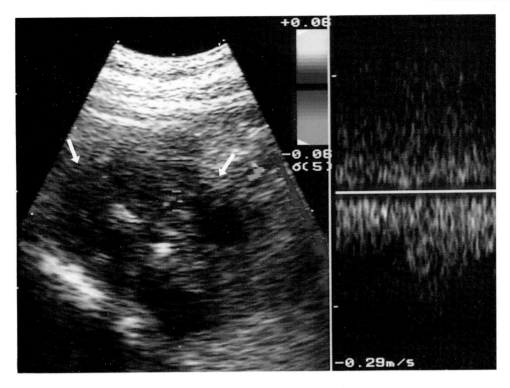

Fig. 6.13 Parathyroid carcinoma (arrow) with irregular margins and inhomogeneous structure.

can be detected, almost entirely filling the surface of the gland (Figs 6.7, 6.15).

Spectral analysis usually demonstrates flow with a high diastolic component, low resistive index and systolic peak values ranging between 5 and 40 cm/s.[40-42] No direct relation apparently exists between the peak velocities measured in the main parathyroid vessels and the degree of hyperfunction of the glands.[42]

On the other hand, in about 10% of cases,[40] according to the technology currently available, the glands apparently are not vascularized. This occurs under the following cir-

cumstances[28]: when the parathyroid glands are small (less than 1 cm in diameter) and deeply located (Fig. 6.16); when there are tumors with wide areas of necrotic degeneration (see Fig. 3.14); in lesions located at the base of the neck, adjacent to large vessels, in which it is technically necessary to increase the PRF beyond 1.5–2.0 kHz in order to eliminate the motion artifacts attributable to vascular pulsatility.

It should also be remembered that hyperplastic thyroid nodules with no hyperfunction (a frequent event in association with HPT), have a vascular pattern that is usually characterized by perinodular flow along with minimal or absent intranodular flow (see chapter 5).[41] Thus, clinically, the use of color Doppler is justifiable for assessment of the thyroid or parathyroid origin of nodules that are questionable on B-mode ultrasonography, as judged by their various vascularization characteristics.

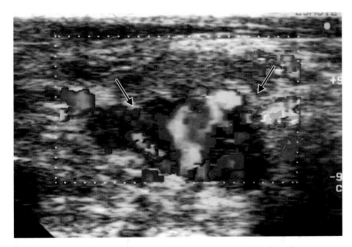

Fig. 6.14 Parathyroid adenoma (2.5 cm) (arrow) with abundant intraparenchymal vascularization.

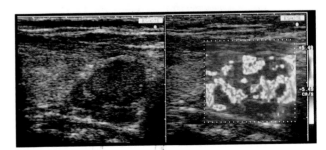

Fig. 6.15 Parathyroid hyperplasia (2.0 cm). With power Doppler (right) the lesion appears to be completely filled with blood vessels.

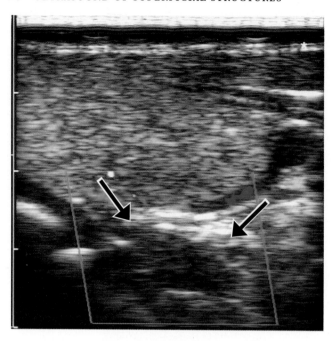

Fig. 6.16 Small, deeply located parathyroid tumor (arrow): no flow signals are detectable.

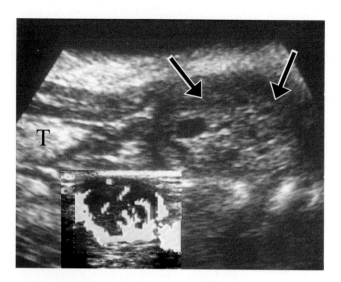

Fig. 6.17 Ectopic parathyroid adenoma (arrow) within the thyro-thymic ligament. Small box: power Doppler representation of the same tumor showing caudally located hilum. T: lower pole of the thyroid lobe.

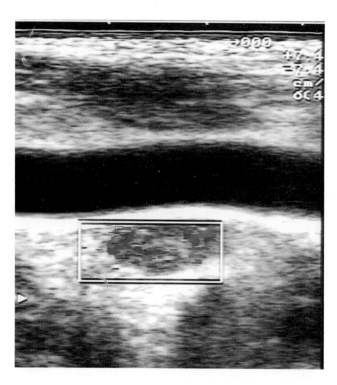

Fig. 6.18 Undescended parathyroid gland (hyperplasia) located behind the carotid artery and with flow signals.

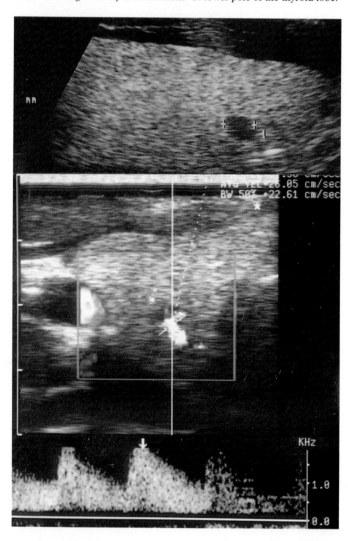

Fig. 6.19 Tiny (7 mm) intrathyroidal parathyroid hyperplasia (top). With color Doppler (bottom) the gland displays a hypervascular pattern with high diastolic component.

Diagnostic potentials and limits

Sensitivity

The ability of B-mode US to detect pathologic parathyroids depends on various factors including the location of the glands (typical or atypical), the lesion size and number (single or multiple), the simultaneous presence of thyroid goiter and a history of previous neck surgery.

Location of lesions. The detection of glands in a typical site is easier than that of glands in an atypical site.

Glands in a typical site. The superior glands have to be searched for behind the upper to middle third of the thyroid lobe, whereas the inferior glands can be located behind the lower thyroid pole (usually), but also anteriorly, behind the prethyroidal muscles (see Fig. 6.3) or within the thyrothymic ligament, 1–2 cm caudally to the lower thyroid pole (Fig. 6.17).

Glands in an atypical site. These include the following:

1. Undescended parathyroid glands or glands located along the common carotid artery:[43,44] on B-mode US they appear to be almost superimposable on the hyperplastic nodes of the jugular chain. The only suspect features are the missing hyperechoic hilum on B-mode US, as well as the vascular pattern on color Doppler sonography (Fig. 6.18).[28] The definite diagnosis is achieved, nevertheless, only with percutaneous US-guided FNAB; this is very important, as these lesions are frequently missed on surgical exploration;[45] in particular, when the glands are located in the carotid sheath, they are overlooked on operation if the surgeon does not specifically open the sheath and dissect within it.[6]
2. Parathyroid glands of the cervical thymus: these are fairly easily detectable on scans performed during swallowing, as already described (see Fig. 6.17).
3. Intrathyroidal parathyroid glands: these are easily detected, mostly in the middle to inferior portion of the thyroid lobe, completely surrounded by thyroid tissue; they are ovoid and usually homogeneously hypoechoic, with the main axis oriented in the cephalad–caudad direction.[30]

   Although their identification is easy, the differentiation from thyroid nodules is difficult:[46,47] the only grounds for suspicion are the presence of a peripheral hyperechoic capsule on B-mode US as well as a hypervascular pattern on color Doppler sonography (Fig. 6.19).[28] However, in this case also, percutaneous FNAB enables the diagnosis to be made with confidence. These lesions can be missed at surgery owing to their soft consistency, indistinguishable from that of thyroid tissue; nevertheless intraoperative diagnosis (Fig. 6.20) calls for either thyroidotomy or subtotal thyroid lobectomy.[4,6] The pathologic parathyroid glands located below the thyroid capsule as well as those within a sulcus of the thyroid gland, are not considered to be true

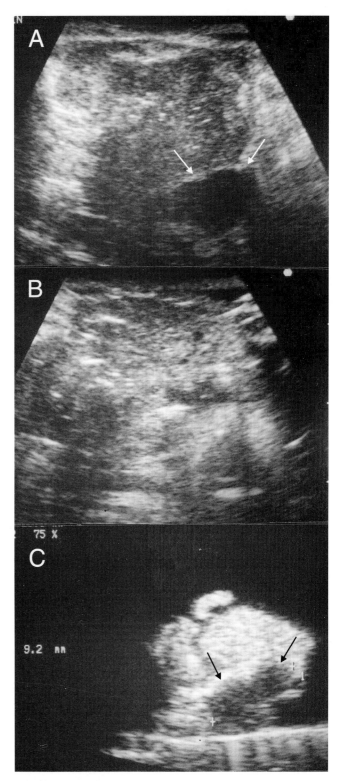

Fig. 6.20 Intraoperative scans. **A** Small, deeply located parathyroid hyperplasia (arrow) in patient with history of three previous surgical explorations with removal of six parathyroid glands. Following US-guided surgical ablation (**B**), US confirms the absence of residual parathyroid tissue. **C** The gland removed (arrow) is visible in the surgical specimen, surrounded by fatty tissue.

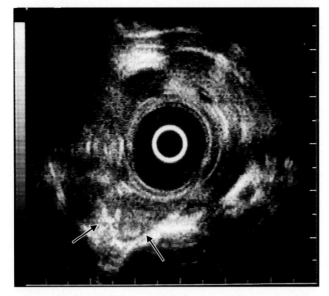

Fig. 6.21 Endo-esophageal sonography with 12 MHz probe. Retro-esophageal adenoma. The hypoechoic lesion (arrow) is demonstrated on the right posterior aspect of the esophagus. (Courtesy of Dr A. Fratton, Verona.)

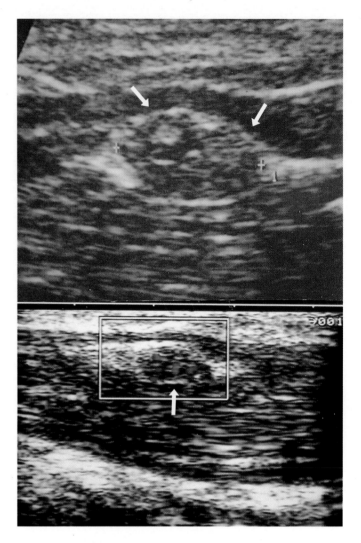

Fig. 6.22 Hyperplastic (top) and hypervascular (bottom) fragments (arrow) of parathyroid gland autotransplanted into the forearm.

intrathyroidal glands. These lesions – not always easily detected at surgery – have sonographic features similar to those of the extracapsular glands;[30] however, not uncommonly, the echogenic band separating the parathyroid from the thyroid gland cannot be recognized, thus causing problems of differentiation from the thyroid nodules.

4. Retroesophageal and retrotracheal cervical parathyroid glands: these are only rarely detected, when they have become quite large, slightly protruding on one side of the trachea or esophagus; their demonstration is made easier by contralateral head rotation movements which increase the protrusion, thus allowing a better exploration of the retrotracheal area.[30]

5. Mediastinal parathyroid glands: those located within the anterior mediastinum, caudally to the superior sternal notch cannot be visualized. Those located within the posterior–superior mediastinum (located para-esophageally or paratracheally) can sometimes be imaged with the technique described above for retro-tracheal or retroesophageal cervical parathyroid glands. Sometimes, it may be useful to employ low-frequency probes (5 MHz), angled caudally, for maximal penetration.[30]

Cervical or mediastinal lesions, with retroesophageal location or within the tracheo-esophageal groove, can be easily demonstrated employing *endo-esophageal US* (Fig. 6.21). The experience achieved so far with this modality is limited; moreover, owing to its invasiveness (albeit limited), its use is suggested only in patients with persistent or recurrent HPT.[48]

6. Hyperfunctional glandular fragments, autotransplanted in the forearm: these fragments, responsible for recurrent HPT, are recognized as hypoechoic, round or oval, sharply marginated structures localized between muscular fascicles;[49,50] in these cases color Doppler sonography may be useful in order to confirm the findings of B-mode US (Fig. 6.22).

Size of lesions. US is able to detect lesions that have a major axis less than 1 cm in length (see Fig. 6.19), especially when the glands are in their usual location and the thyroid is of normal size and structure. However, it must be emphasized that there are significant variations in sensitivity depending on the size of the lesions; in the series by Reading[32] the sensitivity, which is only 29% for glands weighing between 40 and 100 mg, increases for larger glands (being about 95% in glands more than 1000 mg in weight).

Number of lesions. The diagnosis of multifocal path-

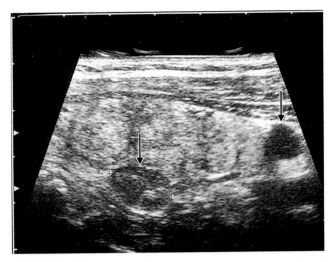

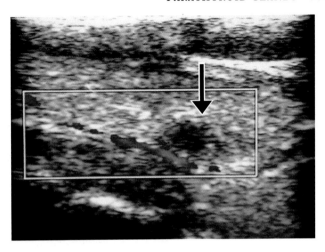

Fig. 6.23 Two parathyroid hyperplasias (arrow) in patient with thyroid multinodular goiter. One gland is posteriorly located, the other is caudal to the lower thyroid pole.

Fig. 6.24 Small, posteriorly located hypoechoic nodule (arrow) of the thyroid gland, mimicking a parathyroid tumor. The complete absence of flow signals with color Doppler rules out the possibility of a parathyroid lesion.

ology (hyperplasias, multiple adenomas) is often diffi-cult,[29,51] bearing in mind that hyperplastic glands do not have a regular increase in volume. Notably, some glands may have a volume that is normal (or only slightly greater than that of a normally functioning gland).[8]

Associated thyroid goiter. In cases of goiter (diffuse or multinodular), the thickness of the thyroid parenchyma can require the use of lower-frequency probes, with conse-quent reduction in spatial resolution. Moreover, the inhomogeneous echo texture, as well as the irregular and lobulated margins of goiter, may hide pathologic para-thyroid glands, especially if these are small (Fig. 6.23).[30]

Previous neck surgery. The search for pathologic glands is easier in patients with no previous neck operation than in those who have already undergone surgery, such as those operated on for thyroid pathology and (much more frequently) those patients who have undergone surgery for primary or secondary HPT and who have displayed persistent or recurrent symptoms.

In patients with no previous surgery, sonography has a sensitivity ranging between 65 and 75%, with a mean value of 72%;[52–54] on the other hand, in previously operated patients with persistent or recurrent HPT it is less sensitive (ranging between 50 and 65%, with mean value about 60%). This decrease is mainly due to the fact that, in such patients, the anatomic landmarks are more difficult to recognize (owing to fibrosis following operation) and they have a very high incidence of ectopic glands and of multigland disease.[55]

Specificity

The sonographic specificity is greater than 90%, as the incidence of false positives is further reduced by the use of high-frequency probes.

Dilated thyroid veins, adjacent to the lower thyroid pole may mimic enlarged parathyroid glands; however, the tubular pattern, the increase in diameter with Valsalva's maneuver and the demonstration of flow on color Doppler sonography allow a correct differentiation.[30]

Thyroid nodules, especially if hypoechoic and located pos-teriorly, as well as (more rarely) *pathologic cervical nodes*, notably if belonging to the recurrent chain, can be difficult to differentiate from parathyroid lesions.[11,29,32,46,47] In these circumstances (i.e. differentiation between thyroid and parathyroid nodules), color Doppler sonography is cur-rently recommended;[40,41] the parathyroid glands usually display signs of intraglandular flow, whereas hyperplastic non-hyperfunctional thyroid nodules usually display peri-nodular flow and a nearly complete lack of intranodular flow (see Ch. 5) (Fig. 6.24). However, color Doppler does not always permit this differentiation, since hyperplastic hyperfunctional nodules, as well as thyroid adenomas and carcinomas, show hypervascularization features similar to those usually observed in the parathyroid glands. Fur-thermore there are – although rarely (about 10% of cases) – parathyroid glands that do not show signs of intraglandular flow, at least with the technologies currently employed. The cases not clearly assessed by color Doppler sonography may be resolved by US-guided FNAB.

Percutaneous fine needle aspiration biopsy (FNAB)

Percutaneous FNAB is currently the most reliable modality to characterize nodules that are doubtful both on US and with the other imaging modalities, thus increasing their specificity. As the lesions are usually small, the procedure requires accurate US guidance so that the needle hits the target precisely (Fig. 6.25). CT guidance can be employed in those rare instances in which atypically located lesions

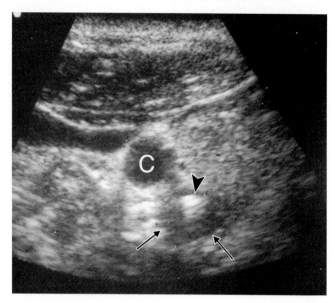

Fig. 6.25 US-guided fine-needle aspiration biopsy of parathyroid tumor (arrow). The tip of the needle (arrowhead) is clearly visible in the middle of the nodule. C: carotid artery.

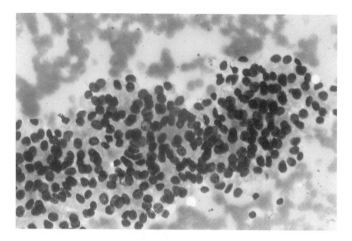

Fig. 6.26 Cluster of closely packed parathyroid cells resulting from fine-needle aspiration biopsy. (Courtesy of Dr C. Ravetto, Department of Pathology, Busto Arsizio.)

cannot be demonstrated by US.[56] Non-cutting 21–22 G needles are usually employed, permitting the preparation of cytologic specimens or radioimmunological PTH assay.

When fine-needle aspirated material is densely cellular, either cytology or immunocytochemistry can be used. Cytological examination, performed with the common stains for morphological evaluation (Papanicolaou, May–Grunwald–Giemsa), can be conclusive, owing to the typical appearance of clusters of closely packed parathyroid cells (Fig. 6.26). However, three main problems can occur:

- it is impossible to differentiate between parathyroid and thyroid tissue when few cells are aspirated, in the absence of colloid or macrophages[57,58]
- it is difficult to differentiate between follicular tumors of the thyroid gland and parathyroid adenomas[59–61]
- it is possible to misdiagnose parathyroid adenomas as papillary carcinomas of the thyroid gland, as reported in a few cases.[51,60,62]

To overcome these drawbacks it is convenient to combine routine staining with the Grimelius cytochemical method, which demonstrates argyrophilic granules within the cytoplasm of the parathyroid cells, that are absent in the follicular thyroid cells.[63,64] Argyrophilic granules are present in medullary carcinoma of the thyroid, but cytologic discrimination is possible in routinely stained cytologic smears, prepared previously.[63]

Nevertheless the Grimelius method is time consuming and based on a comparative quantitative analysis. Hence, nowadays it has been replaced routinely by the highly accurate immunocytochemical stains for intracellular PTH,[58,65] using either specific anti-PTH antibodies or, more commonly, antibodies for neuroendocrine tissues.

When the aspirated material is sparsely cellular, the radioimmunologic PTH assay is routinely employed. The aspirated material is diluted in 1 ml saline and frozen, in order to maintain the stability of PTH;[66,67] two aspirates are usually taken from the suspected lesion. A reference aspirate for PTH can be taken from the ipsilateral thyroid lobe, in addition to a plasma sample obtained on the same occasion.[57,66] The PTH content of a parathyroid lesion is higher than that of the corresponding thyroid aspirate and the respective serum value. More commonly, two different radioimmunoassays are performed for each target, one for PTH and one for thyroglobulin (TG), assuming that PTH is specific for parathyroid tissue and TG for thyroid tissue.

Accuracy

From a review of the literature, cytology (146 cases reported between 1983 and 1992)[57–59,61,62–65,68,69] shows a sensitivity of 86.9%; of the false negatives, a few are due to an incorrect target, others to inadequate material, and yet others are due to incorrect diagnoses of thyroid tumors. These last errors[59,61,62] were observed in samples for which only routine stains for morphological evaluation had been used; such errors could have been avoided by the use of cytochemical or immunocytochemical methods. The specificity in the series considered is 100%; that is, there is no thyroid nodule wrongly interpreted as a pathologic parathyroid gland although in theory this possibility should not be excluded according to the previous remarks.

Conversely, the radioimmunologic PTH assay (in the 60 cases reported in the literature between 1983 and

1992)[12,56,57,66,67,70] shows a sensitivity of 96% (the false negatives probably caused by an incorrect target) with a specificity of 100%.

At present, immunocytochemistry of the aspirated cells and radioimmunologic PTH assay are preferred, whenever available, as they are almost completely diagnostically accurate, provided that the target is hit correctly.

Microhistology

The results (regarding both cytology and PTH assay) achieved with non-cutting needles do not justify the use of cutting needles for preparation of microhistologic samples;[71] these do not have a high degree of sensitivity owing to the dearth of material obtained (in 45% of cases): one reason appears to be the difficulty of obtaining tissue cores when dealing with cystic and/or necrotic tumors or tumors with a soft consistency.[71]

Indications

The procedure is almost without risks: in the literature one single case of transient hematoma has been described;[67] another patient, who experienced cervical discomfort and mild dysphagia for some days, was normocalcemic 6 months after aspiration (the therapeutic effect of FNAB was probably attributable to hemorrhagic necrosis of the adenoma).[56]

Nevertheless, FNAB is routinely performed only in patients with persistent or recurrent HPT who are candidates for re-operation or in patients with secondary HPT who are going to be treated by US-guided PEI.[72] The indications are greatly limited in primary HPT at the first diagnostic work-up: in the patients in whom surgery is scheduled, the procedure may be justified only in cases where there are atypical US data (e.g. suspicion of parathymic or intrathyroidal parathyroid glands);[67] FNAB is also recommended in the rare cases in which US-guided PEI is chosen instead of surgery,[73] as already described for secondary HPT.

OTHER IMAGING MODALITIES

Non-invasive imaging

The imaging modalities usually employed as alternatives to US are CT, MRI and scintigraphy. Like US, these modalities are not able to visualize the normal parathyroid glands; furthermore, the previous comments regarding the use of US for differentiation between adenomas, hyperplasias and carcinomas apply equally to US. Nevertheless CT, MRI and scintigraphy have the advantage of permitting exploration of both neck and mediastinum (Figs 6.27C, 6.28).

Computed tomography

The CT study must be performed with contiguous scans, 5 mm thick, between the hyoid bone and tracheal bifurcation.[74] Administration of intravenous contrast material is necessary in order to discriminate correctly between vascular structures and parathyroids, the latter appearing homogeneous or slightly inhomogeneous in density, less than that of the vascular structures and of the thyroid gland (Fig. 6.27). The thyroid is often separated from the parathyroids (in their typical location) by a thin fatty layer.[74–76] Sometimes, variations in density are apparent on CT, similar to the echo texture variants already mentioned for US. These variations are explicable in terms of the changes in the internal structure of the glands, such as

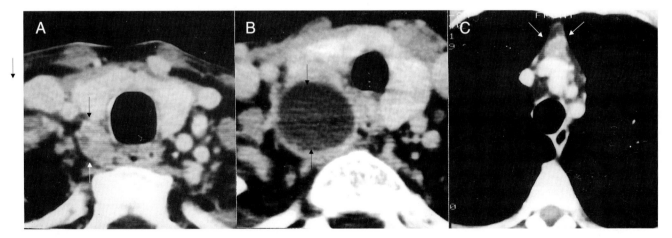

Fig. 6.27 Parathyroid glands: CT features. **A** Adenoma. The lesion (arrow), located behind the right lobe of the thyroid gland, presents (after intravenous administration of contrast material) a slightly inhomogeneous density, less than that of the neck blood vessels and of the thyroid, from which it is separated by a thin fatty plane. **B** Cystic carcinoma. The lesion (arrow), located behind the inferior pole of the right thyroidal lobe, is of low density with a peripheral rim of higher attenuation. **C** Mediastinal adenoma. The lesion (arrow) is in the anterior mediastinum, in front of the left innominate vein, close to its confluence with the right innominate vein.

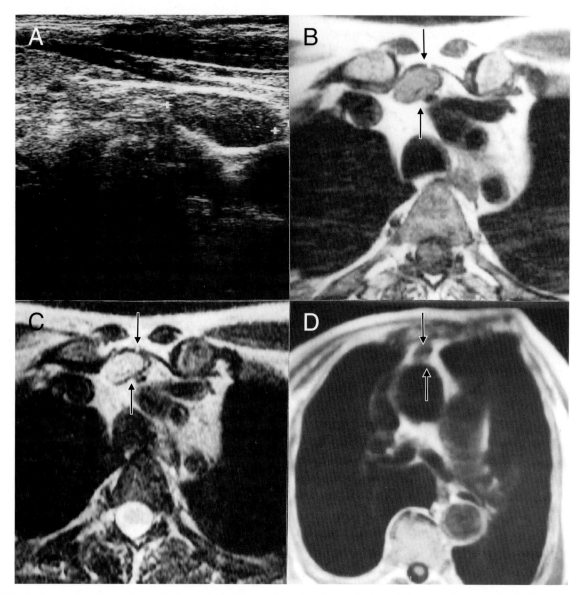

Fig. 6.28   Parathyroid glands: MR features. **A–C** Adenoma located at the cervicothoracic junction. **A** US longitudinal scan showing the hypoechoic tumor (+) located caudally to the lower thyroid pole. On MRI the lesion (arrow), located in front of the innominate veins, shows a fairly low signal intensity on the T_1-weighted image (**B**) and higher signal intensity on the T_2-weighted image (**C**). **D** Mediastinal adenoma: the lesion (arrow) is situated behind the sternum, in front of the ascending aorta (T_1-weighted image). (Courtesy of Dr A. Del Maschio, Milan.)

necrotic or hemorrhagic degeneration,[74] cystic adenomas or true cysts (Fig. 6.27B),[35] glandular calcifications,[36] or lipoadenomas.[77]

Magnetic resonance imaging

MRI is routinely performed with axial scans, 4–5 mm thick, each separated by a 0.5 mm gap.[78,79] If neck exploration proves negative, the mediastinum must be evaluated with particular care. Scans on additional planes (coronal and sagittal) may sometimes solve diagnostic problems that are not resolved by the preliminary axial scans.[80] At present, the intravenous administration of paramagnetic contrast material does not appear to increase significantly the potential of the modality; it has, therefore, to be suggested only in selected cases.[78]

It is appropriate to use T_1- and T_2-weighted sequences (the fast spin echo technique is now preferred to diminish motion artifacts),[81] since on the T_1-weighted images (allowing a better anatomic detail) pathologic glands often display a fairly low signal intensity, not very different from that of the thyroid gland. On the T_2-weighted images most lesions show a marked increase of the signal intensity compared with that of the thyroid gland (Figs 6.28, 6.29).[82,83]

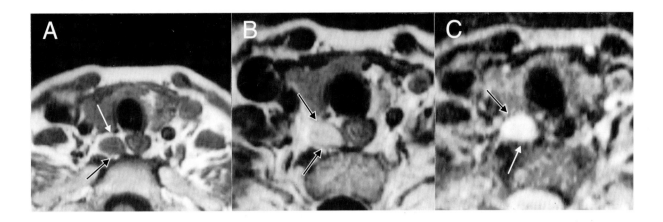

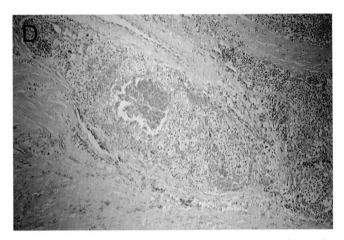

Fig. 6.29 Parathyroid glands: MRI features. Adenoma located behind the right thyroidal lobe. On the T_1-weighted image (**A**) the lesion (arrow) has a fairly low signal intensity, not very different from that of the thyroid gland. Following intravenous administration of gadolinium–diethylene-triaminepentaacetic acid (DTPA) (**B**) the tumor shows considerable enhancement on the T_1-weighted image. On the T_2-weighted image (**C**) the lesion demonstrates a high signal intensity. This behaviour on MRI is due to a high degree of cellularity and sinusoidal dilatation of the glands (see the histological specimen in **D**). (Courtesy of Dr A. Giovagnoni, Ancona.)

However, this behaviour is not constant: sometimes the signal intensity is fairly low on both T_1- and T_2-weighted images, probably because of acute intralesional hemorrhage and/or degenerative fatty changes (Fig. 6.30). However, to date these different patterns have not been explained convincingly in all cases.[84,85]

Scintigraphy

Scintigraphy is performed using a double isotope, thallium (^{201}Tl) and technetium, using a subtraction technique;[86,87] recently, [^{99m}Tc] methoxyisobutylisonitrile ([^{99m}Tc]MIBI) – which involves greater energy (140 keV compared with 80 keV for ^{201}Tl) – has been proposed as an alternative to ^{201}Tl.[88,89] It is recommended that the patient is injected in sequence with first ^{201}Tl (or [^{99m}Tc]MIBI) and then technetium. ^{201}Tl (or [^{99m}Tc]MIBI) is in fact concentrated in both thyroid and parathyroid glands, whereas technetium is concentrated in the thyroid gland only; using computerized subtraction of the two images, only the hyperfunctioning parathyroids remain visible (Figs 6.31, 6.32).[90] The uptake of ^{201}Tl and MIBI is mainly affected by the cellularity of the lesion; thus, highly cellular nodules of the thyroid gland can also show increased uptake of these radioisotopes and mimic the behaviour of the parathyroid glands.[90]

Subtraction scintigraphy with [^{99m}Tc]sestamibi and ^{123}I has been introduced fairly recently: it seems to provide a significantly greater degree of sensitivity in the detection of both normally located and ectopic glands.

Diagnostic potential of non-invasive imaging

CT, MRI and scintigraphy are not more reliable than US in the detection of glands in their normal location – in fact, US can sometimes be superior. On the other hand, they are more sensitive for the study of glands in an atypical location (for example retrotracheal, retroesophageal and, in particular, mediastinal glands); with regard to the mediastinum, MRI is currently the most sensitive non-invasive modality.[91]

The three modalities have limits similar to those of US in the detection of small lesions, of multifocal lesions, and of lesions associated with thyroid goiter.[51,76,80,83,85,92–94]

Review of the literature[52–54] in patients with a 'virgin neck' (i.e. without previous surgery) reveals that *sensitivity* values (Fig. 6.33) are not very different among the various modalities (CT: 63–78%, mean 71%; scintigraphy: 55–

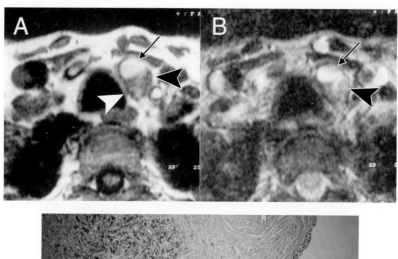

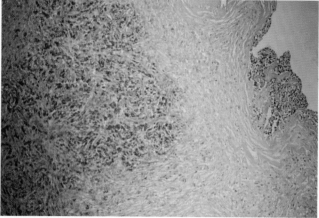

Fig. 6.30 Parathyroid glands: MRI features. Spin echo T_1-weighted (**A**) and T_2-weighted (**B**) images of parathyroid adenoma. The lesion shows hyperintensity in the anterior portion (arrow) on both T_1 and T_2 images, due to acute hemorrhage (see the histological specimen in **C**) and/or fatty changes, whereas in the posterior portion it is low in signal intensity (arrowhead) because of the presence of fibrosis. (Courtesy of Dr A. Giovagnoni, Ancona.)

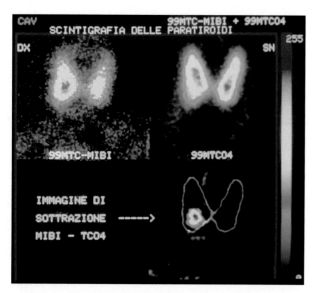

Fig. 6.31 Parathyroid glands: scintigraphy. Adenoma situated at the lower pole of the right thyroid lobe ([99mTc]MIBI–technetium subtraction scanning). The lesion is clearly demonstrated only after subtraction of the two previous images.

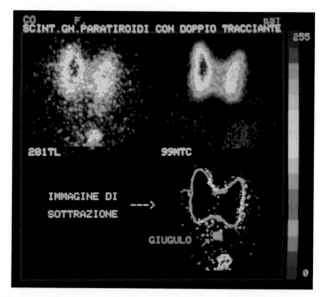

Fig. 6.32 Mediastinal adenoma (thallium–technetium subtraction scanning). In this case the subtraction technique is not necessary to demonstrate the lesion, already identified after 201Tl administration (top left).

IMAGING SENSITIVITY

NON OPERATED PATIENTS

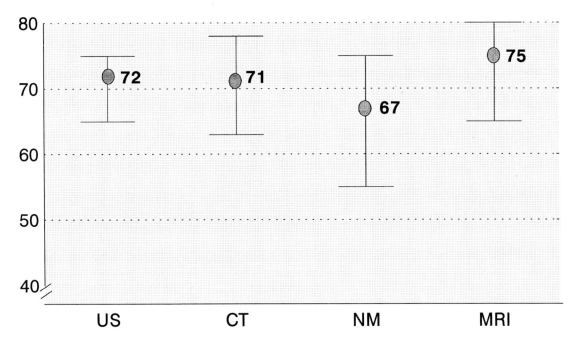

Fig. 6.33 Ranges and mean values of sensitivity of ultrasound (US), computed tomography (CT), scintigraphy (NM) and magnetic resonance imaging (MRI) in the detection of parathyroid lesions in non-operated patients.

75%, mean 67%; MRI: 65–80%, mean 75%). These values are not very different from those of US.

In patients who have previously undergone surgery,[53,54,95] a decrease in sensitivity (Fig. 6.34) can be recognized, similar to that observed with US (CT: 47–57%, mean 53%; scintigraphy: 49–60%, mean 55%; MRI: 66–74%, mean 70%). Moreover, it should be noted that in this group of patients the loss of sensitivity for MRI is about 5% (from 75 to 70%), but ranges between 12 and 18% for US, CT and scintigraphy. MRI is in fact less impaired by scar tissue from previous surgery, because of its superb contrast resolution;[95] furthermore, MRI is more reliable in the detection of lesions situated mediastinally.[91]

With regard to the *specificity*, CT, MRI and scintigraphy are almost identical to US, presenting the same limits: pathologic cervical nodes and, in particular, thyroidal nodules may mimic pathologic parathyroid glands, thus causing false positives.[46,54,85,94,96–98]

Invasive imaging

The angiographic techniques (selective arteriography, selective venous sampling)[99] are currently used only in selected cases, when non-invasive modalities fail. The venous approach must be preceded by the arterial approach: indeed, arteriography, even if negative, provides a detailed map of the venous system, which facilitates sampling and correct interpretation of the PTH profile, bearing in mind the anatomic variability of the veins as well as the changes often induced by previous surgery.[99,100] The combined use of arteriography and venous sampling permits location of 80–85% of the glandular lesions.[53,100]

CLINICAL USE OF IMAGING MODALITIES

Secondary hyperparathyroidism

Imaging modalities in secondary HPT are of very limited use[85] in those patients destined for both medical and surgical treatment: indeed, both subtotal parathyroidectomy and total parathyroidectomy with autotransplantation gain only minimal advantages from imaging modalities that are rarely able to demonstrate all the hyperplastic glands. However, US is necessary in those cases in which PEI (as an adjunct to medical treatment) is scheduled:[72] initial location of the lesions is necessary, perhaps in conjunction with FNAB, in order to confirm that the lesions identified involve the parathyroid glands.

IMAGING SENSITIVITY

PERSISTENT OR RECURRENT HYPERPARATHYROIDISM

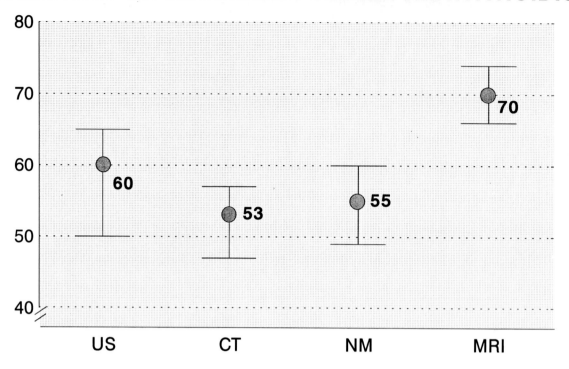

Fig. 6.34 Ranges and mean values of sensitivity of US, CT, NM and MRI in the detection of parathyroid lesions in patients with persistent or recurrent hyperparathyroidism following surgery.

Primary hyperparathyroidism

In patients with no previous surgery, imaging modalities are useful but not mandatory; in fact, the sensitivity of the different modalities ranges between 67 and 75% (Fig. 6.33), whereas surgical exploration not guided by imaging is successful, in experienced hands, in 90–95% of cases.[2,11,101,102] A few recent studies have demonstrated, moreover, that preliminary assessment by imaging neither simplifies surgery nor reduces operating time significantly.[52,103]

The only examination to be used routinely is US,[85] owing to its low cost and fairly good diagnostic reliability. The other imaging modalities are not recommended, because of their poor cost–benefit ratio, except in two unusual circumstances:[104] for those patients with previous thyroid surgery (who have to be considered in the same way as those who have undergone surgery for HPT), and those patients with severe hypercalcemic crises in whom the risk of persistent symptoms due to unsuccessful surgery may be unacceptable, thus justifying several attempts to locate lesions before operation.

Persistent or recurrent hyperparathyroidism

In persistent or recurrent HPT surgical exploration is difficult, owing to postoperative fibrosis and to the greater incidence of ectopic glands. Without the information provided by imaging modalities its success rate is lower than that reported for the initial surgery;[105] furthermore, there is also an increasing rate of complications such as hypocalcemia and injury to the recurrent laryngeal nerve.[104] Preliminary pinpointing of the glands facilitates re-operation, increasing its positive outcome to over 90%.[2,11,23,101]

In the diagnostic work-up, US is scheduled as first examination, complemented by FNAB in doubtful cases and followed by the other non-invasive imaging modalities. Of the latter, MRI is more reliable than either CT or scintigraphy (Fig. 6.34). Should the diagnostic problem not be solved, the use of angiographic techniques is still advisable.

INTERVENTIONAL PROCEDURES: PERCUTANEOUS ETHANOL INJECTION (PEI)

PEI in secondary hyperparathyroidism

The pharmacological treatment of secondary hyper-

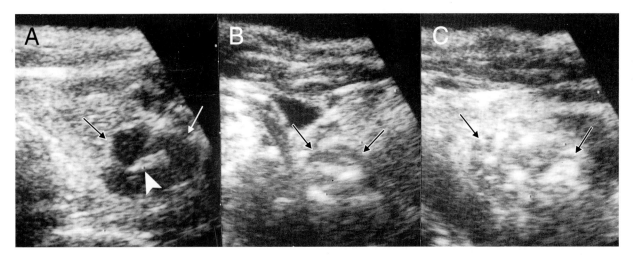

Fig. 6.35   PEI of parathyroid hyperplasia (arrow). **A** The needle tip is visible (arrowhead) in the center of the lesion. **B** During the injection the gland increases its echogenicity (arrow) and at the end of the procedure (**C**) it is somewhat enlarged and hyperechoic (arrow).

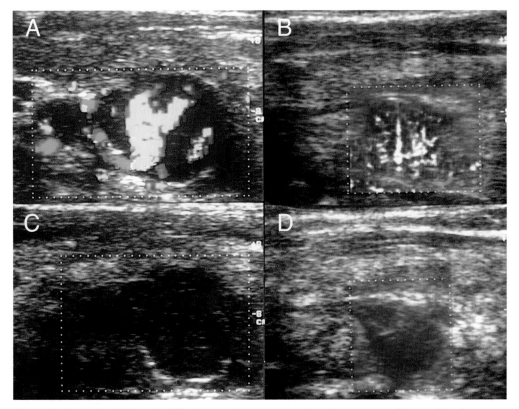

Fig. 6.36   Immediately following PEI, drastic reduction or complete disappearance of intranodular flow signals is featured, both with color Doppler (**A**, **B**) and with power Doppler (**C**, **D**).

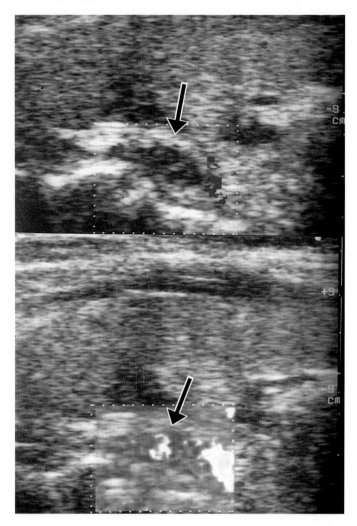

Fig. 6.37 Following three PEI procedures, the parathyroid hyperplasia (arrow) does not display remaining blood flow signals with conventional frequency-based color Doppler (top), whereas power Doppler (bottom) shows persistent signals throughout the gland.

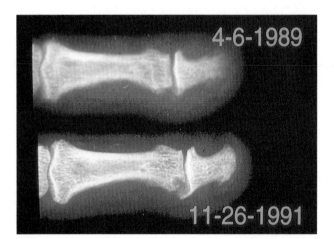

Fig. 6.38 Partial restoration of bony structure of fingers 2 years after PEI treatment.

parathyroidism (SHPT) usually includes administration of phosphate binders, active vitamin D sterols and, more importantly, calcitriol pulse therapy, which can suppress PTH hypersecretion.[106] In patients refractory to medical therapy and with severe progression of osteitis fibrosa, surgery is mandatory, consisting of either subtotal parathyroidectomy or total parathyroidectomy with auto-transplantation of parathyroid tissue fragments.

Resistance of SHPT to calcitriol therapy occurs in severe SHPT and is probably due to the reduction in numbers of calcitriol receptors:[107] this occurs mostly in large parathyroid glands, which display nodular hyperplasia, a higher rate of cell proliferation[108] and a higher rate of recurrence of SHPT when they are autotransplanted. Injection of ethanol into these glands reduces the parathyroid mass and restores the response to calcitriol therapy.

PEI of the parathyroid glands was first introduced by our group in 1985[109] and has subsequently been performed in many centers in the world.[110–112] PEI is indicated in patients presenting no more than two enlarged glands, neither exceeding 2–2.5 cm in maximum diameter. Where there are three or four larger glands surgery is mandatory.

Sterile 95% ethanol is injected percutaneously using either 22 G non-cutting spinal needles or, more recently,

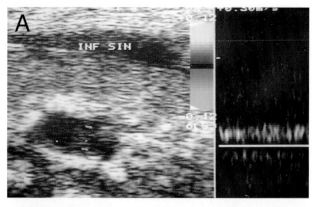

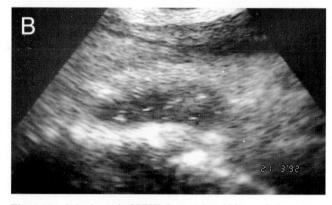

Fig. 6.39 **A** At the end of PEIT the parathyroid hyperplasia (recurrence) appears to be completely avascular. **B** 14 months later, the gland becomes newly hyperfunctional and intranodular flow signals reappear.

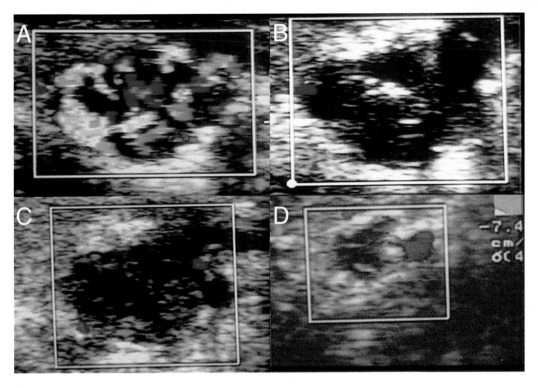

Fig. 6.40 Successful PEIT of large parathyroid hyperplasia: from **A** to **D** the progressive decrease in vascularization and size is clearly seen.

21 G needles with a closed conical tip and three small sideholes within 3.5 mm of the tip (PEIT needle, Hakko, Japan). Injections are performed slowly, with the patient lying supine with his neck hyperextended on a pillow. The amount of ethanol to be injected during each session ranges from 70 to 100% of the calculated gland volume, care being taken to avoid needle 'overpenetration' which could cause posterior leakage of ethanol around the recurrent laryngeal nerve. The number of PEI sessions for each patient is variable, depending on serum PTH levels, the initial size of the target, and the structural and vascular changes induced by ethanol.

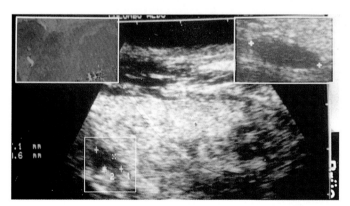

Fig. 6.41 On 5-year follow-up the PEI-treated gland (small box) remains appreciably smaller (5 mm) than before PEI (top right box). FNAB reveals only fibrotic changes (top left box).

US guidance is obtained with 7.5–13 MHz small-parts mechanical annular probes or 7.5 MHz intraoperative linear probes with lateral biopsy adaptors or 3.5 MHz convex probes with central biopsy canal for a perpendicular approach. The former are preferred for small, superficial targets, the latter (3.5 MHz) for large deep glands. PEI can easily be monitored by US because of the abrupt increase in volume and echogenicity (due to air microbubbles mixed with ethanol) of the glands (Fig. 6.35) and the rapid disappearance of the intranodular flow signals with color Doppler (Fig. 6.36). Color Doppler or, preferably, power Doppler (a better indicator of parenchymal perfusion) permits detection of those intranodular areas with persistent blood flow signals, i.e. those areas still functioning (Fig. 6.37), and guidance of further injections into these areas. In such cases PEI is terminated only when flow signals are no longer detectable in the target.

The serum levels of PTH are the best indicators of the efficacy of PEI: in successful cases PTH starts to decrease 7–15 days following the first injection. When the serum levels have decreased significantly, conventional medical therapy can be restarted. Simultaneously, serum levels of calcium and bone alkaline phosphatase also progressively decrease, followed by remission of the radiological signs of osteitis fibrosa and restoration of normal bony structure in 60–70% of cases (Fig. 6.38).[113]

Recurrences following PEI may occur due to parathyroid tissue proliferation within the fibrotic remnant of the previously treated gland (usually assessable with color Doppler) (Fig. 6.39) or to the development of a new hyperplastic gland on follow-up studies (in approximately 30% of cases).[110,113,114] If the latter occurs, additional ethanol should be injected into the new targets, according to the same protocol.

Different rates of good clinical results are achievable in patients with no history of parathyroid surgery and in subjects with previous parathyroidectomy. In the former group, on a mean 2-year follow-up complete remission of SHPT (decrease in PTH levels by more than 50% of the initial values) is achieved in 35–40% of patients and significant reduction of SHPT (PTH decrease between 30 and 50%) in 60% of cases.[113] Even better results have been reported in other studies.[112] In previously operated patients, complete remission is observed in 72% of cases and partial remission in 81%, over the same follow-up period.[114] This marked discrepancy between results in the two groups of subjects is probably due to the presence of functioning parathyroid tissue in different locations, that is undetectable by imaging methods. In fact, the effects of PEI on the treated glands do not differ in the two groups: there is a considerable reduction in the sonographically assessed gland volume (from 0.88 ± 0.56 ml to 0.26 ± 0.22 ml) of all the lesions (Fig. 6.40)[113,114] and in most cases this 'shrinkage' is permanent (Fig. 6.41).

With regard to side effects, moderate and rapidly disappearing local pain during the injections is usually reported. In 5–10% of patients, transient unilateral vocal cord paralysis has been reported,[109–113] lasting 7–90 days, but always with complete spontaneous remission. Vocal cord paralysis is probably due to functional damage to the laryngeal recurrent nerve, caused either by simple compression by the 'swollen' gland after injection or (most likely) by diffusion of ethanol to periglandular tissues. Even though these events are not totally unavoidable, in our personal experience the rate of occurrence can be drastically reduced by avoiding needle overpenetration into the target before injecting ethanol, by employing needles with sideholes and by reducing the amount of ethanol for each treatment.

US-guided PEI, originally developed as an adjunct to medical therapy for the treatment of low-grade SHPT, is currently considered to be the therapy of choice in SHPT recurrence after surgery, and is a useful strategy for control of SHPT in non-operated uremic patients, by reducing the calcitriol-resistant parathyroid cell mass. Where PEI is unsuccessful and patients subsequently undergo surgery, the ethanol-induced fibrotic changes in the neck tissues can complicate surgical exploration: however, easier identification of partially fibrotic glands can be achieved by color Doppler.

PEI in primary hyperparathyroidism

Surgery is generally considered to be the therapy of choice in primary hyperparathyroidism (PHPT), being radical and conclusive in most cases. However, PEI can be a useful alternative to surgery in selected cases, such as when there are acute severe hypercalcemic symptoms, high surgical risk and refusal of surgery.[115,116]

The treatment schedule is the same as that described above for SHPT. According to the limited series reported in the literature, complete remission (normocalcemia and normal serum levels of PTH) is achievable in 55–65% of patients; partial remission (slightly elevated PTH levels)

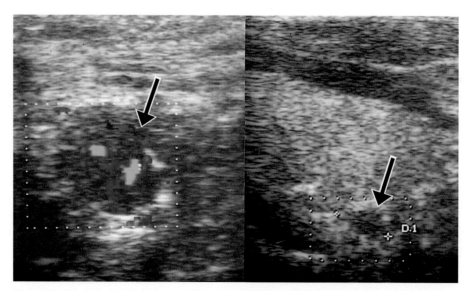

Fig. 6.42 Parathyroid adenoma (2 cm) in primary HPT (arrow) successfully treated with PEI.

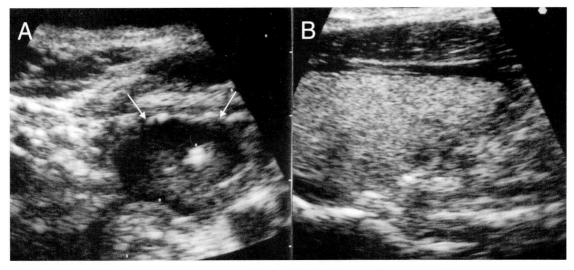

Fig. 6.43A Parathyroid cyst (arrow) treated with PEI; **B** complete disappearance of cyst 15 months later.

can be achieved in a further 10–25% of cases (Fig. 6.42).[116,117]

Unilateral vocal cord paralysis is the only significant side effect reported, accounting for 7–15% of patients and always transient, apart from two cases of patients in whom it was permanent.[116,117]

Even parathyroid cysts can be successfully treated with PEI: following near-total needle aspiration of the fluid content, ethanol is injected in an amount corresponding to 30–35% of the volume of fluid aspirated and is generally re-aspirated within 1–2 days. This procedure can be repeated in two or three sessions, with a final success rate of 100% (Fig. 6.43).

REFERENCES

1. Wang C A 1976 The anatomic basis of parathyroid surgery. Ann Surg 183: 271–275
2. Kaplan E L, Yashiro T, Salti G 1992 Primary hyperparathyroidism in the 1990s. Choice of surgical procedures for this disease. Ann Surg 215: 300–317
3. Akerström G, Malmaeus J, Bergström R 1984 Surgical anatomy of human parathyroid glands. Surgery 95: 14–21
4. Sarfati E, De Ferron P, Gossot D, Assens P, Dubost C 1987 Adénomes parathyroïdiens de sièges inhabituels, ectopiques ou non. J Chir (Paris) 124: 24–29
5. Hooghe L, Kinnaert P, Van Geertruyden J 1992 Surgical anatomy of hyperparathyroidism. Acta Chir Belg 92: 1–9
6. Thompson N W, Eckhauser F E, Harness J K 1982 The anatomy of primary hyperparathyroidism. Surgery 92: 814–821
7. Wang C A, Gaz R D, Moncure A C 1986 Mediastinal parathyroid exploration: a clinical and pathologic study of 47 cases. World J Surg 10: 687–695
8. Dubost C, Lecharpentier Y, Bouteloup P Y 1984 Chirurgie des glandes parathyroïdes. Traitement de l'hyperparathyroïdie. Encycl Med Chir Techniques chirurgicales, Thorax. Editions Techniques, Paris. 42070, 4.10.06.
9. Dubost C, Bouteloup P Y 1988 Explorations médiastinales par sternotomie dans la chirurgie de l'hyperparathyroïdie. J. Chir (Paris) 125: 631–637
10. Scholtz D A, Purnell D C, Woolner L B, Clagett O T 1973 Mediastinal hyperfunctioning parathyroid tumors: review of 14 cases. Ann Surg 178: 173–178
11. Duh Q Y, Sancho J J, Clark O H 1987 Parathyroid localization. Acta Chir Scand 153: 241–254
12. Silverman J F, Khazanie P G, Norris H T, Fore W W 1986 Parathyroid hormone (PTH) assay of parathyroid cysts examined by fine-needle aspiration biopsy. Am J Clin Pathol 86: 776–780
13. Uden P, Berglund J, Zederfeldt B, Aspelin P, Ljungberg O 1987 Parathyroid lipoadenoma: a rare cause of primary hyperparathyroidism. Case report. Acta Chir Scand 153: 635–639
14. Bruining H A 1983 Operative strategy for primary hyperparathyroidism. In Kaplan E L (ed) Surgery of the thyroid and parathyroid glands. Churchill Livingstone, Edinburgh, pp 158–167
15. Kay S, Hume D M 1973 Carcinoma of the parathyroid gland: how reliable are the clinical and histological features? Arch Pathol 96: 316–319
16. McKeown P, McGarity W C, Sewell C W 1984 Carcinoma of the parathyroid gland: is it overdiagnosed? A report of three cases. Am J Surg 147: 292–298
17. Jacobi J M, Lloyd H M, Smith J F 1986 Nuclear diameter in parathyroid carcinomas. J Clin Pathol 39: 1353–1354
18. Smith J F, Coombs R R H 1984 Histological diagnosis of carcinoma of the parathyroid gland. J Clin Pathol 37: 1370–1378
19. Fujimoto Y, Obara T, Ito Y, Kanazawa K, Aiyoshi Y, Nobori M 1984 Surgical treatment of ten cases of parathyroid carcinoma: importance of an initial en bloc tumor resection. World J Surg 8: 392–400
20. Schantz A, Castleman B 1973 Parathyroid carcinoma: a study of 70 cases. Cancer 31: 600–605
21. Muller H 1975 True recurrence of hyperparathyroidism: proposed criteria of recurrence. Br J Surg 62: 556–559
22. Dubost C, D'Acremont B, Gossot D, Sarfati E 1990 Vicissitudes de la chirurgie de l'hyperparathyroïdie primaire. Presse Méd 19: 21–25
23. Levin K E, Clark O H 1989 The reasons for failure in parathyroid operations. Arch Surg 124: 911–915
24. Cheung P S Y, Borgstrom A, Thompson N W 1989 Strategy in reoperative surgery for hyperparathyroidism. Arch Surg 124: 676–680
25. Fitko R, Roth S I, Hines J R, Roxe D M, Cahill E 1990 Para-

thyromatosis in hyperparathyroidism. Hum Pathol 21: 234–237

26. Reddick R L, Costa J C, Marx S J 1977 Parathyroid hyperplasia and parathyromatosis. Lancet 1: 549

27. Brunt L M, Sicard G A 1990 Current status of parathyroid auto-transplantation. Semin Surg Oncol 6: 115–121

28. Solbiati L, Pravettoni G, Ierace T 1993 Collo In: SIUMB (ed) Trattato Italiano di Ecografia, Vol. 1, Poletto Edizioni, Milan, pp 80–115

29. Gooding G A W 1993 Sonography of the thyroid and parathyroid. Radiol Clin North Am 31: 967–989

30. Reading C C 1991 The parathyroid. In: Rumack C M, Wilson S R, Charboneau J W (eds) Diagnostic ultrasound. Mosby, St Louis, pp 524–539

31. Simeone J F, Mueller P R, Ferrucci J T Jr et al 1981 High-resolution real-time sonography of the parathyroid. Radiology 141: 745–751

32. Reading C C, Charboneau W J, James E M et al 1982 High resolution parathyroid sonography. AJR 139: 539–546

33. Graif M, Itzchak Y, Strauss S, Dolev E, Mohr R, Wolfstein I 1987 Parathyroid sonography: diagnostic accuracy related to shape, location and texture of the gland. Br J Radiol 60: 439–443

34. Randel S B, Gooding G A W, Clark O H, Stein R M, Winkler B 1987 Parathyroid variants: US evaluation. Radiology 165: 191–194

35. Krudy A G, Doppman J L, Shawker T H et al 1984 Hyperfunctioning cystic parathyroid glands: CT and sonographic findings. AJR 142: 175–178

36. Lineweaver W, Clore F, Mancuso A, Hill S, Rumley T 1984 Calcified parathyroid glands detected by Computed Tomography. J Comput Assist Tomogr 8: 975–977

37. Obara T, Fujimoto Y, Ito Y et al 1989 Functioning parathyroid lipoadenoma: report of four cases. Clinicopathological and ultrasonographic features. Endocrinol Jpn 36: 135–139

38. Edmonson G R, Charboneau J W, James E M, Reading C C, Grant C S 1986 Parathyroid carcinoma: high-frequency sonographic features. Radiology 161: 65–67

39. Daly B D, Coffey S L, Behan M 1989 Ultrasonographic appearances of parathyroid carcinoma. Br J Radiol 62: 1017–1019

40. Solbiati L, Rizzatto G, Ballarati E, Ierace T, Crespi L 1993 Practical implications of Color Doppler Sonography of parathyroid glands: study of 203 tumors. Radiology 189 (P): 210

41. Solbiati L, Cioffi V, Ballarati E 1992 Ultrasonography of the neck. Radiol Clin North Am 30: 941–954

42. Calliada F, Sala G, Conti M P et al 1993 Applicazioni cliniche del color-Doppler: le ghiandole paratiroidi. Radiol Med 85 (suppl 1): pp 114–119

43. Doppman J L, Shawker T H, Krudy A G et al 1985 Parathymic parathyroid: CT, US and angiographic findings. Radiology 157: 419–423

44. Fraker D L, Doppman J L, Shawker T H, Marx S J, Spiegel A M, Norton J A 1990 Undescended parathyroid adenoma: an important etiology for failed operations for primary hyperparathyroidism. World J Surg 14: 342–348

45. Edis A J, Purnell D C, Van Heerden J H 1979 The undescended 'parathymus': an occasional cause of failed neck exploration for hyperparathyroidism. Ann Surg 190: 64–68

46. Funari M, Campos Z, Gooding G A W, Higgins C B 1992 MRI and ultrasound detection of asymptomatic thyroid nodules in hyperparathyroidism. J Comput Assist Tomogr 16: 615–619

47. Karstrup S, Hegedüs L 1986 Concomitant thyroid disease in hyperparathyroidism. Reasons for unsatisfactory ultrasonographical localization of parathyroid glands. Eur J Radiol 6: 149–152

48. Henry J F, Audiffret J, Denizot A et al 1990 Endosonography in the localization of parathyroid tumors: a preliminary study. Surgery 108: 1021–1025

49. Takebayashi S, Matsui K, Nozawa T, Fujioka E, Hidai H Hyperplasia of autotransplanted parathyroid in the forearm. Clin Nucl Med 15: 354–355

50. Winkelbauer F, Ammann M E, Längle F, Niederle B 1993 Diagnosis of hyperparathyroidism with US after autotransplantation: results of a prospective study. Radiology 186: 255–257

51. Stark D D, Gooding G A W, Moss A A, Clark O H, Ovenfors C O 1983 Parathyroid imaging: comparison of high-resolution CT and high-resolution sonography. AJR 141: 633–638

52. Doppman J L, Miller D L 1991 Localization of parathyroid tumors in patients with asymptomatic hyperparathyroidism and no previous surgery. J Bone Miner Res 6 (suppl 2): pp 153–159

53. Eisenberg H, Pallotta J, Sacks B, Brickman A S 1989 Parathyroid localization, three-dimensional modeling, and percutaneous ablation techniques. Endocrinol Metab Clin North Am 18: 659–700

54. Higgins C B, Auffermann W 1988 MR imaging of thyroid and parathyroid glands: a review of current status. AJR 151: 1095–1106

55. Fugazzola C, Solbiati L, Bergamo Andreis I A 1993 Parathyroid imaging with ultrasonography (US) and computed tomography (CT). Eur Radiol 3 (suppl): p 232

56. Doppman J L, Krudy A G, Marx S J et al 1983 Aspiration of enlarged parathyroid glands for parathyroid hormone assay. Radiology 148: 31–35

57. Karstrup S, Glenth J A, Torp-Pedersen S, Hegedüs L, Holm H H 1988 Ultrasonically guided fine needle aspiration of suggested enlarged parathyroid glands. Acta Radiol 29: 213–216

58. Sardi A, Bolton J S, Mitchell W T Jr, Merritt C R B 1992 Immunoperoxidase confirmation of ultrasonically guided fine needle aspirates in patients with recurrent hyperparathyroidism. Surg Gynecol Obstet 175: 563–568

59. Layfield L J 1991 Fine needle aspiration cytology of cystic parathyroid lesions. A cytomorphologic overlap with cystic lesions of the thyroid. Acta Cytol 35: 447–450

60. Löwhagen T, Sprenger E 1974 Cytologic presentation of thyroid tumors in aspiration biopsy smear. A review of 60 cases. Acta Cytol 18: 192–197

61. Mincione G P, Borrelli D, Cicchi P, Ipponi P L, Fiorini A 1986 Fine needle aspiration cytology of parathyroid adenoma. A review of seven cases. Acta Cytol 30: 65–69

62. Friedman M, Shimaoka K, Lopez C A, Shedd D P 1983 Parathyroid adenoma diagnosed as papillary carcinoma of thyroid on needle aspiration smears. Acta Cytol 27: 337–340

63. Halbauer M, Crepinko I, Tomic Brzac H, Simonovic I 1991 Fine needle aspiration cytology in the preoperative diagnosis of ultrasonically enlarged parathyroid glands. Acta Cytol 35: 728–735

64. Rastad J, Johansson H, Lindgren P G, Ljunghall S, Stenkvist B, Åkerström G 1984 Ultrasonic localization and cytologic identification of parathyroid tumors. World J Surg 8: 501–508

65. Gutekunst R, Valesky A, Borish B et al 1986 Parathyroid localization. J Clin Endocrinol Metab 63: 1390–1393

66. Bergenfelz A, Forsberg L, Hederström E, Ahrén B 1991 Preoperative localization of enlarged parathyroid glands with ultrasonically guided fine needle aspiration for parathyroid hormone assay. Acta Radiol 32: 403–405

67. Mäkäräinen H, Raija T, Matti V K, Pasi S 1992 Cervical ultrasound combined with parathyroid hormone assay prior to parathyroid exploration. Eur Radiol 2: 194–198

68. Verbanck J, Clarysse J, Loncke R, Segaert M, Van Aelst P, Theunynck P 1986 Parathyroid aspiration biopsy under ultrasonographic guidance. Arch Otolaryngol Head Neck Surg 112: 1069–1073

69. Gooding G A W, Clark O H, Stark D D, Moss A A, Montgomery C K 1985 Parathyroid aspiration biopsy under ultrasound guidance in the postoperative hyperparathyroid patient. Radiology 155: 193–196

70. Prinz R A, Peters J R, Kane J M, Wood J 1990 Needle aspiration of nonfunctioning parathyroid cysts. Am Surg 56: 420–422

71. Karstrup S, Glenth J A, Hainau B, Hegedüs L, Torp-Pedersen S, Holm H H 1989 Ultrasound-guided, histological, fine-needle biopsy from suspect parathyroid tumours: success-rate and reliability of histological diagnosis. Br J Radiol 62: 981–985

72. Giangrande A, Castiglioni A, Solbiati L, Allaria P 1992 Ultrasound-guided percutaneous fine-needle ethanol injection into parathyroid glands in secondary hyperparathyroidism. Nephrol Dial Transplant 7: 412–421

73. Karstrup S, Holm H H, Glenth J A, Hegedüs L 1990 Nonsurgical treatment of primary hyperparathyroidism with sonographically

guided percutaneous injection of ethanol: results in a selected series of patients. AJR 154: 1087–1090

74. Cates J D, Thorsen M K, Lawson T L et al 1988 CT evaluation of parathyroid adenomas: diagnostic criteria and pitfalls. J Comput Assist Tomogr 12: 626–629

75. Belin X, Cyna-Gorse F, Lacombe P et al 1993 Imagerie de l'hyperparathyroïdie primaire. Encycl Med Chir, Radiodiagnostic Coeur-Poumon. Editions Techniques, Paris. 32–700-G-10. Paris

76. Sommer B, Welter H F, Spelsberg F, Scherer U, Lissner J 1982 Computed tomography for localizing enlarged parathyroid glands in primary hyperparathyroidism. J Comput Assist Tomogr 6: 521–526

77. Frennby B, Nyman U, Aspelin P, Udén P, Ljungberg O 1993 CT of a parathyroid lipoadenoma. Acta Radiol 34: 369–371

78. Seelos K C, De Marco R, Clark O H, Higgins C B 1990 Persistent and recurrent hyperparathyroidism: assessment with gadopentetate dimeglumine-enhanced MR imaging. Radiology 177: 373–378

79. Von Schulthess G K, Weder W, Goebel N, Buchmann P, Gadze A, Augustiny N, Largiad R F 1988 1.5T MRI, CT, ultrasonography and scintigraphy in hyperparathyroidism. Eur J Radiol 8: 157–164

80. Spritzer C E, Gefter W B, Hamilton R, Greenberg B M, Axel L, Kressel H Y 1987 Abnormal parathyroid glands: high-resolution MR imaging. Radiology 162: 487–491

81. Higgins C B 1993 Role of magnetic resonance imaging in hyperparathyroidism. Radiol Clin North Am 31: 1017–1028

82. Auffermann W, Gooding G A W, Okerlund M D et al 1988 Diagnosis of recurrent hyperparathyroidism: comparison of MR imaging and other imaging techniques. AJR 150: 1027–1033

83. Kier R, Blinder R A, Herfkens R J, Leight G S, Spritzer C E, Carroll B A 1987 MR imaging with surface coils in primary hyperparathyroidism. J Comput Assist Tomogr 11: 863–868

84. Auffermann W, Guis M, Tavares N J, Clark O H, Higgins C B 1989 MR signal intensity of parathyroid adenomas: correlation with histopathology. AJR 153: 873–876

85. Von Schulthess G K, Baumann R, Weder W, Duewell S 1993 MRI, CT, sonography and thallium–technetium subtraction scintigraphy for the detection of parathyroid disease: a four-year experience. Eur Radiol 3: 71–76

86. Ferlin G, Borsato N, Camerani M, Conte N, Zotti D 1983 New perspectives in localizing enlarged parathyroids by technetium–thallium subtraction scan. J Nucl Med 24: 438–441

87. Okerlund M D, Sheldon K, Corpuz S et al 1984 A new method with high sensitivity and specificity for localization of abnormal parathyroid glands. Ann Surg 200: 381–388

88. Coakley A J, Kettle A G, Wells C P, O'Doherty M J, Collins R E C 1989 99Tcm sestamibi – a new agent for parathyroid imaging. Nucl Med Commun 10: 791–794

89. O'Doherty M J, Kettle A G, Wells P, Collins R E C, Coakley A J 1992 Parathyroid imaging with technetium-99m-sestamibi: preoperative localization and tissue uptake studies. J Nucl Med 33: 313–318

90. Kim D Y, Fine E J, Silver C E 1987 Preoperative localization of lesions of the parathyroid gland using thallium–technetium scintiscanning. Surg Gynecol Obstet 165: 212–216

91. Kang Y S, Rosen K, Clark O H, Higgins C B 1993 Localization of abnormal parathyroid glands of the mediastinum with MR imaging. Radiology 189: 137–141

92. Drouillard J, Philippe J C, Érésué J et al 1983 Place de la scanographie dans le diagnostic des adénomes parathyroïdiens. A propos de 27 cas. J Radiol 64: 381–390

93. Hauty M, Swartz K, McClung M, Lowe D K 1987 Technetium–thallium scintiscanning for localization of parathyroid adenomas and hyperplasia. A reappraisal. Am J Surg 153: 479–486

94. Price D C 1993 Radioisotopic evaluation of the thyroid and the parathyroids. Radiol Clin North Am 31: 991–1015

95. Stevens S K, Chang J M, Clark O H, Chang P J, Higgins C B 1993 Detection of abnormal parathyroid glands in postoperative patients with recurrent hyperparathyroidism: sensitivity of MR imaging. AJR 160: 607–612

96. Stark D D, Gooding G A W, Clark O H 1985 Noninvasive parathyroid imaging. Semin Ultrasound CT MR, 6: 310–320

97. Fugazzola C, Caudana R, Franco F, Morana G, Semeraro M V 1992 Contributo diagnostico della tomografia computerizzata e della risonanza magnetica nell' iperparatiroidismo. In: Rovelli E, Samori G (eds) L' iperparatiroidismo primitivo e secondario. Wichtig, Milan, pp 45–49

98. Winzelberg G G 1987 Parathyroid imaging. Ann Intern Med 107: 64–70

99. Doppman J L 1976 Parathyroid localization. Arteriography and venous sampling. Radiol Clin North Am 14: 163–188

100. Miller D L, Doppman J L, Krudy A G et al 1987 Localization of parathyroid adenomas in patients who have undergone surgery. Part II. Invasive procedures. Radiology 162: 138–141

101. Salti G I, Fedorak I, Yashiro T et al 1992 Continuing evolution in the operative management of primary hyperparathyroidism. Arch Surg 127: 831–837

102. Thompson N W 1988 Localization studies in patients with primary hyperparathyroidism. Br J Surg 75: 97–98

103. Serpel J W, Campbell P R, Young A E 1991 Preoperative localization of parathyroid tumors does not reduce operating time. Br J Surg 78: 589–590

104. Miller D L 1991 Pre-operative localization and interventional treatment of parathyroid tumors: when and how? World J Surg 15: 706–715

105. Satava R M Jr, Beahrs O H, Schjolz D A 1975 Success rate of cervical exploration for hyperparathyroidism. Arch Surg 110: 625–628

106. Fukagawa M, Okazaki R, Takano K et al 1990 Regression of parathyroid hyperplasia by calcitriol-pulse therapy in patients on long term dialysis. N Engl J Med 323: 421–422

107. Korkor A B 1987 Reduced binding of (3H) 1,25-dihydroxyvitamin D3 in the parathyroid glands of patients with renal failure. N Engl J Med 316: 1573–1577

108. Fukuda N, Tanaka H, Tominaga Y, Fukagawa M, Kurokawa K, Seino Y 1993 Decreased 1,25-dihydroxyvitamin D3 receptor density is associated with a more severe form of parathyroid hyperplasia in chronic uremic patients. J Clin Invest 92: 1436–1443

109. Solbiati L, Giangrande A, De Pra L, Bellotti E, Cantú P, Ravetto C 1985 Percutaneous ethanol injection of parathyroid tumors under US guidance: treatment for secondary hyperparathyroidism. Radiology 155: 607–610

110. Akizawa T, Fukagawa M, Koshikawa S, Kurokawa K 1993 Recent progress in management of secondary hyperparathyroidism of chronic renal failure. Curr Op Nephrol Hypertens 2: 558–565

111. Page B, Zingraff J, Souberbielle J C et al 1992 Correction of severe secondary hyperparathyroidism in two dialysis patients: surgical removal versus percutaneous ethanol injection. Am J Kidney Dis 19: 378–381

112. Takeda S, Michigishi T, Takakura E 1992 Successful ultrasonically guided percutaneous ethanol injection for secondary hyperparathyroidism. Nephron 62: 100–103

113. Giangrande A, Castiglioni A, Solbiati L, Allaria P 1992 Ultrasound-guided percutaneous fine-needle ethanol injection into parathyroid glands in secondary hyperparathyroidism. Nephrol Dial Transplant 7: 412–421

114. Giangrande A, Castiglioni A, Solbiati L, Ballarati E, Caligara F 1994 Chemical parathyroidectomy for recurrence of secondary hyperparathyroidism. Am J Kidney Dis, in press

115. Charboneau J W, Hay I D, Van Heerden J A 1988 Persistent primary hyperparathyroidism: successful ultrasound-guided percutaneous ethanol ablation of an occult adenoma. Mayo Clin Proc 63: 913–916

116. Karstrup S, Holm H H, Glenthoj A, Hegedus L 1990 Non surgical treatment of primary hyperparathyroidism with sonographically guided percutaneous injection of ethanol: results in a selected series of patients. AJR 154: 1087–1090

117. Jacob D, Cercueil J P, Krause D, Verges B, Thibaud J C, Mabille J P 1993 Ultrasonically guided percutaneous ethanol injection into parathyroid adenomas: technique and long term results. Abstr 8th Eur Cong Radiol (ECR '93), Vienna, 12–17 Sept 1993. Springer-Verlag, Berlin, p 364

7

Masses of the neck and oral cavity

J. N. Bruneton   A. Geoffray

CYSTS

Thyroglossal duct cyst

The thyroglossal duct cyst is the most frequent non-odontogenous cyst of the neck and accounts for about 70% of congenital masses.[1]

During embryogenic development, the thyroid follows the heart and neck vessels down into the mediastinum, leaving an epithelial lining that represents the thyroglossal duct; this becomes atrophic between weeks 5 and 10. Occasionally, its caudal component may persist, and this gives origin to the pyramidal lobe of the thyroid.

No significant sex predominance has been reported in literature; the diagnosis is made before the patient is 10 years old in 30% of cases and after 30 in 35% of patients.[2]

In 75% of cases the cyst is located in the anterior cervical zone, along the midline; only 10–24% of cysts have a lateral location.[3] Up to 60–80% of cysts are caudal to the hyoid bone.

The clinical findings are of a fluctuating, painless cervical mass, that becomes painful when inflamed. At surgery the contents are mucoid or purulent. The differential diagnosis is with adenopathies, laryngoceles, central branchial cysts, dermoid cysts, ectopic thyroids, sebaceous cysts and lipomas.[4] The most frequent complication is the formation of a fistula, usually after trauma or infection.

Only 1% of thyroglossal duct cysts are complicated by a carcinoma, usually a papillary adenocarcinoma. The prognosis, however, is good because metastases are rare.[5]

Studies obtained with CT, showing both the cyst and its surroundings, have been reported.[6] Sonography is the main imaging modality, showing a typical cystic lesion, with posterior enhancement and well-defined margins. Septations or a solid structure are sometimes seen and this complicates the differential diagnosis with infection, thyroid tissue or a tumoral mass. Echogenic thyroid tissue may be found inside the cyst and FNAB is mandatory to confirm normal thyroid tissue.[7,8] Sonography can demonstrate the relationship between the cyst and the hyoid bone, and show a fistula to the tongue or towards the skin.[8] Sonography is also important to demonstrate small, non-palpable, recurrent cysts (Figs 7.1–7.3).

Sonography permits a thorough evaluation of the thyroid; a nuclear scan to evaluate function will be necessary in case of surgery.[9,10]

Branchial cysts

Branchial cysts are the most frequent cystic masses in the lateral cervical region; they develop from the first or second branchial clefts. They may be represented by a sinus (a small non-communicating skin orifice), by fistulas, or, more frequently, by cysts that originate from an incomplete obliteration of the branchial clefts and that are easily demonstrated by sonography. Anomalies originating from the first branchial cleft are cysts, generally located in the lower pole of the parotid gland, and detected in middle age.

Differential diagnosis includes tumoral masses of the parotid gland. Anomalies originating from the second branchial cleft represent 80–90% of branchial cleft pathology and are located between the mandibular angle and the supraclavicular fossa. According to their location, there are four different types of cysts: these are superficial cysts (in front of the sternocleidomastoid muscle), cysts underneath

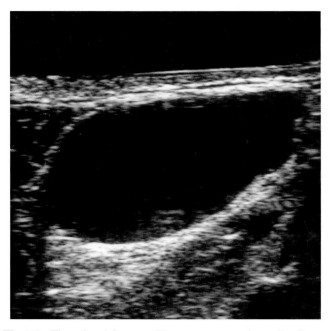

Fig. 7.1 Thyroglossal duct cyst. Transverse scan on the median line.

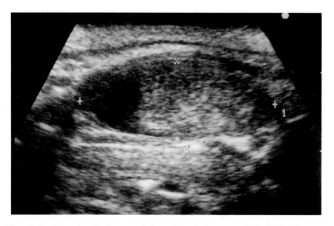

Fig. 7.2 Longitudinal scan of thyroglossal duct cyst. The lesion has mixed echo structure due to the presence of debris (superimposed inflammatory process).

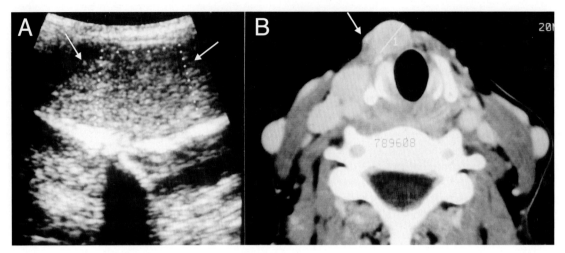

Fig. 7.3 12 mm adenoma of the thyroglossal duct (arrowhead), featuring solid texture on US (**A**) and thyroid-like contrast enhancement on CT scan (**B**). Aspiration biopsy yielded thyroid cells.

the medial cervical fascia and anterior to the carotid artery and jugular vein (the most frequent type), cysts extending to the pharynx and, finally, those extending between the vessels and the lateral wall of the pharynx (Fig. 7.4).

Anomalies of the third and fourth branchial cleft are uncommon. They are usually represented by fistulas of the pyriform sinus and by lateral masses – adenophlegmons – that frequently relapse after medical treatment (Fig. 7.5). Differential diagnosis of these lateral masses is not simple and includes cystic hygromas, laryngoceles, adenopathies, epidermoid cysts and abnormalities of the salivary glands.[7]

CT is used to evaluate these masses.[11,12] Sonography gives the most interesting information.[7,9,10,13] A typical cystic pattern is observed in most cases; a solid mass, due to mucoid or cholesterol contents, is rarely seen and can mimic an adenopathy. Fistulas can be demonstrated towards the skin or the tonsillar tissues. When the diagnosis is uncertain, FNAB becomes necessary and has a sensitivity

of 86%.[14] The specimen shows amorphous debris, cholesterol crystals, a benign squamous lining and rare lymphocytes.

Branchial cysts can become infected, turning into a solid mass, sometimes surrounded by lymph nodes. The possibility of a malignant change is still the subject of debate.[15]

Other cystic lesions

A laryngocele is a dilatation of the saccule of the laryngeal ventricle and represents a rare abnormality (less than 300 cases reported in the literature up to 1977).[15] Laryngoceles are frequently associated with a laryngeal tumor or with occupations that call for forceful expiration through the mouth. They are classified into three types – the internal type, confined inside the larynx, the external type, extending to the neck and the mixed type, which combines both. The sonographic pattern of the internal type is a cystic mass inside the thyroid cartilage.[4] These cystic images suggest the diagnosis of a laryngocele, whereas all solid masses in the same area are attributable to carcinomas.[4] In the mixed type, cystic masses are seen on both sides of the cartilage. CT shows capsulated cystic images close to the hyoid bone. The sonographic diagnosis of a laryngocele filled with air is more difficult because of artifacts that may mimic air contained in the larynx.

Cystic lymphangiomas are discovered in 90% of cases before the patient is 2 years old; they develop from an anomalous sequestration of embryonic tissue into one or more of the five clefts that give origin to the lymphatic system. A hemangiomatous component is mostly present; hence, they are termed 'hemolymphangiomas'.

There is a localized form, in the laterocervical region, and a diffuse form, at the level of the floor of the mouth, the tongue and the parotid region, that can cause respiratory

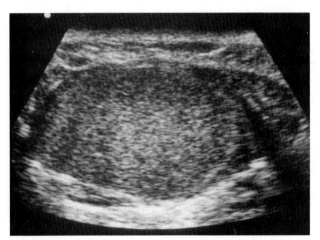

Fig. 7.4 Lateral branchial cyst with echogenic content due to inflammatory changes.

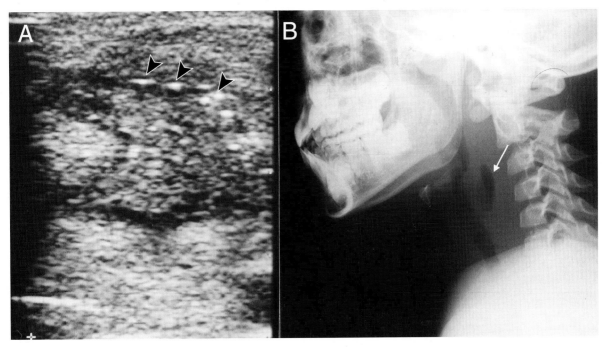

Fig. 7.5 Adenophlegmon. **A** US shows a solid mass with bright spots representing air bubbles (arrowhead) caused by a fistula. **B** On X-ray, air in soft tissues of the neck is detected (arrow).

complications. The clinical findings are a soft mass in the laterocervical region, mobile under the skin, and adherent to the deep planes; complications are due to inflammation and hemorrhage. Spontaneous regression is rare; malignant changes are exceptional.[16] Sonography shows a multicystic mass, with thin septations, and with regular margins in most cases (Fig. 7.6). It is usually located on the right side and behind the sternocleidomastoid muscle. Color Doppler shows flow signals in the septations and in the feeding vessels. CT and MRI show a possible mediastinal extension: contrast-enhanced CT improves the visibility of

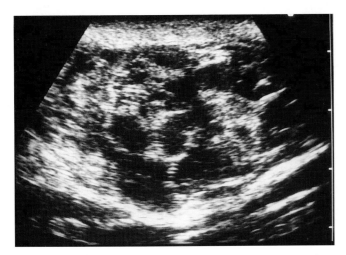

Fig. 7.6 Cervical cystic lymphangioma in a 25-year-old patient: multicystic mass with septations.

septations. With MRI, T_1-weighted images show a mass that is isointense to the muscle; in T_2-weighted images the signal is more intense than fat.[17,18]

Dermoid cysts are described in Chapter 13. They lie on the midline or close to it and correspond to an epidermic inclusion during the process of fusion of the branchial clefts. They are localized at the hyoid level.[19] The presence of dense contents complicates the differential diagnosis with a thyroglossal duct cyst, although the latter is more frequent. In a series of 75 cystic masses of the neck, located on the midline and in children, only 11 were dermoid cysts.[20]

NON-CYSTIC MASSES

Neural masses

Neural masses are rare abnormalities, that can be classified into two groups:

- tumors found anywhere in the body and described also in Chapter 15 (schwannoma, neuroma, neurofibroma, ganglioneuroma)
- tumors characteristic of the cervicofacial region (esthesioneuroma, paraganglioma, glioma, meningioma).

The most frequent neural masses in the neck are schwannomas, neurofibromas in von Recklinghausen's disease, paragangliomas or chemodectomas.[21]

Schwannomas can be found at any age and grow very slowly, so that spontaneous neurological symptoms are exceptional. 25% are situated in the head and neck. Superficial lesions are solitary, painless masses that give symptoms when they develop in areas with many nervous fibres. Recurrences may occur but they are always benign. Malignant schwannomas are extremely rare; in 75% of cases they appear in von Recklinghausen's disease.[22]

The sonographic pattern of neurofibromas and schwannomas is represented by a solid mass with posterior enhancement, that mimics a solitary lymph node (Fig. 7.7). Large tumors and malignant schwannomas displace vessels and muscles; CT is often required to evaluate the extent, especially when the mass grows towards the face or the chest.[23]

Carotid body tumors, also known as chemodectomas, are rare abnormalities located at the level of the common carotid bifurcation. They develop from chemoreceptor tissue and belong to the group of non-chromaffin paragangliomas. Other possible localizations, i.e. the jugular glomus, tympanic glomus, vagal glomus, aortic glomus and masses of the retroperitoneal region, can be detected by other imaging modalities. Carotid body tumors grow slowly and are first seen as a palpable, non-tender lateral neck mass.

Sonographic imaging and color Doppler are important for diagnosis.[24] Ultrasound shows a solitary, well-defined mass, localized close to the carotid bifurcation; they are usually less than 5 cm in diameter, with a solid, hypoechoic and inhomogeneous structure. Color Doppler clearly shows the vascularized pattern of the lesion and of the adjacent vessels (Fig. 7.8). A pseudocystic pattern has also been reported.[24] Contrast-enhanced CT shows marked tumor enhancement. MRI reveals a non-homogeneous mass, because of the large number of vessels and because of blood flow. After gadolinium injection there is an obvious enhancement, similar to that seen with CT.[25]

In conclusion, only chemodectomas can be adequately diagnosed with sonography alone, because of the distinctive features offered by color Doppler. All other neural masses need CT, MRI and FNAB for a definite diagnosis.

Muscular abnormalities

Hematomas of the sternocleidomastoid muscle are usually due to a difficult delivery. The clinical finding is a lateral cervical mass in a neonate. High-frequency sonography confirms the clinical finding and shows a more of less well circumscribed mass, with a variable structure, but usually hypoechoic, localized inside the muscle (Fig. 7.9).[10,26]

Foreign bodies located in the soft tissues of the neck can easily be demonstrated with high-resolution probes, whatever their nature (wood, glass, metal, etc). Foreign bodies appear as echogenic reflections, with posterior shadowing; an echo-poor halo suggests the development of inflammation. Sonography can guide the removal of these foreign bodies.[27]

Tumors originating from the soft tissues of the neck are rare. They usually are sarcomas (fibroid malignant histiocytoma, fibrosarcoma, neurofibrosarcoma, rhabdomyosarcoma, leiomyosarcoma).[28] Sonography shows an ill-defined, echo-poor lesion (Fig. 7.10). When the tumor is not localized in the neck only, CT and MRI are recommended to improve diagnosis.[29]

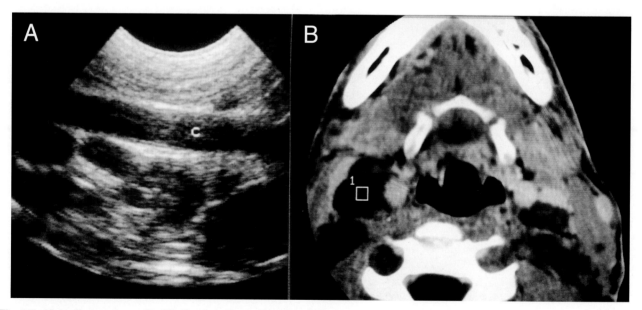

Fig. 7.7 Neurofibromas in von Recklinghausen's disease. **A** Multiple, solid, oval or roundish masses are shown around the carotid artery (C) in the sonogram. **B** Contrast-enhanced CT scan displaying neurofibromas invading both laterocervical regions.

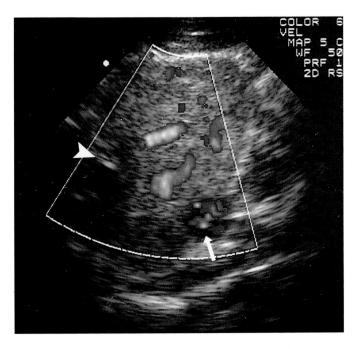

Fig. 7.8 Transverse scan of the left side of the neck. Typical hypervascularized mass between the proximal tracts of the internal (arrow) and external (arrowhead) carotid arteries.

Cervical myositis is easily detected by CT: contrast enhancement is inhomogeneous and suggests inflammatory changes of the muscle. These abnormalities may be due to localized inflammation or represent a paraneoplastic syndrome (Fig. 7.11).

Cancers of the oral cavity

Tumors of the lower portion of the oral cavity can be studied adequately by sonography, by scanning underneath the chin. Sonography may have some limitations, but offers interesting features when the largest diameter of the lesion is less than 3 cm. Lymph node involvement can easily be assessed.

Cancer of the tongue is a squamous-cell carcinoma, that develops in 10% of cases on pre-existing mucosal alterations, such as leukoplakia, lichen, chronic glossitis or exophytic keratosis. Cancer of the tongue represents about 1% of all cancers and 20% of upper respiratory and digestive tract malignancies. Cancer of the tongue is classified according to its location – the base of the tongue (one-third of cases) and the mobile tongue (two-thirds of cases). The more posterior the lesion, the worse the prognosis. Lesions

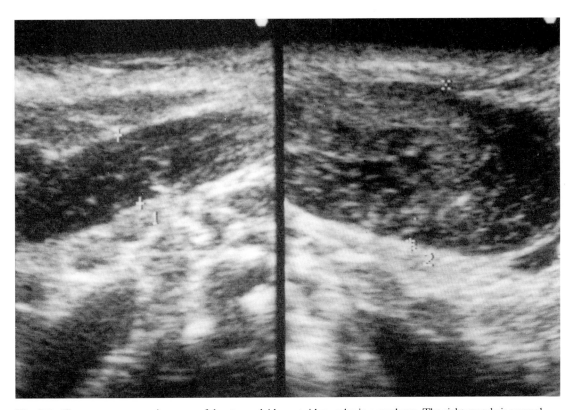

Fig. 7.9 Transverse comparative scans of the sternocleidomastoid muscles in a newborn. The right muscle is normal, whereas the left is thickened and inhomogeneous (fibrosis following hematoma at delivery).

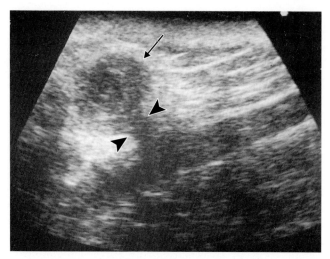

Fig. 7.10 Small cervical recurrence of rhabdomyosarcoma (arrow) infiltrating the wall of the jugular vein (arrowhead).

are usually discovered when very large, with lymph node involvement in up to 40–60% of cases, and it is bilateral in 10–15%.[30] Lymph nodes are more often located in the submandibular region, followed by sublingual and jugular nodes. In recent years, CT has been replaced more and more by MRI as far as staging is concerned.[25,31,32]

Clinical examination of cancer of the mobile tongue must consider the following factors: invasion of the midline; tumor extension towards the floor and the mandible, and extension to the base of the tongue and to the tonsils. In cases of cancers of the base, clinical examination must determine extension towards the mobile tongue, extension

backwards to the valleculae and suprahyoid epiglottis, and lateral invasion of the glossotonsillar sulcus, of the tonsils and pharyngoepiglottic folds.

Sonography reveals cancer of the tongue as an heterogeneous mass, less echogenic than adjacent normal muscles. Small lesions can appear homogeneous, but internal inhomogeneous structure is easily shown when the largest diameter of the tumor exceeds 2 cm. Ulcerations smaller than 5 mm cannot be visualized, unless they contain liquid or air. It is important to identify the tumor's borders, which are usually well defined in T2 cancers (the largest diameter of which is 2–4 cm); it is more difficult to do so for larger cancers. Sonography must always demonstrate anterior, lateral and posterior extension, as well as invasion of the midline. Sonography has some limitations: T1 lesions are too small for ultrasound detection; some cancers of the mobile tongue may be difficult to image; very extensive cancers do not allow a convenient evaluation of their borders and of peripheral invasion; changes due to therapy may not be easily differentiated from recurrences.[33,34]

Cancer of the floor of the mouth is less frequent than carcinoma of the tongue, and represents about 10% of all upper respiratory and digestive tract cancers. Submental scanning can show the tumoral mass, but it is specific for bone involvement. The role of sonography in this type of pathology is the detection of lymph node metastases.

Tonsillar cancer is more frequent than carcinoma of the oral cavity. It is squamous-cell carcinoma in 90% of cases; the incidence of lymphomas is less than 10%. Chronic alcoholism and tabagism are predisposing factors for all these cancers. Tonsillar cancer extends towards the midline, through the base of the tongue, to the lateral pharyngeal wall, to the soft palate, to the retromolar tri-

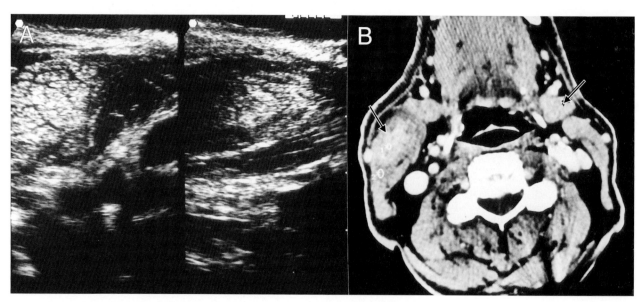

Fig. 7.11 Cervical myositis. **A** Longitudinal scans of both sides of the neck showing abnormal development of muscle fibers. **B** Contrast-enhanced CT scan: myositic lesions are hyperdense (arrow).

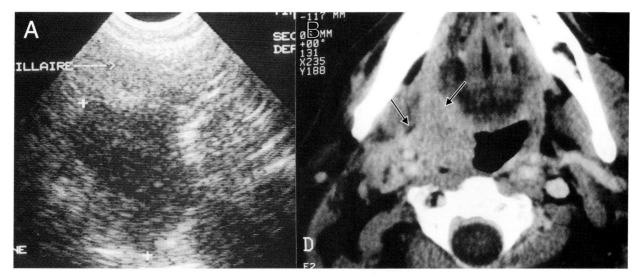

Fig. 7.12   Carcinoma of the tonsil. **A** Hypoechoic mass (4.2 cm) (+) situated behind the submandibular gland (arrow). **B** Contrast-enhanced CT scan permitting better definition of the outlines of the lesion (arrow).

gonus and oral mucosa and to the gums. Sonography may easily demonstrate tumor size and borders; it can show forward extension along the midline, but it cannot delineate upper and posterior diffusion. Ultrasound examinations include evaluation of lymph nodes in the lateral cervical region (Fig. 7.12).[9]

REFERENCES

1. Faerber E N, Swartz J D 1991 Imaging of neck masses in infants and children. CRC Crit Rev Diagn Imaging 31: 283–314
2. Allard R H B 1982 The thyroglossal cyst. Head Neck Surg 5: 134–136
3. Ward G E, Henrick J W, Chambers R G 1949 Thyroglossal tract abnormalities, cysts and fistulas. Surg Gynecol Obstet 89: 727–734
4. Baatenburg de Jong R J, Rongen R J, Lameris J S, Knegt P, Verwoerd C D A 1993 Ultrasound in the diagnosis of laryngoceles. ORL J Otorhinolaryngol Relat Spec 55: 290–293
5. Jacques D A, Chambers R G, Oertel J E 1970 Thyroglossal tract carcinoma: a review of the literature and addition of eighteen cases. Am J Surg 120: 439–446
6. Ward R F, Selfe R W, St Louis L, Bowling D 1986 Computed tomography and the thyroglossal duct cyst. Otolaryngol Head Neck Surg 95: 93–98
7. Baatenburg de Jong R J, Rongen R J, Lameris J S, Knegt P, Verwoerd C D A 1993 Evaluation of branchiogenic cysts by ultrasound. Otorhinolaryngol Relat Spec 55: 294–298
8. Baatenburg de Jong R J, Rongen R J, Lameris J S, Knegt P, Verwoerd C D A 1993 Ultrasound characteristics of thyroglossal duct anomalies. J Otorhinolaryngol Relat Spec 55: 299–302
9. Bruneton J N 1987 Ultrasonography of the neck. Springer Verlag, Berlin
10. Geoffray A, Lagrange A S, Chami M 1993 Echographie des masses cervicales chez l'enfant. Méd Infant 5: 413–426
11. Byrd S E, Richardson M, Gill G, Lee A M 1983 Computed tomographic appearance of branchial cleft and thyroglossal duct cysts of the neck. Diagn Imag Int 52: 301–312
12. Marsot-Dupuch K, Levret N, Chabolle F 1990 Formations kystiques cervicales de l'adulte. Feuillets Radiol 30: 347–361
13. Badami J P, Athey P A 1981 Sonography in the diagnosis of branchial cysts. AJR 137: 1245–1248
14. Engzell U, Zajicek J 1970 Aspiration biopsy and cytologic findings in 100 cases of congenital cysts. Acta Cytol 14: 51–57
15. MacCarthy S A, Turnbull F M 1981 The controversy of bronchogenic carcinoma. Arch Otolaryngol 107: 570–572
16. Canalis R F, Maxell D S, Homenway W C 1977 Laryngocele: an update review. J Otolaryngol 6: 191–199
17. Siegel M J, Glazer H S, St Amour T E, Rosenthal D D 1989 Lymphangiomas in children; MR imaging. Radiology 170: 467–470
18. Som P M, Sacher M, Lanzieri C F et al 1985 Parenchymal cysts of the lower neck. Radiology 157: 399–406
19. Katz A D 1974 Midline dermoid tumors of the neck. Arch Surg 109: 822–823
20. De Mello D E, Lima J A, Liapis H 1987 Midline cervical cysts in children. Arch Otolaryngol Head Neck Surg 113: 418–420
21. Cernea P, Brocheriou C, Guilbert F et al 1977 Schwannomes cervico-faciaux. In: Leroux-Robert J (ed) Tumeurs nerveuses ORL et cervico-faciales. Masson, Paris, pp 85–92
22. Monje Gil F, Gonzales Estecha A, Naval Gias L, Diaz Gonzalez F J, Gil-Diel J L 1989 Tumeur maligne des gaines nerveuses (schwannome malin). Rev Stomatol Chir Maxillofac 90: 20–23
23. Mayer J S, Kulkarni M V, Yeakley J W 1987 Craniocervical manifestations of neurofibromatosis: MR versus CT studies. J Comput Assist Tomogr 11: 839–844
24. Derchi L E, Serafini G, Rabbia C et al 1992 Carotid body tumors: US evaluation. Radiology 182: 457–459
25. Lenz M 1993 CT and MRI of head and neck tumours. Thieme, Stuttgart
26. Crawford S C, Harnberger H R, Johnson L, Aoki J R, Giley J 1988 Fibromatosis colli of infancy: CT and sonographic findings. AJR 151: 1183–1184
27. Shiels W E II, Babcock D S, Wilson J L, Burch R A 1990 Localization and guided removal of soft-tissue foreign bodies with sonography. AJR 155: 1277–1281
28. Weber R S, Benjamin R S, Peters L J, Ro J Y, Achon O, Goepfert H 1986 Soft tissue sarcomas of the head and neck in adolescents and adults. Am J Surg 152: 386–392
29. Gilles R, Couanet D, Chevret S et al 1991 Importance of a post-therapeutic residue in prognosis of head and neck rhabdomyosarcoma in children. Eur J Radiol 13: 187–191
30. Vandenbrouck C, Gerard-Marchant R, Micheau C, Pierquin B, Cachin Y 1970 L'envahissement ganglionnaire des épithéliomes de

la langue mobile et du plancher buccal. A propos de 367 cas traités à l'Institut Gustave Roussy de 1960 à 1965. Ann Otolaryngol 87: 779–790

31. Cooke J, Parsons C 1989 Computed tomographic scanning in patients with carcinoma of the tongue. Clin Radiol 40: 254–256

32. Muraki A, Mancuso A, Harnsberger H, Johnson L, Meads G 1983 CT of the oropharynx, tongue base, and floor of the mouth: normal anatomy and range of variations, and applications in staging carcinomas. Radiology 148 725–731

33. Bruneton J N, Roux P, Caramella E, Manzino J J, Vallicioni J, Demard F 1986 Ultrasonography of cancer of the tongue and tonsil. Radiology 158: 743–746

34. Fruhwald F 1988 Clinical examination, CT and US in tongue cancer staging. Eur J Radiol 8: 236–241

8

Salivary glands

F. Candiani   C. Martinoli

Ultrasound is able both to image all three major salivary glands (i.e. parotid, submandibular and sublingual glands) and to detect most of the lesions affecting them.[1-6]

The availability of small-parts transducers (7.5–15 MHz with built-in water path) has improved the visualization of subtle anatomical and pathological details of superficial structures and allowed recognition of certain structures close to the salivary glands (for example the facial nerve) that were not previously identified. In addition, the development of high-frequency linear arrays with the capacity to obtain high-quality color Doppler images has improved the evaluation of vessels running adjacent to or crossing the salivary glands, thus helping conventional sonography to specify the vascular landmarks of focal lesions and to characterize a number of salivary diseases.

NORMAL ANATOMY

This section describes the normal ultrasonographic anatomy of the three major salivary glands as assessed with small-parts high-frequency probes and color Doppler.

The parotid gland is the largest and most posterior of the salivary glands. It is irregularly shaped and like an inverted pyramid, lying in the posterior portion of the prestyloid (parapharyngeal) space, between the mastoid process posteriorly and the ramus of the mandible anteriorly (Fig. 8.1A) It has an anterior process extending over the masseter muscle, and two posterior processes, one between the mastoid and the sternomastoid muscle and the other in front of the styloid process, in the retropharyngeal space.[7]

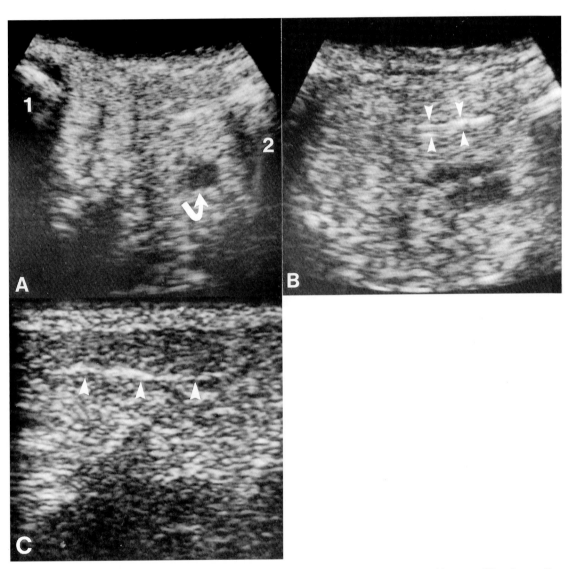

Fig. 8.1   10 MHz ultrasound scan of normal parotid gland. **A** Parotid gland lies between mastoid process (1) and ascending ramus of the mandible (2). It has undefined margins and homogeneous structure, and is crossed by the retromandibular vein (curved arrow). Both facial nerve (**B**) and Stenson's duct (**C**) are shown in their intraglandular course (arrowheads).

From superficial to deep, the structures of the parotid bed revealed by high-resolution ultrasound include the following: (1) the skin; (2) the subcutaneous tissue containing fat and extracapsular lymph nodes; (3) the superficial cervical fascia, depicted sonographically as an highly echogenic band that runs from the sternocleidomastoid muscle posteriorly and the masseter anteriorly, like a superficial parotid capsule; (4) the parotid gland; (5) a deep vascular plane, in which run the internal carotid artery and jugular vein.

Sonographically, the parotid gland has a homogeneous appearance,[3,4] comprising fine, dense parenchymal echoes that are more echogenic than the structures forming the boundaries of parotid spaces and quite similar to those of the normal thyroid. However, the parotid echotexture has a higher grade of attenuation of the ultrasound beam than the thyroid, so that the deep portions of the gland are usually difficult to visualize. Throughout the parotid par-

enchyma, a number of thin hyperechoic lines parallel to the skin can be detected with high-resolution probes. These lines represent normal intraglandular ducts and become brighter and ill-defined after injection of 1–2 ml air into the main excretory duct.[8] The parotid margins are not well defined. To improve visualization of the relationships between the anterior process of the parotid and the masseter muscle, the gland should be evaluated during both contraction and relaxation of the muscle.[5,6] The retropharyngeal portion of the parotid is never detectable because it is masked by the acoustic shadow of the mandible.

The parotid gland is crossed by a number of structures of clinical significance, and primarily by the facial nerve, the excretory duct and the large vessels of the neck.

The facial nerve emerges from the skull through the stylomastoid foramen and divides into temporofacial and cervicofacial branches. The facial nerve and its branches, including the auricolotemporal nerve, enter the superior deep portion of the parotid gland, between the posterior belly of the digastric and sternocleidomastoid muscle, and form a nerve plane separating the parotid into superficial and deep lobes.[7] Along the extraparotid course, the facial nerve is never visible by ultrasound. The intraglandular portion of the facial nerve can be recognized in about 30% of subjects, when examined at a frequency of 10–13 MHz (Fig. 8.1B). The nerve is enveloped by a fibrous sheath and can be detected as a thin hyperechoic fibrillar structure appreciable for a distance of 1–2 cm at 8–10 mm from the skin in the anterior and superficial part of the gland, occasionally as an echo-poor structure.[6] Alternatively, facial branches can occasionally be detected in the central part of the gland as thin linear interfaces of higher reflectivity. The sonographic identification of the facial plane can be of value in predicting the relationship of parotid tumors to the nerve, so that the surgical approach and potential morbidity of operation may be better assessed preoperatively.

The excretory duct of the parotid (Stenson's duct) originates in the anterior portion of the gland, runs on the surface of the masseter with a straight course, then enters through the buccinator muscle to open into the mouth opposite the second upper molar. Occasionally, the main duct can be detected on sonograms as a tubular hyperechoic structure located superficially in the anterior process of the gland (Fig. 8.1C).[8] Both in basal conditions or during salivation it has collapsed walls.

The most superficial vessel detectable with color Doppler in the parotid is the retromandibular vein, which infolds within the parotid near the auricular lobule, crosses the superficial lobe of the gland longitudinally and emerges from it at the inferior margin to continue in the external jugular vein (Fig. 8.2A). The external carotid artery has the same orientation as the retromandibular vein but appears to be larger and runs in a deeper plane, close to the medial

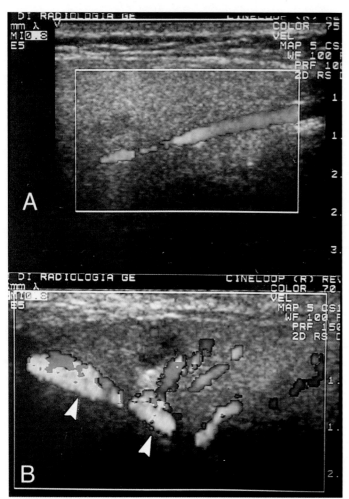

Fig. 8.2 Color Doppler image of normal parotid gland. **A** Retromandibular vein crosses the gland longitudinally and continues as external jugular vein after exiting the lower pole of the parotid. **B** In the upper third of the gland, arterial branches originate from the external carotid artery (arrowheads) to supply parotid parenchyma.

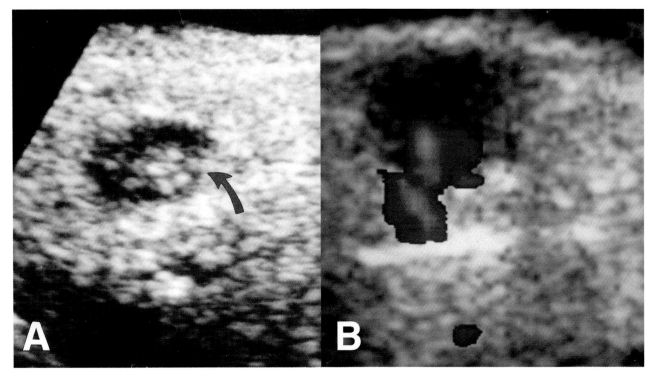

Fig. 8.3 Parotid lymph nodes. Small intraglandular lymph nodes (**A**) have an eccentric echogenic hilum (curved arrow) in which color flow signals are generally detectable (**B**).

borders of the gland or inside the deep portion of the parotid parenchyma. Both vessels are large and represent a constant finding during color Doppler examination of the parotid gland.[9] in the upper third of the gland, the retromandibular vein receives from the parotid parenchyma a number (two to six) of small veins running at right angles to its longitudinal axis and characterized by an orderly arrangement (Fig. 8.2B). Corresponding arterial branches that arise from the external carotid artery may be associated with these veins. On the contrary, in the middle and lower third of the gland, branches supplying parotid parenchyma are rarely shown to originate from large vessels and thus distal intraparenchymal vessels appear mostly as spot signals randomly scattered within this portion of the gland. In a number of cases, the retromandibular vein is joined to the facial vein by an anastomotic trunk running inferior to the margin of the mandible.

In a number of subjects, normal lymph nodes can be appreciated within the parotid as small hypoechoic nodules. When lymph nodes present with an eccentric echogenic hilum (Fig. 8.3A), a diagnosis of parotid lymphadenopathy can be made safely.[4,6] Usually, color Doppler detects the vessel pedicle running in the hilum of the lymph node (Fig. 8.3B).

The submandibular gland is about half the size of the parotid gland and lies in the suprahyoid region, between the body of the mandible and the mylohyoid muscle.[7] It has an almond-shaped body oriented obliquely downward,

anteriorly and medially (Fig. 8.4). The submandibular gland can be separated from the parotid by the interposition of the superior digastric lymph node (Kuttner's node) or alternatively connected to it.[3,10] In contrast to the parotids, the submandibular glands are fully detectable with ultrasound; they have an echostructure similar to that of the parotids, although without attenuation of the beam (because of their smaller size) and with a more complex

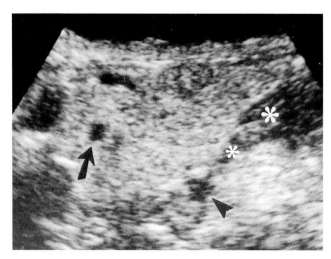

Fig. 8.4 10 MHz ultrasound scan of normal submandibular gland. The gland has an almond-shaped body and appears close to the facial (arrow) and lingual (arrowhead) vessels. Asterisks denote the mylohyoid muscle.

vasculature, sharing as they do a close relationship with the facial and lingual vessels. On color Doppler it can be seen that the facial artery arises from the external carotid artery, either in common with the lingual artery or immediately superior to it, passes superiorly under cover of the mandibular angle and then loops anteriorly, entering a deep groove or perforating the submandibular gland (Fig. 8.5A). Within the gland, the facial artery runs superficially, matched to the corresponding vein, and provides a number of branches supplying the parenchyma and characterized by regular peripheral subdivisions.[9] The facial artery subsequently leaves the gland anteriorly, originates submental vessels and loops around the inferior border of the mandible to enter the face. The lingual vessels can easily be identified with color Doppler as running between the deep margin of the submandibular gland and the muscular floor of the mouth (Fig. 8.5B). They are imaged as paired longitudinal vessels crossing the mylohyoid muscle to supply the tongue.[9]

The submandibular duct (Warthon's duct) emerges from the inferior surface of the gland and terminates at the side of the frenulum of the tongue. When normal, it is not appreciable sonographically cither inside or outside the gland. An intraparenchymal branch of the facial vein can often mimic the appearance of the excretory duct, owing to its longitudinal course and thick, highly reflective walls (Fig. 8.6A,B).[9]

The sublingual glands are the smallest of the three paired salivary glands and are the most deeply situated. Each gland lies in the floor of the mouth between the mandible and the genioglossus muscle, close to the submandibular duct. The sublingual glands may be joined to form a unique horseshoe-shaped glandular mass around the lingual frenulum or connected with the submandibular glands posteriorly.[7] The sublingual glands cannot always be demonstrated with ultrasound.[6] Using submental scans, they appear as small amounts of hyperechoic salivary tissue located between the mylohyoid and genioglossus muscles.

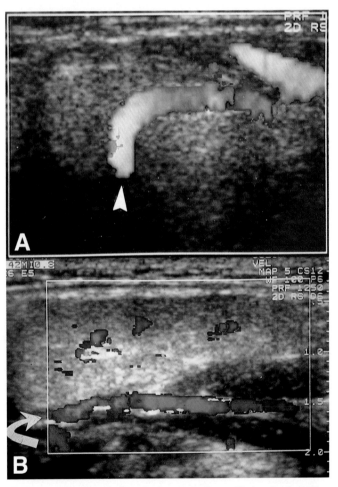

Fig. 8.5 Color Doppler image of normal submandibular gland. **A** The facial artery (arrowhead) loops anteriorly within the gland. **B** The lingual artery (curved arrow) runs between the deep margin of the submandibular gland and the muscular floor of the mouth. Color signals from distal vessels are detected in the submandibular parenchyma.

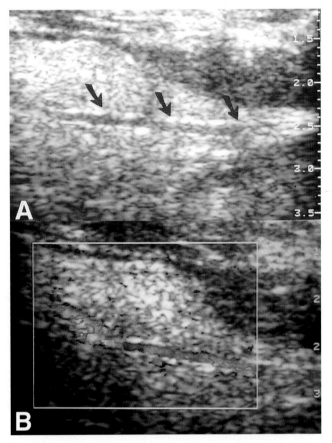

Fig. 8.6 Normal submandibular gland. Corresponding ultrasound (**A**) and color Doppler (**B**) images. A vein, similar in appearance to the excretory duct, with echogenic walls (arrows), is often recognized crossing the anterior portion of the gland longitudinally.

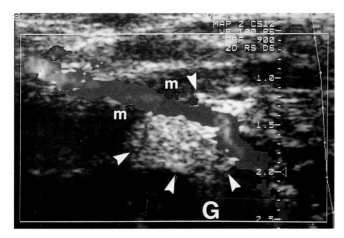

Fig. 8.7   Sublingual gland (arrowheads) lies in the floor of the mouth, between mylohyoid (m) and genioglossus (G) muscles. The lingual vein is seen crossing the gland towards the tongue.

The lingual vessels appear close to the sublingual glands and frequently infold within them (Fig. 8.7). A number of parenchymal branches arising from the lingual vessels can be demonstrated with color Doppler to subdivide the sublingual glands in a regular manner.[9]

VASCULAR CHANGES DURING SALIVARY STIMULATION

No significant changes in parenchymal and ductal appearance are observed with high-resolution ultrasound in the salivary glands during the act of salivation. However, physiologic studies report that an intense hyperemia accompanies the secretion of saliva,[11] with blood perfusion of the salivary glands increasing more than fivefold over the basal value of 0.1–0.6 ml/min.g. Functional hyperemia is a complex response involving not only local mechanisms, but also parasympathetic nervous control. Through direct cholinergic terminations, the arteriolar resistance of the salivary vessels is controlled by the nervous system and is reduced following appropriate stimulation.

Color Doppler is an ideal approach by which to study physiologic changes in the vasculature of the salivary glands, as it allows imaging of the parenchymal vessels and estimation of their resistance by a simple calculation of the resistive index. During color Doppler examination, lemon juice can be used to elicit maximal stimulation of salivation, with concurrent dramatic vascular changes as detected with color Doppler. Specifically, a marked increase in color signals and the development of aliasing artifact within the vessels, due to increasing flow velocities, occurs abruptly on administration of lemon (Fig. 8.8A,B). Such physiologic changes can be detected also by spectral analysis, with a fall in resistive index and a marked increase in systolic peak velocities within the parenchymal vessels.[9] Changes in both resistive index and systolic peak velocity are transient and

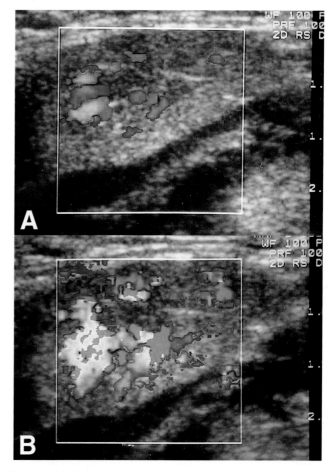

Fig. 8.8   Physiologic changes in vasculature of the submandibular gland during salivary stimulation. **A** Before stimulation with lemon juice. **B** During lemon juice stimulation. A diffuse increase in color flow signals and development of aliasing artifact is observed during lemon stimulation due to a fall in arterial impedance and increase in flow velocity.

tend to normalize within 20 s after the juice has been swallowed.

SALIVARY GLAND DISEASES

A wide variety of pathologic conditions, including diffuse and focal inflammatory, obstructive, traumatic and neoplastic diseases, may affect the major salivary glands and in most of them ultrasound can have an important diagnostic role. This section indicates both the potential applications and the limitations of ultrasound for each salivary gland disease.

Simple hypertrophy

An enlarged parotid gland of normal shape and echostructure is observed in simple hypertrophy. This condition may be due to obesity or to racial factors (Egyptians, North Africans) and may be observed as a consequence of alcoholism, diabetes, thyroid diseases and uremia. Occasionally, parotid hypertrophy may compensate for resected glands.

Acute inflammation

Acute inflammation of salivary glands may have a bacterial (pyogenic streptococci and staphylococci) or viral (mumps) etiology. When the condition is bacterial in origin, it usually develops from infections of contiguous structures (dental, auricular, cutaneous), pre-existing systemic diseases causing immunosuppression (such as neoplastic disease and AIDS) or salivary stasis associated with lithiasis.[3] Clinically, the orifice of the parotid duct is red and secretes pus; there may be signs of peripheral facial nerve paralysis. Acute inflammation of the salivary glands can be studied advantageously with ultrasound, as the use of sialographic contrast media is contraindicated as a source of ascending infections. The inflamed glands are painful when pressed with the transducer and are generally enlarged at presentation, with an echo-poor and slightly heterogeneous structure as a consequence of reactive edema.[4,6] Recurrence and complications may cause damage to the parenchymal structure of increasing extent and severity. Micro-abscesses may occur as small echo-free foci and evolve into large abscesses, which are visible as fluid-filled collections with irregular borders and internal debris (Fig. 8.9A). In these cases, a frequency of 13 MHz may reveal skin thickening over the inflamed gland, as a result of extraglandular reac-

tive involvement, and ultrasound can be used as a guide for percutaneous aspiration and drainage of abscesses.[5,12] Occasionally, parotid abscesses may develop into simple cysts (Fig. 8.9B).[5] When antibiotic therapy has been established, the ultrasound changes that occur in acute inflammation may be moderate and require confirmation by comparative evaluation of the glands on each side. In most cases, the inflamed glands revert to a normal appearance and ultrasound can be used to monitor the healing process.[6]

Mumps (infectious parotitis) and acute recurrent sialectatic parotitis are the most frequent causes of painful parotid swelling in children. The diagnosis of mumps is made clinically and imaging studies are usually unnecessary. However, ultrasound shows unilateral or bilateral enlargement of the parotid glands, with a decrease in parenchymal echogenicity and with multiple lymphadenopathies along the retroauricolar and jugular chains.[3,5] In children with acute recurrent sialectatic parotitis, ultrasound typically identifies multiple small hypoechoic areas within the parotid parenchyma, attributable in part to punctate duct dilation. In clinical practice, ultrasound has been suggested as the method of choice to document the recurrence of parotid swelling and to demonstrate its resolution with therapy.[13]

Chronic inflammation

A variety of chronic inflammatory processes of non-specific and autoimmune origin may affect the salivary glands.

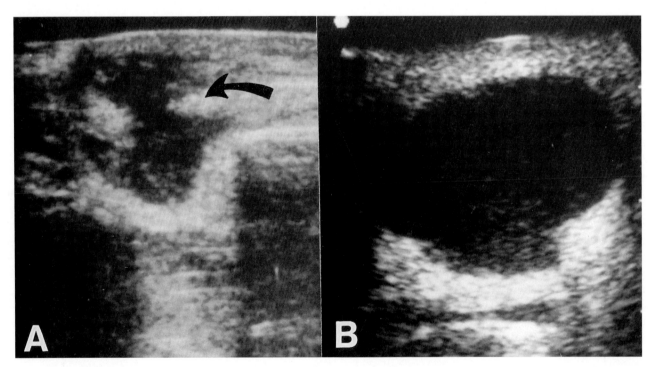

Fig. 8.9 Parotid changes following acute inflammation. **A** Intraglandular abscess (curved arrow) with irregular borders and internal debris. **B** Cyst that has developed from an abscess.

Histopathologically, they cause diffuse damage to the parenchymal structure, inducing progressive atrophy of the acinar tissue and ectatic changes in the ductal system. Clinical features include parotid swelling, decreased secretion of saliva up to xerostomia and secondary infections due to salivary stasis. Sonographic signs of chronic inflammation are usually moderate and mainly consist of a slight decrease in parenchymal echogenicity, cyst-like ectasia of the peripheral ducts and the presence of small reactive intraglandular lymph nodes with an eccentric echogenic hilum.[4,6]

Among the chronic disorders of salivary glands, Sjögren's syndrome presents with the typical triad of keratoconjunctivitis sicca, xerostomia and associated autoimmune disorder, most commonly rheumatoid arthritis.[14] On the basis of imaging findings alone, Sjögren's syndrome is difficult to differentiate from chronic non-specific inflammation and its early changes can be overlooked by ultrasound.[4,6,15] The typical sonographic pattern in Sjögren's syndrome is based on the presence of multiple cystic areas scattered throughout the salivary glands as a result of peripheral non-obstructive sialectasia (Fig. 8.10A). These areas range from multiple, apparently simple cysts to complex, multiseptated cystic masses with well-defined but irregular margins.[16] In the late stages of disease, the heterogeneity of the salivary glands becomes more evident following progressive fibrotic and infective changes.

Theoretically, the recent introduction of high-frequency probes could ameliorate the sensitivity of ultrasound in identifying minimal changes and small cyst-like dilations of the intraglandular ducts. However, a normal sonogram cannot rule out the presence of a diseased gland and sialography currently remains the most sensitive diagnostic approach to detect the early stages of disease.[14,17] In fact,

the sialographic findings correlate well to the histologic severity of Sjögren's syndrome and permit its classification according to a four-point graded scale from 0 to 3, based on increasing signs of damage to the ductal system.[18] Recently a four-point scale of ultrasound findings,[5] corresponding to the sialographic scale, has been proposed: grade 0, no parenchymal changes; grade 1, occasional microcysts (below 2 mm in diameter) and minimal heterogeneity; grade 2, diffuse cysts (over 2 mm) suggesting a microareolar texture (Fig. 8.10A); grade 3, large confluent cysts with septations (complex masses) and highly heterogenous structure; grade 4, disappearance of parenchymal texture in atrophic glands with undefined margins and reduced volume (Fig. 8.10B). In fact, further experience with a large series of patients is still needed to validate the clinical use of sonographic classification for grading the histologic severity of Sjögren's syndrome.

A diffuse increase in parenchymal flow signals and decrease in arteriolar resistance can be observed with color Doppler in glands affected by Sjögren's syndrome (Fig. 8.10B).[19] Generally, the increased vascularization correlates well with morphologic changes such as decreased echogenicity and the presence of cyst-like structures scattered within the gland.[9,20] Similar vascular changes have been already described in other autoimmune diseases, such as Hashimoto's thyroiditis and Graves' disease, and probably represent common, although non-specific, findings in this class of autoimmune disorders, as an expression of the hyperemia associated with inflammation. Unfortunately, the hypervascular pattern has not been observed in those patients with proved Sjögren's syndrome and minor parenchymal changes,[9,20] and thus color Doppler seems unable to predict the presence of disease before major sonographic changes occur in the salivary glands.

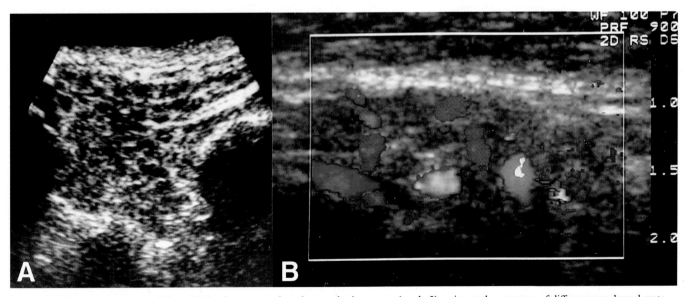

Fig. 8.10 Sjögren's syndrome. **A** Parotid gland appears to be microareolar in texture (grade 2) owing to the presence of diffuse parenchymal cysts. **B** A hypervascular color flow pattern is recognized in a small submandibular gland displaying atrophic parenchymal changes (grade 4).

Sialolithiasis

Sialolithiasis is much more common in the submandibular glands (approximately 80–85%) than in the parotid (10–15%) or sublingual (2–3%) glands, primarily because of the higher mucin content of the saliva. Mucin increases the viscosity of saliva, thus slowing salivary flow from the submandibular gland, and facilitates precipitation of calcium salts. Most salivary stones are radiopaque (80% in the submandibular and 60% in the parotid glands), because they contain calcium carbonate and calcium phosphate and can be detected on plain films. Non-opaque stones are composed of urates. Clinical features include recurrent swelling of the affected gland and pain, which is made worse by eating. Submandibular stones are frequently palpable.

According to Gritzmann,[4] ultrasound has 94% sensitivity, 100% specificity and 96% accuracy in identifying salivary stones and proves superior to plain film in its ability to detect non-opaque stones. Sonographically, salivary stones present as highly echogenic images with posterior acoustic shadow (Fig. 8.11). Shadowing can be appreciated also in 1–2 mm stones when transducers of higher frequency than 10 MHz are used. Generally, detection of salivary stones is more difficult in the parotid than in the submandibular glands, owing to superimposition of the

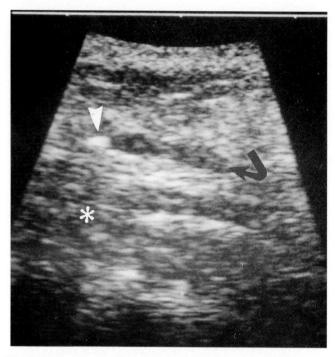

Fig. 8.11 Intraglandular lithiasis. A salivary stone (arrowhead) associated with proximal ductal ectasia (curved arrow) is detected in the submandibular gland. Asterisk denotes posterior acoustic shadow of the stone.

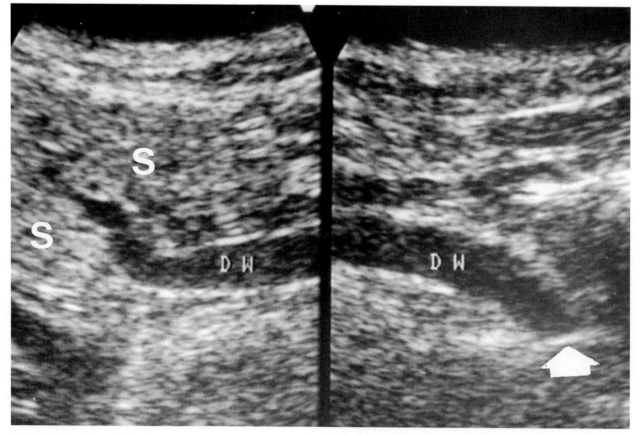

Fig. 8.12 Intraductal lithiasis. A salivary stone (arrow) located at the terminal end of the excretory duct (DW), makes it markedly ectatic. S: submandibular gland.

mandible, whereas intraglandular stones are more easily identified than those that are intraductal. Precise localization of the stone (intraductal or intraglandular) is important to determine therapy (ductal incision or removal of the gland). When the stone causes ductal blockage, concomitant ectasia of the proximal ducts can be easily visualized as tubular hypoechoic structures branching within the gland (Figs 8.11, 8.12). Ductal ectasia becomes more evident if ultrasound evaluation is conducted during salivary stimulation. Consequently, ultrasound coupled with salivary stimulation by lemon juice may have a diagnostic role in identifying salivary obstruction, mainly in those patients with salivary colics and no stone detected sonographically.

Ascending infection can develop from an obstructive stone and spread to the glandular tissue. In these cases, the ductal walls become ill-defined and the parenchyma near the stone becomes hypoechoic as a consequence of acute inflammation (Fig. 8.13A,B).[5] When the obstruction persists, abscesses (see Fig. 8.9A) may be observed within the gland. In these cases, ultrasound can guide percutaneous aspiration and drainage of these collections.[12] In the event

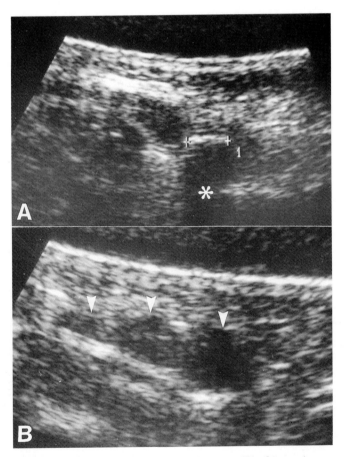

Fig. 8.13 Infected lithiasis. An obstructive stone (**A**) of 1 mm size (calipers) has caused the walls of the dilated proximal ducts (arrowheads) to be poorly defined owing to acute inflammatory changes following ascending infection. Asterisk denotes posterior acoustic shadow of the stone.

of a sterile obstruction, pseudodiverticular cysts with sharp echogenic margins and echo-free content can be observed in the gland as a result of the chronic increase of pressure in the obstructed ducts.[3]

Plain films are usually the first diagnostic approach in patients with suspected salivary stones. If these are normal, or when the exact location of the stone is not established, ultrasound is necessary. When there is a high clinical suspicion of salivary stones and both plain films and sonograms are normal, sialography becomes the technique of choice.

Trauma

Most salivary gland trauma occurs in the parotids, because the submandibular and sublingual glands are protected from external injury by the overlying mandible. The clinical significance of salivary trauma is related to the important anatomical structures that lie in the parotid bed, particularly the external carotid artery, the facial nerve and Stenson's duct. Diagnostic assessment of parotid injuries is better carried out with clinical exploration, CT (to depict the extent of damage in the salivary tissue and cervical spaces) and sialography (especially when doubt persists as to the possibility of parotid duct damage and presence of salivary fistulas) than with ultrasound.

In fact, the sonographic exploration of injured glands is of limited interest and can be difficult to perform in penetrating trauma. Occasionally, ultrasound may have a role when a fluid collection is present, following extravasion of saliva (sialocele) from the gland or hemorrhage from damaged vessels. Collections of saliva appear echo-free or filled with small echoes and present enhanced through-transmission of the beam. In such cases, ultrasound can guide percutaneous aspiration of these collections.[12]

Tumors

Tumors of the salivary glands are relatively rare. Their estimated incidence is less than 3 per 100 000 of total population, while representing about 5% of all head and neck tumors. Certain geographic variations have been reported and Eskimos show the highest prevalence of disease. Tumors are more common in the parotid (85%) than in submandibular (12%) and sublingual (3%) glands. Benign lesions, essentially adenomas, account for 85–90% of all parotid tumors. On the other hand, all submandibular tumors should be considered suspicious, as malignancy is more frequent (33%) in the submandibular glands.[21]

Tumors of the salivary glands can be imaged easily by ultrasound. The main objectives of ultrasound examination of a palpable mass are (a) to assess the presence of a nodule, (b) to distinguish between intra- and extraglandular lesions, (c) to predict whether the nodule is benign or malignant, (d) to indicate, if possible, the relationship between nodule and facial nerve and (e) to perform a local staging of the mass.

Ultrasound has proven high sensitivity (nearly 95–98%) in identifying parotid tumors, even when they are small and non-palpable on presentation.[4] Nevertheless, space-occupying lesions may be overlooked when sited in the retropharyngeal portion of the parotid gland (5%), because they are masked by the acoustic shadow of the mandible, or when they are contiguous to the base of the skull. In these cases, CT or MRI can identify the nodule better than sialography.[22] It must be noted that the specificity of ultrasound is lower than its sensitivity, as inflamed lymph nodes, abscesses and a number of chronic diseases of the salivary glands – including tuberculosis, sarcoidosis and Sjögren's syndrome – can present with non-neoplastic nodules that cannot be differentiated from neoplasms on the basis of imaging findings alone.[4,23]

The correct localization of a palpable mass, either within or outside the salivary gland, is easy to perform with ultrasound (98% accuracy), except for nodules located in the jugulodigastric region, because the capsular outlines of the glands are rarely seen.[4] For this purpose, color Doppler supports conventional ultrasound through the demonstration of the source of feeding vessels entering the nodule.[9] It must be noted that nodules located outside salivary glands are most commonly enlarged lymph nodes.

Identification of the nature of a salivary tumor may be more difficult and ultrasound has not always proved to be conclusive in differentiating benign from malignant lesions and in correlating histopathology with a specific imaging appearance of the tumor. Generally, this reflects the fact that benign and malignant tumors may share similar features and benign tumors cannot be easily distinguished from low-grade malignancies. However, some features that may help to narrow the differential diagnosis have been reported already in the literature and the combined use of high-frequency probes and color Doppler has the potential to improve the predictive values of ultrasound in characterizing salivary nodules.

The most common (60–70%) tumor of salivary glands is the pleomorphic adenoma, also termed 'mixed tumor'. It is a benign, sometimes multicentric, slow-growing tumor composed of epithelial cells and varying proportions of mucoid, chondroid and myxoid tissue. Approximately 90% of these tumors occur in the superficial lobe of the parotid gland and thus ultrasound is an ideal method by which to image it. Sonographically, pleomorphic adenoma presents with a homogeneous solid hypoechoic structure, sharp margins and discrete posterior acoustic enhancement (Fig. 8.14A).[5,6,11] It is never associated with enlarged cervical lymph nodes. In a number of cases, the tumor surface is lobulated and peripheral echo-free areas can be observed as a consequence of hemorrhagic or cystic degeneration.[3] Pleomorphic adenomas present on color Doppler with a peripheral 'basket-like' pattern of flow (Fig. 8.14B), consisting of a fine vascular network surrounding the nodule with various extensions, from which many fine branches direct centripetally.[9] The basket-like pattern of flow has been also described in a variety of either benign or malignant tumors of other organs and has been related to the growing tumors, which continually incorporate the vasculature of the host within themselves.[24] Alternatively, some pleomorphic adenomas do not show any detectable peripheral or intranodular signals. The absence of tumor signals seems unrelated to nodule size. The possibility of malignant transformation of a pleomorphic adenoma

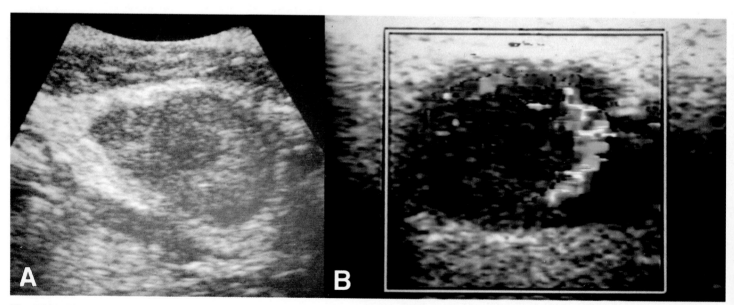

Fig. 8.14 Pleomorphic adenoma. Typically, this tumor presents with homogeneous hypoechoic structure, well-defined margins (**A**) and peripheral color flow pattern (**B**).

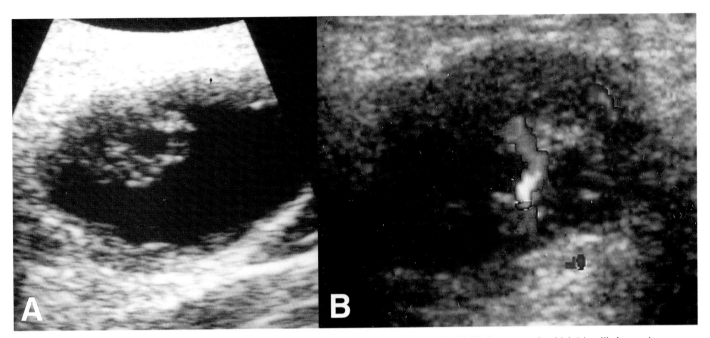

Fig. 8.15 Different aspects of parotid adenolymphoma. **A** Mixed structure with prevalence of fluid-filled spaces and a thick 'ring-like' septation. **B** Solid structure, with a single vessel pedicle entering the nodule at the echogenic hilum.

remains controversial. However, the occurrence of blurred margins, internal heterogeneity and changes of growing rate in a bioptically confirmed pleomorphic adenoma must raise the suspicion of malignancy and consequently needs further biopsies.[3] After resection, pleomorphic adenomas tend to recur locally. In these cases, sonographic examination may be difficult, owing to postoperative scarring and remodelling of salivary tissue.

Adenolymphoma, also termed cystadenoma lymphomatosum or Warthin's tumor, accounts for 6–10% of all salivary tumors. Bilateral presentation of this benign tumor is relatively rare (5%) in the parotids and recurrences are uncommon: both elements are typical of this tumor.

Sonographically, parotid adenolymphoma is hypoechoic with sharp margins but appears less homogeneous than pleomorphic adenoma. Commonly, it has a mixed structure because it contains one or more cystic areas which produce a well-defined posterior acoustic enhancement (Fig. 8.15A).[4–6,11] When cystic areas are prevalent, septations can be demonstrated. A hilar disposition of flow signals, consisting of vessels that enter the nodule through a single or multiple pedicles and that are distributed regularly within the tumor, is most commonly observed (Fig. 8.15B).[9] When the tumor has a mixed structure, flow signals are obtained from the solid portions of the nodule and within septations. A peripheral disposition of tumor vessels, similar to that observed in pleomorphic adenomas, occurs rarely.

Among the rare benign tumors of salivary glands, lipomas and hemangiomas present with a typical sonographic appearance. Lipomas are compressible oval or elliptical masses with regular margins and the typical striped and feathered echotexture (Fig. 8.16). They are more echogenic than the other salivary tumors and in most cases ultrasound suffices for correct diagnosis.[4] However, the suggestion of lipoma can easily be confirmed by CT or MRI, owing to the fat content of the mass. Ultrasound may be helpful in defining whether the mass is located inside the gland or superficial to it, within the subcutaneous tissue. Similar to findings in other sites, no flow signals are usually detected with color Doppler in lipomas of salivary glands.[9] This finding is in accordance with the relative histologic paucity of vascularization in this kind of lesions. Hem-

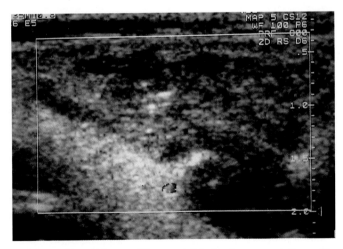

Fig. 8.16 Parotid lipoma. The mass is lobulated on presentation, with sharp margins and the typical striped echostructure. No intratumor flow signals are detectable with color Doppler.

angiomas are mainly observed in children. Sonographically, they are compressible masses with ill-defined margins and may have a complex 'honeycomb' appearance.[5] Color Doppler can identify slow flow within the lacunar portions of the mass.

A variety of malignant tumors can develop in the salivary glands. Most are primitive epithelial lesions including different histologic types, such as mucoepidermoid carcinoma, adenoid cystic carcinoma (cylindroma), epidermoid (squamous cell) carcinoma, acinic cell tumor, adenocarcinoma and undifferentiated carcinoma. Metastases and lymphomas occur rarely. Clinically, all malignant tumors present as fixed, hard masses possibly associated with ipsilateral cervical lymphadenopathies and facial nerve paralysis. Mucoepidermoid carcinoma has a marked tendency to spread into adjacent tissues; adenoid cystic carcinoma tends to infiltrate facial nerve and its branches; undifferentiated carcinoma tends to massive invasion of cervical spaces and encasement of large vessels of the neck. Generally, the malignant nature of advanced (>2 cm) lesions is easily assessed by ultrasound.[4] Large masses have a heterogeneous structure and occasionally a complex internal pattern due to irregular, fluid-filled spaces caused by necrosis or hemorrhage.[3] However, the best indication of their malignant and infiltrative nature is the absence of sharply defined margins (Fig. 8.17A,B).[3,4] Analysis of this feature is possible with small-parts transducers in almost every case, except for those involving deeply located tumors and small nodules. When the tumor is close to adjacent structures (i.e. muscles, skin layers), it may be attached to them as a sign of extraglandular infiltration.

According to Gritzmann,[4] the combination of clinical and ultrasound features has 94% accuracy in differentiating benign from malignant salivary tumors. However, up to 28% of all malignant tumors, and mainly metastases and lymphomas, have distinct margins and thus cannot be differentiated from benign lesions on the basis of the ultrasound appearance only. In addition, early cancers (<2 cm) may appear well encapsulated and homogeneous. In these cases, a careful correlation with clinical findings and meticulous search for enlarged cervical nodes may be helpful to identify malignancy. Recently, color Doppler has been proposed as an additional tool for predicting malignancy.[9,25] In fact, with the exception of non-Hodgkin lymphomas which show a single vessel pedicle which enters and branches into the nodule through a single hilum, most primary and metastatic malignancies of the salivary glands are hypervascular on presentation, with multiple feeder vessels entering the mass and branching irregularly within it. The extent of internal flow is usually much greater than in benign lesions and the arterial velocity can be markedly higher (Fig. 8.17C). Prospectively, in small tumors presenting without definite malignant changes at ultrasound, a hypervascular pattern could alert the clinician that malignancy could be present, regardless of both clinical and morphological presentation. Furthermore, it may be argued that the use of color Doppler could mean that, in the future, FNAB would be used in the assessment of hypervascular lesions only. However, further experience is needed to establish the ultimate utility of color Doppler in this field.

Local staging of malignant tumors can be efficiently carried out by ultrasound in most cases. Difficulties should be encountered only when evaluating the spread of large tumors to deep structures that ultrasound cannot image effectively.[3,6] In these cases, CT and MRI are the modalities of choice.[22,26] Color Doppler may be helpful to perform

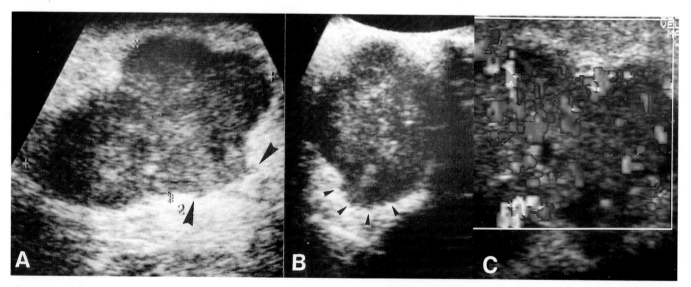

Fig. 8.17   Malignant tumors of parotid gland. **A, B** Mucoepidermoid carcinoma presents with heterogeneous structure and irregular margins (arrowheads). **C** Adenocarcinoma shows internal hypervascularity with diffuse and irregularly distributed color flow signals.

vascular staging, since the growing mass can displace or incorporate large vessels running inside the gland or located close to it, thus causing them to become stenotic or occluded.[9,27] In parotid tumors, evaluation of the relationship between the mass and the intraglandular portion of facial nerve may be possible with high-resolution probes.

Although nerve infiltration can be demonstrated occasionally, it seems much more difficult to rule out involvement of the nerve entirely.[6] However, gadolinium-enhanced MRI seems able to give better results than ultrasound in this respect.[26]

REFERENCES

1. Gooding G A W 1980 Gray scale ultrasound of the parotid gland. AJR 134: 469–472
2. Ballerini G, Mantero M, Sbrocca M 1984 Ultrasonic patterns of parotid masses. JCU 12: 273–277
3. Bruneton J N, Normand F, Santini N, Balu-Maestro C 1987 Salivary glands. In: Bruneton J N (ed) Ultrasonography of the neck. Springer-Verlag, Berlin, pp 64–80
4. Gritzmann N 1989 Sonography of the salivary glands. AJR 153: 161–166
5. Candiani F, Sponga T 1985 Ghiandole salivari. In: Rizzatto G, Solbiati L (eds) Ecografia clinica delle strutture superficiali. Masson Italia, Milan, pp 35–46
6. Derchi L E, Solbiati L 1993 Salivary glands. In: Cosgrove D, Meire H, Dewbury K (eds) Abdominal and general ultrasound. Churchill Livingstone, Edinburgh, pp 677–681
7. Moore K L 1985 Clinically oriented anatomy, 2nd edn. Williams and Wilkins, Baltimore
8. Bradley M J, Ahuja A, Metreweli C 1991 Sonographic evaluation of the parotid ducts: its use in tumour localization. Br J Radiol 64: 1092
9. Martinoli C, Derchi L E, Solbiati L, Giannoni M 1994 Color Doppler imaging of salivary glands. Proc Am Roentgen Ray Soc New Orleans, 24–29 April 1994 (in press)
10. Bartlett L J, Pon M 1984 High-resolution real-time ultrasonography of the submandibular salivary glands. J Ultrasound Med 3: 433–437
11. Cardinale A, Lagalla R, Sanna G, Laconi A 1989 Diagnostica per immagini delle ghiandole salivari. Idelson, Napoli
12. Maragam D, Gooding G A W 1981 Ultrasonic guided aspiration of parotid abscesses. Arch Otolaryngol 107: 546–549
13. Rubaltelli L, Sponga T, Candiani F, Pittarello F, Andretta M 1987 Infantile recurrent sialectatic parotitis: the role of sonography and sialography in diagnosis and follow-up. Br J Radiol 60: 1211–1214
14. Vitali C, Bombardieri S, Moutsopoulos H M et al 1993 Preliminary criteria for the classification of Sjögren's syndrome. Arthritis Rheum 36: 340–347
15. De Vita S, Lorenzon G, Rossi G, Sabella M, Fossaluzza V 1992 Salivary gland echography in primary and secondary Sjögren's syndrome. Clin Exp Rheumatol 10: 351–355
16. Bradus R J, Hybarger P, Gooding G A W 1988 Parotid glands: US findings in Sjögren's syndrome. Radiology 169: 749–751
17. Takashima S, Morimoto S, Tomiyama N, Takeuchi N, Ikezoe J, Kozuka T 1992 Sjögren's syndrome: comparison of sialography and ultrasonography. JCU 20: 99–103
18. Blatt I M, Rubin P 1956 Secretory sialography in diseases of the major salivary glands. Ann Otol 65: 295–317
19. Gritzmann N 1994 Sonography of the extrathyroidal cervical soft tissues, the salivary glands and floor of the mouth. Eur J Ultrasound 1: 9–21
20. Steiner E, Lakitis A, Mostbeck G, Hitzelhammer J, Graninger W, Franz P 1993 Color Doppler of the parotid gland in Sjögren's syndrome. Proc 8th Eur Congr Radiol, Vienna, 12–17 Sept 1993. Eur Radiol 3 (suppl.): 196, Abstract 794
21. Thackray A C, Lucas R B 1974 Tumors of the major salivary glands. Atlas of tumor pathology, 2nd series. AFIP, Washington DC
22. Whyte A M, Byrne J V 1987 A comparison of computed tomography and ultrasound in the assessment of parotid masses. Clin Radiol 38: 339–343
23. Iko B O, Chinwuba C E, Myers E M, Teal J S 1986 Sarcoidosis of the parotid gland. Br J Radiol 59: 547–552
24. Tanaka S, Kitamura T, Fujita M, Nakanishi K, Okuda S 1990 Color Doppler flow imaging of liver tumors. AJR 154: 509–514
25. Schick S, Steiner E, Turetschek K, Grasl M, Franz P, Mostbeck G 1993 Color Doppler sonography of parotid tumors. Proc 8th Eur Congr Radiol Vienna, 12–17 Sept 1993. Eur Radiol 3 (suppl.): 196. Abstract 793
26. Vogl T J, Dresel S H J, Späth M et al 1990 Parotid gland: plain and gadolinium-enhanced MR imaging. Radiology 177: 667–674
27. Ajayi B A, Pugh N D, Carolan G 1992 Salivary gland tumours: is color Doppler imaging of added value in their preoperative assessment? Eur J Surg Oncol 18: 463–469

9

Breast

R. Chersevani   H. Tsunoda-Shimizu

G. M. Giuseppetti   G. Rizzatto

TECHNIQUE FOR PERFORMING BREAST SONOGRAPHY

The technology available for diagnostic ultrasound is discussed in Chapter 1. This chapter therefore starts with some suggestions on how to perform a correct ultrasound examination of the breast.[1-3]

The patient is supine, with arms extended behind her head. The breast is flattened over the chest wall and must not be shifted by the probe during scanning. Where the breasts are large, the outer and inner quadrants can be scanned by rolling the patient to either side – to the left to examine the outer quadrants of the right breast and to the right to examine the outer quadrants of the left breast. Conversely, the inner quadrants of large breasts are better scanned by rolling the patient on to the same side as the breast to be examined. The extended arms raise the breast and allow a better examination of the lower quadrants and of the inframammary fold. The sitting position has also been suggested, not only for its similarity to the craniocaudal view in mammography, but also to avoid nipple attenuation masking the subareolar region. The supine position is widely used, except for upper quadrant masses that are occasionally more evident in the sitting position. A supine patient is more relaxed, moves less and the examiner has a better control of the hand-held probe while scanning. The subareolar region can be adequately imaged also in the supine patient by using a greater amount of coupling gel, by applying compression to the nipple and with oblique scans alongside the nipple.

The whole breast is examined, from the anterior/midaxillary line and the axillary tail to the lateral portion of the sternum, and from the inframammary fold to the peripheral portions of the upper quadrants. Sonography has no limitation in examining the peripheral portions of the breast, that may not be easily imaged with conventional mammographic views. Longitudinal and transverse scans are coupled with radial scanning, around the areola, for a better demonstration of breast ducts, along the line of their main axis. Gain and focus must be adjusted to the area of interest.

Probe rotation, along different scanning planes, is important for the evaluation of both normal and abnormal findings (Fig. 9.1); furthermore, orthogonal scanning

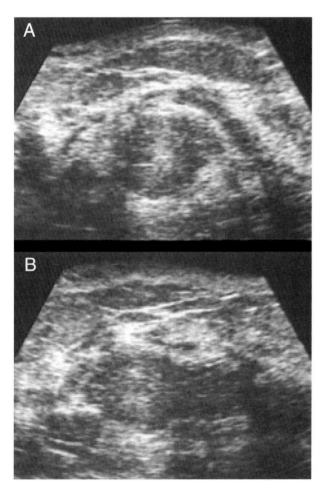

Fig. 9.1 With probe rotation a pseudonodule (**A**) elongates and is a fat lobule in a fatty breast (**B**).

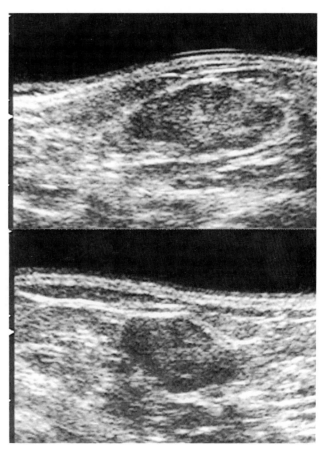

Fig. 9.2 Orthogonal scans of a fibroadenoma to evaluate shape and size.

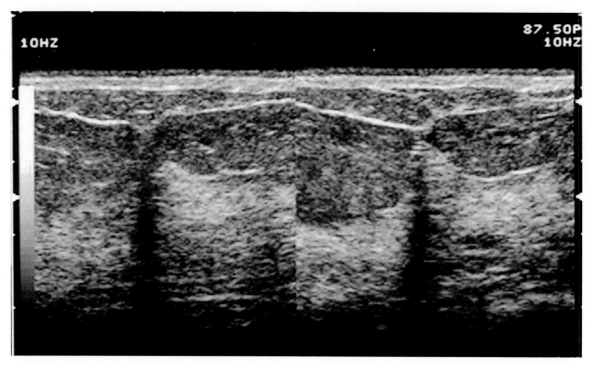

Fig. 9.3 Compression modifies acoustic shadowing due to Cooper's ligaments (from left to right).

allows complete morphologic evaluation and accurate measurement of the size of a lesion (Fig. 9.2). Rotation also allows a thorough examination of the tissues at the periphery of a mass, in order to assess the type of growth, i.e. if a mass simply pushes the surrounding tissues or causes infiltration.

Another important point is compression. Compression, together with the coupling gel, allows contact between skin and probe, reduces the thickness of the area examined, so that deep lesions can be imaged, and prevents false acoustic shadowing (Figs 9.3, 9.4). Compression is also used to detect changes in shape of a lesion, for example whether a cyst becomes flattened (Fig. 9.5), or whether it appears to move while compressed inside the surrounding tissues, as

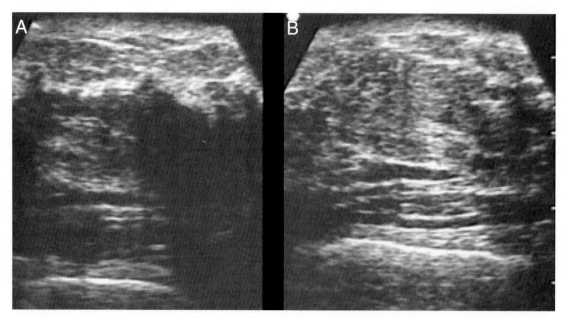

Fig. 9.4 Intense shadowing at the interface between subcutaneous fat and underlying breast parenchyma (**A**) is reduced by increasing compression (**B**).

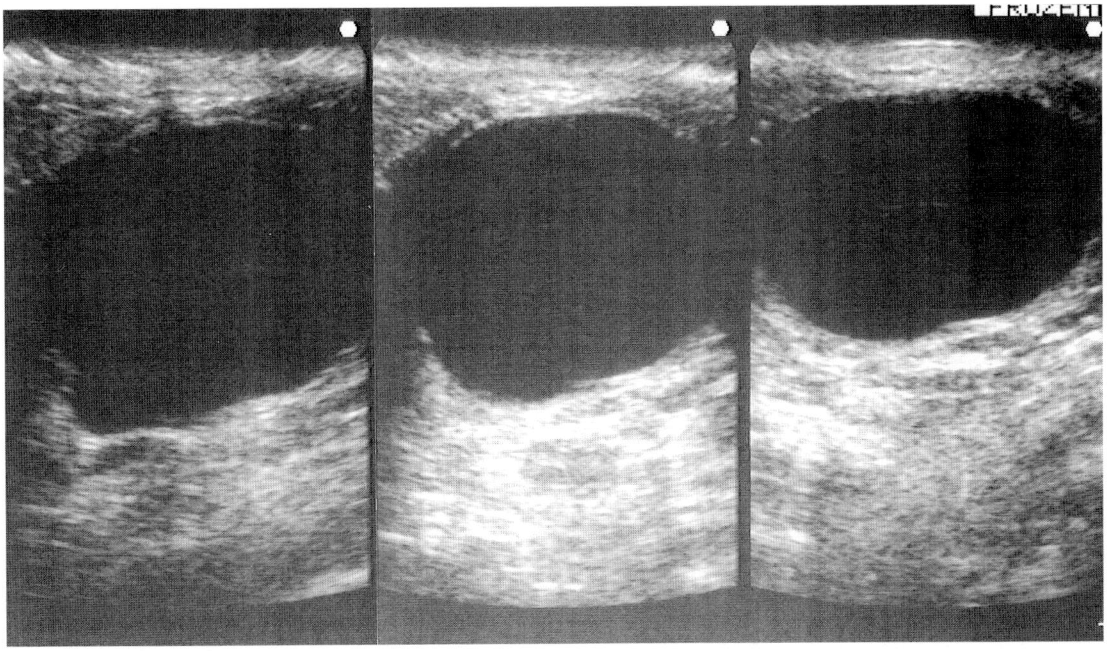

Fig. 9.5   Compression flattens a cyst.

in the case of a non-infiltrating mass such as a fibro-adenoma. Compression allows a better demonstration of tissue characteristics and shows moving echoes inside cysts with echogenic contents.

One final consideration is who should perform sonography. Breast sonography requires not only skill but also interest on the part of the examiner, who must have full knowledge of the patient's history and of the physical and mammographic findings. In our opinion, radiologists should conduct the ultrasound examinations, not merely supervise them, because they can coordinate all the information acquired previously and decide on further procedures.[1,4]

NORMAL SONOGRAPHIC ANATOMY AND PHYSIOLOGY

The breast is made up of 15–20 irregular lobes of branched tubuloalveolar glands. The lobes radiate from the nipple and subdivide into lobules. The gland is surrounded by subcutaneous connective tissue that forms septa between lobes and lobules, providing a support for the glandular elements. These septa, known as Cooper's ligaments, run from the dermis down to the pectoral fascia. Adipose tissue is also present among the lobes. All macroscopic breast structures can be easily imaged with adequate sonographic equipment.

The breast can be divided into four regions:[5]

- skin, nipple, subareolar tissues
- subcutaneous region
- parenchyma (between the subcutaneous and retro-mammary regions)
- retromammary region.

The skin is the superficial component of the breast and requires, for a correct evaluation, the use of high-resolution dedicated probes, associated with a stand-off pad where lower frequencies are employed. The sonographic pattern is a more or less homogeneous band that is more echogenic than the underlying fat tissue (Fig. 9.6). The normal skin thickness varies between 0.5 and 2 mm, and is usually maximum in the lower quadrants, toward the infra-mammary fold.

The nipple may be visualized as a rounded well-defined nodule, of medium echogenicity. Distal attenuation is due

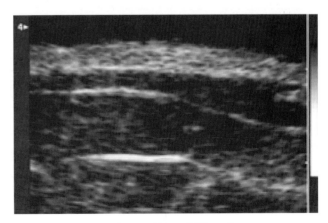

Fig. 9.6   Normal skin imaged with a 20 MHz probe.

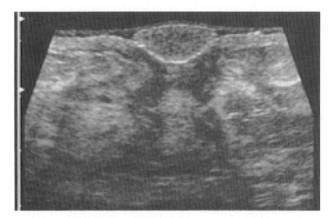

Fig. 9.7 Nipple with distal attenuation.

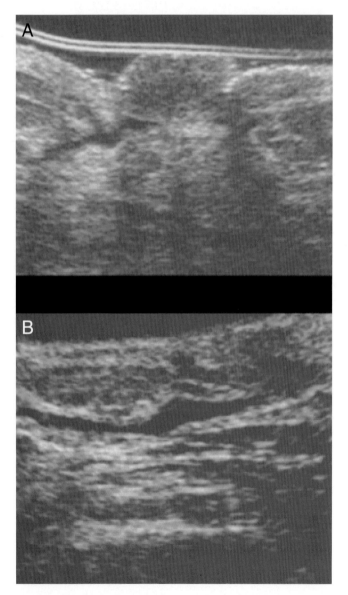

Fig. 9.8 Main ducts coming to the nipple (**A**) and dilatation at the level of the lactiferous sinus, close to the nipple (**B**).

to some degree to its fibrous structure, but also to the uneven surface of the nipple–areola complex, that precludes efficient contact with the scanning surface of most probes. Probes that have a soft rubber surface in contact with the skin result in less attenuation. With a correct examination, the subareolar tissues are usually echogenic, because subcutaneous fat is interrupted at this level (Fig. 9.7). Main ducts running to the nipple may be visualized as anechoic bands, with a progressively increasing diameter. The lactiferous sinus is the widest (up to 3 mm) portion of normal ducts and is located just behind the nipple (Fig. 9.8).

The subcutaneous region contains fat and lymphatics. Fat tissue is a normal component of the breast. It is localized in the subcutaneous layers, inside the breast parenchyma and in the retromammary area. No matter where it is situated, breast fat is always hypoechoic; that is, it is less echogenic than breast parenchyma. Subcutaneous fat is thicker than retromammary fat, up to 2 or 3 cm in thickness. It may be very thin or absent in patients with

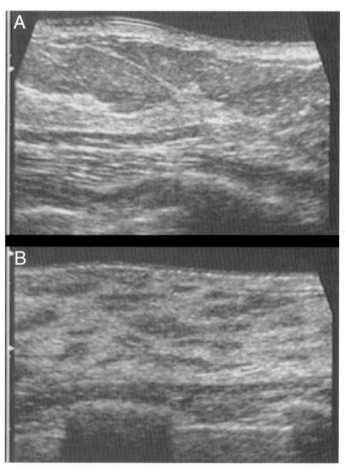

Fig. 9.9 Subcutaneous fat crossed by Cooper's ligament, a hyperechoic oblique line that disappears inside echogenic parenchyma; retromammary fat is thinner (**A**). Very dense, echogenic breast with no subcutaneous fat; echogenic pleural line between two ribs, that give attenuation (**B**).

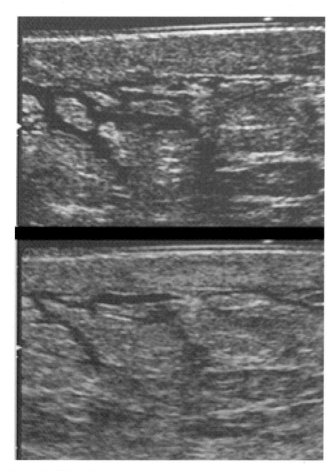

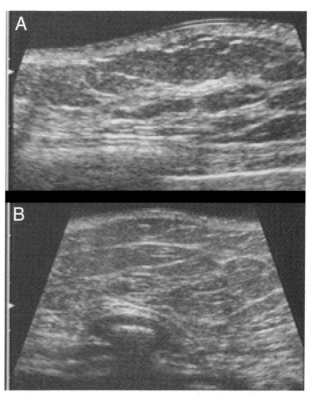

Fig. 9.11   Hypoechoic subcutaneous fat and lobules inside echogenic breast parenchyma (**A**). Fatty involution and totally hypoechoic breast crossed by Cooper's ligaments; axial scan over rib cartilage with shadowing due to calcifications (**B**).

Fig. 9.10   Dilated lymphatics in inflammatory carcinoma: thin, hypoechoic lines forming a network parallel and perpendicular to the skin.

very dense breasts. The subcutaneous fat is crossed by thin, echogenic lines, oblique to the skin surface, that represent Cooper's ligaments. These ligaments run from the skin to the pectoral fascia and are well visualized both in subcutaneous fat and in fatty breasts, with a regular orientation and in contrast with hypoechoic fat. They disappear inside the hyperechoic structure of breasts with a fibroglandular pattern (Fig. 9.9). Breast lymphatics form a microscopic network in the superficial areas of the breast, mainly between the skin and subcutaneous tissues and also along ducts. Normal lymphatics cannot be visualized, but in case of dilatation – caused by inflammation or carcinomatous infiltration as in inflammatory carcinoma – they can be visualized as hypo/anechoic thin lines, parallel and perpendicular to the skin, forming a network (Fig. 9.10).

The breast parenchyma is triangular in shape, with the apex towards the nipple and the base at the chest. The sonographic pattern varies with age and subject, and depends on the amount and type of contents, such as fatty, fibrous and glandular tissues. The fibrous and glandular components are variably echogenic, whereas fat is hypo-echoic, with the result that the breast parenchyma is not homogeneous. Fat may be represented as hypoechoic lobules inside echogenic fibroglandular tissue, and be rounded or oval, or it may be the main breast constituent in fatty involution, imaged as a completely hypoechoic breast crossed by the echogenic ligaments (Fig. 9.11). A breast with a predominantly fibrous structure is echogenic; a breast with a fibroglandular structure is inhomogeneous because of hypoechoic bands, coursing in a radial array around and towards the nipple, which represent the ductal pattern (Fig. 9.12). In younger women with a rich glandular component, the hypoechoic bands contain echogenic lines, better demonstrated when the longitudinal scan is along the main axis of the duct (Fig. 9.13). As the nipple is approached these lines progressively separate and delineate the peripheral ducts (Fig. 9.14). Breast ducts are visualized more easily with radial scans around the nipple as they branch in a dichotomous pattern (Fig. 9.15), and progressively increase in size, towards the lactiferous sinus, the widest portion of normal ducts (3 mm), located in the subareolar tissues (Fig. 9.8).

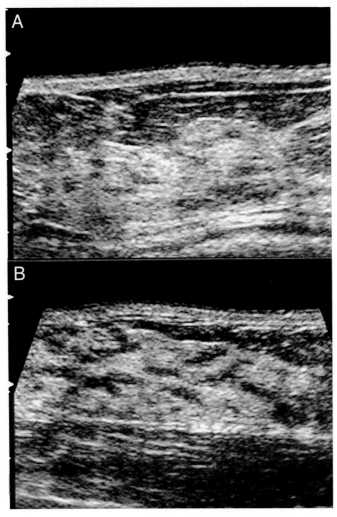

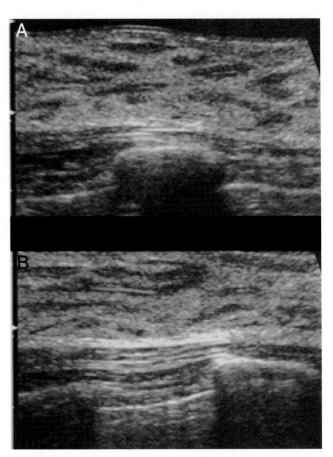

Fig. 9.13 Echogenic lines inside the ductal pattern of younger women (**A**). Longitudinal scan along the main axis of the duct; the pectoralis muscle, the shadowing ribs and the pleural line are clearly visible in the retromammary region (**B**).

Fig. 9.12 Echogenic breast with predominant fibrous structure (**A**). Inhomogeneous breast parenchyma with ductal pattern, very thin subcutaneous fat and fibrillary pattern of pectoralis muscle (**B**).

The blood supply to the breast originates from the intercostal, internal and external mammary, and subscapular arteries. Intramammary breast vessels can occasionally be visualized as tubular anechoic structures, with a more or less echogenic wall; veins have a more superficial location, parallel to the skin, and disappear if compression is too great (Fig. 9.16). There is a deep and superficial venous network with a variable individual pattern, although this is quite symmetrical in the two breasts. Color Doppler sonography can detect flow signals in the superficial portions of normal breasts in young women, and the signal has been reported to be more intense at the time of ovulation. The advent of very sensitive equipment, able to detect slow flows, has permitted the demonstration of vessels located at the periphery of the gland in a greater number of patients. The more recent method of power

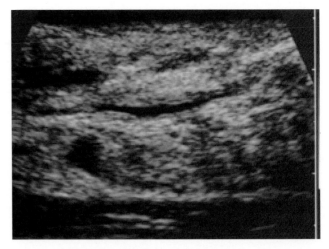

Fig. 9.14 Thin duct delineated by echogenic lines.

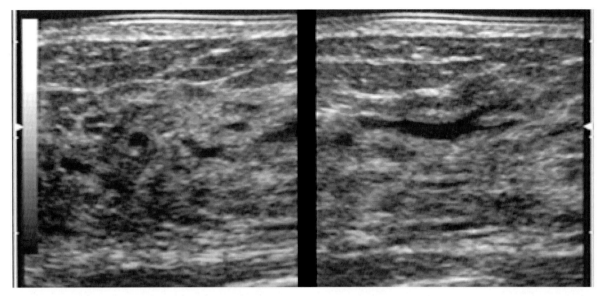

Fig. 9.15 Orthogonal scans on normal branching ducts.

Doppler, which images blood flow by mapping the density of blood cells rather than their velocity, and which is angle independent, permits a more spectacular demonstration of normal flow signals in the most superficial regions of the breast parenchyma, where a richer network of intersecting vessels can be demonstrated. Power Doppler is sensitive enough to detect blood flow signals in the deeper areas of breast parenchyma also (Figs 9.17–9.20). Visualization of the axillary vessels requires adequate scanning of the axilla. The internal mammary artery and vein can be visualized through longitudinal scans of the first and second intercostal spaces, parallel to the sternum (Fig. 9.21).

Intramammary lymph nodes can be demonstrated with sonography, and are more often located in the upper quadrants of the outer breast. Normal lymph nodes are elongated, with a hypoechoic rim surrounding an echogenic center which is the hilum of the node. The greatest diameter is usually less than 1 cm. Morphology changes according to the scanning plane. Although pathology remains the gold standard to rule out malignancy, ultrasound examination can provide some information on the size, shape and structure of the lymph nodes (Fig. 9.22). Color Doppler imaging can add information by showing blood flow at the hilum. Lymphatic drainage is to the axillary, subclavicular and internal mammary chain nodes, through penetrating lymphatics (Fig. 9.23); all these nodes can be easily demonstrated when enlarged.

The retromammary region consists of retromammary

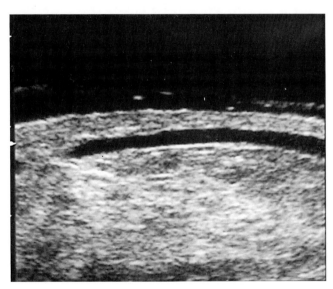

Fig. 9.16 A peripheral vein imaged with B-mode sonography.

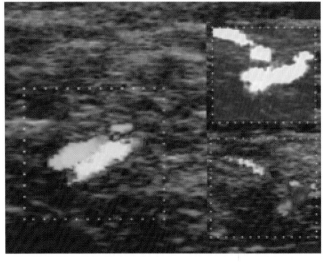

Fig. 9.17 Vessels imaged with color and power Doppler. Color Doppler shows different flow direction.

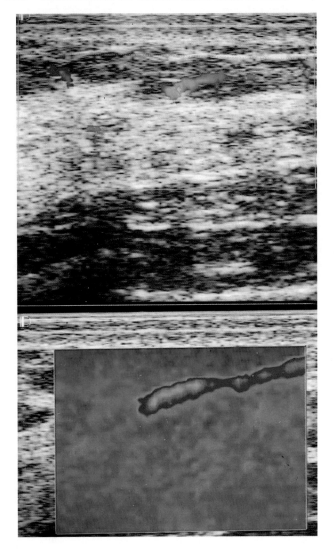

Fig. 9.18 Color Doppler and power Doppler of superficial vessels. The signal is much more intense with power Doppler.

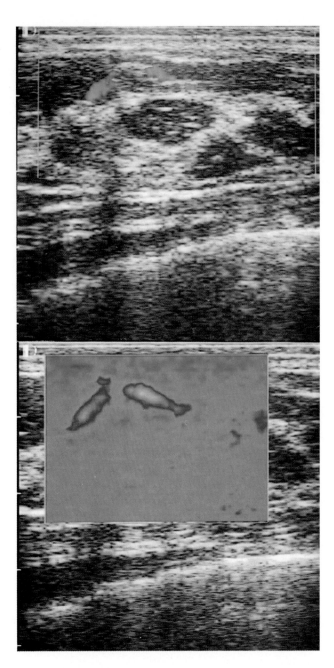

Fig. 9.19 Superficial vessels imaged with color and power Doppler.

fat, the pectoralis muscle, ribs, intercostal muscles and the pleural reflection.

Retromammary fat tissue is a hypoechoic band, having a structure similar to that of subcutaneous fat tissue, but thinner. The deep fascia cannot be visualized. The pectoralis muscle lies just behind the retromammary fat and has a fibrillary pattern. The identification of this muscle is a guarantee that the whole depth of the gland is being examined. The ribs are easily identified by their location and morphology, which changes according to the scanning plane. An axial scan on a rib shows an oval, hypoechoic formation, that cannot be mistaken for a nodule because it

is located underneath the muscle. Even the cartilaginous portion of the ribs produces some distal attenuation that increases where calcification has taken place, resembling a target. The intercostal muscles can be identified in the spaces among the ribs and show a muscular pattern. The echogenic reflection of the pleural line, which shifts during respiration, is the deepest structure that can be identified (Figs 9.9, 9.11–9.13).

The sonographic pattern of breast parenchyma varies with age and parity, and differs among individual subjects, in the same condition, according to the amount of fat, glandular and connective tissue, as previously mentioned.

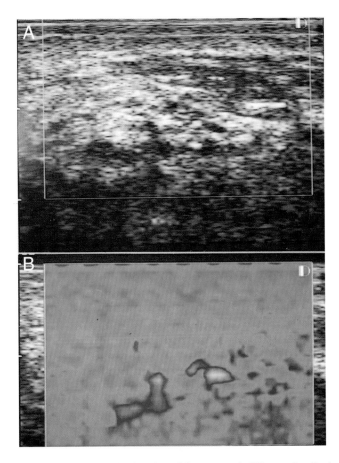

Fig. 9.20 Power Doppler imaging of deeper vessels (B), not visualized with B-mode sonography.

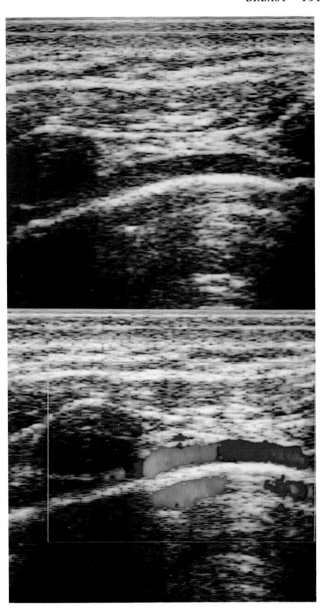

Fig. 9.21 Internal mammary artery imaged with B-mode (A) and color Doppler. The pleural line is clearly visible underneath the vessel.

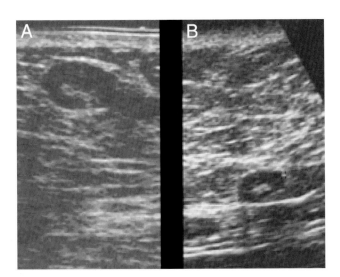

Fig. 9.22 Superficial (A) and deeply located lymph nodes (B), with echogenic hilum.

In addition, the mammary gland is stimulated by a variety of hormones at different times of life.

At puberty, estrogens stimulate the development of ducts, and of glandular and connective tissue: a circumscribed, hypoechoic area may be demonstrated, and it may be asymmetric with the contralateral breast (Fig. 9.24). The changes that occur during the menstrual cycle, i.e. an increase in size, density, nodularity and tenderness of the breast in the second half of the cycle, do not have a significant effect on the sonographic pattern, although increased echogenicity due to edema is sometimes detected, and improves the visualization of solid or liquid masses.

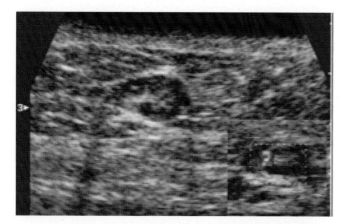

Fig. 9.23 Axillary lymph node imaged also with color Doppler.

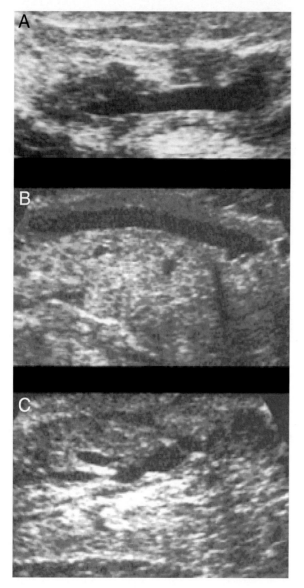

Fig. 9.25 Sonographic pattern of lobules surrounding ducts during pregnancy (**A**). During lactation, breast parenchyma is very echogenic, with no fat and increased vascularization; (**B**): reduced compression to show the vein causes superficial artifacts; dilated ducts (**C**).

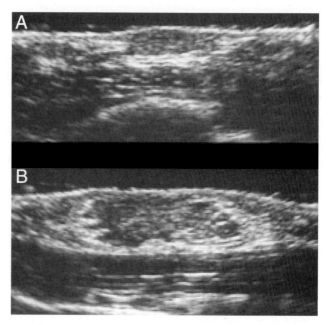

Fig. 9.24 Asymmetric breast development at puberty: the young patient was referred for a palpable lump of the left breast (**B**).

A more thorough change occurs during pregnancy, with the development of alveoli and tubules. A lobular pattern is seen around ducts that are enlarging. During lactation the breast parenchyma becomes intensely and diffusely echogenic, with thinning of subcutaneous fat; dilated ducts, slightly echogenic owing to their milk content, can be visualized (Fig. 9.25).

Fatty involution cannot be considered a condition typical of menopause. Glandular atrophy and increase in fat content is very often encountered in elderly women, but it is also a frequent and therefore a normal variant of the reproductive period. In the latter cases no macroscopic glandular tissue can be identified, either by mammography or by ultrasound examination; with pregnancy an increase in the glandular component replacing fat, takes place. After lactation, fatty involution may again occur in these patients. It may be that the term involution should not be used, and we should describe the breasts only as fatty, glandular or fibroglandular.

Sonography can easily define the type of breast and can predict the mammographic pattern we shall find in the case of young women undergoing mammography after sonography.

ABERRATIONS OF NORMAL DEVELOPMENT AND INVOLUTION (ANDI) AND BENIGN BREAST CHANGES (BBC)

A number of clinical presentations, such as excessive breast development, cyclical nodularity and generalized or discrete mastalgia, represent a frequent cause of the referral of patients for breast imaging. The mammographic pattern usually associated with these clinical findings is that of increased density of the breast and the radiologist normally will relate this increased density to the patient's physical findings and symptoms. However, other patients with the same type of dense breast may be asymptomatic. Furthermore, the same clinical findings and symptoms may be present in women that do not present with a dense breast or that display different breast patterns. A second consideration is that, besides the 'normal' mammogram, there are several quite distinct variants, that must represent normal and not pathological phenomena, as they can be found to some degree in 80–90% of women.[6] The need to provide a morphological explanation for these patients' symptoms has prompted the use of terms taken from pathology, such as dysplasia, adenosis, mastosis, mastopathy, fibrocystic disease, fibroadenosis, chronic cystic mastitis and so on, that have been termed 'a ragbag'.[6] The proposal of the generic term ANDI – aberrations of normal development and involution[7] – has explained many breast conditions, offering a spectrum of changes from an ideal normal appearance, through minor variations, to situations so far from normality as to be considered as benign breast changes (BBC). Although the exact point of separation between disease and non-disease in not easy to define, the diagnosis of a benign breast abnormality or of a variant is important, first because it rules out cancer, and secondly because it gives the patient an explanation of her breast problems. Indeed, every breast consultant (senologist) knows that a symptomatic patient shows relief when she is told that she does not have cancer, but at the same time she wants to know what is wrong with her breast, and is gratified by some sort of diagnosis.

The following is a description of ANDI and BBC according to age.[6]

In the early reproductive period (15–25 years), the aberration in the normal process of lobule formation can produce fibroadenomas, that can result in a disease state if they are multiple or giant. In the same age group, an aberration of stroma formation may cause excessive breast development or juvenile hypertrophy.

In the mature reproductive period (25–40 years), the cyclical hormonal effects on glandular tissue and stroma can become exaggerated and cause cyclical nodularity, with generalized or discrete mastalgia.

In the involution phase (35–55 years), the normal process of lobular involution (that includes pathologic findings such as microcysts, apocrine changes, fibrosis and adenosis) can produce aberrations that result in macrocysts and sclerosing lesions. The latter include conditions such as radial scar, sclerosing adenosis and complex sclerosing lesions. The clinical presentation of these changes includes palpable lumps and masses, mastalgia, and frequent X-ray abnormalities.

In the same age group, the aberration of ductal involution causes duct dilatation and periductal fibrosis due to periductal infiltrates: the clinical presentation is nipple discharge and retraction. The resulting disease state is breast inflammation (periductal mastitis), with bacterial infection and abscess formation.

Another normal process of the involution phase is an epithelial turnover, aberration of which results in a mild or moderate epithelial hyperplasia, and a consequent disease state of florid epithelial hyperplasia and epithelial hyperplasia with atypia. The significance of hyperplasia has been clearly assessed by the American College of Pathology's Consensus Statement of 1986.[8] No matter what attempts are made to correlate these histologic reports to macroscopic findings of breast imaging, hyperplasia can be ascertained only with histology.

Hormonal replacement therapy is frequently prescribed in postmenopausal women, to reduce symptoms and prevent osteoporosis. An increase in the risk of breast cancer has not been shown, but hormonal replacement therapy can cause mammographic changes, which decrease the sensitivity of mammography in the early detection of breast carcinoma and require additional evaluation to exclude malignant changes. The mammographic changes in women on hormonal replacement therapy are a diffuse increase in density, due to an increase of fibroglandular tissue, asymmetric densities, and enlargement or development of fibroadenomas and of cysts.[9,10]

Sonography has a fundamental role in defining breast alterations both in the early reproductive period, when US represents the main and sometimes only imaging modality, as well as in the mature reproductive period and during involution, when it is a useful adjunct to mammography.

As already mentioned, patients of the mature reproductive period that display mastalgia and cyclical nodularity usually show a mammographic pattern of more or less homogeneous increased density. In such cases sonography can evaluate the area of tenderness and palpable masses, guided by the previous mammographic findings. The sonographic pattern is that of increased echogenicity, due to an increase in the fibrous component of the breast (Fig. 9.26). Increased echogenicity may be diffused or localized, and more or less homogeneous. The hyperechoic area may have well circumscribed borders, corresponding to a palpable mass and to a dense well-circumscribed opacity on the mammogram. The finding corresponds to what has been defined as a plaque, more often located in the upper–outer quadrants (Fig. 9.27). These hyperechoic areas may be homogeneous or contain a ductal pattern. The association of mammography and sonography is helpful in these patients as it rules out a palpable carcinoma and explains these patients' symptoms as exaggerated hormonal cyclical effects. The hyperechoic breast may be inhomogeneous because of small cysts – anechoic, well-defined formations, with increased sound through-transmission – and also because of similar formations with an elongated

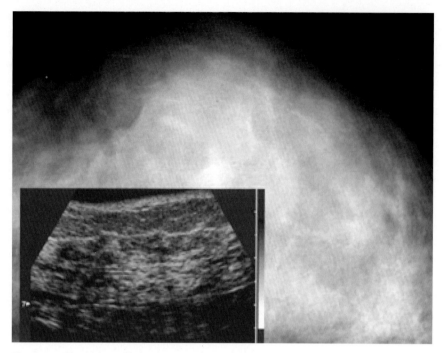

Fig. 9.26   The increased breast density on the mammogram corresponds to an echogenic pattern.

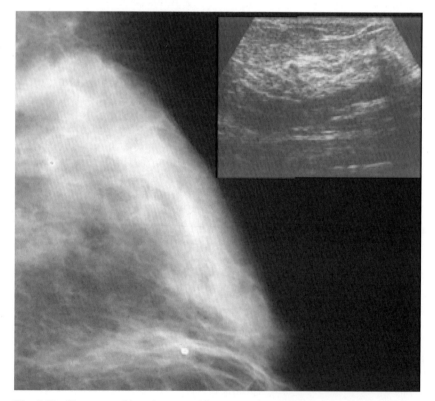

Fig. 9.27   Mammographic and sonographic pattern of a palpable lump that corresponds to a well-circumscribed plaque of echogenic fibroglandular tissue.

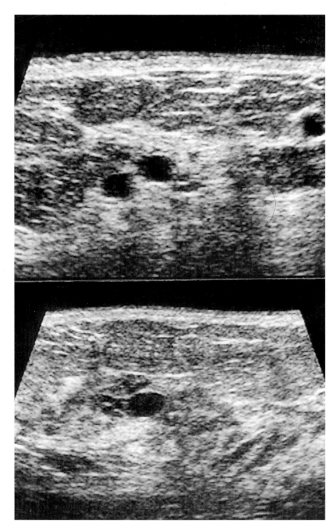

Fig. 9.28 Tiny cysts and slightly dilated ducts in patient with mastalgia.

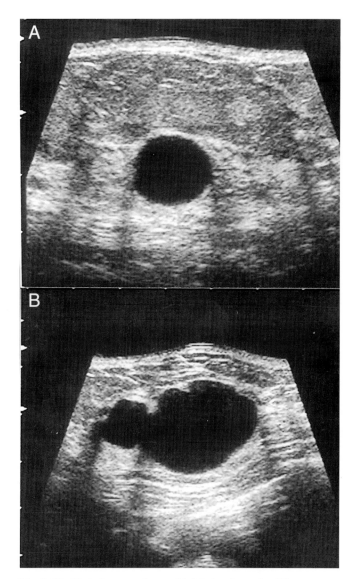

Fig. 9.29 Typical cysts and cyst with lobulated margins (**B**).

shape, that represent initially dilated ducts (Fig. 9.28). It is difficult to determine the boundary between this pattern and the cysts and dilated ducts present in the involution phase. Further discussion of cysts and dilated ducts is found later in this Chapter. Hypoechoic, rounded nodules, with variable sound transmission, are frequently found in these breasts. They represent either small cysts, with echogenic contents, or hypoechoic fat lobules inside the fibrotic breast parenchyma, or the ductal pattern of normal breast parenchyma, scanned axially, end-on. In such cases probe rotation can identify the ductal pattern (Fig. 9.12).

Cysts

Cysts are a very common finding in women during the involution phase (35–50 years of age), but are very rare in women younger than 25 or older than 60 years. Cysts usually regress after menopause, but may increase in number and size during hormone replacement therapy.

The size of cysts varies from a few millimeters up to 5–6 centimeters. Cysts are more often multiple and bilateral, and may develop or regress in a very short time. When visible on the mammogram, the pattern is that of a well-circumscribed opacity; otherwise, they may show as areas of increased, often asymmetric opacity.

The sonographic pattern of a cyst is very well known. The first enthusiastic findings in breast sonography were of cysts and for a long time the only role for this technique has been the solid/liquid differentiation of a mammographic opacity or of a palpable mass.

The criteria for the sonographic diagnosis of a typical or simple cyst are a rounded or oval, compressible, anechoic lesion, with well-defined borders, a bright posterior wall and enhanced sound transmission (Fig. 9.29). When all

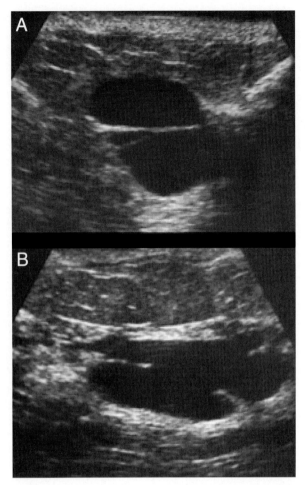

Fig. 9.30 Cysts compressing one another (**A**) and with septations (**B**).

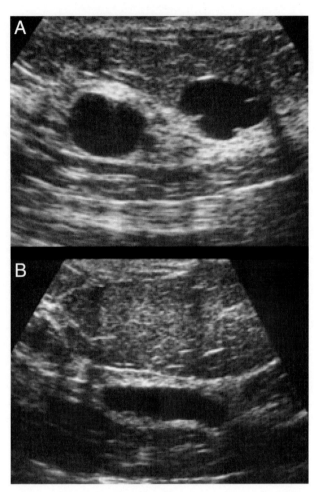

Fig. 9.31 Cysts of different shapes. The upper one (**A**) has echogenic contents and no enhanced sound transmission; deep flattened cyst (**B**).

these criteria are fulfilled, the accuracy of diagnosis is 100% and no further diagnostic procedures are required unless the cyst is symptomatic. Cysts are compressible and this is particularly true with cysts that are not under tension, and the shape of which is modified not only under the pressure of the probe, but also by other nearby cysts. The shape becomes polygonal and the cystic walls may be mistaken for septations. Cysts may also be loculated and contain septations (Fig. 9.30). In some conditions there is no enhancement of sound transmission: these include small cysts with low-level echoes, cysts located close to the pectoral muscle, cysts with a fibrotic wall, or cysts situated in tissues having an increased echogenicity (Fig. 9.31). Lateral shadows may form from the beam's refraction along the lateral borders of a rounded cyst.

A few technical considerations are important before approaching the differentiation between a typical and an atypical, or complex cyst. To avoid troublesome artifacts, gain and power settings must be adjusted and the area of interest must be correctly focused. Very superficial cysts may require a stand-off pad, to avoid near-field rever-

berations, and power or gain settings that are too high must be corrected, to reduce echoes in the anterior portion of a cyst. The same adjustments are useful to ascertain sound transmission.

The sonographic finding of cysts associated with dilated ducts is quite common: both conditions are typical of the involution phase (Fig. 9.32).

Atypical, complex cysts are characterized by a thickened wall and an echogenic content. Types of complicated cyst that can still be included among the aberrations of involution are cysts of long standing, cysts that redevelop after aspiration and those containing milk of calcium. Long-standing cysts are usually hypoechoic, with low-level echoes, some sound enhancement and a more or less thickened wall. Only the demonstration of moving echoes inside the cyst can ascertain a liquid nature. Otherwise the sonographic pattern is undistinguishable from that of a solid, homogeneous, non-attenuating, well-defined mass, and only FNAB will allow differentiation between a solid or liquid mass (Fig. 9.33). Cysts may redevelop after aspiration; this occurs in about 25% of cases and more often if

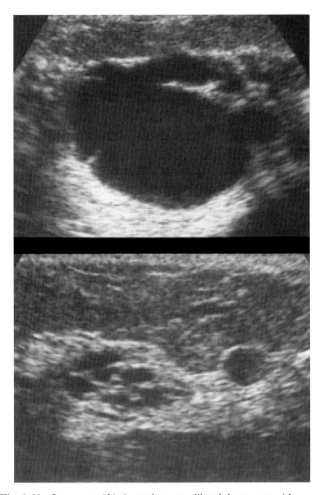

Fig. 9.32   Large cyst (**A**) situated among dilated ducts; cyst with echogenic contents (**B**) and dilated ducts.

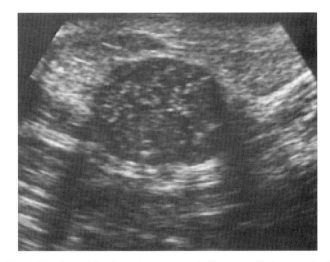

Fig. 9.33   Cyst with echogenic contents, similar to a well-circumscribed solid nodule.

aspiration is not complete. Recurrent cysts may also show a thickened blurred wall and an echogenic content. Another typically benign condition is that of cysts containing milk of calcium, that shows as bright, layering echoes (Figs 9.34, 9.35). Sedimented calcium is a benign entity that has a typical appearance also on the mammogram, where the shape of the calcifications changes according to the view: on the cranio-caudal view, milk of calcium is seen as an ill-defined smudge, that becomes linear, curvilinear or like a teacup on the lateral view. Milk of calcium can be found in cysts of any size and has been reported also in lipid cysts.[11]

Simple cysts can be left alone unless they are large, painful, palpable or are a cause of concern to the patient. In such cases aspiration is indicated.

The diagnosis of an atypical cyst is important because it represents abnormalities that require a totally different therapeutic approach. Atypical, complex cysts may be associated with inflammation, papilloma, or cancer, and are discussed later with these topics. Cancer may grow in a breast that has cysts, grow on the wall of a cyst or simply invade it from the outside. The cancer/cyst association is rare (0.5% of carcinomas) but must always be kept in mind in case of intracystic vegetations. Intracystic vegetations are benign in 75% of cases and usually represent papillomas, malignant in 20% of cases or due to borderline abnormalities, e.g. phyllodes, in the remaining 5%. An adequate US examination allows a correct evaluation not only of cystic contents and wall, but also of the surrounding tissues, so pneumocystography is not necessary. Nevertheless, it may be requested by the surgeon, who usually is more familiar with conventional imaging (Fig. 9.36). FNAB of the solid vegetation and examination of the cytologic specimen are the gold standard.

Sclerosing lesions

Sclerosing lesions represent an aberration of lobular involution, presenting with X-ray abnormalities. Breast sclerosing changes include conditions that are referred to as radial scar, sclerosing adenosis, obliterative mastitis and complex sclerosing lesions. These abnormalities are not correlated to trauma or inflammation. On the mammogram, radial scar is seen as a stellate area of density, with a radiolucent center or no central core. It usually occurs on one plane on the mammogram. Calcifications may be present. Sonography is fairly aspecific and may show sound attenuation due to the fibrous component or an echogenic area (Fig. 9.37). Biopsy differentiates the lesion from a stellate carcinoma.

Fibroadenoma

Fibroadenoma – a growth of fibrous and glandular tissue – is the most common benign tumor of the female breast.

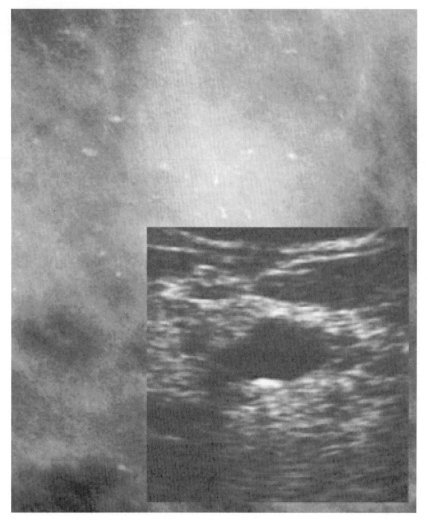

Fig. 9.34   Tiny intracystic echoes due to milk of calcium, with characteristic linear calcifications on the lateral mammographic view.

Although it may occur at any time in the reproductive period, fibroadenoma is more common before 25–30 years of age, resulting from an aberration of lobule formation in the early reproductive period. Fibroadenomas account for 95% of all benign abnormalities in young women. Lactating adenoma is the term used for fibroadenomas that appear or grow during pregnancy and lactation. When found in older women they usually represent a long-standing abnormality. However, new development or enlargement of already known fibroadenomas has been reported in premenopausal and postmenopausal women on hormone replacement therapy.[9,10] In fact, fibroadenomas depend on estrogen stimulation to develop and grow.

The mammographic pattern is that of a well-circumscribed, bulging, homogeneous opacity, with round, oval or lobulated borders. Margins may be completely defined, or masked by overlying fibroglandular tissue. Fibroadenomas may be completely invisible in dense breasts, as is the case in young women. Long-standing fibroadenomas undergo necrosis and hyalinization, resulting in coarse, 'pop-corn' calcifications, that allow an easy and accurate diagnosis on the mammogram. When calcifications are absent, mammography cannot differentiate fibroadenomas from cysts.

Fibroadenomas are multiple in 10–20% of patients, often bilateral, located in the upper outer quadrant in about half the cases. Fibroadenomas usually grow to 2–3 cm in diameter. Giant fibroadenoma is the term used for nodules larger than 6 cm. The shape is mostly oval, with prevalence of the long axis (L), or transverse diameter, parallel to the skin, on the short axis, or anteroposterior diameter (A). The ratio L/A quantifies the degree of elongation of the tumor, indicating the growth of fibroadenoma along the natural tissue planes of the breast. The ratio $L/AP>1.4$ has been reported in 86% of fibroadenomas, and $L/AP<1.4$ in 100% of carcinomas.[12] The typical fibroadenoma is a solid, homogeneous well-defined nodule, with regular borders, an elongated shape, a very sharply marginated posterior

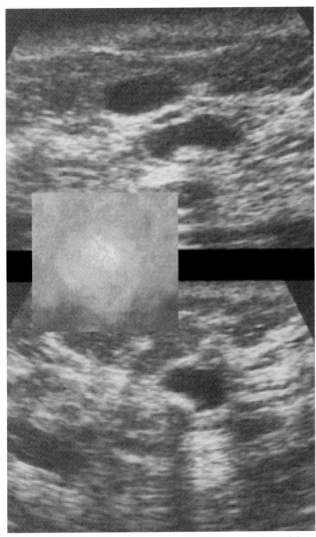

Fig. 9.35 Milk of calcium with coarse calcifications: craniocaudal mammographic view and intracystic echoes shifting with patient movement.

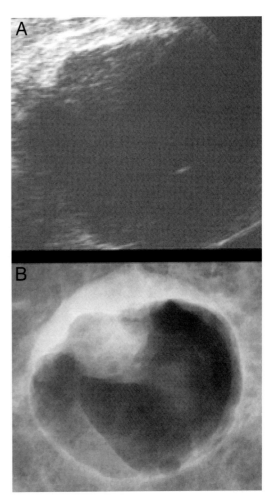

Fig. 9.36 Intracystic carcinoma. The solid vegetation is imaged with sonography (**A**), which reveals irregular wall thickening, and with pneumocystography (**B**).

wall and intermediate distal attenuation (Figs 9.2, 9.38). The nodule simply expands into the nearby tissues, pushing them, with no infiltration. Variations of probe pressure can show a certain gliding movement, that confirms the absence of infiltration, and corresponds to the physical finding of a mobile, non-infiltrating, palpable nodule. These sonographic findings in a young girl with a palpable mass allow a confident diagnosis. Mammography is not performed, because of young age and dense breasts, and sonographic follow-up may be indicated, to monitor size variations. Fibroadenomas may be isoechoic with breast tissues, hypoechoic, or echogenic, according to a prevalent adenomatous or fibrous component, and depending also on the echogenicity of the surrounding tissues. Hypoechoic fibroadenomas can be difficult to detect in a fatty breast. Other causes of an inhomogeneous structure are calcifications, that cause shadowing when large enough, or

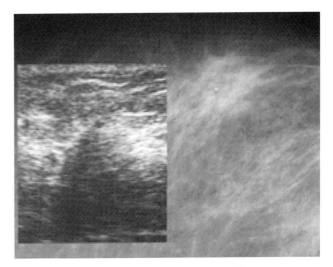

Fig. 9.37 Aspecific mammographic and sonographic patterns in a sclerosing lesion. The star-shaped opacity on the mammogram is a hypoechoic attenuating lesion on the sonogram.

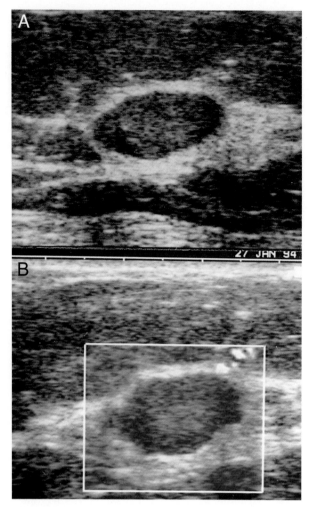

Fig. 9.38 Sonographic pattern of a typical fibroadenoma, with an elongated shape, well-defined margins, homogeneous structure, and no change in sound transmission (**A**). With power Doppler there is only one vascular pole and no flow signals inside the nodule (**B**).

flow, has been reported in recent years in fibroadenomas, with the presence of vessels being correlated to size.[14] We have recently concluded a study on 111 solid nodules – 61 benign, mostly fibroadenomas, and 50 carcinomas. Vascularization was present in 36.1% of benign lesions, and absent in 63.9%. Vascularized lesions were found in younger women (mean age 38.5 years), compared with non-vascularized nodules (mean age 48.7 years). Vessels were located at the periphery of the nodule in 81.8%, and all over the nodule in 13.6%, with an irregular distribution in only one case (4.6%). In vascularized fibroadenomas, the vascularized area was monotone and covered less than 10% of the total area of the nodule. The number of vascular poles, considered in fewer cases (24 carcinomas and eight fibroadenomas) was less in fibroadenomas (mean number 1.5) than in carcinomas (mean 2.1). Our conclusion was that the parameters considered could help to differentiate benign from malignant nodules, with a considerable overlap for large fibroadenomas in young women, showing an active proliferation (Fig. 9.42). Another recent report has concluded that color Doppler signals in a lesion otherwise thought to be benign should prompt a biopsy, whereas the absence of signals in an indeterminate lesion is reassuring.[15]

Phyllodes tumor

Phyllodes tumor is a rare fibroepithelial breast tumor, with a more cellular myxoid stroma than fibroadenoma. It is characterized by a rapid growth, producing bulging lumps on the breast. Patients' mean age is greater than that for fibroadenoma (50–60 years). Phyllodes tumors can degenerate into sarcomas in up to 10% of cases. Only histology can give a differential diagnosis by showing an increased mitotic activity for sarcomas. The tumor may recur locally and metastasize to the lungs via the bloodstream.

The mammographic pattern is that of a benign-looking round or lobulated opacity. The sonographic pattern is of a solid hypoechoic well-defined nodule, with no distal attenuation, resembling a fibroadenoma (Fig. 9.43). The echo structure may be inhomogeneous, because of clefts. Intramural cysts have been reported.[16]

Breast imaging gives aspecific findings and cannot differentiate between benign and malignant phyllodes tumors (Fig. 9.44). Furthermore, a differentiation may be impossible even between inhomogeneous fibroadenomas and phyllodes tumors. The stromal proliferation typical of phyllodes is not always demonstrated on cytologic specimens, so core biopsy may prove more useful.

Lipoma

Lipomas are a proliferation of fat cells, which form an encapsulated mass. They are usually found on the

liquid areas (Fig. 9.39). Distal attenuation is reported in about 30% of fibroadenomas.[2] Attenuation is explained by a predominant fibrous component.[13]

Sonographic patterns are fairly variable and FNAB is currently employed to confirm diagnosis. The shape can be rounded, polygonal, or lobulated. Inhomogeneous areas can be encountered. Sound transmission cannot be evaluated when the lesion is located deeply, close to the pectoral muscle. Fibroadenomas may be multiple, sometimes close together, forming what appears to be a single nodule, of bizarre shape (Fig. 9.40). Fibroadenomas can be mistaken for fat lobules, but fat lobules can also mimic fibroadenomas. The structure of fat lobules is similar to that of subcutaneous fat, but some lobules may be very obvious and stand out from the echogenic parenchyma so that they may mimic a nodule (Fig. 9.41).

Vascularization is another important parameter and has already been discussed in Chapter 3. No flow, or minimal

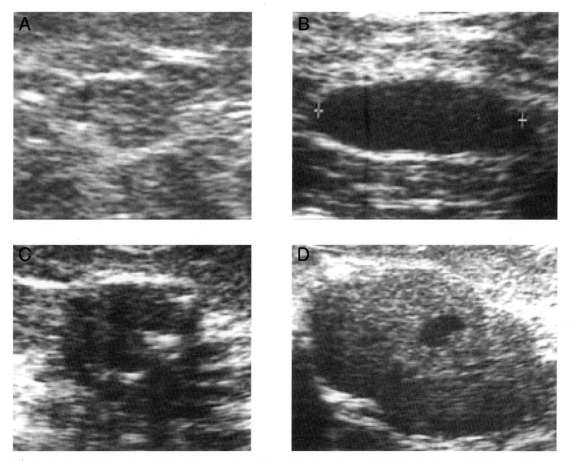

Fig. 9.39 Surgically confirmed fibroadenomas. Isoechoic nodule, barely recognizable in fatty breast (**A**); hypoechoic nodule with a significant L/AP ratio (**B**); gross calcifications causing shadowing (**C**); small anechoic liquid area, probably representing a duct (**D**).

mammograms of elderly women as radiolucent areas, with a thin, dense, fibrotic capsule. Lipomas cannot be differentiated in a fatty breast if the capsule is not seen. The patient is usually asymptomatic, because lipomas are fairly soft.

The sonographic structure of a lipoma is similar to that of breast fat – hypoechoic, homogeneous and compressible. When some fibrous tissue is present lipomas may be less homogeneous, with an echogenic component (Fig. 9.45). A hyperechoic rim may be depicted. Sonography is not necessary to diagnose these masses, which are clearly seen on the mammogram, and aspiration biopsy can be avoided. A correlation with mammography is always necessary because a hypoechoic fat nodule can mimic a mass (Fig. 9.41)

Hamartoma

Hamartomas are benign breast tumors, composed of variable amounts of fat, fibrous tissue and glandular tissue. The varying composition accounts for a characteristic mammographic finding of a well-defined, encapsulated, inhomogeneous mass, in which radiolucent fat tissue is mixed with dense fibroglandular tissue. The appearance is that of a breast inside the breast, with a sausage-like structure.[17] Hamartomas are also referred to as fibro-adenolipomas, lipofibroadenomas and adenolipomas, according to the main component.

The sonographic pattern reflects the different components: fat is hypoechoic, fibroglandular tissue is echogenic. Distal attenuation or enhancement correlates with the type of tissue present. Because of wide sonographic variability, a minimal role has been given to US examinations in the diagnosis of breast hamartomas.[18] Nevertheless, the sonographic pattern of an encapsulated, inhomogeneous mass, with variable attenuation, can be correlated to the mammographic findings to confirm mammographic diagnosis, obviating the need for biopsy (Fig. 9.46).

Duct ectasia

Duct ectasia is included among the aberrations of ductal involution in the years preceding and during menopause.

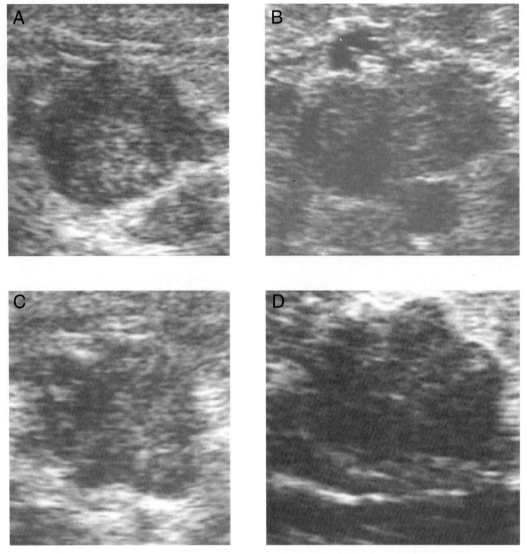

Fig. 9.40 Atypical fibroadenomas. Rounded shape and prevalent AP diameter (**A**); lobulated ill-defined borders and neighboring ducts (**B**); lobulated ill-defined borders and surrounding echogenic tissue (**C**); deeply located nodule, with lobulated borders and distal attenuation, probably due to the adjacent muscle but also to the structure of the node (**D**).

Some degree of dilatation may be found in up to 70% of women over 50 years of age.[6]

In general, rare single ducts of increased caliber can be found in the breast at any age, especially when scanning radially around the nipple–areola complex. The condition of duct ectasia is characterized by a more extensive segmental dilatation of ducts behind the areola, but also elsewhere in the breast.

Sonography has really confirmed the high incidence of this variant, that can be wholly asymptomatic or give nipple discharge and/or retraction, palpable lumps, and burning discomfort, mainly in the nipple area. Nipple discharge is seen in about 25% of cases. It is greenish, serous, sometimes bloody. Duct ectasia is the cause of 30% of nipple discharges.[19]

Dilated ducts contain a yellow, pasty material, due to inspissated secretions: a granular, necrotic debris, with lipid-laden macrophages, desquamated cells and calcifications. The pathologic specimen shows dilated ducts with periductal chronic, inflammatory infiltrates, neutrophils, lymphocytes and also plasma cells. The etiology is unknown. It is generally believed that periductal inflammation damages the ductal wall, destroys the elastic network surrounding the ducts and causes dilatation.[20] Chronic inflammation leads to fibrosis, which produces nipple and skin retraction, and hard masses that may be mistaken for cancer.

Duct ectasia can be wholly undetectable on the dense mammogram, or show as a prominent ductal pattern, mainly starting from the nipple, either opaque, or radio-

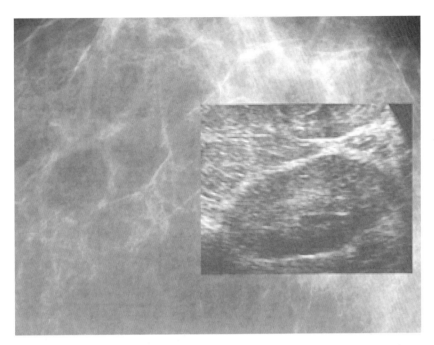

Fig. 9.41 Fat lobules can mimic fibroadenomas. A correlation with mammography shows radiolucent fat.

lucent, when contents are fatty compared with the dense fibrous tissue surrounding them. Rod-like, branching calcifications can also be demonstrated.

Sonography adds anatomic detail and shows multiple, dilated ducts, that may be regular, tortuous and of variable size, or with pseudonodular dilatations. The type of contents (liquid or solid, i.e. amorphous debris, calcifications) can easily be determined with sonography (Figs 9.47, 9.48). The ductal wall, a thick, sometimes irregular,

hyperechoic reflection can also be demonstrated (Fig. 9.49). In case of nipple retraction, sonography can help to rule out cancer of the subareolar tissues.

There are other situations in which sonography can demonstrate dilated ducts:

- dilated ducts containing echogenic milk are a normal finding during lactation (Fig. 9.25)
- dilated ducts may sometimes be found close to cysts;

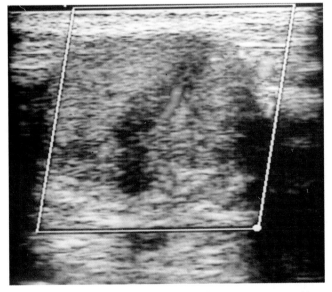

Fig. 9.42 Rapidly growing fibroadenoma, in a young woman, with monotone flow signals inside the nodule. Flow signals are typical of enlarging fibroadenomas.

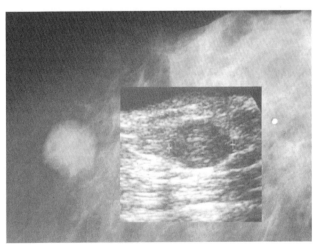

Fig. 9.43 Small phyllodes tumor (11.3 mm) resembling a fibroadenoma.

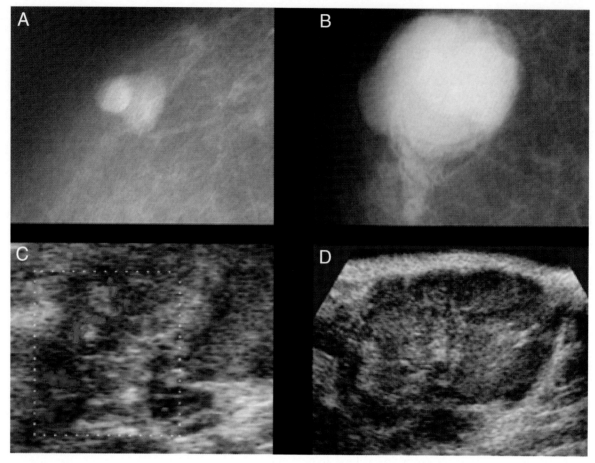

Fig. 9.44 Phyllodes sarcoma. Mammogram obtained 1 year previously (**A**): the nodule was considered to be a probably benign opacity. Rapid growth after 10 months (**B**). The nodule is vascularized (**C**). Margins are well defined and the structure is inhomogeneous (**D**).

these elongated, liquid structures could also represent small, collapsed cysts

- papillomas can be demonstrated with sonography because of associated duct dilatation
- dilated ducts can be demonstrated at the periphery of masses; the contents are liquid in cases of obstruction, or hypoechoic, in cases of ductal spread of carcinoma.

The contemporaneous presence of dilated ducts and cysts is explained by the fact that both conditions are typical of involution processes (Fig. 9.32).

Papillomas

Papillomas are neoplastic papillary growths inside a duct. They are usually solitary, and located inside the principal ducts or the lactiferous sinus. Serous or bloody nipple discharge is the main clinical presentation. The mean age of the affected female population is 40–50 years. The present consensus, although controversial, is that most solitary intraductal papillomas are benign, with a slight increase in the relative risk for invasive breast carcinoma (1.5–2-fold).

The duct should be completely excised to avoid local recurrences.

Multiple, intraductal papillomas should be distinguished from this group: they are located peripherally, affect young women – hence the name juvenile papillomatosis – and can be associated with atypical hyperplasia in up to 40% of cases.[21] This is the reason why multiple peripheral papillomas show a moderately increased risk for breast carcinoma (fivefold) according to the Consensus Statement of 1986.[8] The clinical finding is a palpable mass, that can be mistaken for a fibroadenoma.

Galactography is the main imaging modality in patients with bloody or serous nipple discharge. The injection of contrast agent into the secreting nipple orifice can demonstrate very small filling defects or obstruction of the duct. Papillomas are rarely larger than 1 cm. Accurate sonographic scannings around the nipple can show the following patterns:

- a dilated duct, containing a solid rounded nodule, more or less echogenic in structure, with no distal attenuation (Fig. 9.50)

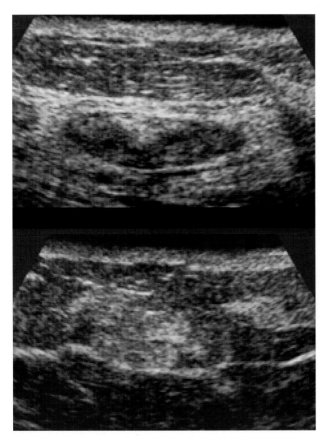

Fig. 9.45 Inhomogeneous lipomas, with a fibrous component.

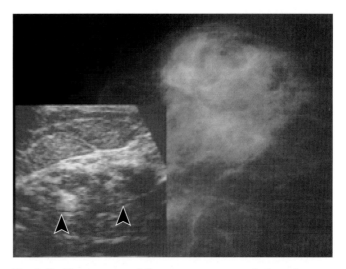

Fig. 9.46 Hamartoma: an inhomogeneous structure both on the mammogram, where radiolucent fat is seen, and on the sonogram (arrows).

● a cyst with a solid growth (Fig. 9.51).

The reported sonographic patterns of juvenile papillomatosis are of an ill-defined, inhomogeneous mass, with no attenuation, and with small echo-free areas at the border of the lesion.[22,23]

Mammography, although quite aspecific because of breast density, may show irregularly shaped calcifications. The gold standard is pathology of the histologic specimen.

Galactocele

A galactocele is a cystic dilatation of a duct in a lactating breast. A single duct may be affected and produces an isolated cyst, but multiple ducts are more often involved. Milk stasis can easily transform galactoceles into breast inflammation. Galactoceles have also been reported in men and in children.

Galactoceles cannot be demonstrated easily with mammography, because the lactating breast is very dense. Radiolucent images of fat density, forming a level in the lateral view have been reported.

Sonography can easily demonstrate galactoceles as cysts with echogenic contents, or as dilated ducts forming a ball (Fig. 9.52).

Acute breast inflammation

Acute breast inflammation is more common in the lactating breast, because of milk stasis and nipple abrasions. Nevertheless, it may also occur in non-lactating women, as a complication of duct ectasia, in patients with diabetes or altered immune response, but also with no apparent cause. *Streptococcus* and *Staphylococcus* are the bacteria more often involved; *Escherichia coli* has been reported, but frequently no micro-organisms are cultured from aspirations of the inflamed breast.

Acute breast inflammations are diagnosed clinically, through symptoms and clinical findings. Mammography shows an aspecific opacity, due to edema and infiltration, sometimes associated with skin thickening and loss of radiolucency of subcutaneous fat. Moreover, as adequate compression of the tender breast is difficult to achieve, mammograms are less diagnostic because of poor quality.

Acute breast inflammation is a condition in which sonography can precede mammography, whatever the patient's age, to confirm a diagnosis that is clinical. Furthermore, sonography can show the extent of inflammation, can demonstrate focal alterations such as abscesses, can anticipate the formation of fistulas before they become apparent on the skin and, finally, can offer a valuable aid to monitor the process up to resolution.

Sonography can also guide aspiration for therapeutic drainage of abscesses and for microbiologic studies. Cytologic examinations may be necessary to differentiate focal alterations in patients with subtle symptoms, and again US can guide the aspiration. Mammography regains its role as the main breast imaging modality in cases of slow or no recovery, and, in any event, after resolution in all patients that are in the age group at risk for carcinoma.[24]

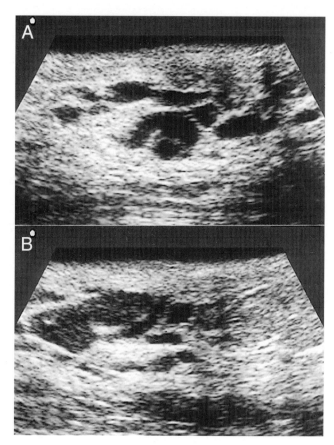

Fig. 9.48 Duct ectasia (same patient as in Figure 9.47). Contents vary: anechoic (**A**) and echogenic (**B**).

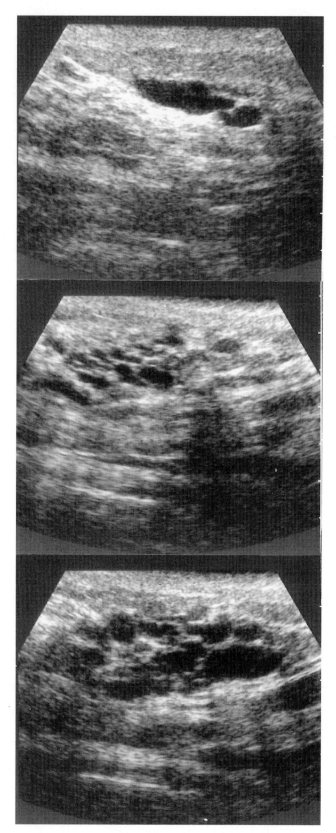

Fig. 9.47 Duct ectasia: different shapes in the same patient.

The sonographic findings in cases of diffuse inflammation are skin thickening, increased echogenicity of subcutaneous fat and of breast parenchyma, with a blurred ill-defined architecture (Fig. 9.53). The sonographic findings in cases of abscess formation are a hypoechoic, irregularly shaped area, that is inhomogeneous because of debris, with borders that may be ill defined, or more evident to form a better-defined wall. The surrounding tissues are echogenic. The purulent contents of an abscess may also be echogenic (Figs 9.54, 9.55).

Inflammation can also occur in pre-existing cysts, dilated ducts and galactoceles (Fig. 9.56). High-resolution sonography can easily demonstrate inflammatory changes in all breast constituents. The skin thickens and becomes hyper- or hypoechoic. Subcutaneous fat shows increased echogenicity and no visualization of Cooper's ligaments; this pattern is quite aspecific because fat changes are similar for both inflammatory and neoplastic infiltration (Fig. 9.57). Breast ducts may also be involved and show a hypoechoic purulent content, which may be associated with a purulent nipple discharge (Fig. 9.54). Dilated lymphatics forming a network in the subcutaneous tissues can also be demonstrated (Fig. 9.55).

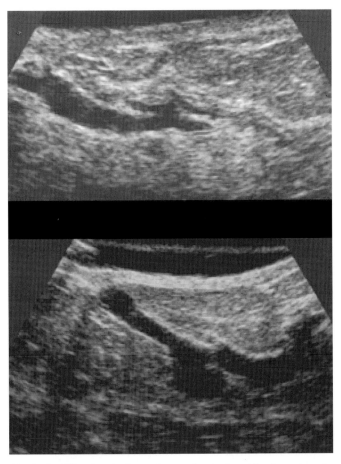

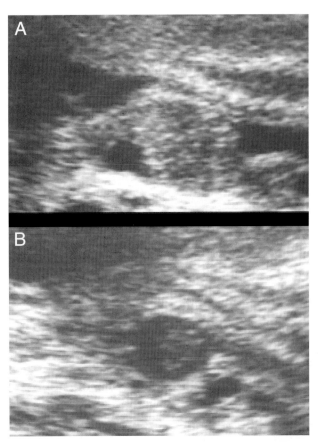

Fig. 9.50 Papillomas: solid masses (**A**, 6 mm; **B** 2 mm); the larger mass is located in a slightly dilated retroareolar duct (**A**).

Fig. 9.49 Dilated main ducts, close to the nipple, with echogenic walls and slightly echogenic contents.

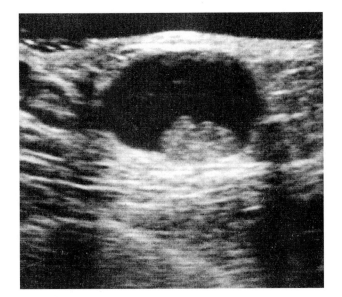

Fig. 9.51 Intraductal papilloma: solid proliferation in a cystic dilatation of a duct running to the nipple.

Breast trauma

This section considers the sonographic patterns of accidental breast trauma; changes related to the trauma of breast surgery are discussed later on.

Although the diagnosis is made with clinical history and physical findings, the referral of patients with breast trauma has progressively increased, thanks to sonography, which, in the acute phase, is the main imaging modality. Sonography can evaluate extent, type and evolution of changes caused by trauma. In the acute phase, as with breast inflammation, edema and bleeding cause an aspecific increase in density on the mammogram; furthermore, the tender and painful breast cannot be compressed adequately to achieve a good-quality mammogram.

The clinical findings are bruises (the extent of which is not necessarily correlated to the type of trauma), skin thickening, hardening of the superficial tissues and painful, palpable lumps.

Sonography has an invaluable role as the first-choice

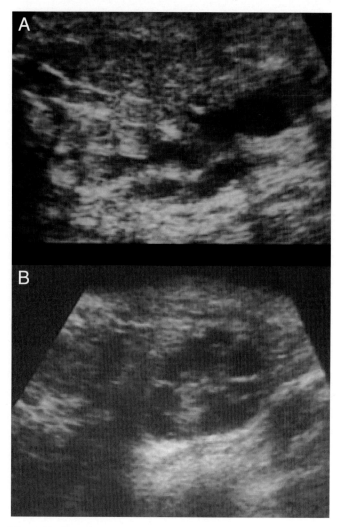

Fig. 9.52 Lactating breast: physiologically dilated ducts (**A**) and a galactocele (**B**).

examination in the first 2–3 weeks. We have arbitrarily defined three phases according to the time that has elapsed after trauma: acute in the first 4–5 days, intermediate after the acute phase and up to 2 weeks, and late phase after a year.[25] This timing is not rigid, as it depends on the type of trauma and on the time necessary for complete resolution, which varies with each patient.

The sonographic findings of acute breast trauma are as follows:

- focal skin thickening and increased echogenicity of subcutaneous fat
- disruption of normal architecture, with increased echogenicity, and loss of differentiation among the different breast constituents
- small echogenic areas due to recent bleeding
- small hypoechoic areas, which probably represent tissue damage due to contusion (Fig. 9.58)

If these changes do not regress, as may be the case in more

severe traumas, the patient enters the intermediate phase. The sonographic patterns of the intermediate phase are those of fluid collections and hematomas.

Fluid collections are inhomogeneous, with ill-defined borders and irregular shape; they are usually located in the superficial portions of the gland. This superficial location is fairly typical of trauma abnormalities. Hematomas resemble complex cysts, with echoes due to clots and inflammatory debris. Both hematomas as well as fluid collections may require interventional procedures that can be guided by sonography, which shows not only where aspiration is needed but also if it is complete.

The findings of the late phase, after a year, are fat necrosis and oil cysts; some scars may also be related to trauma, but the cause is more frequently surgical trauma. Not all patients with breast trauma show this type of evolution: most have a complete recovery. Sequelae are not always related only to the severity of the trauma, but also depend on the individual response of each breast.

Fat necrosis and oil cysts are occasional findings in women undergoing mammography for breast screening. These patients usually have a history of accidental trauma or minor surgery. Sonography has no role in the detection of late sequelae of trauma. Mammography not only regains its role, but is also mandatory from a year after trauma, because of a reported possible increase in breast carcinoma after trauma.[26] To date, trauma has been demonstrated as a predisposing factor only for a low-grade rare breast malignancy – dermatofibrosarcoma protuberans.[27]

Oil cysts are a specific type of fat necrosis. Mammography reveals rounded radiolucent areas, with a thin opaque rim that sometimes is calcified.[28] Sonographic findings are of well-defined hypo- or echogenic nodules, with variable sound transmission. Contents with a different density not only show a variable echogenicity, but may also layer, and form a level (Figs 9.59, 9.60). The mammographic pattern of fat necrosis is quite typical – coarse irregular calcifications bordering radiolucent fatty areas. Sonography can show loss of parenchymal architecture, with areas of attenuation due to the calcifications (Fig. 9.61).

Rare benign conditions

Other, very uncommon, benign breast abnormalities show a very aspecific mammographic and sonographic pattern and require biopsy for a definite diagnosis.

Leiomyomas arising from breast parenchyma are extremely rare, owing to the dearth of smooth muscle in the breast. Mammographic and sonographic patterns are aspecific: leiomyomas are imaged as solid well-defined masses with a homogeneous structure.[29]

Mondor's disease is a rare abnormality, caused by obliterating phlebitis of the thoraco-epigastric vein, sometimes associated with thrombosis. It causes pain, skin retraction

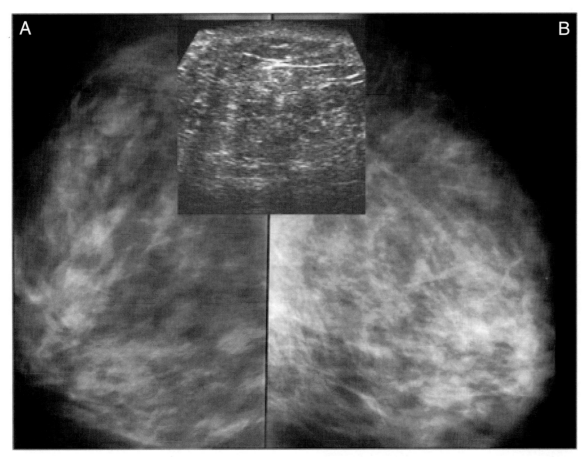

Fig. 9.53 Diffuse inflammation of the left breast. Increased density on the mammogram (**B**), and increased echogenicity of subcutaneous fat and of breast parenchyma, with ill-defined architecture on the sonogram.

and a palpable tender cord, that represents the thrombosed superficial vein. It is an uncommon condition associated with trauma, breast surgery and physical activity. The diagnosis is made through physical findings. Mammography shows a rope-like density, representing the vein, and rules out cancer.[30] Sonography shows the vessel, a hypoechoic tubular structure, that may be inhomogeneous because of thrombus.

Sarcoidosis is a very rare breast abnormality attributable to a granulomatous disease, presenting with axillary lymph nodes and a breast mass causing skin retraction. The breast may be the only organ affected. Mammographic and sonographic findings are totally aspecific.

Breast fibromatosis is an extra-abdominal desmoid that can recur locally. Imaging modalities cannot differentiate this abnormality from carcinoma.

Nipple adenoma is a benign proliferative lesion of the nipple, with a retroareolar nodule, nipple abrasion, retraction and discharge. Malignancy is the diagnosis that is commonly suggested before biopsy.

Diabetic fibrosis may occur in diabetic patients. The physical findings are hard, irregular lumps, which do not adhere to nearby tissues. Mammography shows an aspe-

cific, diffuse opacity. Sonography shows a diffuse, intense shadowing, that origins from the superficial portions of the gland and masks underlying tissues. FNAB is challenging because the masses are very hard and entrap the needle, which cannot be moved freely inside the mass for adequate sampling.

BREAST CARCINOMA AND OTHER MALIGNANCIES

Breast carcinoma

Carcinoma is the main breast disease, to the extent that the diagnosis of all other benign abnormalities becomes significant because it rules out cancer. Mammography is the main diagnostic tool to detect cancers that are not palpable. Pathology is the gold standard to differentiate masses.

The role of sonography is to add more diagnostic parameters to those already found with clinical examination and mammography. As with mammography, many sonographic patterns are non-specific, with a frequent overlap between benign and malignant findings. Nevertheless, the

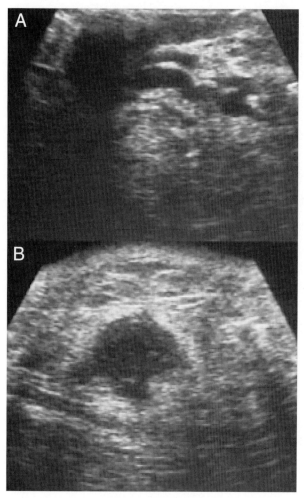

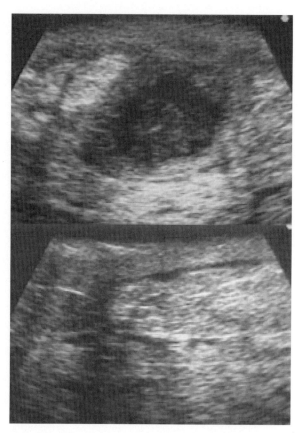

Fig. 9.55 Retroareolar abscess, with skin thickening, ill-defined wall, hypoechoic contents and visible lymphatics.

Fig. 9.54 The same untreated patient develops an abscess (**B**), with ductal involvement and purulent nipple discharge.

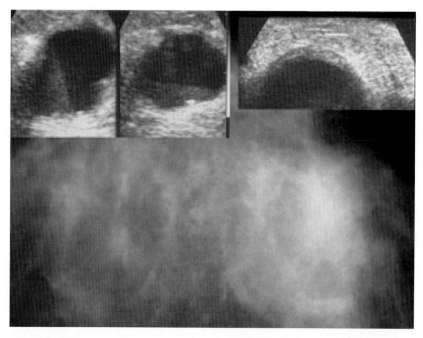

Fig. 9.56 Inflamed cyst: the wall is thickened and blurred. Echogenic debris forms a fluid–fluid level that shifts when the patient moves. Non-specific increased opacity on the mammogram.

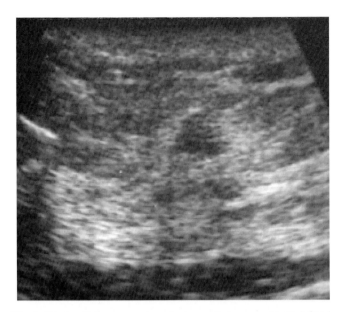

Fig. 9.57 Small abscess: a triangular hypoechoic area, with ill-defined wall and increased echogenicity of surrounding tissues. The sonographic pattern is non-specific, very similar to cancer. The patient showed inflammatory skin changes.

combination of clinical history and physical, mammographic and sonographic findings can be useful to help choose the correct approach and decide on the employment of more invasive biopsy techniques.

The sonographic description of breast masses includes parameters such as location, number, size, type of structure, shape, margins, type of interface, posterior sound transmission and skin changes.[2] The presence and type of vascularization must also be considered, along with the demonstration of microcalcifications and the suggestion of ductal spread and of lymph node involvement.

The most frequent location of breast carcinoma is the upper outer quadrant, which is the site of cancer in 50% of cases. A larger concentration in this area of terminal duct lobular units, where carcinoma is believed to arise, seems to explain this higher rate. The frequency rate for other locations is as follows: upper inner, 15%; outer lower, 10%; inner lower, 5%. The central area, behind the areola, accounts for about 17%, while massive carcinomas represent about 3% of cancers. Cancer may be multifocal, multicentric and bilateral.

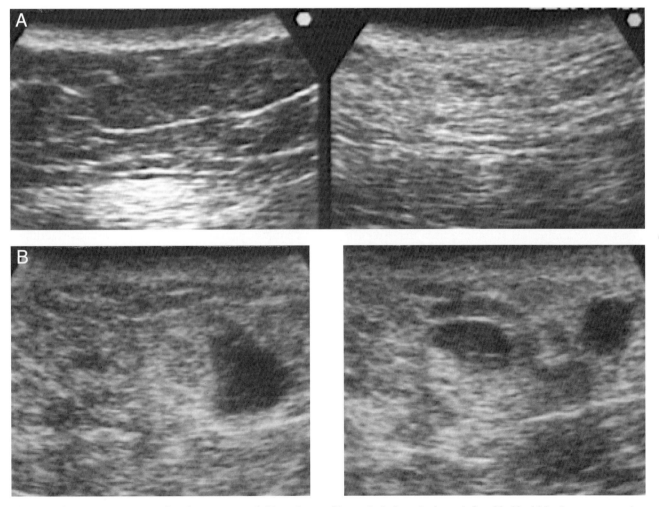

Fig. 9.58 Breast trauma: comparison between normal skin and normal hypoechoic fat and echogenic fat with skin thickening on trauma site (**A**). Hypoechoic areas inside echogenic fat tissue, in the superficial portions of the breast, after trauma (**B**).

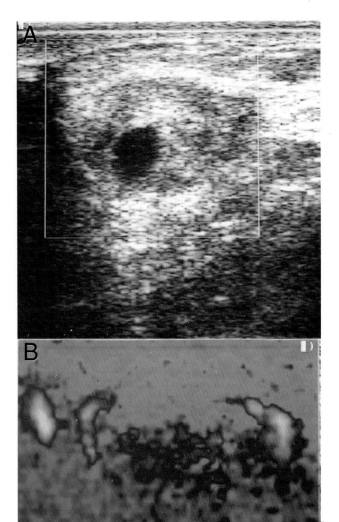

Fig. 9.59 Inflamed fat necrosis: inhomogeneous area, with an echogenic periphery and hypoechoic center; sound transmission is enhanced. Power Doppler signals at the periphery (**B**).

Tumor size varies according to the time of diagnosis. The correct determination of tumor size is important for patient management, particularly for breast conservation therapy. The poor correlation between mammographic and clinical estimates with the size measured on the pathologic specimen is well known. Sonography has shown the best correlation with pathologic cancer size when compared with mammographic and clinical measurements.[31]

Sonography can differentiate the mass from desmoplasia, a fibrous reaction of the neighboring tissues, in an attempt to halt the malignant growth; it is highly echogenic (Figs 9.62, 9.63). Desmoplasia cannot be differentiated by palpation, and is just as dense as cancer growths on the mammogram. Furthermore, mammography may fail to delineate the whole tumor in dense breasts.

Another parameter that is correlated to size and also to shape is the L/AP ratio, where L is the longest diameter, parallel to the skin, and AP is the anteroposterior diameter, which is the growth perpendicular to the skin. The L/AP ratio quantifies the degree of elongation of the tumor. Data reported in the literature are controversial. A certain prevalence of the anteroposterior diameter (L/AP ratio $\leqq 1$) has been reported for 61% of carcinomas smaller than 1 cm^3, compared with only 4% of fibroadenomas.[32] In another series, using the threshold of 1.4, 86% of fibroadenomas had an L/AP diameter >1.4, whereas 100% of carcinomas (28 cases) had a ratio <1.4.[12] The same quantitative analysis applied to a retrospective review by other authors has found no significant difference between benign and malignant lesions.[33] Although fibroadenomas tend to be longer than they are deep, the L/AP ratio should simply be considered as one of the criteria allowing characterization of a mass, along with all the other parameters considered, without forgetting the marked overlap of US findings in benign and malignant nodules (Figs 9.64, 9.65).

Carcinomas are usually hypoechoic masses. The sonographic structure is more or less homogeneous, depending on the homogeneity of the pathologic structure, on the presence of fibrous tissue, calcifications, and tumoral vessels, and on necrosis (Figs 9.66, 9.67). Very heterogeneous histopathologic patterns forming many interfaces are responsible for echogenic growths, more often associated with intense shadowing (Fig. 9.68).[34] There are two main morphologic patterns for malignant masses – stellate and circumscribed. Shape and margins differentiate stellate and circumscribed carcinomas, according to the type of growth, which can be infiltrating or simply expansive.[35,36] An infiltrating growth shows irregular margins, which appear even more irregular because of associated desmoplasia. Well-circumscribed masses have a rounded or oval shape, with slightly blurred or well-defined margins that merely push into the surrounding tissues, causing compression and dislocation, but no distortion. A slight change in shape and a gliding motion inside breast tissues is demonstrated on pressing the probe on a circumscribed, non-infiltrating mass; this is not seen with hard, infiltrating masses in which the interface may be an irregular thick hyperechoic rim, surrounding the mass and representing desmoplasia; there is increased echogenicity of surrounding fat as a reaction to infiltration, and an architectural distortion that pulls on the fibrous stroma of the gland (Figs 9.62, 9.63, 9.68). Conversely, circumscribed carcinomas do not cause changes in the surrounding tissues, apart from compression. The borders are fairly well defined, sometimes only blurred or lobulated (Fig. 9.66).

The type of interface depends also on the skin changes produced by cancer. Superficial masses, as well as causing changes in subcutaneous fat, infiltrate the skin, which thickens or changes its echogenicity (Fig. 9.69). Less superficial cancers may also cause skin changes by pulling on Cooper's ligaments, and by changing their orientation.

For some time, distal attenuation has been considered

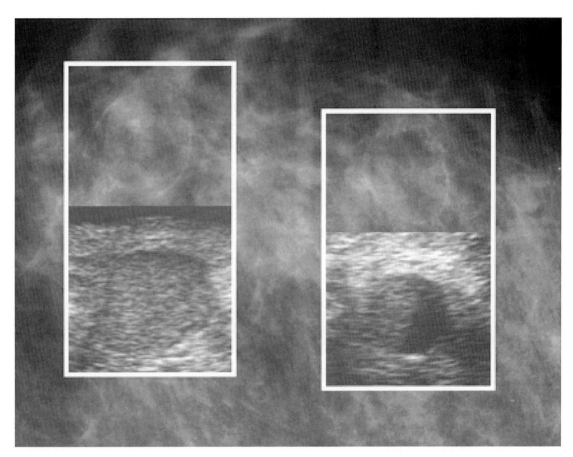

Fig. 9.60 Different patterns of lipid cysts.

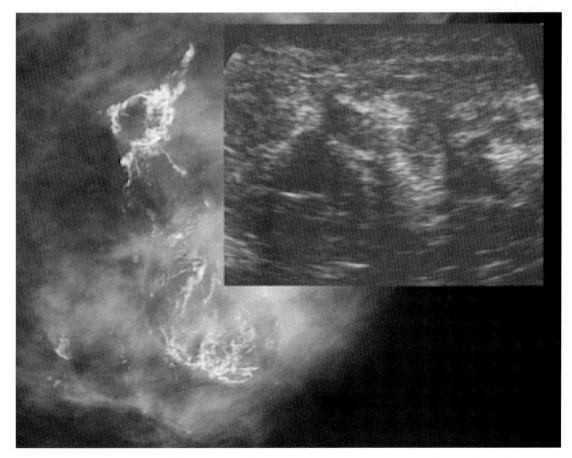

Fig. 9.61 Fat necrosis: coarse calcifications and radiolucent fat tissue on the mammogram. Non-specific shadowing on the sonogram.

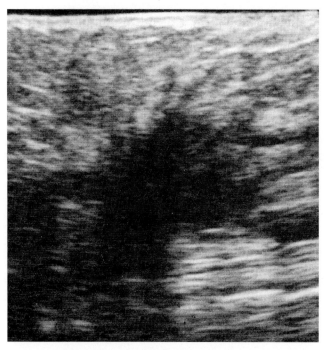

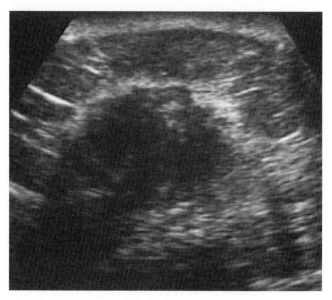

Fig. 9.63 Infiltrating ductal carcinoma: inhomogeneous hypoechoic structure with irregular margins, desmoplasia and some attenuation.

Fig. 9.62 Infiltrating ductal carcinoma: ill-defined irregular margins and increased echogenicity of surrounding tissues.

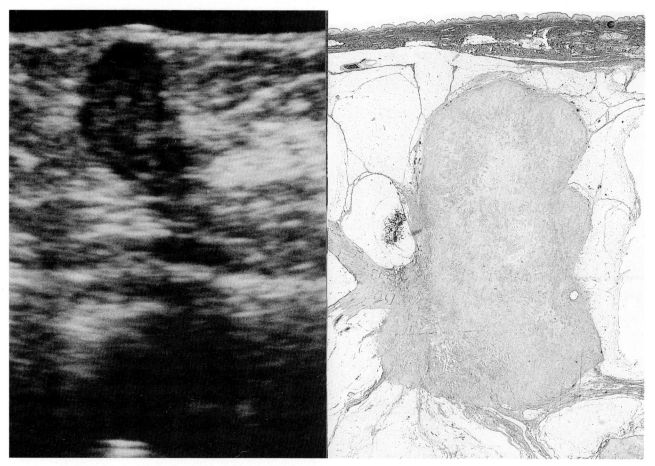

Fig. 9.64 Infiltrating ductal carcinoma: the tumor has a well-defined margin towards the skin and a prevalence of the anteroposterior diameter (15 mm).

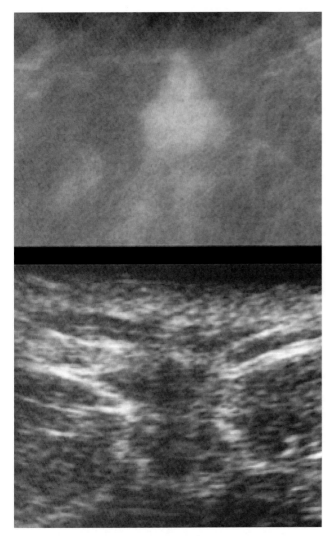

Fig. 9.65 Small infiltrating carcinoma with prevalent anteroposterior diameter (7.3 mm).

characteristic of malignant masses. However, it has been demonstrated that posterior sound transmission depends on the amount of fibrous tissue in the mass.[37] Cancer can produce attenuation in 30% of cases, to the point of obscuring the posterior margin of the lesion (Figs 9.69, 9.70).[38] Nevertheless, no change in posterior sound transmission may occur, or cancer can cause distal sound enhancement, as is the case with medullary and mucinous carcinomas, with carcinomas growing in cysts, and also with some infiltrating ductal carcinomas (Figs 9.71, 9.72).

Sonography can also demonstrate vessels newly produced by tumors. Color Doppler has been considered to be a promising adjunct to ultrasound imaging in the differential diagnosis of breast lesions.[14] Semiquantitative evaluations, based on the average number of vessels per square centimeter and average density of color pixels, have resulted in the demonstration of vessels in and around a large proportion of cancers (Figs 9.66, 9.73), with a larger

area being occupied by vessels in cancers than in benign masses.[15]

In our recent series of 50 carcinomas, color Doppler has shown flow signals in 90% of cases, with bidirectional flow in 93.3%. Flow signals were peripheral in 33.3%, central in 17.8% and irregular in 48.9%. The ratio between vascularized area and nodule size was less than 10% in 44.4% of cases, less than 30% in 40% of cases, and more than 30% in 11.6% of cases. The average size of masses showing flow signals was 1.6 cm, whereas 1.1 cm was the average size of non-vascularized masses. More recently, for the last 24 examples of cancer, we have also considered the number of vascular poles, which was 2.1 for malignant nodules, compared with 1.5 for the benign nodules examined. Among the non-vascularized tumors (5/50) we have found two mucoid carcinomas, containing a great deal of mucin but little stroma.

When attempting to differentiate a benign from a malignant mass with color Doppler the following factors must be borne in mind:

- large proliferating fibroadenomas, in young women, can show flow signals (Fig. 9.42)
- small cancers, and some specific types of cancer, such as mucoid carcinoma, may not be vascularized (Fig. 9.74)
- the sonographic equipment currently available varies drastically in its ability to detect slow flow signals.

Recently, it has become apparent that sonography can suggest the ductal spread of carcinoma. Infiltrating ductal carcinoma may have an extensive intraductal component that causes local recurrence where surgery is very conservative. For this reason it is extremely important that the margins of the resected specimen are free of cancer cells. Pathology is the gold standard to demonstrate cancer cells in ducts at the periphery of cancer. Mammography may have a good predictive value to determine the possibility of an extensive intraductal component. Cancers showing calcifications on the mammogram are associated with an extensive intraductal component in 65% of cases.[39] Stenosis or obstruction of a duct caused by cancer can be demonstrated on the ductogram. Sonography can also have a role in suggesting ductal spread of carcinoma. The sonographic features that can be found at the periphery of a mass are an asymmetric dilated duct, and rigid, stretched, hypoechoic tubular structures at the periphery of the tumor (Fig. 9.75).

The solitary duct associated with cancer obstruction is anechoic, dilated and located proximally to the lesion. The sonographic pattern of hypoechoic tubular structures at the periphery of a mass has been correlated to the pathologic specimen, to explain such images.[40] Multiple parallel scans were performed along the tubular structure representing a duct and its location was marked on the skin before operation. After surgery a series of histologial slides was made,

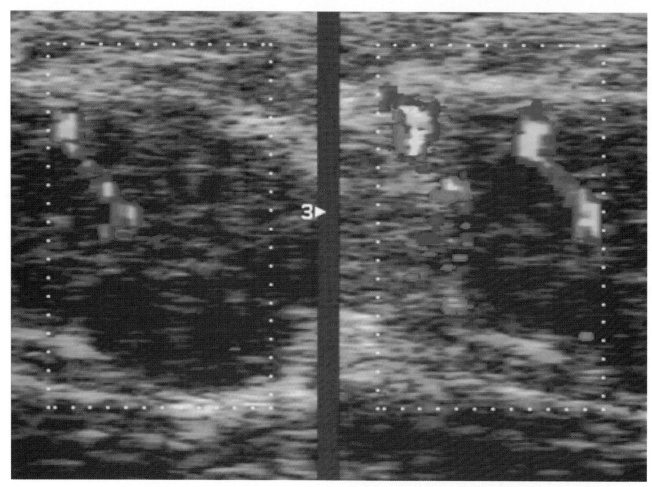

Fig. 9.66 Carcinoma with lobulated, fairly circumscribed borders; large feeding vessels and a mosaic pattern at the periphery of the nodule.

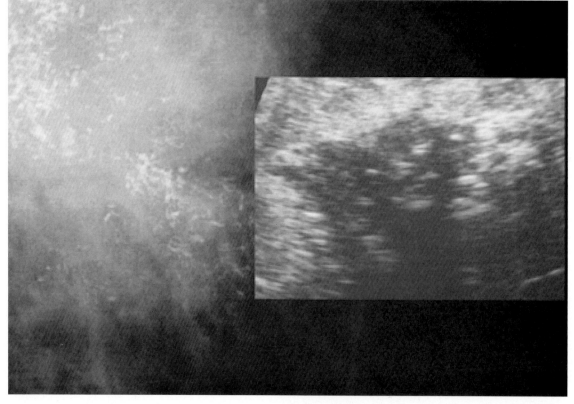

Fig. 9.67 Sonographic demonstration of calcifications inside and outside a mass, on the right lateral border of the sonogram.

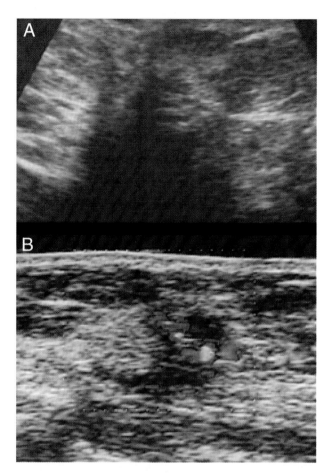

Fig. 9.68 Intense shadowing behind an echogenic distortion of superficial breast parenchyma that represents a carcinoma with echogenic structure (**A**). Another cancer with an echogenic component that has no flow signals (**B**).

aligned with the structure localized, to compare the sonographic pattern with the pathologic findings. The US/pathologic correlation in 33 T_1N_0 cancers has resulted in 11 true positive, 14 true negative, 3 false positive and 5 false negative findings.[41] Sonography cannot predict the existence of cancer cells inside a duct. Nevertheless, the demonstration of tubular structures at the periphery of a mass, along with the size of the nodule, must be considered as invaluable information for the surgeon before conservative surgery. Color Doppler may be employed to differentiate vessels from ducts, as both are tubular structures.

Microcalcifications are associated with cancer in 42% of cases and are easily detected with mammography.[42] Sonography has no role in the detection of microcalcifications, nor in evaluating their morphologic features. Nevertheless, the use of high-resolution correctly focused probes can reveal tiny echogenic spots inside a nodule, which correspond to the mammographic image. Most small calcifications do not produce acoustic shadowing because of their size. Microcalcifications cannot be as easily depicted

when located inside echogenic fibroglandular breast tissue, and there is some difficulty in differentiating them from the echogenic interfaces among tissues. At the moment there is no role for sonography, apart from showing the structure in which calcifications are located, i.e. microcalcifications in a nodule, milk of calcium in microcysts, calcifications inside ducts.

Axillary and supraclavicular nodes are very frequently involved by breast cancer, starting from the outer breast quadrants. Sonography can easily detect enlarged lymph nodes, show their size and shape, and evaluate if the echogenic hilum is maintained. Node enlargement can result from inflammation, hyperplasia, breast cancer or metastases. A rounded shape and loss of the echogenic hilum suggest infiltration. Compared with mammography and clinical examination, sonography has a higher sensitivity in the detection of axillary lymph nodes.[43] These are preoperative indications and, of course, pathologic examination of lymph nodes after surgery is the only way to rule out cancer diffusion. Metastases to the internal mammary lymph nodes, mainly from cancer of the inner quadrants, can be suggested preoperatively by parasternal sonography.[44] Longitudinal and transverse scans are taken from the first to the fourth parasternal rib interspaces. Enlarged lymph nodes can be demonstrated close to the internal mammary vessels. Color Doppler can be useful in the identification and localization of the vessels. These lymph nodes are usually not considered in cancer staging. In cases of enlargement, adequate radiotherapy can be planned on these nodes; sonography can indicate the depth and distance of the nodes from the sternal border, and can be used instead of lymphoscintigraphy. CT can also demonstrate enlarged nodes of the internal mammary chain.

Breast imaging modalities cannot adequately differentiate the histologic type of carcinoma. Invasive carcinomas show a stellate pattern, that has also been called scirrhous carcinoma. Circumscribed carcinomas include medullary, mucinous and papillary carcinomas, but some invasive ductal carcinomas can also have well-defined borders. Medullary carcinomas show posterior sound enhancement and may be identical to a complex cyst, with hypoechoic contents (Fig. 9.76).[45] The same applies to mucinous or colloid carcinoma, because of the high mucin content.

One must always be aware that there is an overlap between benign and malignant sonographic patterns, and that pathology is the gold standard.

Intracystic carcinoma is a rare form of breast cancer. Histologically it represents a papillary carcinoma, arising from the wall of a cyst. The sonographic pattern is that of a complex cyst, showing wall thickening, or a solid vegetation protruding into the cyst (Fig. 9.77). Another condition in which a cyst is associated with carcinoma, is when an adjacent carcinoma invades a cyst. In both situations the

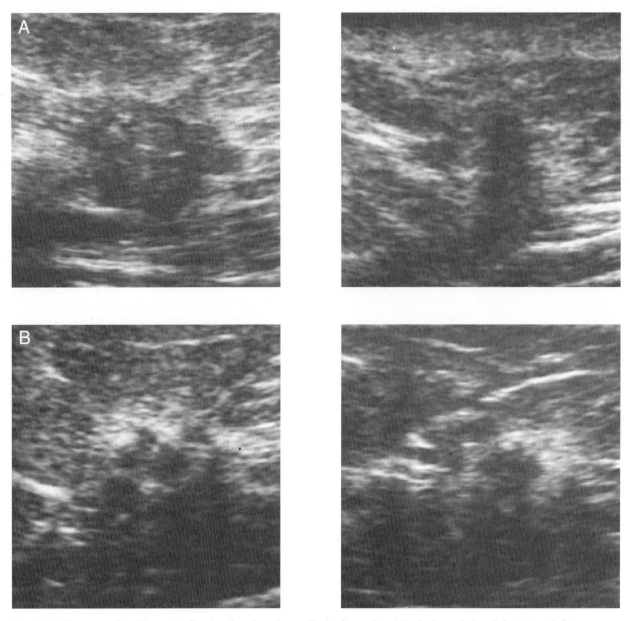

Fig. 9.69   Two cases of multicentric infiltrating ductal carcinoma. In the first patient (**A**), the larger lesion (left, 15 mm) infiltrates surrounding tissues and changes the echostructure of the skin; there is no sound attenuation. The smaller lesion (6 mm) causes attenuation (right). In the second patient (**B**) all the nodules produce attenuation, no matter what their size.

cyst may have echogenic contents due to blood. Aspiration cytology is more rewarding when accomplished on the solid portion of the mass, as there may be few cancer cells in the bloody contents of the cyst. Sonography not only delineates the solid vegetation, obviating the need for pneumo-cystography, but also guides sampling of the solid mass.

Invasive lobular carcinoma, owing to its particular growth pattern, may be as difficult to detect with sono-graphy as it is with mammography. Although a hypoechoic mass may be encountered, the sonographic findings may simply be of inhomogeneous architectural distortion, with no apparent mass (Fig. 9.78).

Inflammatory carcinoma is the result of lymphatics having been infiltrated by cancer cells. Physical findings are reddening and thickening of the skin, which has the appearance of orange peel. Sonography shows marked skin thickening, increased echogenicity of underlying fat tissue and a network of hypoechoic thin bands, parallel and per-pendicular to the skin, which represent dilated, engorged lymphatics. These sonographic images correspond to the dense, blurred network that reduces radiolucency of sub-cutaneous fat on the mammogram. Other sonographic parameters include increased echogenicity of breast par-enchyma, with no differentiation among its constituents.

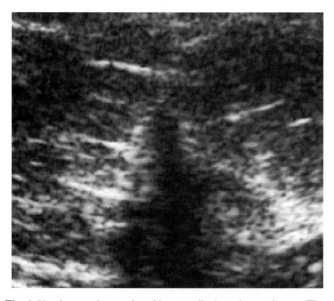

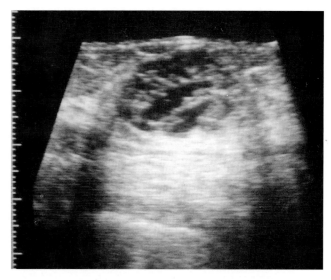

Fig. 9.71 Posterior sound enhancement in mucinous carcinoma.

Fig. 9.70 Attenuation produced by a small triangular carcinoma. The image is magnified.

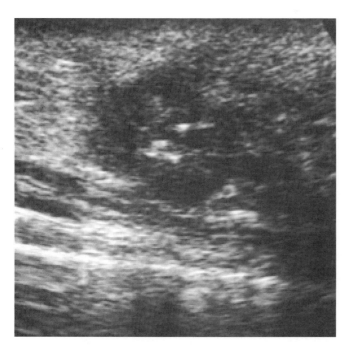

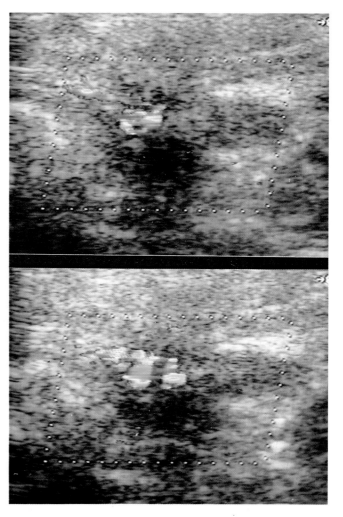

Fig. 9.72 Posterior sound enhancement in infiltrating ductal carcinoma. The lesion is close to the pectoralis muscle. Calcifications inside the nodule are clearly demonstrated.

Fig. 9.73 Mosaic color Doppler signals in carcinoma.

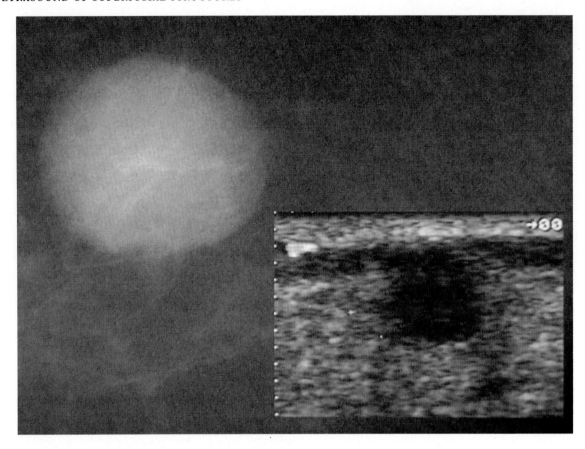

Fig. 9.74 Non-vascularized mucoid carcinoma. Flow signals are demonstrated underneath subcutaneous fat, far from the lesion, that is hypoechoic with distal sound enhancement. Margins are well defined on the mammogram.

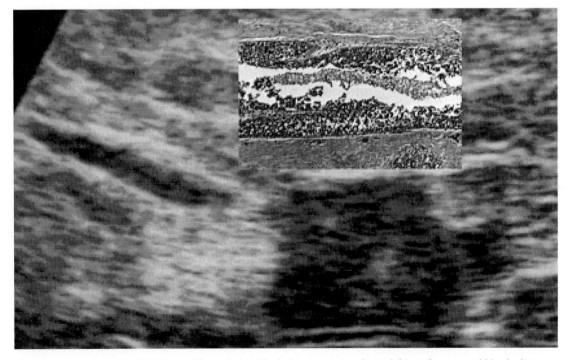

Fig. 9.75 Ductal spread of carcinoma. Hypoechoic stiff tubular structure at the periphery of cancer and histologic specimen.

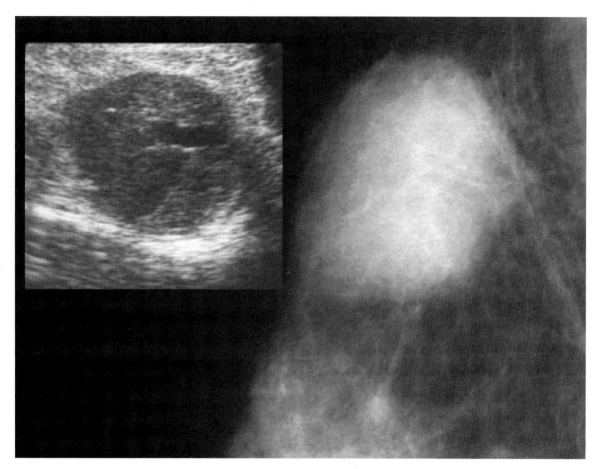

Fig. 9.76   Medullary carcinoma: circumscribed inhomogeneous nodule, with posterior sound enhancement.

Distal sound attenuation may mask underlying masses (Fig. 9.10).

Apart from the mammographic patterns and the use of sonography to give a further characterization, the main modality to differentiate benign and malignant masses is tissue diagnosis. The use of MRI has also been reported. This has been used in breast since 1982, although the first

results were not promising because lesions could barely be differentiated from benign glandular tissues, nor could they be characterized according to the type of signal. The use of contrast agents, such as gadolinium-DTPA, has increased the possible role of MRI in evaluating breast pathology. The features of malignant lesions with MRI are fairly similar to those of mammography, except for microcalcifications, which cannot be imaged. High-contrast resolution shows irregular borders and thin spiculations. After contrast enhancement, both benign as well as malignant lesions show an increased signal compared with the surrounding tissues, but the uptake in malignancy is more rapid (Fig. 9.79).

Other breast malignancies

Metastases to the mammary gland represent 1–6% of all breast malignancies. The primary cancer may be in the lung (oat-cell carcinoma), digestive tract, reproductive system, or in the contralateral breast; melanomas, sarcoma, lymphoma and leukemia may also spread to the breast. Plasmocytoma breast localizations have also been reported.

The metastatic nodule may be single (but more often multiple), palpable or asymptomatic, unilateral or bilateral,

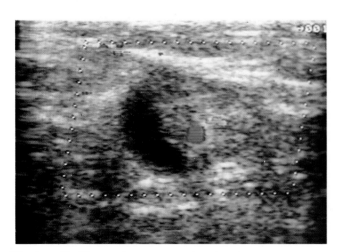

Fig. 9.77   Papillary carcinoma on a cystic wall: color Doppler signals.

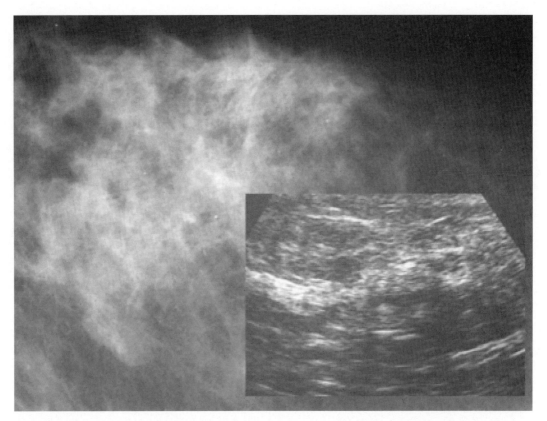

Fig. 9.78 Lobular carcinoma: parenchymal distortion on the mammogram. The sonographic pattern can be deceiving when no hypoechoic nodule is detected.

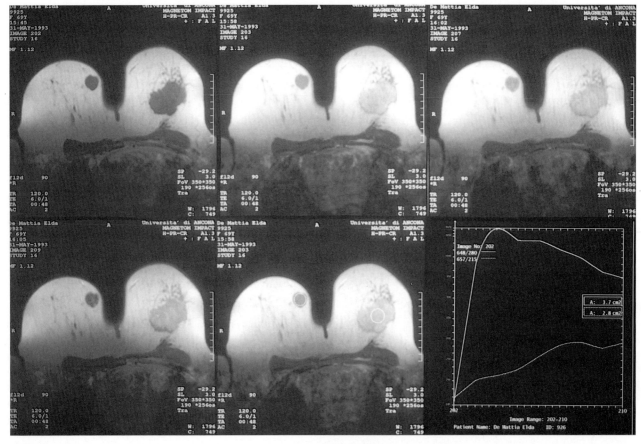

Fig. 9.79 Different MRI patterns for fibroadenoma and carcinoma after Gd-DTPA.

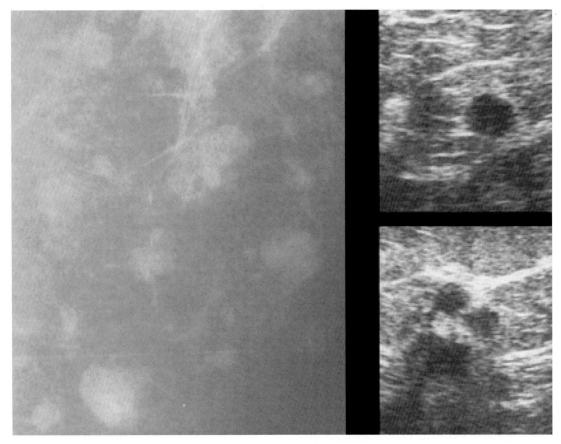

Fig. 9.80   Metastases to the breast: multiple small rounded opacities with slightly blurred margins on the sonogram.

with or without accompanying lymph nodes. Mammography shows multiple well-circumscribed rounded opacities that can be mistaken for cysts. Sonography demonstrates hypoechoic rounded nodules, with slightly blurred margins and no desmoplasia; there is no change in sound transmission (Fig. 9.80).[46] Metastases may be the first finding in patients with no known malignancy, or may appear in the breast after a long-standing disease. In both situations aspiration biopsy is necessary for diagnosis, as mammographic and sonographic findings are non-specific.

Sarcomas are very uncommon breast malignancies. They either arise from mesenchymal elements of benign tumors, such as phyllodes, or from breast stroma. The radiologic description of some cases has been reported in the literature. The mammographic pattern is non-specific. Osteogenic sarcomas containing osseous trabeculae have also been reported.

MALE BREAST

In males the breast is very rudimentary. The normal male breast is made of fat, sparse fibrous septa and vessels. The normal sonographic pattern is that of hypoechoic fat tissue crossed by some echogenic bands (Fig. 9.81). Obese patients may show excess fat, which means that the thick-

ness of the superficial hypoechoic tissues increases. The male breast is usually free from pathologic involvement.

The two main processes that may be found are gynecomastia and carcinoma. Other benign conditions such as trauma and inflammation display patterns that are fairly similar to those noted in the female breast, with the exception that there is no glandular tissue. There have been pathologic reports on mammary duct ectasia, nipple adenoma, intraductal papilloma and myofibroblastoma of the male breast. Another very rare condition, metastatic carcinoma, usually originates from the prostate and may be found after estrogen therapy; metastases from melanomas and lung cancer may also be found.[47]

Gynecomastia is an enlargement of the male breast due to hypertrophy and hyperplasia of both glandular and stromal components. Gynecomastia can be grossly divided into physiologic, pathologic and idiopathic gynecomastia.

Physiologic gynecomastia occurs in infants, adolescent boys and elderly men and is due to hormonal imbalance. Resolution is spontaneous in the first two conditions.

Pathologic gynecomastia may have many causes, including the following:

● deficient production or action of testosterone, for congenital defects (congenital anorchia, Klinefelter syn-

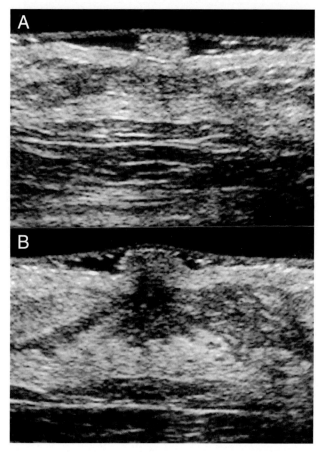

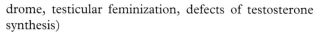

Fig. 9.81 Male breast: normal finding (**A**); gynecomastia (**B**).

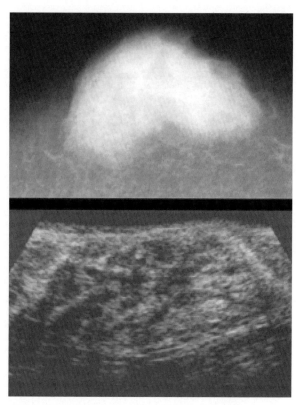

Fig. 9.82 Nodular gynecomastia: a homogeneous opacity on the mammogram, and an inhomogeneous mass on the sonogram: a ductal pattern can be visualized.

drome, testicular feminization, defects of testosterone synthesis)

- deficient production or action of testosterone, secondary to testicular failure (viral orchitis, trauma, castration, neurologic or granulomatous disease, renal failure)
- increased estrogen production: estrogen secretion (true hermaphroditism, testicular tumors, lung carcinoma and other tumors producing hCG)
- increased estrogen production: increased substrate for extraglandular aromatase (adrenal disease, liver disease, starvation, thyrotoxicosis)
- increased estrogen production: increased extraglandular aromatase
- drugs: estrogens (diethylstilbestrol, digitalis, estrogen-containing cosmetics, estrogen-contaminated foods), drugs that enhance endogenous estrogen secretion (gonadotropins, clomiphene), inhibitors of testosterone synthesis and/or action (ketoconazole, metronidazole, alkylating agents, cisplatin, spironolactone, cimetidine), unknown mechanisms (busulfan, isoniazid, methyldopa, tricyclic antidepressants, pencillamine, diazepam, marijuana, heroin).[48]

Physical findings are an enlargement of the gland and a palpable mass, which can be unilateral or bilateral. Mammographic positioning requires a certain skill because of the small breast; automatic exposure control is hardly ever used. Mammographic findings can reveal a diffuse opacity, similar to that in the glandular breasts of women, with a more or less prominent ductal pattern, or a rounded opacity behind the areola; the former is evidence of long-lasting gynecomastia.

The sonographic findings of gynecomastia[49] are a hypoechoic homogeneous area behind the nipple, forming a nodule (Fig. 9.82) and an inhomogeneous fibroglandular pattern, resembling that in the female breast (Fig. 9.81). An increased amount of fat tissue, with no glandular component, can mimic gynecomastia in obese patients; palpation may not differentiate fat from glandular tissue, and breast imaging is useful in such situations. Color Doppler sonography has shown increased flow signals in patients with gynecomastia on hormone therapy for prostate cancer (Fig. 9.83). A correlation with physical and mammographic findings is important also for the male breast (Fig. 9.84). Aspiration cytology may be needed to rule out the less frequent carcinoma.

Carcinoma of the male breast is a very rare condition of elderly men (60–70 years of age), with a frequency ratio to

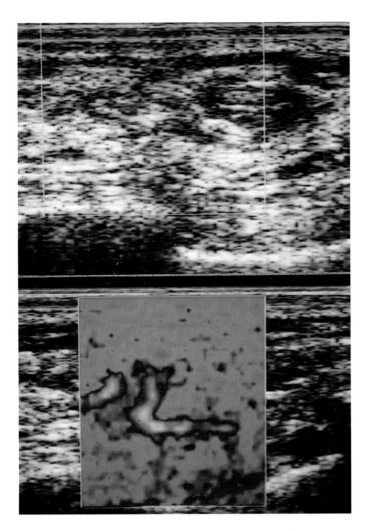

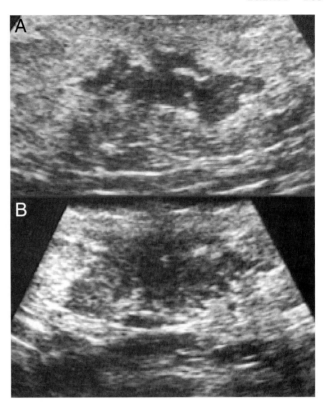

Fig. 9.84 Non-specific sonographic findings in a male breast: acute inflammation (**A**); breast cancer (**B**).

Fig. 9.83 Gynecomastia in a patient on hormone therapy for prostate carcinoma: striking color Doppler signals.

that of female breast cancer of 1:100.[50] A possible relationship between gynecomastia and carcinoma has not yet been completely substantiated, nor has its correlation with estrogen treatment in prostatic carcinoma; nevertheless, 40% of breast carcinomas show microscopic changes consistent with gynecomastia.[47] The most common physical findings are a palpable mass and nipple discharge. Palpable masses are easily detected because of the small breast size. For the same reason early invasion of the chest wall may occur. Mammographic findings are subareolar well-marginated or spiculated masses, that may be obscured by coexisting gynecomastia. Calcifications are variably reported.[51]

There are few reports in the literature on the sonographic patterns of breast carcinoma: findings are similar in males and females. False positive and false negative sonographic findings are corrected by complementing sonography with mammography. The role of aspiration cytology must always be kept in mind.

Inflammation and trauma show the same sonographic patterns as in female patients (Fig. 9.85).

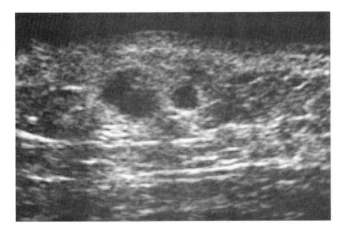

Fig. 9.85 Sonographic findings in a male patient with breast trauma.

BREAST CHANGES AFTER SURGERY AND RADIOTHERAPY

Early diagnosis of breast carcinoma has resulted in an increase in surgical biopsies and in conservative surgery. Both situations account for the great number of breasts currently examined after surgery.

Patients that have had conservative breast surgery for carcinoma have follow-up imaging for several reasons, including the following:

- to confirm cancer removal
- to detect postoperative complications
- to detect recurrences, which may occur close to the surgical scar in 6–9% of cases
- to make a differential diagnosis between the surgical scar and a stellate recurrence
- to rule out new cancers or metastases.

Correct evaluation of the postoperative breast is not possible if all the changes due to surgery or radiotherapy are not thoroughly understood. Such changes include skin thickening, skin retraction, edema, masses, fluid collections, distortions of breast parenchymal architecture (due to scarring and fibrosis) and calcifications. In order to avoid important errors, all these changes must be considered according to the time interval that has passed after surgery or radiotherapy. The most marked changes are found in the first 12 months. The most rapid changes occur in the period from 6 to 18 months. Stabilization, defined as a lack of change on two successive mammograms, takes place from 12 to 36 months after surgery. An increasing frequency of recurrences is noticed after the first 2 years. Skin thickening and edema are slow to regress and may take up to 3 years to resolve. Fluid collections may take up to 2 years to disappear totally. Scarring and calcifications are late findings and progressively increase in time.[52]

The extent of edema depends on the type of surgery, whether axillary lymph nodes are removed or not, and on radiotherapy. It affects skin, subcutaneous tissues and breast parenchyma. Mammography shows skin thickening, mostly around the areola and in the lower and inner quadrants. Subcutaneous tissues are crossed by thin, opaque, rather blurred lines, due to accumulated interstitial fluid and dilated lymphatics. The breast is dense and inhomogeneous, with a trabeculated pattern.

Sonography shows skin thickening, with interruption of the deeper of the two lines that demarcate the skin. A hypoechoic network localized underneath the thickened skin, formed by thin bands parallel and perpendicular to the skin, represents dilated lymphatics. Fat and fibroglandular tissues, that are easily differentiated with US in the normal breast, are blurred and indistinct, diffusely hyperechoic. This increased echogenicity improves contrast resolution and allows a better demonstration of focal lesions. An increase in the number of interfaces in the edematous

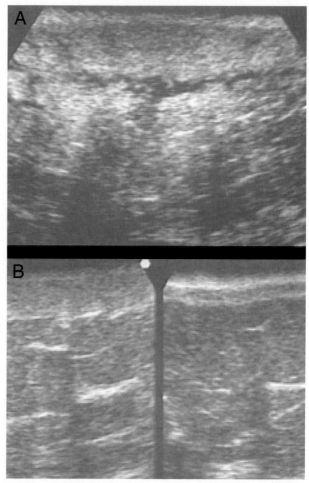

Fig. 9.86 Changes in sonographic patterns at different time intervals after surgery and radiotherapy, in the same patient: skin thickening and lymphatics (**A**) progressively reduce. Comparison between normal and treated breast (**B**).

tissues causes sound attenuation in the deeper tissues (Fig. 9.86).

Fluid collections are frequent findings in the early post-surgical period and represent hematomas, abscesses and lymphoceles. Mammography may not detect them if the breast is dense, or may show non-specific dense asymmetric soft-tissue densities, with ill-defined margins. Sonography can easily identify fluid collections, located in the surgical bed, close to the scar, or migrated because of gravity towards more pendant areas. Sonography can monitor them as they regress slowly, or can guide interventional procedures, in cases of large or inflammatory collections, for a quicker recovery or where large fluid collections may interfere with radiotherapy.

Fluid collections are anechoic or hypoechoic, depending on the type of content – serum, blood or lymph. Recent blood collections have internal echoes due to clots that soon disappear. Margins are ill defined because they are delineated by the surgical excision. Posterior sound enhancement is present. Lymphoceles are frequently encountered as a complication of axillary lymph node dissection and may also show different patterns (Fig. 9.87).

The identification of the area of excision within the breast is important as it may not always correlate with the superficial skin scar. More than 65% of recurrences are found in or close to the excision site. Sonography can demonstrate a hypoechoic line, starting from the skin, crossing the breast tissues and interrupting their architecture; shadowing varies according to the incident beam.

The differentiation of surgical scars and granulomas from a recurrent cancer is difficult. The opportunity to monitor, from the outset, those breast changes that take place after surgery and radiotherapy, may be helpful in detecting physiologic and pathologic processes (Fig. 9.88).

Palpable recurrences appear definitely larger on palpation than with imaging modalities, but not all recurrences are palpable. Tailored mammographic views, tangential to the scar, can demonstrate that an opacity that is suspicious on standard views is connected to the scarred skin, has irregular deep borders and may contain fat tissue that has been enveloped by the scarring process. Stellate recurrences, although close to the surgical scar, are located inside the breast parenchyma, with a dense central core; the recurrent mass maintains its shape in all views.

Sonography, performed with orthogonal scans over the scar, shows that the shape changes with the scanning plane. The scans that are transverse to the main axis of the scar show an irregular hypoechoic superficially located area, which elongates and becomes less well defined in the longitudinal scan along the scar's main axis. Compression and inclination of the probe can reduce to some degree the shadowing produced by the fibrous scar. A recurrence maintains its shape, no matter what scanning plane is used, and shows the morphologic parameters already discussed for carcinoma. Distal shadowing depends on the amount of connective tissue present (Fig. 9.89).

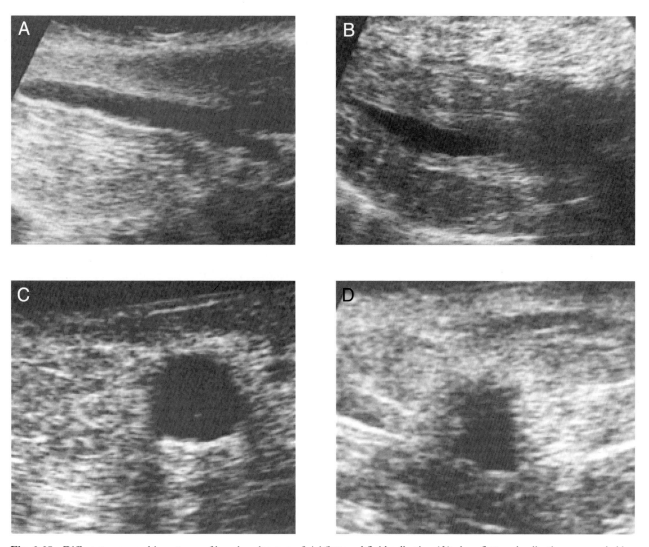

Fig. 9.87 Different sonographic patterns of lymphoceles: superficial flattened fluid collection (**A**); deep flattened collection surrounded by hypoechoic tissue (**B**); rounded fluid collection (**C**); hypoechoic area, with prevalent anteroposterior diameter (**D**).

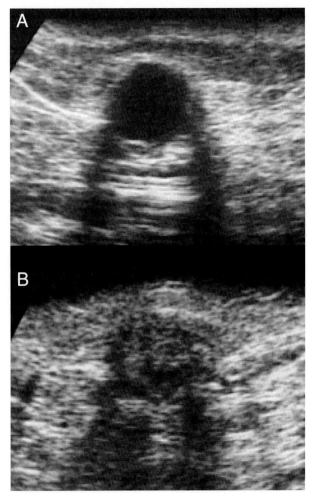

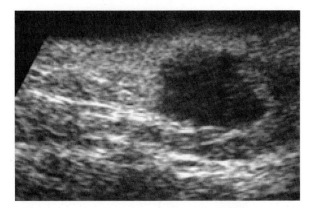

Fig. 9.89 Recurrent cancer, close to the thickened skin.

Fig. 9.88 Sonographic follow-up of a fluid collection (**A**) and granuloma formation (**B**).

MRI of the breast (discussed later) has an important role in differentiating fibrous scar tissue from cancer recurrence. The latter shows a definite enhancement with gadolinium, compared with scar tissue.

Calcifications after surgical procedures are usually attributable to fat necrosis. The mammographic finding is quite characteristic, with irregular coarse calcifications separated by radiolucent fat tissue. The sonographic finding is non-specific. Calcifications, when large enough, cause shadowing. Hypoechoic irregularly shaped areas can be imaged between calcifications (Fig. 9.61). Oil cysts are a particular type of fat necrosis – round, radiolucent images, with a thin, opaque rim, that may calcify. On sonography the cyst may appear homogeneous, or show a mixed, variably echogenic structure (Fig. 90). Fat necrosis and oil cysts appear and stabilize in the first 12–18 months. Any calcification appearing after this period is cause for concern.

Sonography can also be employed to monitor changes in patients receiving endocrine treatment and/or chemotherapy as the initial treatment before local therapy, or as the only treatment for cancer. Very cellular and circumscribed masses, as is the case with ductal and most medullary carcinomas, may disappear; on the other hand, the colloid component of mucinous cancers and stellate masses rarely shows complete regression.[53] Color Doppler imaging can help to assess and predict the response of breast cancer to medical treatment. In a recent report, changes in vascularity paralleled changes in tumor size and could determine the effect of therapy in advance, long before clinical examination and B mode-findings.[54]

Breast imaging is also used to evaluate patients that have had breast reconstruction after mastectomy, or for cosmetic purposes. In both conditions imaging is used to detect early cancer or recurrences, and to demonstrate implant complications.

There are two types of breast reconstruction; these are tissue transfer of autogenous muscle and skin, from the abdomen or the back, to simulate a breast, and the use of implants. The mammographic pattern of the simulated breast using autogenous tissues shows fat, with vessels and connective tissue and no ductal or glandular elements. Augmentation mammoplasty with injections of liquid silicone into the breast has been used in the past, but has now been totally abandoned, because of the development of silicone granulomas. Different types of implants are in use, and studies are in progress to construct prostheses containing a material that is more radiolucent than silicone, such as peanut oil or other types of biologically compatible gels. These materials could improve the results obtained with mammography in the augmented breast.[55]

The types of implants now in use are single lumen (a silicone elastomer shell containing silicone gel), double lumen (gel silicone is contained in an inner lumen, while an outer lumen contains saline) and saline implants (saline is contained within silicone elastomeric capsules). Expanders can also be used as implants (Fig. 9.91). Owing to increasing concern that silicone leakage from implants may be harmful, the use of silicone implants has been restricted, and saline implants are now more used.

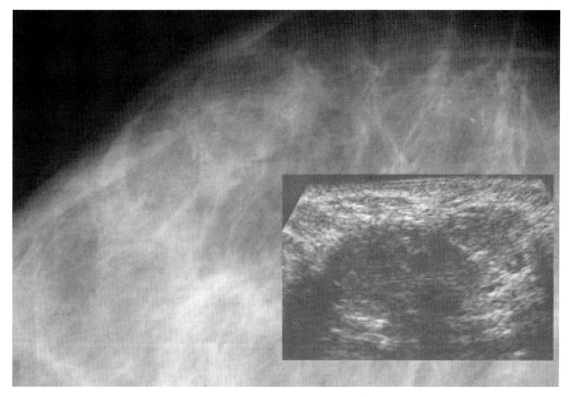

Fig. 9.90 Lipid cysts underneath the surgical scar. The inhomogeneous sonographic patterns of these nodules may be suspect, but a tangential mammographic view is helpful, as it demonstrates rounded radiolucent formations, with a thin rim.

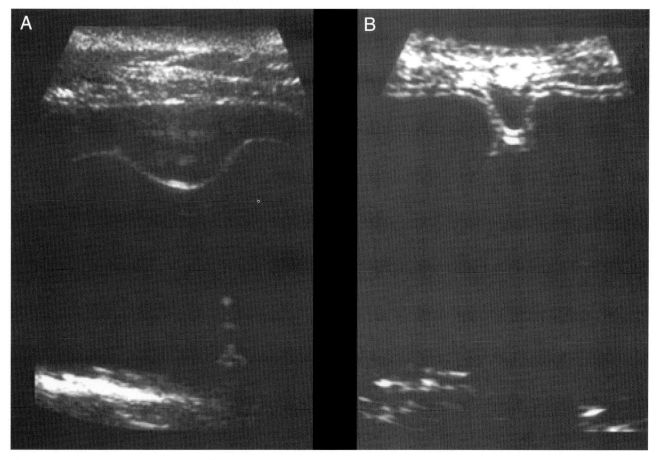

Fig. 9.91 Double lumen implant (**A**); the valve of an expander (**B**).

The normal implant is oval, with smooth rounded margins and a thin-walled shell. On sonography its contents appear anechoic, sometimes with superficial reverberation artifacts of the same thickness. The retromammary or subpectoral location can be easily demonstrated by identifying the fibrillary structure of the pectoralis muscle above the implant. The subpectoral location is preferred to the retromammary, because the implant is less likely to move. Moreover, fewer fibrous reactions take place around the implant, probably because the muscle presses on the implant with a certain massage action, preventing capsule formation. The subpectoral location also interferes less with physical examination and imaging modalities.

Screening for breast cancer in patients with implants requires, besides the usual mammographic views, two modified views, according to Eklund, with the implant displaced posteriorly towards the chest and the breast pulled forward under the compression plate, which keeps the implant back and ensures adequate compression. Sonography is useful to characterize mammographic findings and also palpable abnormalities, differentiating those that originate from the implant.

The complications encountered with implants are dislocation, pericapsular fibrosis, capsular contraction, inflammation, hematoma, implant rupture, implant lobulation and herniation. Human adjuvant disease (HAD), as well as immune and connective tissue disorders, have also been related to silicone.

A fibrous capsule normally forms around the implant, consisting of fibrous and collagen tissue. The capsule and the implant wall appear as an echogenic line. The fibrous tissue may thicken and ultimately shrink, causing contraction. The sonographic pattern of pericapsular fibrosis is that of a thickened hyperechoic capsule surrounding the whole implant, or some portions only. The capsule may calcify. The implant becomes very stiff and spherical. Capsular contraction can also produce lobulation of margins (Fig. 9.92). These complications are more often found in implants located behind the skin or behind the glandular tissue.

Inflammation and hematoma are complications that occur shortly after surgery. The sonographic findings of breast inflammation have already been discussed. Hypoechoic or anechoic areas can be visualized close to the implant, with internal echoes due to debris. The same pattern may be found with hematomas, which are inhomogeneous because of clots and internal membranes.

Implant rupture causes silicone extravasation outside the shell of the implant. The silicone may be contained by the capsule, as is the case in intracapsular rupture, or may pass into the surrounding breast, as is the case in extracapsular rupture, forming granulomas, areas of fibrosis and calcifications. Implants break more easily when they develop wrinkles and folds, which weaken the shell, or when they are old, or (more often) when located behind the gland. Pericapsular fibrosis may prevent silicone diffusion into the breast. Manual procedures to break the capsule – close capsulotomy – may cause extravasation of the silicone that was previously contained by the fibrous capsule. After implant rupture, physical findings are an asymmetric,

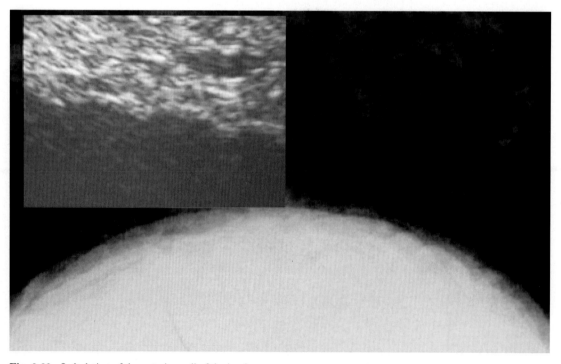

Fig. 9.92   Lobulation of the anterior wall of the implant.

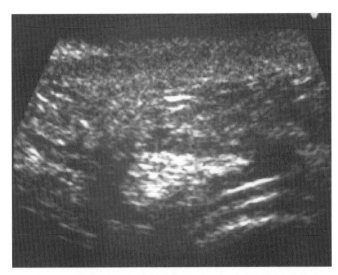

Fig. 9.93 Implant rupture: 'echodense noise' anterior to the implant, causing attenuation.

sometimes deformed breast of a different consistency, or a painful lump. Mammography may reveal lobulation or interruption of the margin of the implant, if this area is included in the field of view of the mammogram. It can also show extrusion of silicone between the implant and the fibrous capsule or outside the capsule, into the breast parenchyma.

Sonography reveals echogenic areas, also termed echodense noise, with posterior shadowing, and hypoechoic masses close to the rupture or in the axillary tissues (Fig. 9.93).[56,57] The margin of the implant is interrupted and

masked by shadowing; echogenic, horizontal lines, forming a 'stepladder', are also present (Fig. 9.94). These lines represent the collapsed implant shell floating inside the silicone gel and must be differentiated from the thin artifacts due to reverberation or the normal folds that cross an anechoic folding implant.[58] Echodense noise represents extruded silicone and may be caused by phase aberration due to the speed of sound, which is slower in silicone than in the soft tissues of the breast.[56]

Calcifications may form on the capsule or on silicone granulomas, associated either with injection of free silicone in the breast or with implant rupture. Calcifications are also associated with fat necrosis, a frequent finding after breast surgery.

Implants with a lobulated border may suggest rupture or merely indicate a herniation (a pouch), which can easily be demonstrated with US (Fig. 9.95). In lobulated implants there is no interruption of the margin of the implant and no noise, because silicone remains in the lumen.

Increasing concern about damage caused by silicone leaks and about the delayed diagnosis of breast carcinoma because of implants is bringing many women to remove intact implants. Bilateral symmetric masses containing coarse calcifications and located behind the glandular tissues have been reported at mammography, following implant removal.[59] The sonographic pattern is nonspecific, with fat and echogenic fibrous tissue and coarse calcifications that cause shadowing.

Sonography has some limitations in the evaluation of implants. The back wall of the implant and the tissues behind it cannot be evaluated. Furthermore, reverberation

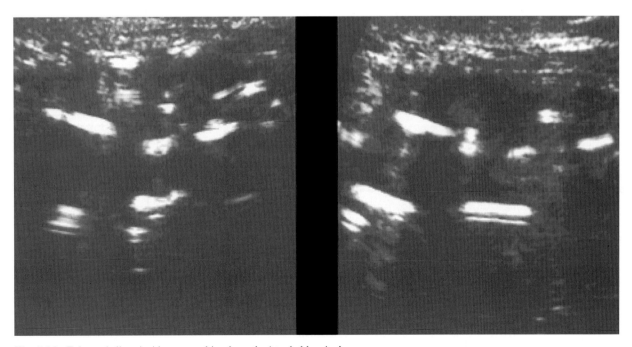

Fig. 9.94 Echogenic lines inside ruptured implant: the 'stepladder sign'.

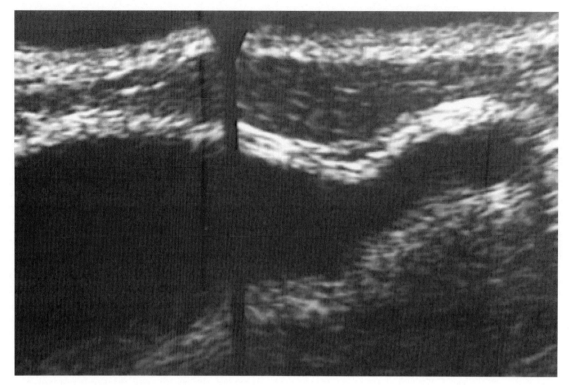

Fig. 9.95   Herniation of an implant, forming a pouch.

artifacts behind the anterior wall can cause some confusion and no study is possible where silicone has been injected previously. MRI can differentiate silicone from surrounding tissues and intracapsular from extracapsular leakage. Implant rupture can also be diagnosed with the demonstration of a free-floating silicone shell within the gel.[60]

SONOGRAPHIC GUIDANCE TO INTERVENTIONAL PROCEDURES

Screening mammography reveals many abnormalities that may need tissue sampling for a definite diagnosis. At the same time, the number of surgical biopsies must not increase, because of costs and because of breast changes caused by surgery. Moreover many of the abnormalities detected are non-palpable, so a guide is needed to sample or localize these findings. Breast imaging can guide interventional procedures both with mammography and with sonography.

Any lesion demonstrated with sonography can be sampled or localized under US guidance if some important rules are followed. A complete US examination must precede biopsy or localization, and it must be correlated with mammography. Correspondence of mammographic and sonographic findings is determined by considering location, depth, morphology, size and acoustic behaviour of a lesion. If sonography detects more than one lesion at

the site of a mammographic abnormality, a mammographic view preliminary to the interventional procedure, with the needle in place, can ascertain that the abnormality sampled or localized correlates with the mammographic finding. The use of a fenestrated mammographic compression plate with markings has been suggested in order to avoid misidentification of mammographic masses with US.[61] The coordinates of the grid pinpoint the mass on the mammogram and guide the probe across the fenestrated plate.

It is obvious that a guide is needed to reach non-palpable abnormalities, but sonographic guidance is useful also for palpable lesions. In such situations US can help to determine the appropriate sampling site, avoiding necrotic or vascularized areas; the needle is directed to the solid portion of atypical cysts with vegetations that may represent carcinoma; aspiration of cysts can be monitored to complete evacuation.

A fundamental rule is to avoid any type of biopsy before imaging, because damage due to biopsy takes a long time to regress and may mimic an abnormality or delay a correct diagnosis.[62]

Before performing any procedure the patient must receive explanations, for better cooperation; it is recommended that informed consent is obtained.

The two types of biopsies used are fine-needle aspiration biopsy (FNAB) or large-core needle biopsy. Equipment has already been described in Chapter 1.

FNAB is currently the most popular technique. Readily

available 20–25 gauge needles, 1.5 inches (38 mm) long are used. A 10 or 20 ml syringe is used for aspiration. A grip pistol on the syringe permits a single-operator technique. No anesthesia is generally required for FNAB. The transducer and skin are carefully cleansed and sterile gel is applied. The use of a biopsy device is not necessary when sampling superficial organs if training has been achieved.

The needle is inserted obliquely, along the short axis of the probe or along the long axis. The former, vertical, approach allows needle tip visualization only when it has reached the scanning plane at the level of the lesion, where a bright echo, with some attenuation, is seen. The latter approach, also called lateral approach, shows the whole length of the needle, so penetration can be monitored more easily. This type of approach is preferred by less-experienced operators, but requires longer needles. During the procedure the lesion must be firmly immobilized underneath the probe, so that it will not shift once the needle is inserted. Probes that have a soft rubber surface towards the skin allow a better hold. Needle guides are available, and may help the beginner. Nevertheless, needle guides prevent repositioning of the needle and samplings in more than one direction; furthermore, longer needles are required, which means a longer needle path and possible needle bending.[63] The freehand technique can be achieved with some training, as soon as the operator begins to correlate the oblique path of the needle and the depth of the lesion. Home-made phantoms are cheap and may prove useful.

Once the tip of the needle is positioned, to-and-fro fanlike movements are applied, so that the needle shaft fills with sampling material. There are two sampling techniques: in the first, aspiration is applied while the needle is moving; in the second, the needle is rotated inside the lesion, without aspiration, and sampling is achieved as a result of capillarity. At the end of sampling the syringe is connected and a brief aspiration is applied.[63] Aspiration is never applied during needle withdrawal.

In order to achieve successful results three requirements must be fulfilled: the needle must be inside the area that has to be sampled; the specimen must be adequate; there must be cooperation between the radiologist and the cytopathologist.

Cytopathologists seldom assist during these procedures. In order to reduce the rate of non-diagnostic sampling, preliminary information must be obtained from the cytopathologists on sample treatment and on the correct preparation of a cytologic smear. Direct demonstration of what to do and what to avoid is more useful than any written instruction.

Core biopsy uses large-bore 14–18 gauge Tru-Cut needles and a spring-activated device. Local anesthesia is necessary to avoid patient discomfort; ethyl chloride spray over the skin or a subcutaneous injection of 2 ml of lido-caine 1% are commonly used. A small skin incision is necessary to allow needle penetration. The tip of the needle is positioned on the surface of the lesion; a lateral approach, in relation to the long axis of the probe, is preferred because it allows a better demonstration of the position of the needle, showing the entire needle shaft. The system is then fired and both the needle and the cutting cannula are propelled forward, inside the lesion; the size of the core and the length of the throw depend on the type of needle. It is advisable not to direct the needle tip towards the chest or implants. This is another reason for choosing the lateral approach, as the needle path is less steep. The large tissue core obtained can be read by any pathologist and sampling is always adequate. Again, the pathologist can give important information on sample treatment.

The decision whether to choose FNAB or core biopsy is fairly controversial and an increasing number of reports have been published on this topic. The choice must be made together with the pathologist or cytopathologist. Core biopsy has definitely reduced the rate of inadequate sampling and does not require an experienced cytopathologist. An oversimplified list of indications to use core biopsy instead of FNAB is that the former can be an alternative to open surgery, can differentiate in situ and invasive carcinomas, and permits more efficient sampling of microcalcifications and a better demonstration of invasive lobular carcinoma, of scars and fibrosis, and of fat necrosis, for example.

Minor complications, such as bleeding, pain or ecchymosis can occur with FNAB or core biopsy. Infections and pneumothorax could be potential complications. Vasovagal reactions have also been reported.[64] A malignant seeding of the needle track has been reported after a large-core biopsy of a mucinous carcinoma.[65] In order to avoid this type of complication, sonography offers a better interventional approach, as it uses the shortest path from the skin to the lesion, so that the needle track will definitely be excised during surgery.

The procedures for localization are the same as those discussed for biopsy. The different methods and needles are discussed in Chapter 1. When non-removable wires are used, two preliminary mammographic views should be obtained to make sure that the abnormality found on the mammogram is being pinpointed. The needle is then withdrawn and the wire can be anchored to the tissues. The mammograms, correlated with the coordinates of the wire tip with respect to the lesion, are also very useful to the surgeon. No matter what guide is used, radiography of the specimen, possibly in a double view and with compression, is fundamental to demonstrate the complete removal of an abnormality.

Both localization and aspiration procedures require the choice of the shortest route from the skin to the abnormality, so that less normal tissue is violated and the lesion is more easily resected by the surgeon. The choice between a mammographic or sonographic guide depends on the operator's skill and personal preference, on the type of equipment available and on the role of sonography in the breast imaging department.

The advantages of a US guide over mammography are as follows:

- shorter route from the skin
- the sonographic approach is very similar to the surgical one, with the patient supine or oblique–supine
- US guide is more comfortable for the patient, as no compression is needed and she is lying down
- sampling or localization can be monitored in real time
- fanlike sampling, in more than one direction, is possible and allows the collection of more material
- the procedure is faster when using US
- US equipment is usually more available than sterotaxis
- US guide is indicated for abnormalities close to chest wall, or implants, or located in the periphery of the breast
- lymph nodes can easily be sampled, no matter where they are situated
- no radiation is used, so US guidance can be chosen in pregnancy and with patients that refuse X-rays
- there is no need to interrupt mammographic screening schedules and use the mammographic stereotaxic equipment
- localization procedures can be performed also in the operating room.

The disadvantages of US when compared with mammographic guidance are as follows:

- it is difficult to depict microcalcifications, which are barely shown if the equipment is inadequate and if they are not located in a nodule
- very small masses may be difficult to demonstrate and to reach
- small, deep masses in a fatty breast may be overlooked.

Biopsy is necessary whenever we need tissue diagnosis. Sonography is useful because it adds further information about the abnormalities shown with mammography and allows a reduction in the number of such abnormalities that require biopsy or surgery. Any abnormality visualized with sonography can be biopsied with an US guide.

CURRENT ROLE OF BREAST ULTRASOUND EXAMINATIONS

Many reports have been written in these last years on the role of ultrasound as a breast-imaging modality.[66–76] The attempt to use sonography as a substitute for mammography for early cancer detection, in order to avoid radiation, has rapidly been abandoned. The concerns of the 1970s about breast irradiation with mammographic screening have totally subsided, because of both the acknowledgement that early cancer detection is important for prognosis and the advent of low dose mammography.

Nevertheless, it is too reductive to use sonography only to differentiate cystic from solid lesions. In our opinion, sonography can play an important part in breast imaging as long as some fundamental rules are kept in mind.

Sonography is highly operator dependent. The person performing the examination must be skilled and have an interest in this technique. The operator must also be aware of normal and pathologic breast findings, of the correct procedures to obtain an adequate examination, and of the physical and clinical findings presented by the patient. When sonography is used to complete a mammographic examination, the mammograms must be viewed in order to correlate the findings of the two imaging modalities. The subsequent report should combine the results of both imaging modalities.

Sonography of soft tissues, and particularly of the breast, depends to a very great extent on the type of equipment used. High-resolution probes allow a better differentiation of normal and pathologic breast tissues. The employment of high-resolution dedicated probes, correctly focussed in the near field, can undoubtedly increase the diagnostic possibilities of this method and its use. Examinations performed with inadequate probes are not only non-diagnostic and time-consuming, but reduce the possibilities of this imaging modality and the confidence that a radiologist may have in its use.

Sonography must always be preceded by a complete record of the patient's history, symptoms and physical findings and must be correlated to these and to other previous examinations, such as mammography.

Sonography is seldom a first-choice examination, except for some particular situations such as the following:

- a palpable mass in a young woman, less than 30 years old, in whom mammographic results are affected by breast density
- pregnant or lactating patients – the former to avoid radiation, the latter because of the mammographically dense breast
- in the acute phase of breast trauma or inflammation, when adequate compression may not be achieved, owing to tenderness and pain, and when preliminary mammographic findings may be totally non-specific, because both processes cause an increase in breast density. In such cases mammography regains its role as a second-choice procedure, once the acute phase has subsided, and in patients in the age range for breast carcinoma.

Sonography is a useful and widely accepted adjunct to mammography in other situations. A palpable abnormality, not clearly delineated on the mammogram – because of breast density, or superimposed adjacent tissues, or peripheral location in areas of the breast that cannot be correctly imaged with mammographic views – can be easily

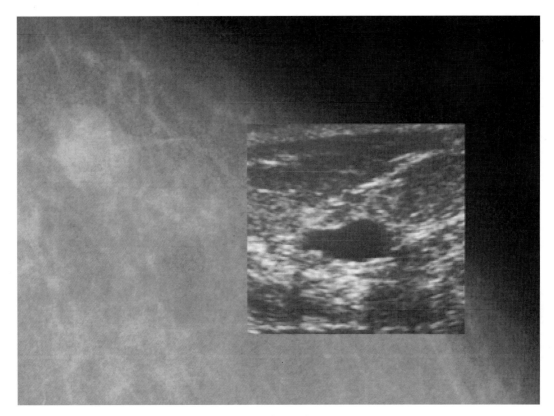

Fig. 9.96   Mass in a fatty breast, that corresponds to a flattened cyst.

examined with sonography. Although a palpable mass can be evaluated clinically and no instrumental guide is needed for aspiration biopsy, we have already touched on the reasons that suggest an approach guided by imaging procedures. Probably benign findings on the mammogram – single or multiple, palpable or occult – can be examined with sonography, and their solid or cystic structure can be defined (Fig. 9.96). Sometimes lesions can be seen only on one mammographic view; the abnormality can then be located either with tailored mammographic views or with sonography.

There are conflicting published reports on the role of sonography in the evaluation of asymmetric breast densities. In our experience, sonography is an invaluable aid to rule out masses that can be obscured by the dense tissues. The demonstration of echogenic breast tissue, or of a cystic mass in the area of increased density, can avoid close mammographic follow-up and biopsy (Fig. 9.97).

Although there is a considerable overlap among the sonographic parameters that may characterize a nodule as benign or malignant, and pathology is the gold standard and the only reliable method for tissue diagnosis, sonography can give further guidance on the patient's management and reduces the number of biopsies necessary. This is particularly true in relation to the cyclical changes shown by many women, such as pain and palpable lumps,

associated with a high rate of dense breasts and no gross mammographic abnormalities. The sonographic evaluation is aimed at the symptomatic area, and may show echogenic fibrous and glandular tissues, or fibrocystic changes, ruling out the presence of masses.

Many other indications for breast sonography are given in the preceding sections, relating to various breast abnormalities.

Sonography can easily monitor postoperative changes, to demonstrate complications, mainly fluid collections, that may be masked by the edematous breast. It can also monitor changes in previously diagnosed benign breast parameters.

Asymptomatic women with normal mammographic findings do not require an ultrasound breast examination. The use of sonography in a completely dense breast, with no significant abnormalities on the mammogram, gives this procedure a screening role with a very low sensitivity.

Mammographically detected masses with the characteristics of carcinoma can also be evaluated with sonography, mainly to confirm sonographic patterns consistent with cancer, to give an accurate evaluation of tumoral extent, and to guide biopsy, allowing a one-step surgical procedure.

Evaluation of node status is achieved more readily with sonography than with physical examination or mam-

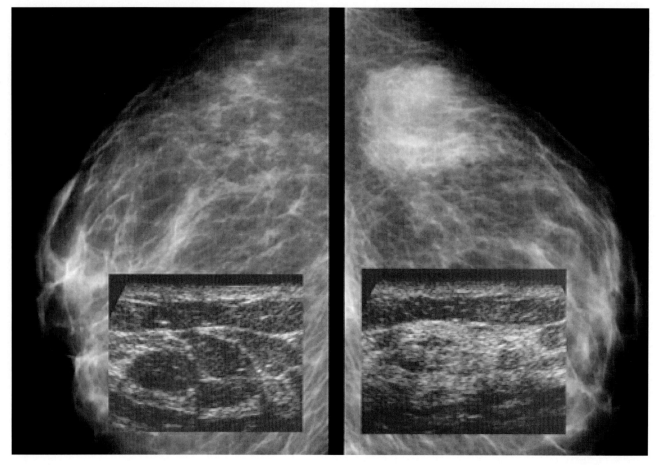

Fig. 9.97   Asymmetric breast density showing echogenic, fibrous tissue on the sonogram.

mography. Although the gold standard to determine node involvement is pathology, and axillary node dissection is part of the surgical treatment of cancer, sonography is helpful to evaluate nodes of the internal mammary chain and of the supraclavicular zone.

Local staging of cancer, accurate size measurement, and the demonstration of muscle infiltration and of metastatic lymph nodes, is today the main role for MRI. Local staging is particularly important in case of conservative surgery. Sonography cannot adequately determine muscle involvement, especially in cases of deeply located cancers, with attenuation that obscures the muscle (Fig. 9.98). MRI can easily differentiate the mass from muscle fibers and the deep fascia and demonstrate muscle involvement (Fig. 9.99).

The detection of multifocal or multicentric carcinoma, present on pathologic specimens in 14–47% of cases, and possible with sonography, is another acknowledged role for MRI.

Interventional breast procedures performed under sonographic guide are discussed above.

No matter how correct the set-up of an ultrasound breast examination, there are some limitations to this imaging modality. Sonography cannot be used to screen occult breast cancer. Although ultrasound detection of asymptomatic carcinomas, not seen on mammograms, has occasionally been reported, the process is time consuming and there is an overall lower sensitivity for sonography than for mammography. Furthermore, microcalcification, an important landmark for early cancer easily demonstrated on state-of-the-art mammograms, cannot be detected with sonography. High-resolution equipment can show calcifications and possibly demonstrate the lesion that harbors them: a solid nodule, a cyst, or ducts. Calcifications situated in nodules are more easily demonstrated than those interspersed in breast tissue, particularly if such tissues are very echogenic. Fatty involution and fatty breasts are poorly examined with sonography because of the diffuse hypoechoic background, corresponding to a favorable radiolucency in mammography. Small, deeply located solid masses are difficult to image; compression must be applied. Cysts are imaged more easily, because of their anechoic structure.

Probes with a higher frequency and a higher spatial and

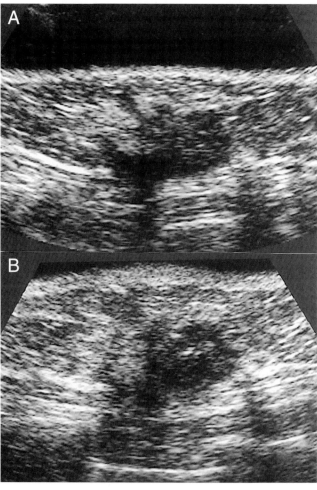

contrast resolution have improved the quality of sonographic images. This technique does not have a role in breast screening, but it has certainly secured a place next to mammography and physical examination for the diagnosis and management of breast abnormalities, reducing the number of biopsies.

Fig. 9.98 Pectoralis muscle involvement: sonography. The mass has a posterior lobulated margin that cannot be differentiated from the muscle (**A**). Hypoechoic mass, containing microcalcifications; shadowing of the posterior border on the left obscures the underlying muscle (**B**). Sonography cannot assess muscle involvement.

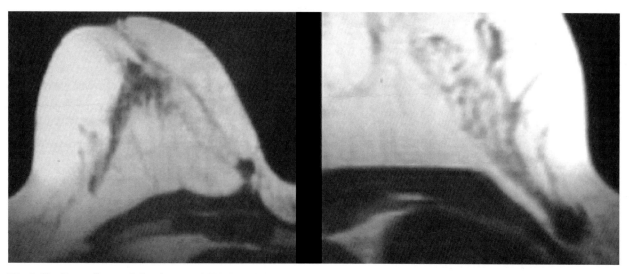

Fig. 9.99 Pectoralis muscle involvement: MRI. Muscle involvement is demonstrated on the left.

REFERENCES

1. Kopans D B 1989 Breast imaging. Lippincott, Philadelphia
2. Mendelson E B 1991 Breast sonography. In: Rumack C M, Wilson S R, Charbonneau I W (eds) Diagnostic ultrasound. Mosby, St Louis, pp 541–563
3. Rizzatto G, Chersevani R, Giuseppetti G M, Baldassarre S, Bonifacino A, Ranieri E 1993 Breast ultrasound. Editoriale Grasso, Bologna
4. Rizzatto G, Chersevani R, Solbiati L 1993 High-resolution ultrasound assists in breast diagnosis. Diagn Imag Int 5: 42–45
5. Bassett W L, Kimme-Smith C 1989 Breast sonography: technique, equipment, and normal anatomy. Semin Ultrasound CT MR 10: 82–89
6. Roebuck E J 1990 Clinical radiology of the breast. Heinemann, Oxford
7. Hughes L E, Mansel R E, Webster D J T 1987 Aberrations of normal development and involution (ANDI): a new perspective on pathogenesis and nomenclature of benign breast disorders. Lancet 2: 1316–1319
8. Consensus Statement 1986 The relative risk for invasive breast carcinoma based on pathologic examination of benign breast tissue. Arch Path Lab Med 110: 171–173
9. Cyrlak D, Wong C H 1993 Mammographic changes in postmenopausal women undergoing hormonal replacement therapy. AJR 161: 1177–1183
10. Meyer J E, Frenna T H, Polger M, Sonnenfeld M R, Shaffer K 1992 Enlarging occult fibroadenomas. Radiology 183: 639–641
11. Linden S S, Sickles E A 1989 Sedimented calcium in benign breast cysts: the full spectrum of mammographic presentation. AJR 152: 967–971
12. Fornage B D, Lorigan J G, Andry E 1989 Fibroadenoma of the breast: sonographic appearance. Radiology 172: 671–675
13. Cole-Beuglet C, Soriano R Z, Kurtz A B, Goldberg B B 1983 Fibroadenoma of the breast: sonomammography correlated with pathology in 122 patients. AJR 140: 369–372
14. Cosgrove D O, Bamber J C, Davey J B, McKinna J A, Sinnett H D 1990 Color Doppler signals from breast tumors. Work in progress. Radiology 176: 175–180
15. Cosgrove D O, Kedar R P, Bamber J C et al 1993 Breast diseases: Color Doppler US in differential diagnosis. Radiology 189: 99–104
16. Buchberger W, Strasser K, Heim K, Muller E, Schrocksnadel H 1991 Phylloides tumor: findings on mammography, sonography, and aspiration cytology in 10 cases. AJR 157: 715–719
17. Baratte B, Teissier J M, Grumbach Y 1990 Les tumeurs bénignes du sein de la femme. (Benign tumors of the breast of the woman). Radiol J CEPUR 10: 33–37
18. Adler D D, Jeffries D O, Helvie M A 1990 Sonographic features of breast hamartomas. J Ultrasound Med 9: 85–90
19. Fabre V, Baratte B, Grumbach Y 1990 Les écoulements mamellonaires. (Nipple discharge). Radiol J CEPUR 10: 57–64
20. Page D L, Anderson T J 1987 Diagnostic histopathology of the breast. Churchill Livingstone, Edinburgh
21. Cardenosa G, Eklund G W 1991 Benign papillary neoplasms of the breast: mammographic findings. Radiology 181: 751–755
22. Kersschot E A J, Hermans M E, Pauweis C et al 1988 Juvenile papillomatosis of the breast: sonographic appearance. Radiology 169: 631–633
23. Le Treut A, Testard S, Trojani M, De Mascarel I, Dilhuydy M H 1991 La papillomatose juvénile. J Le Sein 1: 17–21
24. Auquier M A, Baratte B, Grumbach Y 1990 Conduit à tenir devant un sein inflammatoire. (Inflammatory breast). Radiol J CEPUR 10: 49–56
25. Chersevani R, Rizzatto G 1991 Ultrasound of breast traumas. Clinical report. Eur J Ultrasound 1: 71–75
26. Israel L, Breau J L, Morere J F, Kohn M 1988 Cancers du sein post-traumatiques: 14 cas. Interpretation biologique. Presse Med 17: 592
27. De Wilde Von R, Hesseling M, Holzgreve W, Raas P 1988 Traumatisch bedingtes dermatofibrosarkoma protuberans der mamma. Zentralbl Gynakol 110: 633–635
28. Evers K, Troupin R H 1991 Lipid cyst: classic and atypical appearances. AJR 157: 271–273
29. Manna P, Giuseppetti G M, Latini L, Baldassarre S, Antognoli S 1993 Su un caso di leiomioma della mammella. (Breast leiomyoma: A case report). Radiol Med 86: 155–158
30. Conant E F, Wilkes A N, Mendelson E B, Feig S A 1993 Superficial thrombophlebitis of the breast (Mondor's disease): mammographic findings. AJR 160: 1201–1203
31. Fornage B D, Toubas O, Morel M 1987 Clinical, mammographic, and sonographic determination of preoperative breast cancer size. Cancer 60: 765–771
32. Fornage B D, Sneige N, Faroux M J, Andry E 1990 Sonographic appearance and ultrasound guided fine-needle aspiration biopsy of breast carcinomas smaller than 1 cm^3. J Ultrasound Med 9: 559–568
33. Adler D D, Hyde D L, Ikeda D M 1991 Quantitative sonographic parameters as a means of distinguishing breast cancers from benign solid masses. J Ultrasound Med 10: 505–508
34. Teubner J, Bohrer M, van-Kaick G, Georgi M 1993 Echomorphologie des Mammakarzinoms. Radiologe 33: 277–286
35. Feig S A 1992 Breast masses. Mammographic and sonographic evaluation. Radiol Clin North Am 30: 67–92
36. Jackson V P Sonography of malignant breast disease. Semin Ultrasound CT MR 10: 119–131
37. Cole-Beuglet C, Soriano R Z, Kurtz A B, Goldberg B B 1983 Ultrasound analysis of 104 primary breast carcinomas classified according to histopathologic type. Radiology 147: 191–196
38. Baratte B, Youssef G, Grumbach Y 1991 Apport de l'échographie au diagnostic du cancer du sein. J Le Sein 1: 29–36
39. Stomper P C, Connolly J L 1992 Mammographic features predicting an extensive intraductal component in early-stage infiltrating ductal carcinoma. AJR 158: 269–272
40. Tsunoda-Shimizu H, Ueno E, Tohno E 1990 Echogram of ductal spreading of breast carcinoma. Jpn J Med Ultrason 17: 44–49
41. Tsunoda-Shimizu H, Ueno E, Tohno E, Tanaka H, Aiyoshi Y, Itai Y 1993 Breast conservative therapy: the evaluation of ductal spreading of breast cancer by ultrasound. JSUM Jpn Soc Ultrasound Med Proc May: 459–460
42. Sickles E A 1986 Mammographic features of 300 consecutive nonpalpable breast cancers. AJR 146: 661–663
43. Pamilo M, Soiva M, Lavast E M 1989 Real-time ultrasound, axillary mammography, and clinical examination in the detection of axillary lymph node metastases in breast cancer patients. J Ultrasound Med 8: 115–120
44. Scatarige J C, Hamper U M, Sheth S, Allen H A 1989 Parasternal sonography of the internal mammary vessels: technique, normal anatomy, and lymphadenopathy. Radiology 172: 453–457
45. Meyer J E, Amin E, Lindfors K K, Lipman J C, Stomper P C, Genest D 1989 Medullary carcinoma of the breast: mammographic and US appearance. Radiology 170: 79–82
46. Derchi L E, Rizzatto G, Giuseppetti G M, Dini G, Garaventa A 1985 Metastatic tumors in the breast: sonographic findings. J Ultrasound Med 4: 69–74
47. Rosai J (ed) 1989 Ackerman's Surgical pathology. Mosby, St Louis
48. Wilson J D, Braunwald E, Isselbacher K J et al (eds) 1991 Harrison's Principles of internal medicine. McGraw-Hill, New York
49. Baratte B, Arlot S, Teissier J M, Grumbach Y 1990 Pathologie mammaire masculine. (Breast diseases in male). Radiol J CEPUR 10: 109–114
50. Cotran R S, Kumar V, Robbins S L (eds) 1989 Robbin's Pathologic basis of disease. Saunders, Philadelphia
51. Dershaw D D, Borgen P I, Deutch B M, Liberman L 1993 Mammographic findings in men with breast cancer. AJR 160: 267–270
52. Mendelson E B 1992 Evaluation of the postoperative breast. Radiol Clin North Am 30: 107–138
53. Balu-Maestro C, Bruneton J N, Geoffray A, Chauvel C, Rogopoulos A, Bittman O 1991 Ultrasonographic posttreatment follow-up of breast cancer patients. J Ultrasound Med 10: 1–7
54. Kedar R P, Cosgrove D O, Smith I E, Mansi J L, Bamber J C 1994 Breast carcinoma: measurement of tumor response to primary medical therapy with Color Doppler flow imaging. Radiology 190: 825–830
55. Mendelson E B 1992 Silicone implants present mammographic challenge. Diagn Imag September 70–76
56. Rosculet K A, Ikeda D, Forrest M E et al 1992 Ruptured gel-filled

silicone breast implants: sonographic findings in 19 cases. AJR 159: 711–716

57. Harris K M, Ganott M A, Shestak K C, Losken H W, Tobon H 1993 Silicone implant rupture: detection with US. Radiology 187: 761–768

58. DeBruhl N D, Gorczyca D P, Ahn C Y, Shaw W W, Bassett L W 1993 Silicone breast implants: US evaluation. Radiology 189: 95–98

59. Stewart N R, Monsees B S, Destouet J M, Rudloff M A 1992 Mammographic appearance following implant removal. Radiology 185: 83–85

60. Gorczyca D P, Sinha S, Ahn C Y et al 1992 Silicone breast implants in vivo: MR imaging. Radiology 185: 407–410

61. Conway W F, Hayes C W, Brener W H 1991 Occult breast masses: use of a mammographic localizing grid for US evaluation. Radiology 181: 143–146

62. Svensson W E, Tohno E, Cosgrove D O, Powles T J, Al Murrani B, Jones A L 1992 Effects of fine-needle aspiration on the US appearance of the breast. Radiology 185: 709–711

63. Fornage B D, Coan J D, David C L 1992 Ultrasound-guided needle biopsy of the breast and other interventional procedures. Radiol Clin North Am 30: 167–185

64. Helvie M A, Ikeda D M, Adler D D 1991 Localization and needle aspiration of breast lesions: complications in 370 cases. AJR 157: 711–714

65. Harter L P, Curtis J S, Ponto G, Craig P H 1992 Malignant seeding of the needle track during stereotaxic core needle breast biopsy. Radiology 185: 713–714

66. Jackson V P 1990 The role of US in breast imaging. Radiology 177: 305–311

67. Bassett W L, Kimme-Smith C 1991 Breast sonography. AJR 156: 449–455

68. Reynolds H E, Jackson V P 1991 The role of ultrasound in breast imaging. App Radiol November: 55–59

69. Bassett W L, Ysrael M, Gold R H, Ysrael C 1991 Usefulness of mammography and sonography in women less than 35 years of age. Radiology 180: 831–835

70. Mendelson E B 1991 Ultrasound secures place in breast Ca management. Diagn Imag April: 120–129

71. Flageat J, Vicens J L, Buchon R 1991 Techniques d'imagerie du sein en 1991. J Radiol 72: 645–654

72. Feig S A 1992 Breast masses. Mammographic and sonographic evaluation. Radiol Clin North Am 30: 67–92

73. Kopans D B 1993 Breast imaging and the standard of care for the symptomatic patient. Radiology 187: 608–611

74. Sickles E A, Filly R A, Callen P W 1984 Benign breast lesions: ultrasound detection and diagnosis. Radiology 151: 467–470

75. Jackson V P, Hendrick R E, Feig S A, Kopans D B 1993 Imaging of the radiographically dense breast. Radiology 188: 297–301

76. Catarzi S, Giuseppetti G M, Rizzatto G, Rosselli Del Turco M 1992 Studio multicentrico per la valutazione dell'efficacia diagnostica della mammografia e dell'ecografia nelle neoplasie mammarie non palpabili. Radiol Med 84: 193–197

10

Testis and scrotum

G. Rizzatto   R. Chersevani

TECHNIQUE

Scrotal sonography is generally performed with the patient supine. A towel is put on the penis and the patient can be invited to keep the penis away from the scrotal area. The spermatic cord is studied with the patient standing up and/or with the Valsalva maneuver to investigate minimal varicocele and reflux. To evaluate scrotal blood flow, Doppler parameters are usually adjusted to their most sensitive settings. The PRF should be minimized and the lowest possible wall filter should be used.

NORMAL ANATOMY AND ITS VARIANTS

The testis descends into the scrotum around the seventh month of intrauterine life. Although testicular descent is extraperitoneal, a peritoneal portion, known as the processus vaginalis, enters the inguinal canal with the testis. After birth, the processus vaginalis becomes closed proximally; this obliteration prevents the abdominal contents from entering the scrotum. This also results in an isolated peritoneal pouch, the tunica vaginalis, that encircles the testis, with the exception of the posterior area involving the head of the epididymis.

The tunica vaginalis has two layers – the outer parietal layer and the inner visceral layer, which covers the testis; these are separated by a small volume of fluid. In most patients, this fluid is normally detected around the upper pole of the testis and the head of the epididymis (Fig. 10.1); in some cases it permits visualization of the small appendix testis and appendix epididymis. The visceral layer of the tunica vaginalis is adherent to the tunica albuginea, a fibrous capsule that surrounds the testis; a fold of the tunica albuginea forms the mediastinum testis.

The mature testis consists of approximately 250 cone-shaped lobules, which are separated by thin fibrous septa. This lobular structure usually cannot be identified with ultrasound; it may be imaged when capsular vessels become more evident (Fig. 10.2). There are one to four tortuous seminiferous tubules within each lobule; they join straight seminiferous tubules, the tubuli recti, that connect them to the rete testis. The rete testis is a network of epithelium-lined spaces that are embedded in the fibrous stroma of the mediastinum and drain into the epididymis via 10–15 efferent ductules.

On high-frequency ultrasound, the mature testis appears as a homogeneous ovoid structure of medium echogenicity (Figs 10.1, 10.3). Its size and volume are variable: the longitudinal diameter is 30–45 mm, the transverse diameter is 22–28 mm and the volume ranges from about 16 to 20 ml.[1] The testis usually decreases in size with age.[2] Before puberty, the testis has the same echogenicity as that of the normal adult; the longitudinal diameter is always less than 20–25 mm. The mediastinum of the testis is not always visualized; usually it appears as a peripherally located structure running in a superior–inferior direction (see Fig. 10.16); its echogenicity depends upon the amount of fibrous and fatty tissues present.[3] In addition, the rete testis becomes visible in some patients as a hypoechoic, multiloculated complex adjacent to the head of the epididymis (Fig. 10.4). This benign condition is frequently bilateral and often associated with an ispsilateral spermatocele.[4] Color Doppler may be useful to rule out vascular ectasia or tumors (Fig. 10.5).

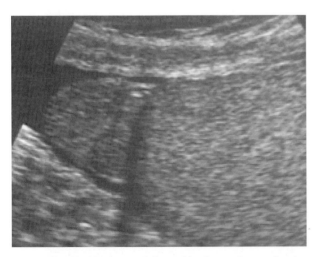

Fig. 10.1 Fluid inside the pouch formed by the two layers of tunica vaginalis usually allows good visualization of the upper pole of the testis and head of the epididymis.

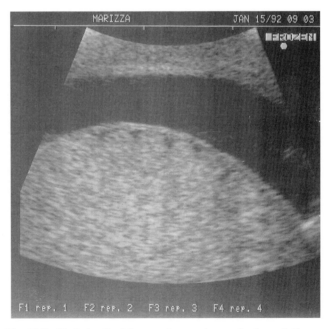

Fig. 10.2 Typical path of the capsular vessels, running beneath the tunica albuginea, suggests the lobular structure of the testis.

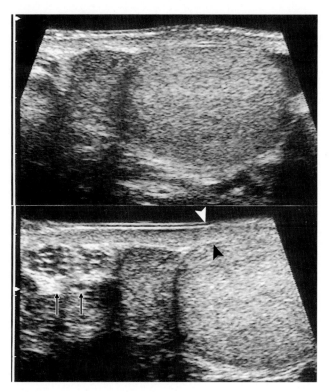

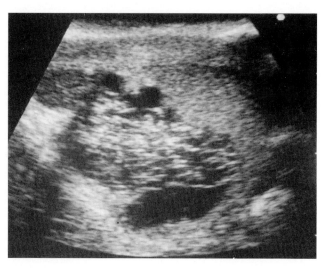

Fig. 10.4   Typical mixed pattern in a patient with a moderate ectasia of the rete testis.

Fig. 10.3   Normal sonographic findings from longitudinal scrotal scan; good visualization of testis and head of epididymis, spermatic cord (arrows) and scrotal wall (arrowheads).

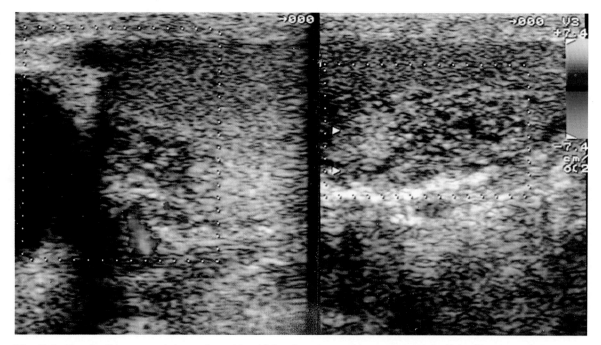

Fig. 10.5   Ectasia of the rete testis in a patient with epididymal cystic area due to spermatocele. Color Doppler excludes presence of an intratesticular varicocele.

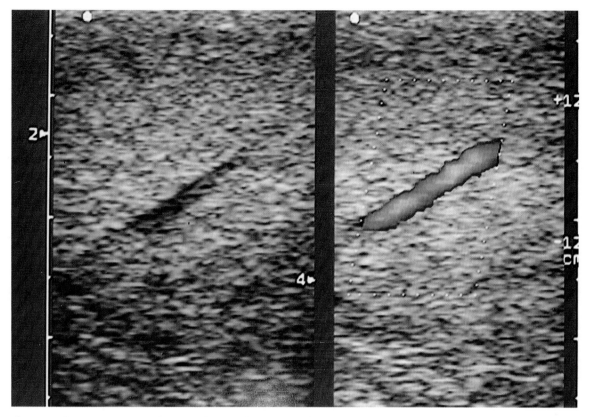

Fig. 10.6 Hypoechoic transtesticular band due to the presence of transtesticular artery.

In other cases discrete hypoechoic bands cross the testis, generally perpendicular to the mediastinum testis (Fig. 10.6). These reflect normal variation of the intratesticular artery and vein and are of no clinical significance.[5] At least 50% of normal testes contain a transmediastinal artery that carries blood away from the mediastinum and towards the opposite edge of the testis (Fig. 10.7).[6] Transmediastinal arteries are usually single and unilateral; adjacent veins are less often seen. Anatomic studies have shown that the typical pattern of arterial flow is from the peripheral capsular arteries, originating from the testicular artery, to centripetal arteries and then to the recurrent rami, also referred to as centrifugal arteries. When a transtesticular artery is present, it gives rise to capsular arteries that travel beneath the tunica albuginea and give rise to centripetal arteries (Fig. 10.8). Using power Doppler, capsular and centripetal arteries are visible in all mature testes (Fig. 10.9); because the pediatric testis and vessels are smaller, identification of vessels is less reliable.[7] The capsular arteries originate from the testicular artery that, after entering the scrotum, runs along the posterior aspect of the testis and penetrates the tunica albuginea. The testicular arteries originate from the aorta, just distal to the renal arteries, and descend in the retroperitoneum to enter the spermatic cord. They lie in the spermatic cord with the cremaster artery (from the inferior epigastric artery) and the deferential artery (a branch of the vesicular artery). There are many ana-

stomoses between these vessels. Nevertheless, the testicular artery primarily supplies the testis; this artery and its branches show a typical low-resistance flow,[7] whereas the deferential and cremasteric arteries supply the high-resistance vascular beds of the epididymis, vas deferens, and peritesticular tissues.

Venous outflow is through the pampiniform plexus that flows into the cremaster and the internal spermatic vein and subsequently into the ipsilateral testicular vein.[8] The

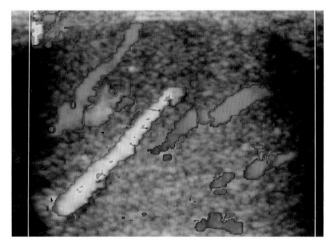

Fig. 10.7 Prominent transtesticular artery running perpendicular to the hyperechoic mediastinum; centripetal arteries and veins.

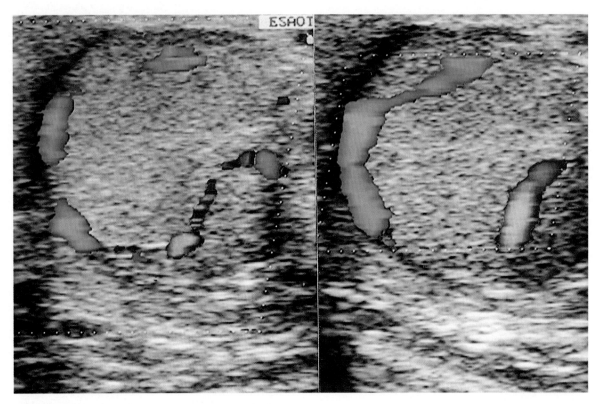

Fig. 10.8 Two different aspects of the capsular arteries.

left testicular vein drains into the left renal vein; the right testicular vein directly joins the inferior vena cava. The cremasteric plexus is posterior to the pampiniform plexus; it is under lower venous pressure and has many anastomoses with the anterior plexus. The cremasteric plexus mainly drains the extratesticular blood; it flows into the cremasteric vein.

The epididymis is composed of extremely convoluted tubules, draining from the testis to the ductus deferens, which ascends superiorly into the spermatic cord. The epididymis consists of a head, body and tail. The head lies on the upper pole of the testis; it is easily seen in most patients (Figs 10.1, 10.3); it is triangular or crescent-shaped. Its echogenicity is variable; normally it is as echogenic as, or slightly less echogenic than, the normal testis.[3] It contains very few vessels, if any. Its size, which tends to decrease with age,[2] varies from 6 to 13 mm in length and from 4 to 12 mm in transverse diameter. The body usually measures less then 4 mm thick and runs along the posterior or posterolateral margin of the testis, decreasing towards the tail. These two portions are usually less echogenic than the normal testis; they drain into the deferent duct that leaves the scrotum through the spermatic cord. Longitudinal scans show a ribbon-like, complex structure (Fig. 10.3); multiple tubular structures (deferent duct, vessels, nerves and lymphatics) run together into the abdomen via the inguinal canal. The Valsalva maneuver in conjunction with color Doppler allow immediate recognition of the venous pampiniform plexus (Fig. 10.10).

The scrotal sac consists of two separate compartments that contain the ipsilateral testicular structures and usually prevent bilateral diffusion of most pathological processes; in addition this facilitates comparative studies. The median septation (Fig. 10.11) is due to a raphe that is continuous with the dartos muscle; this muscle lies just below the scrotal skin and is responsible for its wrinkling. A thin layer of loose connective tissue separates the dartos muscle from the deeper-lying cremasteric muscles; traumatic extravasations and inflammatory edema rapidly increase the thickness of this layer. The fibers of the cremasteric muscle originate from the abdominal wall and extend down from the region of the inguinal ring to enclose the spermatic cord and testis. They are responsible for the cremasteric reflex that retracts the ipsilateral scrotal contents, which is usually absent during testicular torsion.[9] The scrotal wall is variably thick, ranging from 3 to 6 mm; in pathological conditions the thickness of the affected site must always be compared with the contralateral hemiscrotum.

MALPOSITION OF TESTES

Ectopia testis is a rare condition; it is the result of deviation from the normal pathway of descent. The most common sites are pubopenile, femoral triangle and perineal (Fig.

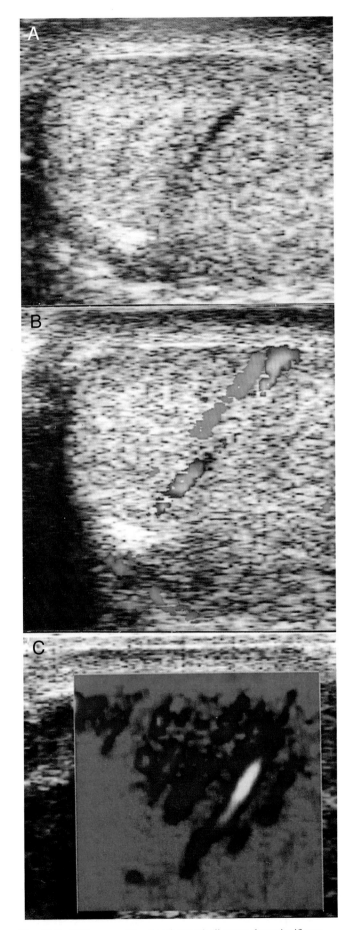

Fig. 10.9 With power Doppler (bottom) all testes show significant vascularity.

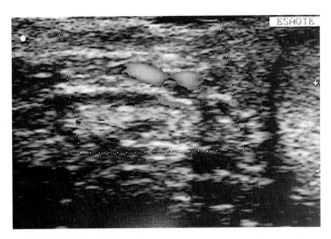

Fig. 10.10 In normal subjects the Valsalva maneuver and a standing position help to demonstrate flow inside the tubular structures of the spermatic cord.

10.12). Ectopia may be also interstitial, on the oblique muscle above the inguinal canal.

Undescended testis is found in 4% of full-term infants; the testis is usually in the scrotum within 4–6 weeks. Only 0.8% of males at the age of 1 year have true cryptorchidism, which is bilateral in approximately 20% of these. The incidence of undescended testis is increasing.[10]

Infertility and cancer of the testis are the major risk for these patients. The risk of cancer is now estimated to be five to 10 times as high as for healthy men. The incidence of infertility is reduced if surgical orchiopexy is carried out before the age of 1–3 years; on the other hand, surgery does not eliminate the risk of malignant change.[11]

In approximately 75–85% of cases the undescended testis is in the inguinal canal or superficial inguinal region; it is easily palpated and identified with ultrasound, unless patients are obese. In about 30% of cases the epididymis cannot be identified as a separate structure; lack of surrounding fluid and compression by the adjacent structures make the testicular margin less defined than in the normally located testis (Fig. 10.13). The testis is homogeneous, slightly less echogenic; color Doppler shows that vascularity is poor. In patients referred after puberty, the undescended testis exhibits different degrees of atrophy; it may be

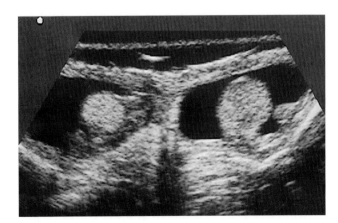

Fig. 10.11 Neonatal hydrocele showing a clear separation between the right and the left hemiscrotum.

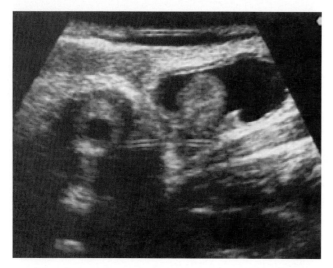

Fig. 10.12 On the left of the rectum the left testis, in perineal ectopic position, is surrounded by hydrocele.

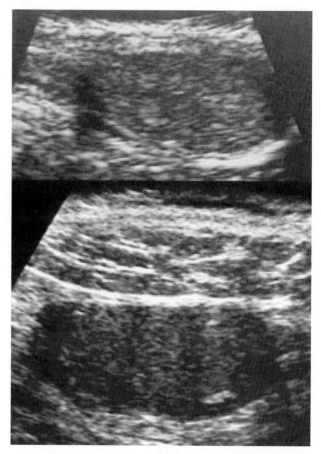

Fig. 10.13 Cryptorchid testes in a 3-year-old child (top) and in a 26-year-old subfertile adult (bottom); the latter testis is atrophic and hypoechoic, with bright calcifications.

affected by different pathological conditions such as varicocele, inflammation or tumors (Fig. 10.14).

In 15–25% of cases the testis is in the abdomen, but in a few patients it lies deep to the abdominal wall or at the level of the kidney. Usually, the testis is near, or only a few centimeters from, the internal inguinal ring; generally, these testes are non-palpable. Although ultrasound examination is performed with a full urinary bladder, it can easily miss abdominal testes;[12,13] false positive diagnoses are not infrequent. In negative or doubtful cases, CT or MRI must be used.

TESTICULAR ATROPHY

Testicular atrophy may be secondary to cryptorchidism, inflammation, torsion or trauma. Less frequent causes include hypothyroidism, estrogen therapy, cirrhosis, renal transplantation, diseases of the pituitary gland and hypothalamus, debility and senility. Ultrasound shows a hypoechoic testis (Figs 10.13, 10.15). Volume and vascularity are reduced; the epididymis is usually normal.

TESTICULAR AND EPIDIDYMAL CALCIFICATIONS

Focal echogenicities, with or without acoustic shadowing, are occasionally seen in the testicular parenchyma; most of them are due to phleboliths, intraluminal calcifications or spermatic granulomas (Fig. 10.16). Calcifications in or adjacent to the epididymis are more frequent; they may be seen in up to 3% of asymptomatic patients, possibly related to previous inflammation.[2]

Diffuse, tiny echogenic foci are characteristic of microlithiasis (Fig. 10.16). This incidental finding increases in frequency as the use of higher frequencies results in better

contrast resolution. The hyperechoic foci give rise to a diffuse speckled appearance, usually associated with reduced vascularity; these foci represent calcified concretions within the lumina of the seminiferous tubules.[14] Degenerate tubular epithelial cells within the lumen, and associated collagenous material serve as a site for dystrophic calcification; up to 30–40% of the seminiferous tubules may be involved and obstructed.

The etiology is uncertain; testicular microlithiasis is frequently associated with cryptorchidism or delayed testicular descent, subfertility, or gonadal dysgenesis. The coexistence of testicular microlithiasis with carcinoma has also been documented.[14,15] Association of microlithiasis and hypoechoic focal areas may be considered to be grounds for suspicion of neoplasm; surgical biopsy or US-guided FNAB are called for. In all other cases, ultrasound is recommended to monitor the testicular texture.[15]

FLUID COLLECTIONS

Hydrocele, hematocele, pyocele and lymphocele

Hydrocele is an abnormal fluid collection between the

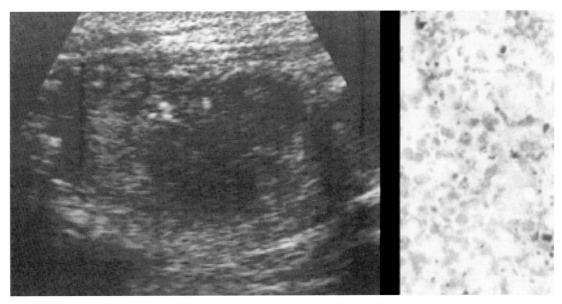

Fig. 10.14 Cryptorchid testis with a small hypoechoic nodule with calcifications, in a 48-year-old patient. Atypical seminoma on FNAB (right).

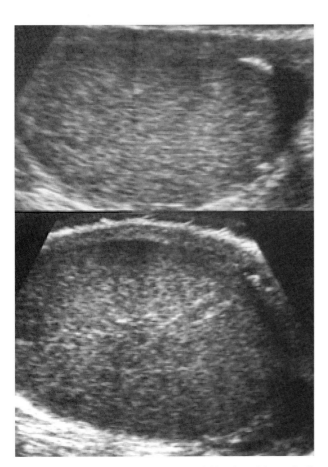

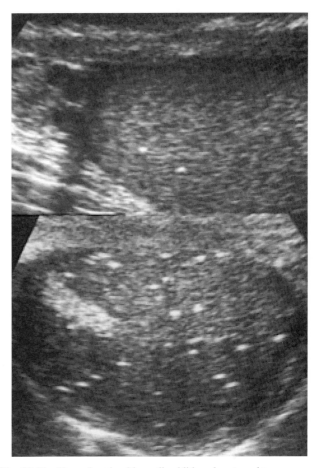

Fig. 10.16 Normal testis with small epididymal cysts and two intratesticular calcifications (top). Diffuse bilateral microlithiasis (bottom): sagittal view of the left testis showing the hyperechoic band of the mediastinum.

Fig. 10.15 Subatrophic adult testes with calcification of the vaginalis (top right) and hyperechoic bands of fibrosis (bottom).

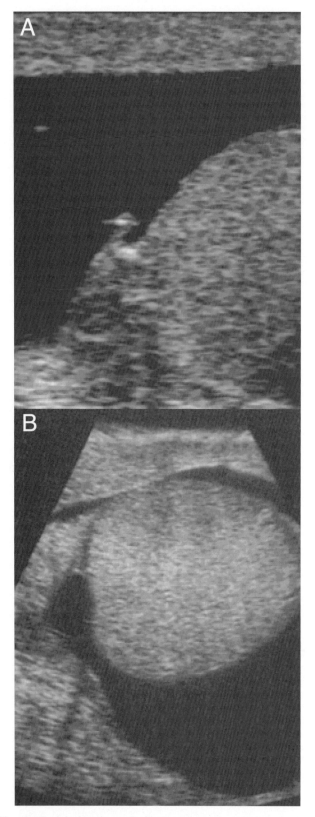

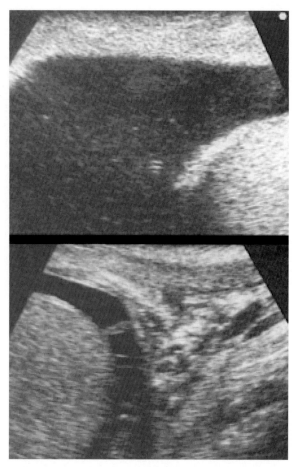

Fig. 10.18 A patient with acute orchitis shows low-level echoes within the fluid collections (top) and small septations at the lower pole of the testis (bottom).

Fig. 10.17 A hydrocele usually displaces the testis posteriorly (top); a hydrocele allows visualization of the small appendix epididymis. A spermatocele is usually septated and displaces the testis anteriorly (bottom).

parietal and visceral layers of the tunica vaginalis. This condition is frequently found in neonates, when the processus vaginalis that connects the scrotal sac and the peritoneum is still open (Fig. 10.11). Normally it closes at or before 18 months of age.

In children or adults, hydroceles are idiopathic or secondary to inflammation, torsion or trauma. Hydroceles in association with tumor are infrequent; in most of these cases they are associated with pediatric tumors and with large non-seminomatous tumors in adults.

Sonographically, hydroceles appear as anechoic fluid collections; they usually displace the testis posteriorly and medially (Fig. 10.17).[3,16] Septations are infrequent, mostly associated with chronic conditions or old hemorrhage and infection. Hydroceles can be usually distinguished from spermatoceles and other cystic masses by the way in which they surround the testis and are relatively mobile. Chronic hydroceles may develop low-level mobile echoes; this is seen more often when higher frequencies are used. These echoes are generally due to cholesterol crystals and cannot be distinguished from echoes caused by inflammatory debris or blood. In chronic hydroceles there may be diffuse

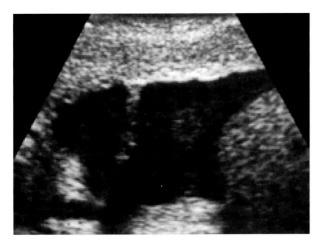

Fig. 10.19   The presence of gas inside a hematocele due to ballistic trauma gives rise to a bright comet tail artifact.

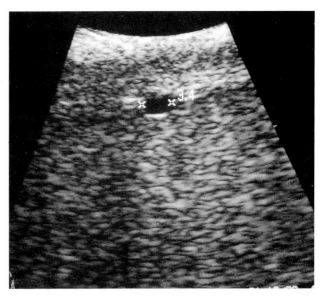

Fig. 10.20   Small cyst of the albuginea (3.4 mm in diameter).

thickening of the scrotal wall, parietal calcifications and even scrotoliths.[17]

Hematoceles and pyoceles usually complicate trauma and inflammation; they are echo free in only a few cases. With high-frequency sonography they usually exhibit low-level internal echoes, fluid debris levels and internal septations (Fig. 10.18); the presence of gas can be identified as a strong reflector with posterior comet tail artifacts (Fig. 10.19).[18] Scrotal lymphoceles have been described following renal transplantation.[19] They may be caused by lymphatic disruption or dissection of a peritransplant lymphocele, with subsequent extravasation of fluid, via the inguinal canal, to the scrotal sac. There can be low-level echoes and septations.

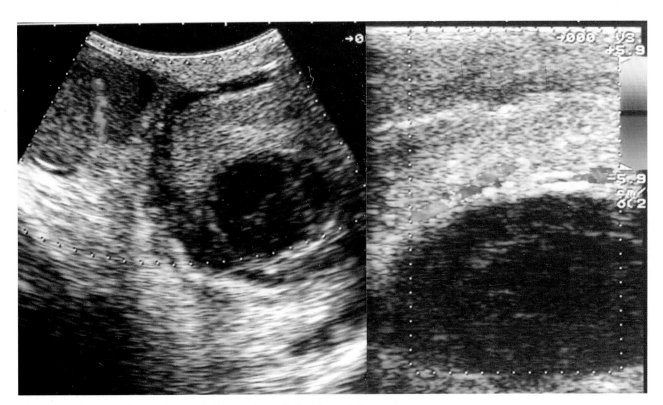

Fig. 10.21   Intratesticular cyst; intratesticular vessels are displaced anteriorly.

Cysts and spermatoceles

Benign cysts of the albuginea and of the testis are not uncommon.[3,20] Cysts of the albuginea generally present as small palpable masses that are echo free on ultrasound (Fig. 10.20); they are marginal, usually located near the rete testis and the epididymis. Intratesticular cysts generally are non-palpable (Fig. 10.21); recent histologic studies suggest that they originate from the rete testis or are secondary to inflammation, trauma and dysgenic predisposition.[20] It is very important to differentiate between benign and neoplastic cysts. Cyst-like structures are usually depicted as portions of malignant, complex tumors. Nevertheless, cystic tumors may be solitary; moreover, they may exhibit ultrasonic patterns, including avascularity, that are typically benign (Fig. 10.21). In these cases, FNAB is a safe and easy method of confirmation.

Epididymal cystic structures are seen in approximately one-third of asymptomatic adults.[3] Spermatoceles are more common. These are cystic collections of seminal fluid, usually within an efferent duct near the head of the epididymis, and may be secondary to inflammation, trauma or vasectomy.[21] Ultrasound shows cystic fluid collections, often multiple (Fig. 10.22). Small collections do not differ from epididymal cysts. Larger spermatoceles often present septations; high gain settings produce slow-moving internal echoes or fluid–fluid levels (Fig. 10.23). These spermatoceles usually displace the testis anteriorly (Fig. 10.17). If aspirated, spermatoceles are found to contain milky, sperm-like fluid; they may be treated with ethanolamine oleate sclerotherapy, with a cure rate higher than 80%.[22] Ultrasound may be used to guide the maneuver and to assess its therapeutic efficacy.

VARICOCELE

Varicocele is a common abnormality occurring in 8–20% of the normal adult population.[8,23] The incompetence of the spermatic vein valves gives rise to most varicoceles: in 85–95% of cases these occur on the left side, because the left spermatic vein drains into the left renal vein which is compressed between the aorta and the superior mesenteric artery; in 10–15% of cases this is bilateral; rare isolated varicoceles occur on the right side.[24] Other causes of varicocele are left renal vein thrombosis or tumoral compression, and neoplastic involvement of the retroperitoneum or of the pelvis.

Varicocele is considered to be a potential cause of male infertility because of retrograde flow in the draining vessels, venous stasis and increased scrotal heat. This association is still controversial; nevertheless, following ligation of spermatic cord venous channels or sclerotherapy, improvement of both sperm quality and conception rate has been reported.[24] Moreover, varicoceles are more common in infertile males and are often associated with changes in semen composition.

Diagnosis of large varicoceles is easy and is usually made by palpating the dilated vessels in the scrotal sac or the spermatic cord. Small or moderate varicoceles require adequate physical examination, with the patient standing and performing a Valsalva maneuver. There is no direct evidence that the size of varicocele influences the degree of sperm abnormality.

Ultrasound allows accurate detection and measurement of even subclinical varicoceles. The spermatic cord is scanned with the patient supine and standing up, both at rest and during the Valsalva maneuver.[8,25] The diameter

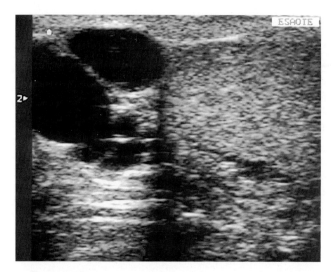

Fig. 10.22 Multiple cysts within the epididymal head and minimal ectasia of the rete testis.

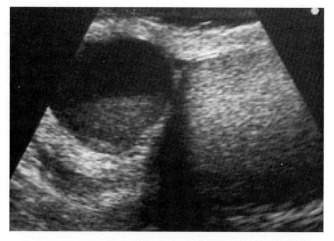

Fig. 10.23 Fluid–fluid level inside a spermatocele of the epididymal head.

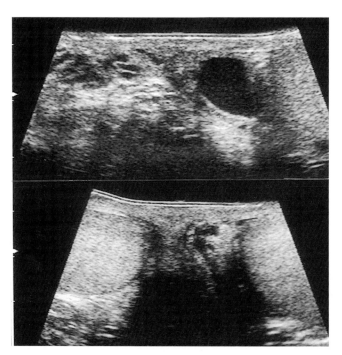

Fig. 10.24 Evidence of dilated veins inside the spermatic cord in a patient with epididymal cyst.

frequency transducers, variable low-level echoes can often be seen inside the dilated veins, moving in the direction of the blood low and giving physiologic evidence of the reflux (Fig. 10.26). The sensitivity of this method, when compared with venography, is 93%.[26] Although it is highly sensitive for subclinical varicoceles, it may suggest a significant prevalence of varicoceles in normal subjects or in postoperative patients.[26] Correlation with sperm parameters and physical findings is therefore required to give clinical sense to the sonographic findings.

Ultrasound can discriminate between unilateral and bilateral varicoceles. Moreover, it is often possible to define the extent of the venous abnormality. Enlarged serpiginous or tubular vessels that assume an anterior position superior to the testis suggest involvement of the pampiniform plexus; those lesions involving the cremasteric plexus are dorsal to the testis (Fig. 10.27).[8] Intratesticular varicocele may appear as a vague hypoechoic area in the testis or mimic tubular ectasia.[27] After ligation or sclerotherapy, blood flow is diverted from the pampiniform plexus into other draining veins; these alternative pathways can give sonographic evidence of the cremasteric plexus and short communicating veins within the scrotal wall (Fig. 10.28).

Doppler sonography can also be used to grade the venous reflux as stasis (grade I), intermittent (grade II) or continuous (grade III).[28]

TESTICULAR TORSION

The normal testis and epididymis are anchored to the scrotal wall. If there is a lack of development of these attachments, the testis is free to twist on its vascular pedicle.

of the dominant vein demonstrating color flow is then measured from the inner walls. A varicocele is diagnosed when the vessel is more than 2 mm in diameter (Fig. 10.24). In addition, color Doppler permits the presence of reflux to be visualized as areas of enlarging and changing color (Fig. 10.25); reflux is considered to be an essential component of clinically significant varicoceles. With high-

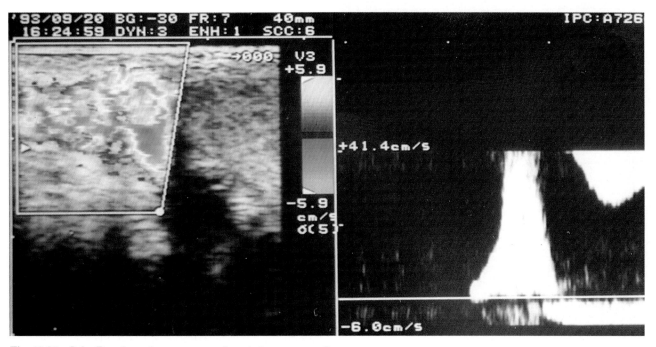

Fig. 10.25 Color Doppler and spectrum reveal an obvious venous reflux.

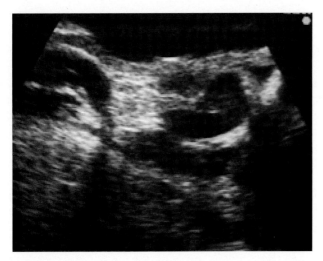

Fig. 10.26 Dilated veins inside the spermatic cord, showing internal echoes, moving on dynamic imaging.

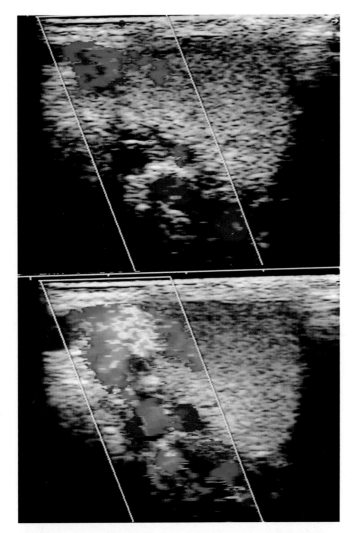

Fig. 10.27 Varicocele involving the cremasteric plexus; progressive evolution of the color Doppler image during the Valsalva maneuver.

This will result in complete, incomplete or relapsing obstruction to venous outflow and, eventually, to arterial inflow.[16] Ischemia may result in testicular infarction and necrosis, leading to either orchiectomy or atrophy (Fig. 10.29).

Testicular torsion occurs most commonly around the onset of puberty and the early teenage years.[29] Neonatal extravaginal torsions are rare.[30] Cord detorsion must be performed as early as possible.[29] Testicular viability is the final outcome when the interval from the onset of symptoms is less than 6 h. If surgery is performed within 24 h there is a 60–70% salvage rate; the proportion of testes saved falls to less than 20% when operation is delayed.[31]

The clinical onset is usually acute, with testicular pain and scrotal swelling in young boys, whereas scrotal masses are more frequent in infants. Most patients have a history of previous episodes of similar transient symptoms. Nausea and vomiting are quite common. The scrotum may be tender on palpation; the testis may be at a higher level owing to shortening of the spermatic cord. The cremasteric reflex is usually absent.[9] Positive urine cultures and fever are present in about 20% of these patients; elevated white blood cell counts occur in 50% of cases.[32] Differential diagnosis with acute epididymitis may be difficult in up to 50% of cases. With lack of adequate information, immediate surgery is preferred; this approach improves both the salvage rate and the rate of unnecessary surgical explorations in patients with epididymitis.

Nuclear medicine scanning is highly accurate; it can detect reduced or absent perfusion in 94–99% of cases.[33] Sonographically, most cases exhibit a normal gray-scale appearance during the critical phase.[16] In some cases of complete torsion the spermatic cord and the epididymis are enlarged and usually hypoechoic (Figs 10.30, 10.31); hydrocele and thickening of the scrotal wall may be associated. Decreased testicular echogenicity is seen only in cases with a poor prognosis.

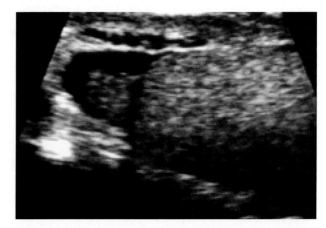

Fig. 10.28 After surgical ligation there is evidence of new alternative pathways within the scrotal wall.

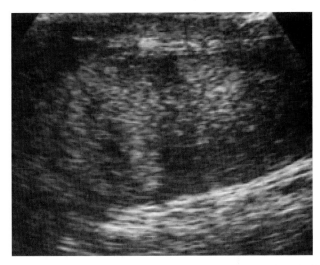

Fig. 10.29 Inhomogeneous atrophy 10 months after delayed surgical detorsion.

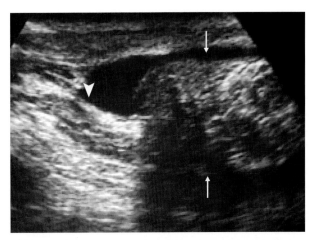

Fig. 10.30 Acute testicular torsion; enlarged epididymis (arrows) and spermatic cord (arrowheads).

Conversely, color Doppler is very sensitive, in case of incomplete torsion as well.[16,34] In most positive cases no flow is detectable; comparison with the contralateral spermatic cord and testis, at the same settings, is always necessary. Color Doppler is also specific; nevertheless, few cases of vascularization in torsional testes have been reported.[34,35] The sensitivity of the instruments available to the low flows, and the time at which patients present for scanning, vary widely; for these reasons surgical decisions cannot be based on sonographic evidence only.

TRAUMA

Testicular injuries are mainly associated with sporting activities, vehicle accidents and ballistic trauma.[3,36,37] Owing to the mobility of the testis and the protective covering of the scrotal wall, true ruptures are infrequent; most injured testes can be treated conservatively. If surgical repair is required, it must be performed within 3 days; early surgery reduces the rate of orchiectomy from 55.5 to 7.4%.[36]

In all such cases physical examination is difficult or impossible because of the severe testicular pain, scrotal swelling, wounds or ecchymosis. The role of sonography is to determine whether the testis is normal or if there is testicular disruption requiring immediate surgery.[3,37–39]

In many cases sonography reveals only involvement of the scrotal wall. The loose connective layer, between the dartos and cremaster muscle layers, is the site of wall thickening as a result of reactive edema, extravasation and hemorrhage (Fig. 10.32). A multilayered pattern is typical of urinary extravasation from bladder rupture; the wall may become up to 4–6 cm thick. Variable amounts of fluid may be associated. In the acute phase, hematoceles are generally echo free; high gain settings reveal low-level moving echoes

(Figs 10.33, 10.34). Echogenic debris and septations are usually identified in chronic hematoceles.

The hematocele may also be echogenic, or have a complex pattern, immediately after the trauma; in these cases the testicular margins must be carefully evaluated to exclude fractures and consequent extrusion of the disrupted testis (Fig. 10.35). In general, early surgical exploration is required. In other cases the traumatized testis shows normal structure or focal areas of variable size and echogenicity, and reduced vascularity (Fig. 10.36). In the latter cases, strict sonographic surveillance is recommended for the first few days, to allow proper selection for surgical repair. As a result of trauma, the epididymis may have an increased volume, reduced echogenicity or abnormal position in relation to the testis (Fig. 10.37).

Foreign bodies can be identified successfully and located precisely (Fig. 10.37); penetrating bullets may leave

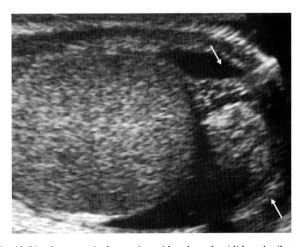

Fig. 10.31 Acute testicular torsion with enlarged epididymal tail (arrows) and wall thickening.

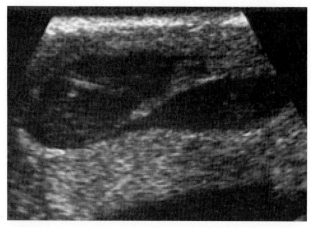

Fig. 10.32 Enlarged view of a thickened wall (24 mm) with internal haematoma.

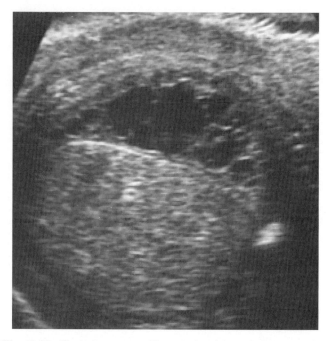

Fig. 10.33 Testicular trauma with normal testis, septated hematocele and wall thickening.

anechoic tracts through the testes[37]; air within the hematocele is seen as bright reflections producing comet tail artifacts (Fig. 10.19).

INFLAMMATORY DISEASES

Acute inflammatory diseases

Epididymitis and epididymo-orchitis are the most common infections involving the scrotum and the most common causes of acute scrotal pain.[16,40] In general, they occur in older patients than those presenting with testicular torsion; nevertheless, there is a marked overlap in the clinical findings.

In 80% of cases cultures are positive for specific micro-organisms – *Neisseria gonorrhoeae* and *Chlamydia trachomatis* in younger patients, *Escherichia coli* and *Proteus*

mirabilis in men above 35 years of age.[41] These infections usually start in the prostate or in the bladder; retrograde spread via the deferens duct is most common. Bilateral involvement is infrequent. In general, orchitis is the result of direct spread from the inflamed epididymis. Most other isolated testicular inflammations are viral in origin.

The clinical symptoms range from severe febrile illness to mild discomfort. Only in 50% of the patients does the pain develop acutely. Urinary symptoms are rare, whereas pyuria is present in over 40% of patients; fever occurs in 30%. On physical examination the epididymis and/or testis

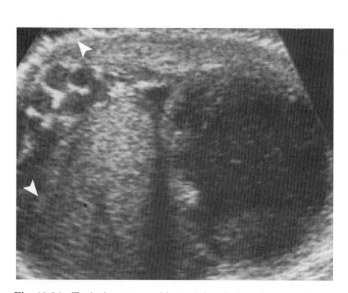

Fig. 10.34 Testicular trauma with normal testis, large hematocele, varicocele (arrowheads) and thickened wall.

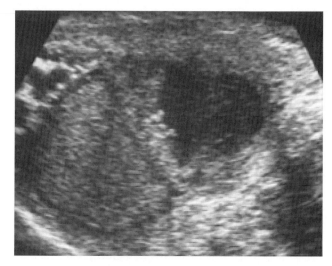

Fig. 10.35 Fractured testis with partial loss of the lower pole.

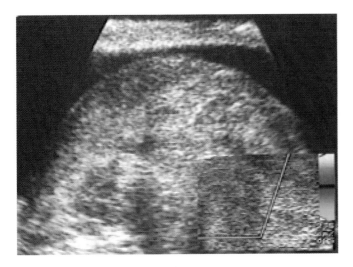

Fig. 10.36 Testicular trauma resulting in diffuse alteration in testicular texture and reduced vascularity.

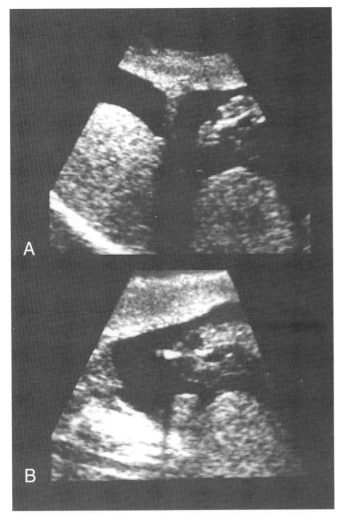

Fig. 10.37 Ballistic injury. The body of the left epididymis is floating in the hematocele (top); a small pellet inside the epididymis gives rise to a bright echo with acoustic shadowing (bottom).

may be swollen and tender; in the most acute cases they may be indistinguishable. Skin edema and erythema may be associated.

In the majority of cases sonography reveals enlargement and decreased echogenicity of the structure.[3,16,41-44] Involvement may be focal (Fig. 10.38) or diffuse (Fig. 10.39). Focal involvement is more frequent in the epididymis; in very acute cases hypoechoic areas, due to small abscesses, are associated with hyperechoic areas caused by hemorrhage and necrosis. Single large hypoechoic areas due to abscess formation may replace the epididymis. All these findings are more frequent at the level of the head of the epididymis; the body and tail usually are normal or slightly hypoechoic and may exhibit a moderate increase in volume (Fig. 10.40). Instruments with adequate sensitivity to low flows are always able to demonstrate an increased number of vessels in the affected area (Figs 10.41–10.43).[34,41,45] The vessels detected have a very low vascular resistance; more venous flow is recognized.[41] These features are the result of the hyperemia that occurs in inflammatory conditions. The presence of vessels in the epididymis is diagnostic; normally, this area is avascular. On the other hand, a focal or diffuse increase in testicular vascularity may also be associated with focal tumors or diffuse infiltration from leukemia or lymphoma.[41]

Wall thickening and hydrocele are usually noted and can be used to differentiate inflammation from a neoplasm;[46] septations, debris, fluid–fluid levels and comet tail artifacts due to gas are the sonographic patterns of an infected hydrocele (Fig. 10.44).[18]

Chronic inflammatory diseases

Chronic inflammatory conditions are usually due to the spread of tuberculosis from the urinary tract.[3,47,48] Involvement from sarcoidosis is rare. Generally, infections start in the epididymis; if left untreated, they will spread to the testes in more than two-thirds of cases.[3]

The most distinctive features are an enlarged epididymis, mostly in the tail portion, and diffuse alteration of the echo texture (Figs 10.45–10.47). Granulomatous nodules often simulate extratesticular neoplasms. Sonographic evidence of testicular involvement consists of a diffusely enlarged hypoechoic testis with indefinite separation from the epididymis. Calcifications may be present in the epididymis, testis and tunica vaginalis (Figs 10.46, 10.47).

SCROTAL HERNIA

A scrotal hernia is secondary to an inguinal hernia; this is mostly indirect, via the inguinal canal, whereas direct hernias, via Hesselbach's triangle, are less common.[3,49]

In general, clinical diagnosis is easy; nevertheless, chronic hernias may be irreducible and often mimic a scrotal mass.

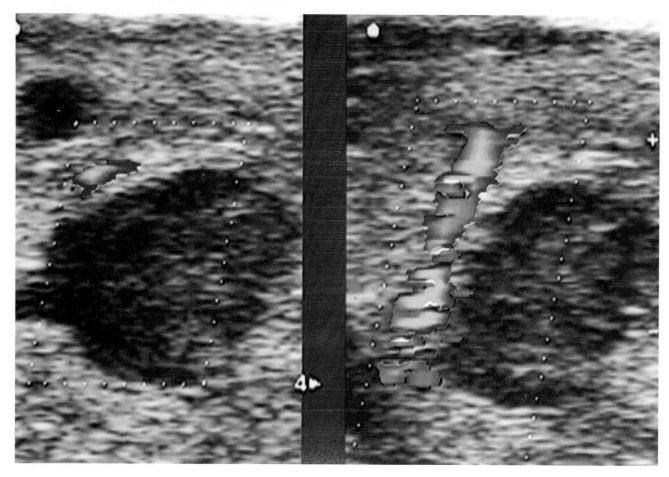

Fig. 10.38   Acute orchitis showing intratesticular focal abscesses with peripheral vascularity.

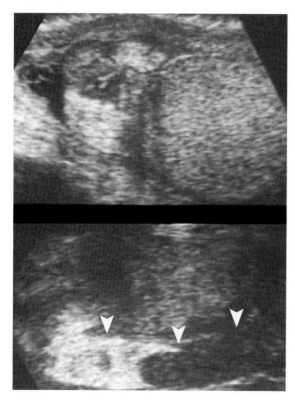

Fig. 10.39   Acute epididymitis with diffuse involvement of the head (top) and body (arrowheads) of the epididymis (bottom).

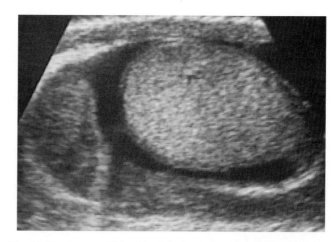

Fig. 10.40   Acute epididymitis of the head. Associated hydrocele is responsible for body and tail visualization; they are slightly hypoechoic and enlarged.

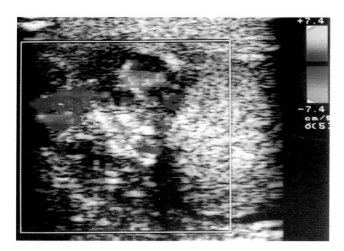

Fig. 10.41 Acute epididymitis showing increased vascularity of the head region.

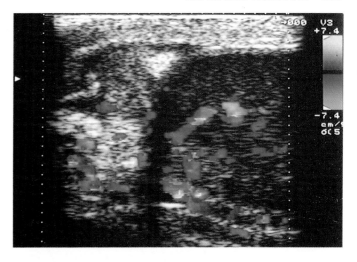

Fig. 10.42 Epididymo-orchitis. Both epididymis and testis exhibit increased vascularity; orchitis decreases testicular echogenicity.

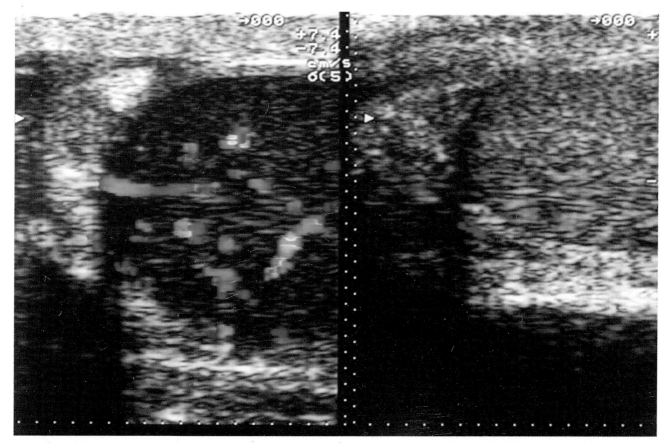

Fig. 10.43 Right orchitis; at the same gain settings, only the right testis exhibits increased vascularity and diffuse hypoechoic texture.

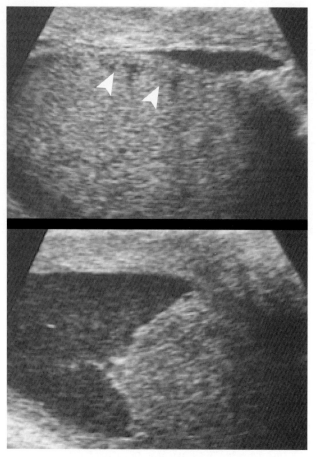

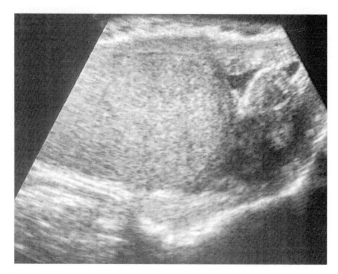

Fig. 10.45 Chronic epididymitis with wall thickening and granulomatous nodule of the epididymal tail.

Fig. 10.44 Diffuse orchitis with wall thickening, low echogenic pyocele (bottom), normal testicular texture with increased visibility of the capsular vessels (arrowheads).

Sonography usually demonstrates a normal testis and epididymis displaced by a heterogeneous mass that can be traced to the inguinal canal. Most of these masses become modified or move during the Valsalva maneuver (Fig. 10.48). Omental hernias appear echogenic; some vessels can be depicted by color Doppler. When bowel is present the pattern is heterogeneous (Fig. 10.49); fluid-filled loops, gas and peristalsis can be evident.

Chronic hernias cause compression of the normal scrotal contents; they can produce testicular atrophy.

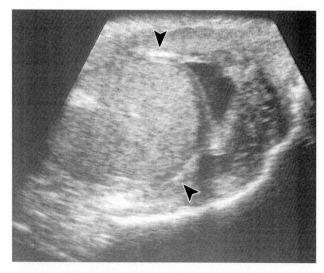

Fig. 10.46 Chronic epididymitis with wall thickening, calcifications within the tunica vaginalis (arrowheads) and nodular increase of the epididymal tail.

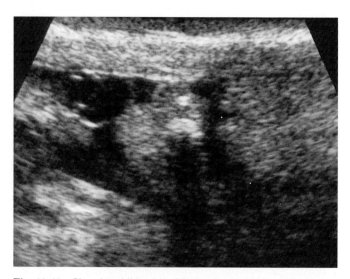

Fig. 10.47 Chronic epididymitis of the head with gross calcifications and septated hydrocele.

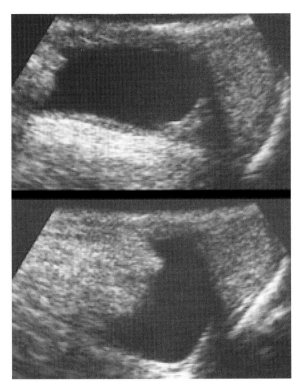

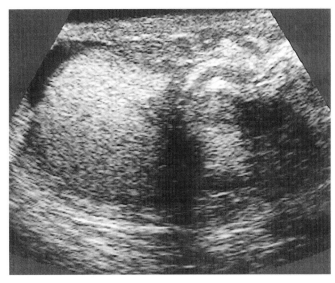

Fig. 10.49   Enlarged scrotum with a complex mass adjacent to the testis, due to hernia with bowel loops.

Fig. 10.48   Hyperechoic omental hernia shifting down towards the testis during the Valsalva maneuver.

TUMORS

Most testicular tumors are malignant germ-cell neoplasms. Only 5% are benign tumors;[3] they may be cystic (epidermoid cyst) or solid (gonadal stromal tumors, adenomatoid tumor, leiomyoma, lipoma, fibroma, hamartoma, neurofibroma) (Figs 10.50, 10.51). These benign tumors are the most frequently occurring epididymal neoplasms (70%); liposarcoma and fibrosarcoma in the adult and rhabdomyosarcoma in the child represent the rare malignancies arising outside the testis.

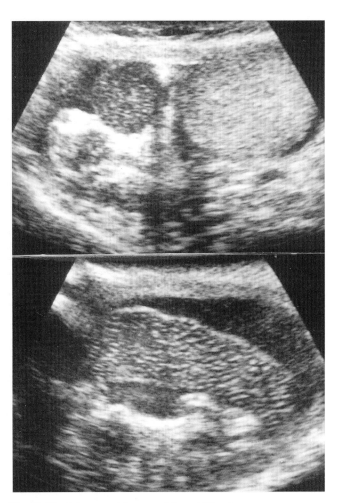

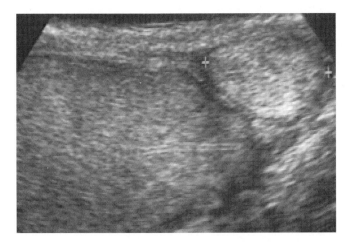

Fig. 10.50   Hyperechoic fibroma of the epididymal tail, 14 mm in diameter.

Fig. 10.51   Adenomatoid tumor of the epididymis.

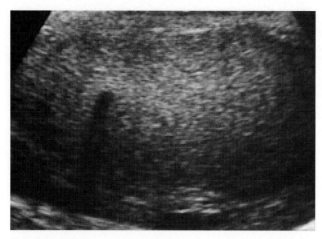

Fig. 10.52 'Burned out' choriocarcinoma of the testis presenting as a pleural metastatic effusion and intratesticular calcified scar with acoustic shadowing.

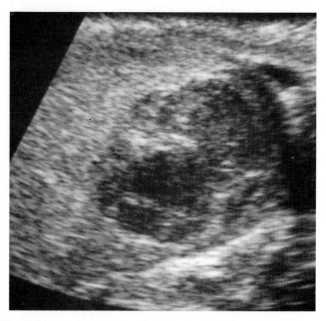

Fig. 10.53 Lower testicular pole: hypoechoic metastases originating from prostatic carcinoma.

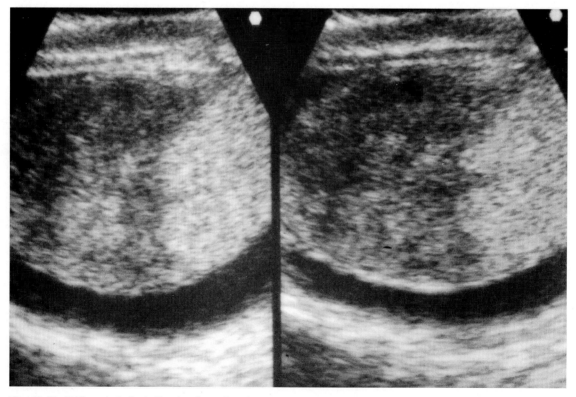

Fig. 10.54 Diffuse testicular infiltration due to lymphoma.

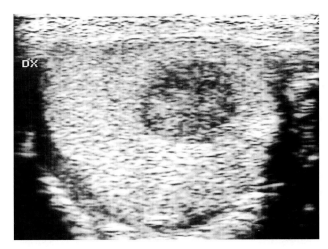

Fig. 10.55 Small hypoechoic seminoma with regular margins and homogeneous texture.

Germ-cell tumors are the most common solid neoplasms in young adult males.[50-52] Seminomas account for 40–50%; the worst prognosis is associated with the anaplastic type (10%). In 10–15% of cases seminoma is mixed with non-seminomatous elements. Among the non-seminomatous tumors, the most aggressive type is the embryonal cell carcinoma (15–20%); it may be mixed with teratoma, giving rise to aggressive teratocarcinomas. Chorio-carcinoma is always a mixed tumor; it can give rise to 'burned out' tumors in which the primary tumor resolves into a fibrous or calcified scar, while major metastatic disease becomes apparent in other regions (Fig. 10.52).[53]

Metastatic tumors comprise 0.6–3.6% of all testicular tumors.[54] They originate from the prostate (34.6%), lung (17.3%), melanoma (8.2%), colon (7.7%) and kidney (5.8%) (Fig. 10.53). Testicular infiltration in patients with lymphoma or leukemia is not uncommon (Fig. 10.54); the testis seems to provide a sanctuary for this disease, owing to an apparent 'gonadal barrier' that inhibits concentration of chemotherapeutic agents.[55,56]

About 60–70% of patients with testicular tumors present with painless testicular masses. Another 10–15% present with mild or progressive pain simulating inflammation. About 15% present with symptoms related to secondary deposits producing pleural effusion or enlargement of retroperitoneal, mediastinal or supraclavicular nodes; in these cases the primitive testicular tumor can be non-palpable or even 'burned out'. In other patients the onset is associated with endocrine alterations, the most frequent being masculinization in children and feminization in adults.

Advances in diagnostic and staging procedures, in addition to innovations in surgery, radiation therapy and chemotherapy, make cure the expected outcome for most patients.[50-52] For patients with stage I seminoma, 5-year survival rates are usually better than 95%, with figures for stage II patients between 85 and 90%. The percentage of patients with advanced non-seminomatous cancer achieving cure has improved to 70–80%. Delayed treatment always results in significant reduction of the cure rate.

Gray-scale sonography permits easy recognitions of testicular focal alterations, with a tumor detection sensitivity approaching 100%.[16,57-59] High-frequency transducers permit detection of nodules less than 5 mm in diameter (Fig. 10.55). Unfortunately, in many cases the patterns of benign and malignant pathologies overlap, resulting in a large number of false positive diagnoses.[60] Not only benign tumors but also infarcts, orchitis and hemorrhage can mimic a testicular tumor.

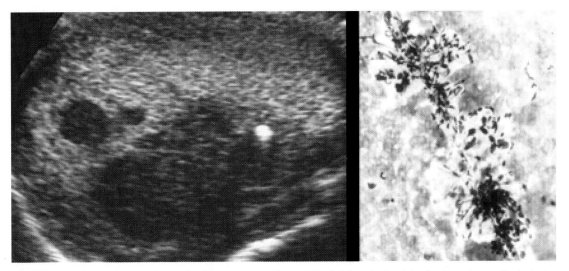

Fig. 10.56 Multiple hypoechoic nodules due to teratocarcinoma. The bright echo is originating from the needle tip during FNAB that resulted in a typical diagnostic smear.

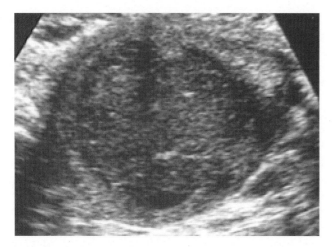

Fig. 10.57   Embryonal cell carcinoma with diffuse involvement of the testis.

Most small neoplasms (under 8–10 mm in diameter) present as hypoechoic homogeneous focal areas embedded in the normal testicular texture; the margin may be very regular. Larger tumors are usually inhomogeneous (Figs 10.56, 10.57); calcifications, necrotic areas, cystic or dysembryogenetic components may be variably associated. In 40% of embryonal cell carcinomas and about 30% of teratomas there are echogenic foci; 90% of teratocarcinomas and teratomas and 20% of embryonal cell carcinomas have cystic components.[58]

In most of these cases current instrumentation shows hypervascularity; power Doppler is able to depict vessels also in tumors less than 15 mm in diameter (Figs 10.58, 10.59). However, differentiation between neoplasms and benign changes is reliable only where there are large focal lesions; changes presenting as small focal lesions or diffuse inhomogeneous testicular enlargement cannot be differentiated. Color Doppler has a limited role;[16] the absence or presence of hydrocele, or epididymal or scrotal wall involvement, cannot be used as decisional criteria.[61] The clinical history may help in the decision but it is often contradictory. The lesion may be monitored for a short period to determine the necessity for orchiectomy;[16] as an alternative, ultrasound can guide FNAB.

FNAB is performed using short 23 gauge needles; no anesthesia is required. The procedure is safe: two rapid passes always enable diagnostic smears to be obtained; color Doppler helps to avoid puncture of vascularized areas (Fig. 10.60). Where malignant cells are detected, early surgery is recommended.

To test the diagnostic accuracy of our procedure we have biopsied 71 testicular lesions (prevalence of malignancy 74%); three patients were biopsied for possible synchronous bilateral tumor. In this series, check procedures did not show any neoplastic recurrence or minor complication: they included a follow-up of at least 26 months with clinical examination, scrotal and abdominal ultrasound, chest X-rays and laboratory tests. The sensitivity for malignancy was 94% with a specificity and a positive predictive value of 100%; the negative predictive value was 87%.

FNAB is very useful in the differentiation of small, nonpalpable testicular lesions, the detection rate of which is increasing owing to better resolution of instruments, and more widespread use of testicular sonography and screening programs. Sonography may constitute a screening technique for patients at risk for testicular tumor;[62] moreover, FNAB may be a safe alternative to open testicular biopsy.

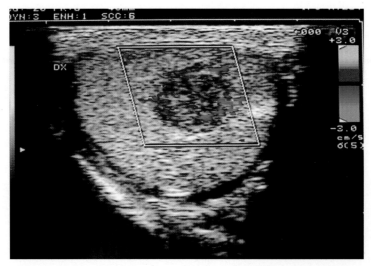

Fig. 10.58   The same seminoma as in Figure 10.55; typical hypervascularity.

Carcinoma in situ of the testis is a precursor of invasive germ cell tumors in a high percentage of cases.[63] Abnormal germ cells are diffusely distributed in 85–100% of the testes affected by seminoma and non-seminomatous tumors, in 5–10% of the contralateral testes, in 100% of patients affected by gonadal dysgenesis and in 33% of those with androgen insensitivity. In addition, cryptorchid testes are at risk: the rates are 25% for abdominal testis, 0.68% for inguinal testis and 0.5–1.5% after early successful orchiopexy. Successful early sonographic detection of small tumors has already been reported in these categories.[62,64] Sonography is particularly recommended in cryptorchidism and for evaluation and follow up of the contralateral testis in patients with testicular tumor. Bilateral neoplasia occur in 1.1–3% of all patients; only 9.5–11% of the tumors present simultaneously. In sequential presentation, 47% of the second tumors are diagnosed within 2 years and 68% within 5 years.[64] Where a focal lesion is detected, FNAB can help to avoid useless orchiectomy.

POSTORCHIECTOMY SCROTUM AND PROSTHESES

Orchiectomies, trans-scrotal or transinguinal, give rise to a potential space within the scrotal sac. Initially, this space is occupied by a small volume of fluid, which gradually resolves.[65] On ultrasound examination, the residual space appears empty or with few echoes; generally, the ipsilateral scrotal wall is thickened. Hematomas are more common after transinguinal orchiectomy; they should generally resolve within 5–6 weeks after surgery. Hematomas often present as septated fluid collections with dependent debris that moves as the patient moves (Fig. 10.61); ultrasound may be useful to guide percutaneous aspiration.[65]

The use of silicone rubber prostheses is increasing in popularity; they do not cause inflammation or hypersensitivity. Sonographically these silicone prostheses appear anechoic;[65,66] they cannot be compressed and the surrounding scrotal wall is usually distended (Fig. 10.62).

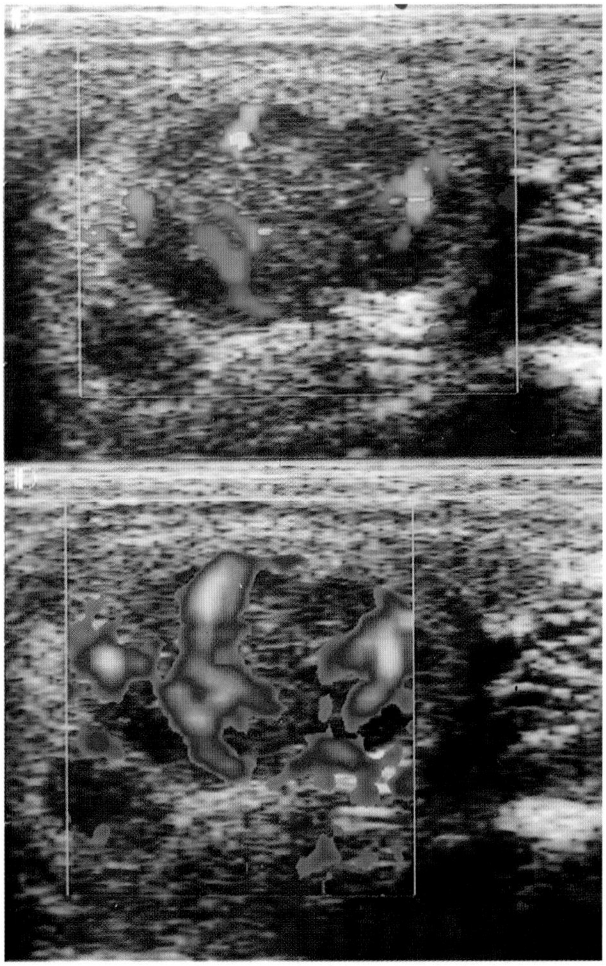

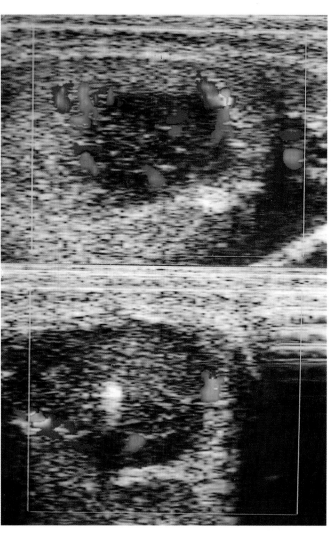

Fig. 10.59 Aggressive teratocarcinoma with irregular hypervascularity; power Doppler enhances vascular morphology.

Fig. 10.60 Color Doppler helps to guide the needle into non-vascularized areas.

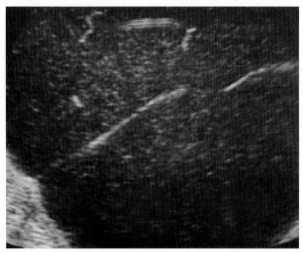

Fig. 10.61 Septated hematocele complicating left orchiectomy.

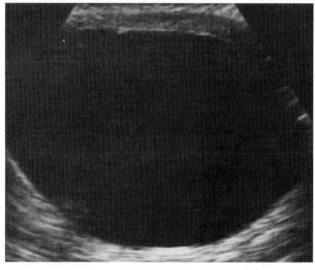

Fig. 10.62 The anechoic space originating from a silicone rubber prosthesis.

REFERENCES

1. Rifkin M D 1990 Measurements of the scrotal contents. In: Goldberg B B, Kurtz A B (eds) Atlas of ultrasound measurements. Year Book Medical, Chicago, pp 180–187
2. Leung M L, Gooding G A W, Williams R D 1984 High-resolution sonography of scrotal contents in asymptomatic subjects. AJR 143: 161–164
3. Hill M C, Sanders R C 1986 Sonography of benign disease of the scrotum. In R C Sanders, M Hill (eds) Ultrasound annual. Raven Press, New York, pp 197–237
4. Tartar V M, Trambert M A, Balsara Z N, Mattrey R F 1993 Tubular ectasia of the testicle: sonographic and MR imaging appearance. AJR 160: 539–542
5. Fakhry J, Khouri A, Barakat K 1989 The hypoechoic band: a normal finding on testicular sonography. AJR 153: 321–323
6. Middleton W D, Bell M W. Analysis of intratesticular arterial anatomy with emphasis on transmediastinal arteries. Radiology 189: 157–160
7. Horstman W G, Middleton W D, Melson G L, Siegel B A 1991 Color Doppler of the scrotum. Radiographics 11: 941–957
8. Rifkin M D, Foy P M, Kurtz A B, Pasto M E, Goldberg B B 1983 The role of diagnostic ultrasonography in varicocele evaluation. J Ultrasound Med 2: 271–275
9. Rabinovitz R 1984 The importance of the cremasteric reflex in acute scrotal swelling in children. J Urol 132: 89–90
10. John Radcliff Hospital cryptorchidism study group 1986 Cryptorchidism: an apparent substantial increase since 1960. Br Med J 293: 1401–1404
11. Desgrandchamps F 1990 Testicles non descendus. État des connaisances actuelles. J Urol (Paris) 96: 407–414
12. Weiss R M, Carter A R, Rosenfield A T 1986 High resolution real-time ultrasonography in the localization of undescended testis. J Urol 135: 936–938
13. Wolverson M K, Houttuin E, Heiberg E, Sundaram M, Shields J B 1983 Comparison of computed tomography with high-resolution real-time ultrasound in the localization of the impalpable undescended testis. Radiology 146: 133–136
14. Janzen D L, Mathieson J R, Marsh J I et al 1992 Testicular microlithiasis: sonographic and clinical features. AJR 158: 1057–1060
15. Patel M D, Olcott E W, Kerschmann R L, Callen P W, Gooding G A W 1993 Sonographically detected testicular microlithiasis and testicular carcinoma. JCU 21: 447–452
16. Middleton W D 1991 Scrotal sonography in 1991. Ultrasound Q 9: 61–87
17. Martin B, Tubiana J M 1988 Significance of scrotal calcifications detected by sonography. JCU 16: 545–552
18. Di Donna A, Rizzatto G 1986 Pyocele of the scrotum: sonographic demonstration of fluid–fluid level and a gas-forming component. J Ultrasound Med 5: 99–100
19. Dierks P R, Moore P T 1985 Scrotal lymphocele: a complication of renal transplant surgery. J Ultrasound Med 4: 91–92
20. Hamm B, Fobbe F, Loy V 1988 Testicular cysts: differentiation with US and clinical findings. Radiology 168: 19–23
21. Jarvis L J, Dubbins P A 1989 Changes in the epididymis after vasectomy: sonographic findings. AJR 152: 531–534
22. Mattila S I, Tammella T L, Makarainen H P, Hellstrom P A 1993 Ultrasound follow-up of ethanolamine oleate sclerotherapy for spermatoceles. Eur Urol 23: 361–365
23. Gonda R L, Karo J J, Forte R A, O'Donnell K T 1987 Diagnosis of subclinical varicocele in infertility. AJR 148: 71–75
24. Belker A M 1981 The varicocele and male infertility. Urol Clin North Am 8: 41–51
25. Civitanic O A, Cronan J J, Sigman M, Landau S T 1993 Varicoceles: postoperative prevalence. A prospective study with color Doppler US. Radiology 187: 711–714
26. Petros J A, Andriole G L, Middleton W D, Picus D A 1991 Correlation of testicular color Doppler ultrasonography, physical examination and venography in the detection of left varicoceles in men with infertility. J Urol 145: 785–788
27. Weiss A J, Kellman G M, Middleton W D, Kirkemo A 1992 Intratesticular varicocele: sonographic findings in two patients. AJR 158: 1061–1063
28. Hirsch A V, Kellett M J, Robertson G, Pryor J P 1980 Doppler flow studies, venography, and termography in the evaluation of varicoceles of fertile and subfertile men. Br J Urol 52: 560–565
29. Cattolica E V, Karol J B, Rankin K N, Klein R S 1982 High testicular salvage rate in torsion of the spermatic cord. J Urol 128: 66–68
30. Zafaranloo S, Gerard P S, Wise G 1986 Bilateral neonatal testicular torsion: ultrasonographic evaluation. J Urol 135: 589–590
31. Donohue R E, Utley W L 1978 Torsion of spermatic cord. Urology 11: 33–36
32. Williamson R C N 1976 Torsion of the testis and allied conditions. Br J Surg 63: 465–476
33. Caldamone A A, Valvo J R, Atebarmakian V K, Rabinovitz R 1984 Acute scrotal swelling in children. J Pediatr Surg 19: 581–584
34. Burks D D, Markey B J, Burkhard T K, Balsara Z N, Haluszka M M, Canning D A 1990 Suspected testicular torsion and ischemia: evaluation with color Doppler sonography. Radiology 175: 815–821
35. Steinhardt G F, Boyarsky S, Mackey R 1993 Testicular torsion: pitfalls of color Doppler sonography. J Urol 150: 461–462

36. Schuster G 1982 Traumatic rupture of the testicle and a review of the literature. J Urol 127: 1194–1196
37. Learch T J, Hansch L P, Ralls P W 1993 US of ballistic scrotal trauma. Radiology 189 (P): 156
38. Schaffer R M 1985 Ultrasonography of scrotal trauma. Urol Radiol 7: 245–249
39. Bhandary P, Abbitt P L, Watson L 1992 Ultrasound diagnosis of traumatic testicular rupture. JCU 20: 346–348
40. Freton R C, Berger R E 1984 Prostatitis and epididymitis. Urol Clin North Am 11: 83–94
41. Horstman W G, Middleton W D, Melson G L 1991 Scrotal inflammatory disease: color Doppler US findings. Radiology 179: 55–59
42. Hricak H, Jeffrey R B 1983 Sonography of acute scrotal abnormalities. Radiol Clin North Am 21: 595–603
43. Rifkin M D, Kurtz A B, Goldberg B B 1984 Epididymis examined by ultrasound. Correlation with pathology. Radiology 151: 187–190
44. Martin B, Conte J 1987 Ultrasonography of the acute scrotum. JCU 15: 37–44
45. Lerner R M, Mevorach R A, Hulbert W C, Rabinowitz R 1990 Color Doppler US in the evaluation of acute scrotal disease. Radiology 176: 355–358
46. Subramanyam B R, Horii S C, Hilton S 1985 Diffuse testicular disease: sonographic features and significance. AJR 145: 1221–1224
47. Scott R F, Bayliss A P 1985 Ultrasound in the diagnosis of granulomatous orchitis. Br J Radiol 58: 907–909
48. Kim S H, Pollack H M, Cho K S, Pollack M S, Han M C 1993 Tuberculous epididymitis and epididymo-orchitis: sonographic findings. J Urol 150: 81–84
49. Subramanyam B R, Balthazar E J, Raghavendra B N, Horii S C, Hilton S 1982 Sonographic diagnosis of scrotal hernia. AJR 139: 535–538
50. Steinfeld A D 1990 Testicular germ cell tumors: review of contemporary evaluation and management. Radiology 175: 603–606
51. Marks L B, Rutgers J L, Shipley W U et al 1990 Testicular seminoma: clinical and pathological features that may predict para-aortic lymph node metastases. J Urol 143: 524–527
52. Hesketh P J, Krane R J 1990 Prognostic assessment in nonseminomatous testicular cancer: implications for therapy. J Urol 144: 1–9
53. Shawker T H, Javadpour N, O'Leary T, Shapiro E, Krudy A G 1983 Ultrasonographic detection of 'burned-out' primary testicular germ cell tumors in clinically normal testes. J Ultrasound Med 2: 477–479
54. Patel S R, Richardson R L, Kvols L 1989 Metastatic cancer to the testes: a report of 20 cases and review of the literature. J Urol 142: 1003–1005
55. Moorjani V, Mashankar A, Goel S, Khandelwal K, Patange V, Merchant N 1991 Sonographic appearance of primary testicular lymphoma. AJR 157: 1225–1226
56. Lupetin A R, King W, Rich P, Lederman R B 1983 Ultrasound diagnosis of testicular leukemia. Radiology 146: 171–172
57. Grantham J G, Charbonneau J W, James E M et al 1985 Testicular neoplasms: 29 tumors studied by high-resolution US. Radiology 157: 775–780
58. Schwerk W B, Schwerk W N, Rodeck G 1987 Testicular tumors: prospective analysis of real-time US patterns and abdominal staging. Radiology 164: 369–374
59. Horstman W G, Melson G L, Middleton W D, Andriole G L 1992 Testicular tumors: findings with color Doppler US. Radiology 185: 733–737
60. Tackett R E, Ling D, Catalona W J, Melson G L 1986 High resolution sonography in diagnosing testicular neoplasms: clinical significance of false positive scans. J Urol 135: 494–496
61. Worthy L, Miller E I, Chinn D H 1986 Evaluation of extratesticular findings in scrotal neoplasms. J Ultrasound Med 5: 261–263
62. Lenz S, Giwercman A, Skakkebaek N E, Bruun E, Frimodt-Møller C 1987 Ultrasound in detection of early neoplasia of the testis. Int J Androl 10: 187–190
63. Reinberg Y, Manivel J C, Fraley E E 1989 Carcinoma in situ of the testis. J Urol 142: 243–247
64. Sanchez S, Mahlin M 1986 Simultaneous bilateral testicular tumors, one side clinically occult: detection by ultrasonography. J Urol 135: 591–592
65. Eftekhari F, Smith J K 1993 Sonography of the scrotum after orchiectomy: normal and abnormal findings. AJR 160: 543–547
66. Hopper K D, Meilstrup J W, Skoog S J 1984 The sonographic appearance of the Heyer–Schulte testicular prosthesis. J Ultrasound Med 3: 267

11

Penile sonography

U. Patel   W. R. Lees

Improvements in gray-scale, duplex and color Doppler ultrasound technology have made penile sonography the initial imaging modality for this organ, particularly for the investigation of erectile dysfunction. High-resolution gray-scale ultrasound allows accurate delineation of the normal and abnormal corporal and vascular anatomy, while the penile erectile physiology can be studied in fine detail and with unique ease by Doppler ultrasound. More recently the penile urethra has also been studied sonographically.

ANATOMY

The anatomy of the penis is arranged to allow both an excretory and an erectile function. The main components are three cylindrical spongy vascular bodies – two dorso-lateral corpora cavernosa overlying a midline, single corpus spongiosum. Each corpus is encircled by a resistant fibro-elastic covering – the tunica albuginea – and all three corpora are bound together and enclosed within two further fascial coverings.[1] Although the tunica separates each corpus cavernosum from its counterpart, distal fenestrations in this lining allow some vascular communication between the two corporal bodies. Proximally the corpus spongiosum expands to form the bulb of the penis, which provides part of the anatomical anchorage of the organ to the body. The proximal segments of the corpora cavernosa, termed the crura, also have an anchoring function. Engorgement and enlargement of the paired cavernosa is solely responsible for penile rigidity and erection. Distally, the corpus spongiosum expands into the glans penis. The glans is not directly involved in the erectile process, but the rigidity of the erect penile shaft probably mechanically interferes with glans drainage, as it does demonstrate some enlargement in the fully erect state.

The urethra is enclosed within the corpus spongiosum and the radiologically defined anterior urethra comprises that part of the urethra encased by the bulb and corpus spongiosum. Empty of fluid, it has no lumen and is not recognizable by ultrasound. The bulbospongiosus and ischiocavernous muscles lie at the base of the penis and assist with erection.

Histologically, the corpora are a network of connected sinusoidal spaces, each sinusoid being fed and drained by a single afferent and efferent vessel.[2] The cavernosal sinusoid is capable of considerable volume enlargement; in the flaccid state the sinusoidal spaces contain little blood and are more or less collapsed. During erection these spaces become engorged and enlarge with blood under pressure. Engorgement is not merely a passive process, as the smooth muscle fibres in the sinusoidal walls actively relax during erection. The ability first, to engorge the sinusoids and second, to maintain this engorgement, forms the fundamental basis of the penile erection.

Vascular anatomy

Arterial supply to the penis is by three branches of the internal pudendal artery: the cavernosal artery (supplying the corpora cavernosa), the dorsal artery of the penis (branches of which supply the corpus spongiosum and the glans penis) and the urethral artery (Fig. 11.1). The internal pudendal artery is itself a branch of the internal iliac artery. Each corpus cavernosum is supplied by a single cavernosal artery alone, which enters the body at the base of the penis, traversing centrally and slightly medially through the length of the cavernosum and giving off helicine branches, each of which terminates in and supplies a single cavernosal sinusoid. Arteriopathy may affect any part of the arterial supply from the aorto-iliac segment to the distal cavernosal artery.

The sinusoids are drained by venules, which in turn communicate with small emissary veins that penetrate through the tunica albuginea and join the dorsal vein of the penis. Compression, and occlusion, of the emissary veins against the stiff tunica by cavernosal distension is believed to constitute the main veno-occlusion mechanism, and is central to the normal penile erectile process. In most men the dorsal vein is the sole conduit of cavernosal

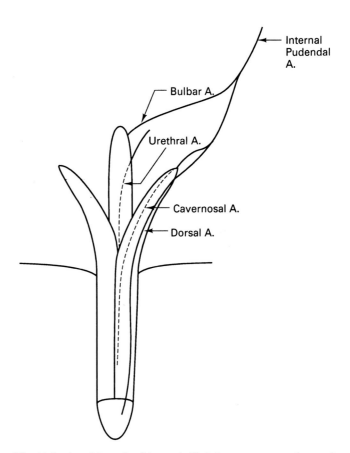

Fig. 11.1 Arterial supply of the penis. Variations are common (see text)

drainage; in a minority blood also leaves directly via the cavernosal and crural veins at the base of the corpora cavernosa.

Variations of vascular anatomy are common (in up to 50% of patients). The most frequent are a common internal pudendal artery origin for both cavernous arteries, an absent dorsal artery and accessory penile arteries.[3] Variations of penile venous anatomy can also occur and on cavernosography some normal men will exhibit cavernosal drainage via veins of the glans and corpus spongiosum. The relevance of vascular anomalies to the penile haemodynamics is unclear.

Neural anatomy

Neural input of the penis is by somatic nerves arising from the sacral plexus (sacral segment levels S_2, S_3 and S_4 via the internal pudendal nerve) and also by the autonomic nervous system. The former provides the sensory supply and also innervates the penile musculature, while the autonomic system richly innervates the smooth muscle of the cavernosal arteries and cavernosal sinusoids.[1] It is still a matter of dispute whether the dorsal vein, which also has some smooth muscle, has an independent neural supply with an active role in venous shutdown.[4]

Effects of aging

Little is known about the effects of aging on the penile anatomy and vascularity. Repeated minor trauma of copulation and age-related changes in the elasticity of the tunica albuginea have been suggested as possible etiological factors with Peyronie's disease and veno-occlusive dysfunction, respectively.[5] On gray-scale ultrasound there is little to distinguish the cavernosa of the young from the aged penis.

PHYSIOLOGY OF PENILE ERECTION

Penile erection is a result of engorgement and enlargement of the corporal sinusoids, secondary to interlinked and cyclical changes in arterial inflow and venous outflow. Although this is purely a hemodynamic event, satisfactory erection is also dependent on endocrine, metabolic and general physical well-being. The initiation of the cycle is also dependent on (as yet poorly understood) neurophysiological and psychosomatic factors.

Lue's division of the erectile cycle into six phases[6] is very useful conceptually as it correlates well with described Doppler waveform pattern changes (see also Fig. 11.8):

1. *Flaccid phase.* The arterial flow is low owing to high resting arteriolar and sinusoidal smooth muscle tone. Outflow via emissary veins equals inflow and sinusoidal flow is continuous. Intracavernosal pressure (ICP) is low and static, but peripheral resistance is high because of smooth muscle contraction.

2. *Latent phase.* On initiation (neurophysiologically or pharmacologically) there is a tenfold or greater increase in both systolic and diastolic arterial inflow secondary to smooth muscle relaxation and marked reduction in peripheral vascular resistance. The cavernosal sinusoids begin to engorge as inflow is very much greater than outflow, but the penis remains soft as ICP continues to be steady.

3. *Tumescence.* Once the sinusoids are fully engorged they gradually distend, the ICP rises and the penis stiffens and lengthens. With this volume and pressure rise the emissary veins are compressed within the tunica and the venous outflow diminishes and finally ceases. As the peripheral vascular resistance increases, the diastolic portion of the arterial flow gradually declines.

4. *Full erection.* This results from increasing sinusoidal distension because systolic inflow continues while outflow has been restricted. As the ICP continues to rise (>100 mmHg), systolic inflow is also gradually restricted.

5. *Rigid erection.* Contraction of the ischiocavernous muscles, activated by unknown factors, elevates the ICP to more than systolic blood pressure and maximal rigidity and erection occurs. Arterial inflow may cease completely at this stage.

6. *Detumescence.* Venous drainage is gradually re-established. ICP diminishes and the normal flaccid state is restored.

ULTRASOUND OF THE PENIS

With high-frequency transducers (5–10 MHz, with 7.5 MHz being ideal) the penis can be examined with ease and in great detail. Linear array probes are more convenient to use because of the circular cross-section of the penis. Evaluation of erectile impotence requires both duplex and color Doppler facility. Color Doppler is essential, in our opinion, as the cavernosal arteries can be impossible to identify with a gray-scale alone, and sampling factors, such as angle correction and accurate Doppler gate placement, must be optimal for consistent and reproducible results.

The penis should be scanned in both longitudinal and transverse sections. The corpora cavernosa and corpus spongiosum are both of homogeneous hypoechogenicity, and the surrounding tunica stands out as a thin echodense linear structure (Figs 11.2, 11.3). The tunica should be less than 2 mm thick in the flaccid state and less than 0.5 mm thick with erection. The cavernosal sinusoids are visible on engorgement only as echo-poor cystic spaces, whereas the cavernosal arteries may be identified in either the flaccid or erect penis by their linear echogenic arterial walls. On erection a hypoechoic periarterial rim may

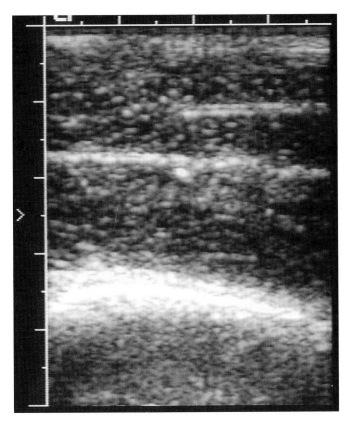

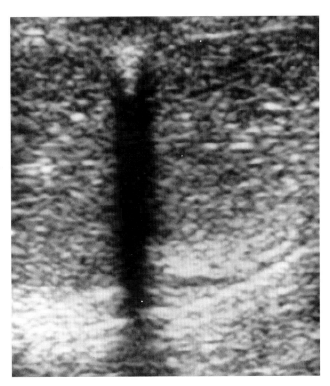

Fig. 11.3 Transverse view of the paired dorsolateral corpora cavernosa showing homogeneous echogenicity.

Fig. 11.2 Longitudinal view of the paired corpora cavernosa, with the highly echogenic midline tunica albuginea. Normally, the two cavernosa are of similar dimensions and echogenicity. The parallel echogenic walls of the cavernosal artery are seen within the cavernosa nearest to the transducer.

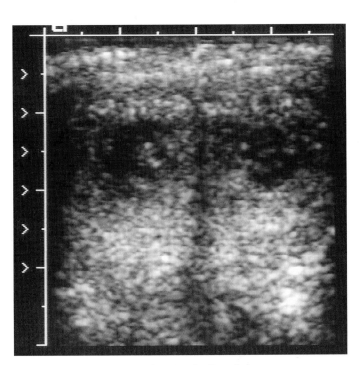

Fig. 11.4 Transverse view of maximally distended corpus cavernosum. Note the periarterial hypoechogenicity due to sinusoidal distension.

become apparent (Fig. 11.4). Measurement of the cavernosal artery diameter is too imprecise and non-specific to be recommended. In the flaccid state the diameter range is 0.2–1 mm, and after papaverine can display up to a twofold increase.[7] Calcification of the cavernosa or the tunica is always abnormal, and we have not yet seen penile arterial calcification.

The anterior urethra can be properly studied by ultrasound only after retrograde or antegrade urethral distension.[8] Retrograde filling is preferable, using sterile saline, water or anesthetic gel injection through a Knuttson clamp. By transcutaneous scanning the entire penile portion of the anterior urethra can be examined. Imaging of the more proximal portion of the anterior urethra, including the bulbous portion, requires the transperineal approach. Strictures can be identified, their length and diameter measured and the presence of calculus or sludge determined. Unlike contrast urethrography, this method also allows assessment of the urethral mucosa and peristricture soft tissues.

Penile vasculature is evaluated with both duplex and color Doppler imaging.[6,7,9–11] After pharmacostimulation, flow can always be recorded in the dorsal and cavernosal

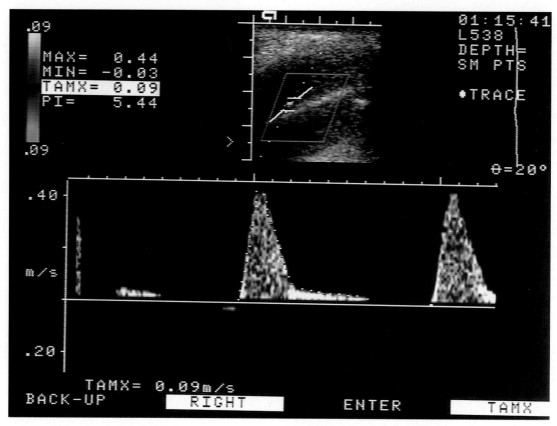

Fig. 11.5   Cavernosal artery waveform recording, from a segment of the artery close to the base of the penis. The velocity and pulsatility index values are diagnostic of a normal penile hemodynamic response (see Figs 11.6–11.9).

arteries. Helicine artery and dorsal vein flow may or may not be seen in the normal patient. Careful attention paid to the rudiments of Doppler sampling (such as beam steering, accurate Doppler gate placement, angle correction, etc.) is always worth while. Spectral waveforms should be measured from the cavernosal artery close to the base of the penis, as velocities are highest here and angle correction will be optimal (Fig. 11.5). Inappropriate sampling (both site and temporal – see below) is the probable source of much of the conflict in published data so far. The penile vasculature can also be mapped using color Doppler, and vascular anomalies and abnormalities can be detected.

EVALUATION OF ERECTILE IMPOTENCE

Currently, it is believed that impotence results from a failure of initiation (psychogenic or neurogenic impotence), poor arterial inflow (arteriogenic impotence) or an inadequate venous closure mechanism.[6] This mechanistic approach fails to take into account the many other factors (psychological, metabolic, etc.) that are known to be relevant; however it is a useful way of approaching the problem.

Aetiology of erectile failure (Table 11.3)

How exactly psychogenic or neurogenic dysfunction results in impotence is unclear, as our understanding of the neurochemistry of erectile initiation is still poor. Hemodynamically, it presents as failure of initial relaxation of smooth muscle tone. This situation is also seen with pharmacological antagonism or receptor failure.

Arterial inflow may also fail to augment because of structural disease, such as proximal arterial stenosis or diffuse cavernosal artery disease, and there is an association between arteriogenic impotence and generalized peripheral arteriopathy. Anatomical anomalies of the penile arteries may also be a causal association. A small group of, usually young, patients develop impotence secondary to stenosis or rupture of the internal pudendal artery after blunt or penetrating pelvic trauma. It is important to identify these patients as they generally have a good result from arterial reconstruction. The etiology of venous leakage is still poorly understood. Postulated causes of failure of emissary vein closure include decreased penile tissue elasticity and tunical stiffness due to aging, trauma, Peyronie's disease, penile surgery or vascular disease. A further possible cause is the failure of a proposed active neuromuscular veno-occlusive mechanism operating at the sinusoidal or dorsal vein level.

Lack of sinusoidal distension may also cause impotence, a situation seen with intracorporal fibrosis, Peyronie's disease, small vessel arteriopathy and possibly with aging. Finally, some patients may have more than one cause of impotence and, in particular, arteriogenic impotence and venous leakage may coexist.

The penile Doppler study (PDS) is capable of categorizing patients into the broad groups as above.[7] Table 11.3 summarizes the aetiological and mechanistic factors of erectile failure. The Table also indicates the diagnostic features of each category as seen on PDS and this is explained further below. However, initial outpatient assessment should be conducted to select those patients who would benefit from detailed study. In particular, patients with hormonal imbalance or typical psychogenic impotence of recent origin should be selected.

Penile Doppler study

The test should be carried out in quiet, private surroundings to allay patient anxiety as much as possible. The penis should initially be examined with a gray-scale ultrasound, and areas of fibrosis and Peyronie's plaques noted. Baseline vascular assessment is imprecise, can be time consuming and is of no value. We favor papaverine pharmacostimulation because of its general availability and most reported experience is with this drug, used singly or in combination with an adrenogenic drug (e.g. phentolamine). Prostaglandin may become the drug of choice in the future as its pharmacological and side effect profile is superior to that of papaverine. Some advocate physical or photographic stimulation in addition to pharmacostimulation;[8] we do not use them routinely. The dosage used is 40 mg for those below 40 years of age, and 1 mg/year of life for those who are 40 or more years old. In patients with probable neurogenic impotence we start with 20 mg as these patients can be exquisitely drug sensitive. The drug is injected intracavernosally through a 25 G needle close to the base of the penis, and massaged in. A short-lived (<1 min) stinging sensation is common; significant complications (e.g. priapism) are rare (<1%). Significant systemic side effects, because of a more generalized peripheral vasodilatation, are very uncommon and usually are seen in patients with venous leakage given more than 80 mg papaverine.

Initial vasodilatation occurs within 30–60 s and can be assessed by the degree of diastolic flow elevation in this phase. Cavernosal artery waveforms should then be recorded every 2 min or so, until peak systolic velocity (around 5 min after injection) and minimal end-diastolic velocity (around 9 min after injection) have been achieved. The range for the time of peak response is wide (between 1 and 20 min, see Fig. 11.6) and prolonged sampling may be necessary. Dorsal artery flow is not influenced by intracavernosal pressure changes and its velocity is gen-

erally higher than in the cavernosal artery, but measurement of dorsal artery peak velocity is a poor diagnostic discriminator.[11] The two cavernosal arteries can demonstrate a marked asymmetry of velocity rise, independent of the site of injection. The clinical relevance of this asymmetry to erectile function is still a matter of dispute.[12,13] The strength of the erection achieved can be graded adequately on a subjective scale; Table 11.1 shows the scale that we use. Maximal pharmacostimulation is central to a properly conducted PDS and some patients may require a further dose of papaverine; we have used up to 120 mg papaverine safely.

Many waveform measures and indices have been studied. Table 11.2 is a review of the relative value of each of these. Measurement of systolic and diastolic velocities is most reliable; diagnostic classification should be based on these values, and all other measures used as supportive or ancillary assessments. It is important to remember that the PDS is a dynamic investigation requiring a stepwise evaluation, as illustrated in Table 11.3. Thus, only if an adequate initial relaxation is seen can the arterial inflow be assessed accurately; and only once arterial adequacy has been confirmed should the characteristics of sinusoidal distension be evaluated before, finally, the integrity of the venous occlusion mechanism can be confirmed.

Normal and abnormal waveform profiles

The temporal evolution of velocities and waveform profiles is a reflection of the changes in cavernosal artery flow and intracavernosal pressure. A distinct normal pattern has been identified both quantitatively (velocity curves) and qualitatively (waveform profile evolution),[12,14,15] and are shown in Figures 11.6–11.8. Normal waveform evolution and velocity measures identify an intact penile hemodynamic circuit and are seen with psychogenic and neurogenic impotence, as well as in normal men.

Patients with abnormality of inflow (arteriogenic impotence) will fail to increase their arterial inflow sufficiently to engorge the sinusoids and activate emissary vein closure. The waveforms will show poor velocities and diastolic flow will persist throughout the test period, albeit at a low level (Fig. 11.8). The level of systolic velocity separating the normal from abnormal arterial response is still disputed; proposed cut-off levels have ranged widely

Table 11.1 Grade of erection*

Grade	Strength of erection
1	No change, or tumescence and penile elongation but no significant rigidity on palpation
2	Tumescence, penile elongation and rigidity achieved. Erection less than 90 degrees while in the supine position
3	Greater than 90 degrees erection while in the supine position

* Maximal pharmacological stimulation should be ensured

Table 11.2   Quantitative assessments during the penile Doppler study, with reported diagnostic values

Assessment	Normal range	Diagnostic value	Reference
Peak systolic velocity (V_{max})	>35–25 cm/s	If >30 cm/s taken to be normal. Sensitivity 82% and specificity 96% for identifying a normal hemodynamic response	7,12
Minimal end-diastolic velocity (V_{min})	<5–7 cm/s	If <7 cm/s taken as cut-off for normal. Sensitivity 94% and specificity 69% for identifying faulty venous closure mechanism	7,12
Dorsal vein flow (DVF)	Early DVF is normal, late flow is abnormal	Sensitivity 80% and specificity 100% for diagnosis of venous leak. Not confirmed by others	15,32
Pulsatility index (PI)	>300 (mean 600)	<300 (mean 200) seen only with arteriogenic impotence	12,33
Resistivity index (RI)	>0.80	Good correlation with strength of erection achieved (does not differentiate arterial from venous malfunction)	21
Systolic rise time (ΔT)	0.02–0.08 s	>0.1 s seen only with arteriogenic impotence. May help to identify patients with proximal arterial disease (not yet proven)	12,33
Cavernosal artery diameter	0.2–1 mm	Patients with poor arterial response have <50% diameter increase post stimulation. Diagnostically imprecise as there is large overlap between normal and abnormal	9,16,34
Vascular asymmetry	5–25%	Reported to be greater with arterial disease. Not proven in larger studies	12,13
Cavernosal body diameter	Up to 80% increase	Increase reported greater with normal vascular function. Diagnostic value unproven	37
Acceleration index (AI)	>400	Sensitivity 100% but specificity poor at 46%. Claimed to be useful as an assessment additional to V_{max}	35
Calculated penile blood flow index	—	Incorporates both velocity and diameter change. Reported to be more discriminating than either velocity or diameter change used alone	36

Table 11.3   Aetiologies of erectile impotence and their Doppler patterns

Causes	Mechanistic fault	Doppler/ultrasound characteristics after maximal pharmacostimulation
Hormonal Psychogenic Neurogenic }	→ Failure to initiate →	Normal waveform evolution
Receptor antagonism Receptor failure Fibrosis }	→ Failure of initial relaxation →	Persistent high-resistance waveforms
Atheroma Proximal arterial stenosis Anatomical anomalies }	→ Failure of arterial inflow →	Low peak systolic velocities
Peyronie's disease Intracorporal fibrosis Small vessel disease }	→ Failure to distend →	Morphological changes on gray-scale ultrasound. Focal arterial or arteriolar stenosis with velocity gradients
Failure of venous closure Peyronie's disease Idiopathic, etc. }	→ Venous leakage →	Persistent high diastolic velocity

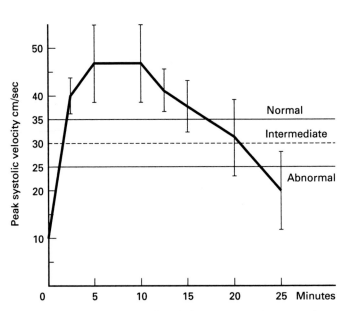

Fig. 11.6   The time/peak systolic velocity curve seen with a normal penile hemodynamic system. The points on the curve refer to mean population values and the error bars represent ± 2 SEM. Systolic velocity is maximal at 5·2 min after stimulation, with a range of between 1 and 20 min after injection. The clearly normal and abnormal ranges are shown with an appreciable intermediate zone.

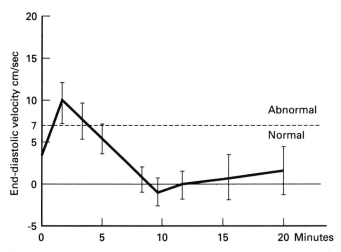

Fig. 11.7 The time/end-diastolic velocity curve as seen with a normal penile venous occlusion mechanism. End-diastolic velocity reaches a nadir at a mean of 9 min after injection (values are means ± 2 SEM). To diagnose an intact venous occlusion mechanism, the systolic velocities should be unequivocally normal and the end-diastolic velocity should remain below the threshold point (7 cm/s on this graph) for at least 5 consecutive minutes.

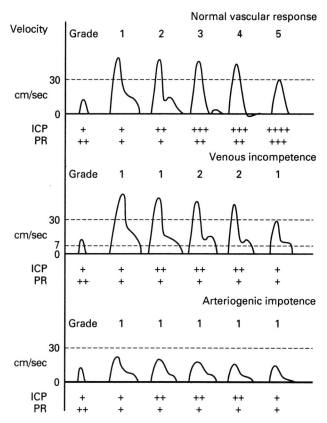

Fig. 11.8 Pattern of Doppler waveform evolution as seen with a normal penile circulation, defective venous occlusion and arterial failure. Grade refers to the waveform grading system devised by Schwartz et al.[14] ICP: intracavernosal pressure, PR: peripheral resistance.

between 20 and 40 cm/s. Recent work has been more in agreement and current views are that a significant intermediate zone exists between the clearly normal and abnormal peak systolic velocity. In our view, peak velocities between 25 and 35 cm/s occupy this gray area (Fig. 11.9), but it is probable that each team should evolve its own velocity range as local variations in practice will always continue.

Patients with normal arterial inflow and inadequate veno-occlusion (the 'venous leakers') will demonstrate normal peak systolic velocities but will not demonstrate waveform progression towards the high peripheral resistance forms (Fig. 11.8). Throughout the hemodynamic response the end-diastolic velocity will continue to be high. There is much more agreement about the cut-off level between the normal and the raised end-diastolic velocity: most authors choose either less than 5 or less than 7 cm/s as being abnormal. Local preference probably influences the choice. Two items worth noting are, first, that reversed

velocity at any stage is seen only with a normal venous closure mechanism and, second, that to diagnose venous leakage the end-diastolic velocity should remain elevated above cut-off level for at least 5 min of sampling and the systolic velocity should be unequivocally normal (Fig. 11.10).

Diagnostic gray areas with PDS

To conduct an accurate PDS, attention must be paid to technical factors, as emphasized above, and maximal pharmacological stimulation must be ensured. However, anxiety (via the adrenergic circuit) can attenuate the pharmacological response by interfering with smooth muscle relaxation, and in patients with borderline abnormal velocity response (either arterial or venous) it is often impossible to be certain that anxiety was not a confounding influence. Clinical indicators of anxiety may be present and can help to identify these patients; such patients often

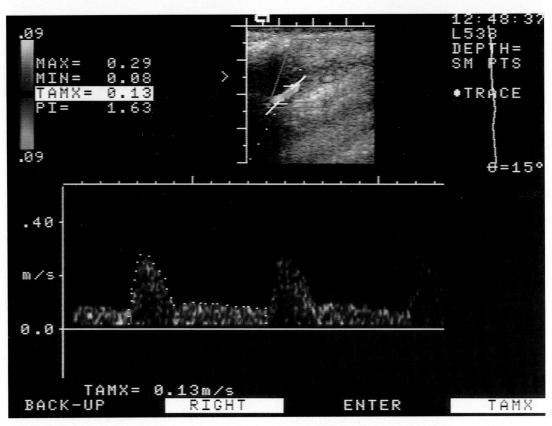

Fig. 11.9 Arterial failure of a mild degree. A slight dicrotic notch can be seen occasionally with arterial failure, as in this case. This waveform was recorded with a longitudinally held transducer. If recorded close to the base of the penis and with beam steering, angle correction should be optimal.

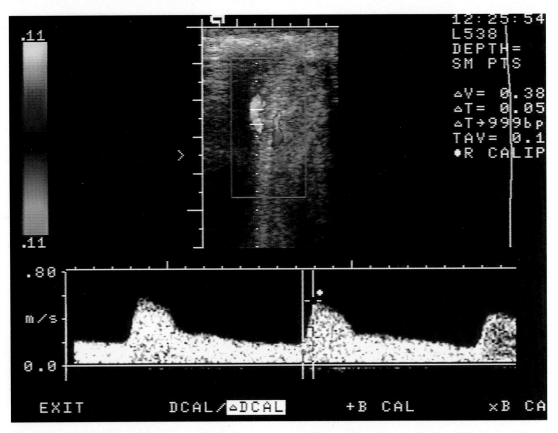

Fig. 11.10 Typical cavernosal artery waveform of venous leakage. The systolic velocity is clearly within the normal range. This waveform was recorded with a transversely held probe close to the root of the penis.

report a fuller erection after leaving the anxiety-generating environment of the hospital. Anxiety overlay is currently the largest source of diagnostic confusion with this test. Maneuvers to reduce anxiety are only partially effective and there is a great need for a drug that is more predictable in its pharmacological effect. Some patients have only a brief hemodynamic response to apparently maximal pharmacostimulation; this may also be due to anxiety or, alternatively, may reflect receptor resistance to papaverine.

A further area of difficulty is the patient with combined arterial and venous disease.[12,16] It is, perhaps, safest to say that at the moment these patients cannot be differentiated reliably from those with pure arteriogenic impotence. In practice, this differentiation is not crucial, as patients with combined vascular disease have a poor response to vascular surgery.

Validity of the penile Doppler study

The precise validity of the PDS is difficult to establish, for two reasons: first, the penile hemodynamic response is a complex phenomenon and to consider it in a purely mechanistic way is probably simplistic and limited; second, the reference standard investigations with which PDS is compared and evaluated are, themselves, not ideal. The diagnosis of psychogenic impotence is often by exclusion. Arteriography has not yet been evaluated thoroughly and the normal cavernosal arteriogram remains to be defined fully because technical factors, most importantly time of injection in relation to papaverine dose, can be difficult to control.[17] Even pharmacocavernosography can give rise to a false positive result.[18]

In spite of these limitations, the PDS has become the method of choice for evaluation of erectile impotence.

Pooling of data from large published series suggests that venous leakage can be diagnosed with a specificity of 56–88% and sensitivity of 55–100%; and arterial failure with a specificity of 64–94% and sensitivity of 82–100%.[5,7,9,12–15,19,20] In both categories the respective figures are dependent on the choice of cut-off value; this choice represents a trade-off between the sensitivity and specificity demanded of the test. It is preferable to ensure a high specificity for the diagnosis of arteriogenic impotence and high sensitivity for the diagnosis of venous leakage, because the treatment options for the former group are limited whereas in the latter group surgery requires careful patient selection.[7] Undoubtedly, the situation will change when, and if, arterial reconstruction becomes feasible.

Vascular mapping

This can be incorporated easily into the PDS. The poor diagnostic value of continuous dorsal vein flow has been mentioned already (Table 11.2). The relevance of arterial anomalies, arterial shunts and arterial narrowing, all of which are seen regularly during PDS, is unclear (Figs 11.11, 11.12). In selected cases such information can be of value but, in general, vascular mapping is of limited use.[9,21] With improvements in three-dimensional ultrasound reconstruction and availability of ultrasound contrast media, a true dynamic penile sonographic arteriogram may well be feasible in the future.

PENILE URETHRA AND ULTRASOUND URETHROGRAPHY

Without distension the urethra is difficult to evaluate, although rare conditions such as urethral cysts or divert-

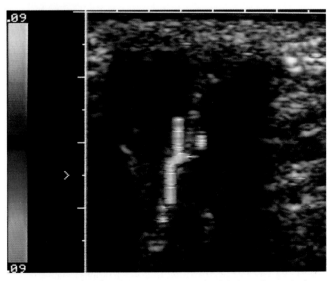

Fig. 11.11 Longitudinal view showing an arterial shunt between the two cavernosal arteries.

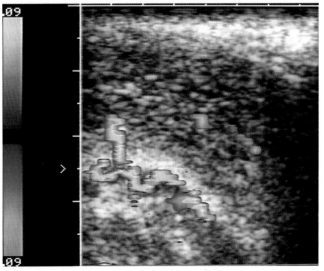

Fig. 11.12 Transverse view of a single dorsal artery supplying both cavernosal arteries.

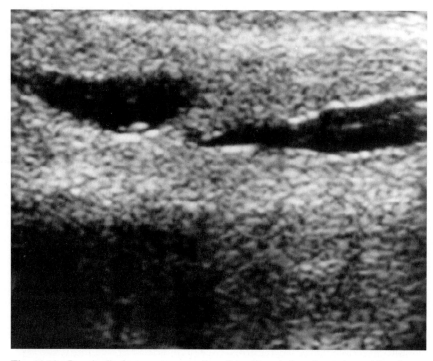

Fig. 11.13 Longitudinal transcutaneous view of the distended penile urethra, with a short stricture. The peristructural soft tissues are of reduced echogenicity (with acknowledgements to Dr D. Rickards).

icula may be recognized. Strictures, calculi and foreign bodies can be studies with precision, only on distension.

Urethral strictures are almost always benign, and the result of previous infection, instrumentation, surgery or trauma. In the anterior urethra, infection and instrumentation are the common causes of stricturing. Strictures may be associated with periurethral abscess, sinus, fistula, calculus and urethral diverticulum.

Studies have shown that a well-performed ultrasound urethrogram can be as informative as a contrast study.[22,23] An advantage of ultrasound is that the degree of peristricture fibrosis (Fig. 11.13) can also be assessed, although it has not yet been shown that this extra information is of clinical value.[24,25] Where ultrasound fails is in its inability to demonstrate the entire urethra. Demonstration of fistulae and false passages is also unreliable. At the moment, ultrasound urethrography is best restricted for follow-up of those patients with known anterior urethral strictures alone.

A further possible area of ultrasound superiority may be in the assessment of the urethral mucosa. This has not been systematically studied and reported as yet. In many cases we have noted irregularity of the mucosal surface

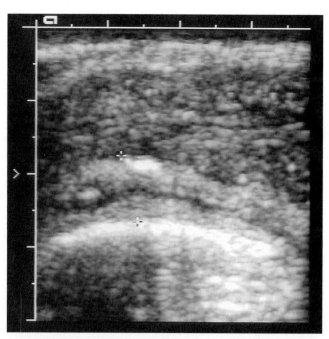

Fig. 11.14 Greatly thickened tunica albuginea (calipers) with an area of calcification denoting Peyronie's disease. The underlying corpus cavernosum is distorted with unequal cavernosal distension.

with marginal elevation of color Doppler signals. This, we believe, represents active inflammation, compared with the thin avascular mucosa of the normal urethra or the avascular smooth mucosa of the epithelialized lumen of a metal stent.

PEYRONIE'S DISEASE AND PENILE FIBROSIS

Peyronie's disease is a localized fibrotic induration of the tunica, of unknown etiology. In its mild variety it may be asymptomatic and recognizable only by careful palpation of the erect penis. More extensive thickening may result in a penile curvature with erection, which may be painful. Pain itself may cause impotence or there may also be an associated vascular malfunction.[26]

On ultrasound, classic Peyronie's plaques present as asymmetric focal echogenic thickening of the tunica, often calcified (Fig. 11.14). This typical appearance is seen in only a minority of patients (<25%) with clearly observable curvature on erection. More commonly we have found a diffuse, mildly echogenic, thickening of the tunica (>2–10 mm thick), with indistinct and blurred margins. This is more readily appreciated in the dorsal aspect of the penis.[26]

The relationship between Peyronie's disease and erectile failure is still a matter of dispute.[26–28] From 1.3–20% of patients referred for assessment of impotence will also have Peyronie's disease. The higher figure applies to selected populations and when patients with the clinically and sonographically subtle form of the disease are included. In our experience almost half the patients with Peyronie's disease will also have either venous leakage or arteriogenic failure on PDS. In some of these patients the plaque can be seen distorting cavernosal arteries or emissary veins and this may directly interfere with vascular function. Further proposed mechanisms are interference with emissary vein drainage as a result of tunical thickening or plaque-related local neuronal demyelination.[26]

Intracavernosal fibrosis, a separate entity from Peyronie's disease, is the result of some form of trauma and is characterized by echogenic foci within the hypoechoic cavernosa. Overt penile trauma is uncommon and currently the most common cause is repeated papaverine (and, less frequently, prostaglandin) injection.[29] Cavernosal fibrosis may also be a sequela of priapism.[30] Significant cavernosal fibrosis and stiffness will undoubtedly interfere with cavernosal distension, leading to impotence. In patients with declining effect of intracavernosal papaverine, it is usually impossible to disentangle the effects of cavernosal fibrosis from increasing pharmacological resistance or the progression of any underlying vascular malfunction.

PRIAPISM

This is defined as a persistent painful erection, although some consider an erection of longer than 6 h as abnormal, irrespective of whether it is painful. There are many causes, of which the most important are sickle cell disease, trauma and the prolonged action of intracavernosal therapy (usually papaverine).[30] Recently, a clearer classification has been proposed, based on pathophysiology.[31] The cause of priapism is persistent sinusoidal engorgement; this could be caused by either a blocked outflow (low-flow priapism, due to either dorsal vein or sinusoidal thrombosis) or a persistently raised cavernosal artery inflow (high-flow priapism, usually after penile revascularization or trauma).[30] Treatment of the two conditions differs significantly and accurate diagnosis is important.

The rarity of the condition means that there are few published data, particularly in the radiological journals. Our limited experience suggests that PDS can make an important contribution to both the assessment and research of this condition. Gray-scale scanning may demonstrate distended sinusoids, and dorsal vein or intracavernosal thrombosis. With persistent priapism, intracavernosal fibrosis will develop and is recognizable as cavernosal hyperechogenicity. With Doppler the cavernosal artery velocity and flow can be assessed; in the high-flow state, velocity will be elevated to between 20 and 30 cm/s, with a low-resistance waveform. Continuous dorsal vein flow may also be seen and we have also noted prominent AV shunts. Low-flow priapism, in contrast, will demonstrate high-resistance, low-velocity cavernosal artery waveforms.

REFERENCES

1. Wein A J, Van Arsdalen K, Hanno P M, Leven P M 1991 Anatomy of male sexual function. In: Jonas U, Thon W F, Stief C G (eds) Erectile dysfunction. Springer-Verlag, Berlin, p 3
2. Clemente C D (ed) 1985 Gray's Anatomy. Lea and Febiger, Philadelphia, p 1559
3. Breza J, Aboseif S R, Orvis B R, Lue T F, Tanagho E A 1989 Detailed anatomy of penile neurovascular structures: surgical significance. J Urol 141: 437–443
4. Wespes E, Depierreux M, Schulman C C 1987 Penile deep dorsal vein cushions and erection. Br J Urol 60: 174–177
5. Benson G S, McConnell J A, Schmidt W A 1981 Penile polsters: functional structures or atherosclerotic changes? J Urol 125: 800
6. Batra A K, Lue T F 1991 Penile erection: circulatory physiology. In:

Kirby R S, Carson C, Webster G D (eds) 1991 Impotence: Diagnosis and management of male erection dysfunction. Oxford : Butterworth-Heinemann, p 19
7. Patel U, Kirby R S, Rickards D 1994 Impotence: the radiologist's role. Clin Radiol (in press)
8. Lee B, Sikka S C, Randrop E R, Vellemarette P, Baum N, Hower J F, Hellstrom W J 1993 Standardization of penile blood flow parameters in normal men using intracavernous PgE1 and visual sexual stimulation. J Urol 149: 49–52
9. Mueller S C, Lue T F 1988 Evaluation of vasculogenic impotence. Urol Clin North Am 15: 65–76
10. McAninch J W, Laing F C, Jeffrey R B 1988 Sonourethrography in the evaluation of urethral strictures: a preliminary report. J Urol 139: 294–297
11. Hwang T I, Liu P Z, Yang C R 1991 Evaluation of penile dorsal

arteries and deep arteries in arteriogenic impotence. J Urol 146: 46–49

12. Patel U, Amin Z, Friedman E, Vale J, Kirby R, Lees W R 1993 Colour flow and spectral Doppler imaging after papaverine induced penile erection in 220 impotent men: study of temporal patterns and the importance of repeated sampling, velocity asymmetry and vascular anomalies. Clin Radiol 48: 18–24

13. Benson C B, Vickers M A 1989 Sexual impotence caused by vascular disease: diagnosis by duplex sonography. AJR 153: 1149–1153

14. Schwartz A N, Wang K Y, Mack L A et al 1989 Evaluation of normal erectile function with colour flow Doppler sonography. AJR 153: 1155–1160

15. Fitzgerald S W, Erickson S J, Foley W D 1991 Colour flow Doppler sonography in the evaluation of erectile dysfunction: patterns of temporal response to papaverine. AJR 157: 331–336

16. Benson C B, Vickers M A, Aruny J 1991 Evaluation of impotence. Semin US CT MR 12: 176–190

17. Rosen M P, Greenfield A J, Walker T G et al 1990 Arteriogenic impotence: findings in 195 impotent men examined with selective internal pudendal arteriography. Radiology 174: 1043–1048

18. Desai K M, Gingell J C 1988 Saline induced artificial erection without papaverine: a potential source of error in diagnosing cavernosal venous leakage. Br J Urol 62: 176–178

19. Quam J P, King B E, Jarne E M et al 1989 Duplex and colour Doppler sonographic evaluation of vasculogenic impotence. AJR 153: 1141–1147

20. Gilbert H W, Desai K M, Gingell J C 1991 Non-invasive assessment of arteriogenic impotence: a comparative study. Br J Urol 67: 512–516

21. Broderick G A, Anger P 1993 Duplex Doppler ultrasonography: non-invasive assessment of penile anatomy and function. Semin Roentgenol 28: 43–56

22. McAninch J W, Laing F C, Jeffrey R B 1988 Sonourethrography in the evaluation of urethral strictures: a preliminary report. J Urol 139: 294–297

23. Gluck C B, Bundy A L, Fine C, Loughlin K R, Richie J P 1988 Sonographic urethrogram: comparision to roentgenographic techniques in 22 patients. J Urol 140: 1404–1408

24. Garcia-Medina V, Berner J D, Llerena J, Garcia-Medina J, Genoves J L 1992 Urethral sonography in the diagnosis of penile and bulbar urethral strictures. Eur J Radiol 14: 31–36

25. Doubilet P M, Benson C B, Silverman S G, Gluck C D 1991 The penis. Semin US CT MR 12: 157–175

26. Amin Z, Patel U, Friedman E P, Vale J, Kirby R, Lees W R 1993 Colour Doppler and duplex ultrasound assessment of Peyronie's disease in impotent men. Br J Radiol 66: 398–402

27. Metz P, Ebbehoj J, Uhrenholdt A, Wagner G 1983 Peyronie's disease and erectile function. J Urol 130: 1103–1104

28. Gingell J C, Desai K M 1989 Review. Peyronie's disease. Br J Urol 63: 223–236

29. Benson G S 1987 Intracavernosal injection therapy for impotence. J Urol 138: 1262

30. Carson C C 1991 Priapism and post-priapism potency problems. In: Kirby R S, Carson C, Webster G D (eds) Impotence: diagnosis and management of male erectile dysfunction. Butterworth-Heinemann, Oxford, p 204

31. Witt M A, Goldstein I, Saenz de Jajeda I 1990 Traumatic laceration of intracavernosal arteries: the pathophysiology of non-ischaemic high flow arterial priapism. J Urol 143: 129

32. Vickers M R, Benson C B, Riches J P 1990 High resolution and pulsed wave Doppler for detection of corporovenous incompetence in erectile dysfunction. J Urol 143: 1125–1127

33. Patel U, Amin Z, Lees W R 1992 Can quantitative waveform analysis improve diagnostic accuracy of penile colour Doppler imaging? Proc R Coll Radiol Ann Sci Meet p 54 (Abstract)

34. Chiang P H, Chiang C P, Wu C C et al 1991 Colour duplex sonography in the assessment of impotence. Br J Urol 68: 181–188

35. Valji K, Bookstein J J 1993 Diagnosis of arteriogenic impotence: efficacy of duplex sonography as a screening tool. AJR 160: 65–69

36. Lopez J A, Espeland M A, Jarow J P 1991 Interpretation and quantification of penile blood studies using duplex sonography. J Urol 146: 1271–1275

37. Chen K K, Chen Y H, Chang L S, Chen M T 1992 Sonographic measurement of penile erectile volume. JCU 20: 247–253

12

Eye and orbit

G. Serafini A. Cavallo

The sonographic study of the ocular globe is performed with high-frequency small-parts transducers (10–13–15 MHz)[1] with water bath, placed directly on the closed eyelid with a significant amount of gel. A transducer of lower frequency (7.5 MHz) is necessary to perform the study of the retro-ocular space.

The examination is performed with the patient in a supine or sitting position with the patient's gaze oriented towards a fixed light; this facilitates the examination of all ocular areas and helps in evaluating the mobility of the pathologic image (e.g. vitreous hemorrhage, retinal detachment).[2] The sonographic examination should consist of axial, sagittal, and oblique views. When penetrating injuries are being examined, it is necessary to place a sterile cover over the transducer.

In order to perform a complete and proper examination the following conditions must be met:

1. Identify the orbital anatomic structures
2. Establish, in the case of pathologic findings, their location and relationships with the anatomic structures
3. Evaluate morphology, dimensions, echo pattern and mobility of the lesions.

Echo Doppler and color Doppler have recently been introduced in ophthalmology.[3–5] Transducers with a B-mode frequency of 7.5 MHz and Doppler frequency of 5 MHz are required. The examination is performed with the eyelid closed, avoiding excessive pressure of the transducer on the ocular globe as this may cause a number of artifacts. Since in orbital globe examinations the ultrasonic band closely parallels the vascular flow, the arteries are distinguishable from the veins by their color (arteries in red and veins in blue). Due to their small dimensions, the vessels exhibit a slow flow which requires the use of small sample volume and low PRF. Moreover, in studies of the venous eye system the wall filter must be set at a minimum of 50 Hz.

ANATOMY OF THE OCULAR GLOBE

The ocular globe (Fig. 12.1) appears ultrasonically (Fig. 12.2) as an echo-free spheroid with anteroposterior, transverse and longitudinal diameters (in adults) of 24.2 mm, 23 mm, and 23.6 mm respectively; it is surrounded by a highly reflective, 1.5 mm thick wall.[6] The ocular cavity appears macroscopically to be subdivided into two parts. The anterior part represents the anterior chamber (approximately 3.5 mm thick) and the posterior part represents the vitreous body. The highly reflective structures which subdivide the orbital globe into two parts are anatomically divided into two portions:

- The lateral portion consists of the iris plane and the zonular fibers, located between the globe wall and the lateral margin of the lens (lens equator).
- The central portion consists of the lens itself and the echographic interface between the lens and the vitreous body.[7,8]

The posterior chamber, which is located between the iris plane and the zonular fibers, is so small that conventional ultrasound equipment cannot adequately examine it.

The walls of the ocular globe consist of the following three membranes:

1. The external membrane is partly ($\frac{1}{6}$) anterior to the cornea and transparent, and partly ($\frac{5}{6}$) posterior to the sclera and opaque. Due to the large amount of connective tissue, the external membrane is sonographically highly reflective. The corneal wall is very thin (0.5 mm); it is visible in its entirety as a highly reflective structure with anterior convexity.

Adequate examination of the corneal plane and the anterior chamber requires transducers with water baths which allow optimal focalization of the superficial layers of the external membrane. Thorough visualization of the corneal plane permits accurate ocular biometry.

The sclera is also highly echogenic.[1,9] The correct measurement of its thickness (between 0.3 and 1.5 mm) is, however, very difficult since it can hardly be differentiated from the hyperechoic surrounding fatty tissue.

2. The middle membrane (uvea) is a highly vascularized tissue. The portion between the head of the optic nerve and the edge of the ciliary bodies is called the choroid. The ciliary bodies represent the anterior portion of the uvea itself.[6] The meeting point between the choroid and the ciliary bodies is called the 'ora serrata' and identifies the anterior limit of the extension of the choroidal detachment.

Anteriorly, the diaphragmatic membrane formed by the uvea and surrounding the pupil is called the iris. The ciliary bodies are ultrasonically visible only with the use of high frequency transducers (15 MHz) (Fig. 12.3) whereas the detection of neoplasms of the ciliary bodies (melanomas) is much easier.

The choroid, due to its rich vascularization, is the section of ocular membrane most visible with color Doppler.

3. The internal membrane is a nervous membrane (retina) extending from the optic papilla to the edge of the ciliary body (ora serrata). Under normal conditions the retina is not detectable as a discrete entity; however, in pathologic conditions such as detachment it is appreciable with color Doppler as a thin, highly vascularized membrane.

The lens, 3.5–4.5 mm thick, is convex shaped with posterior curvature and is usually anechoic. Only its posterior capsule is highly reflective, because of the difference in acoustic impedance with the vitreous body.

ANATOMY OF THE RETRO-OCULAR ORBITAL SPACE

The retro-ocular orbital space, pyramidal in shape, consists of hyperechoic adipose tissue and is demarcated by the bony structures of the orbit. The optic nerve and the extra-ocular muscles are easily identifiable within the fatty tissue.

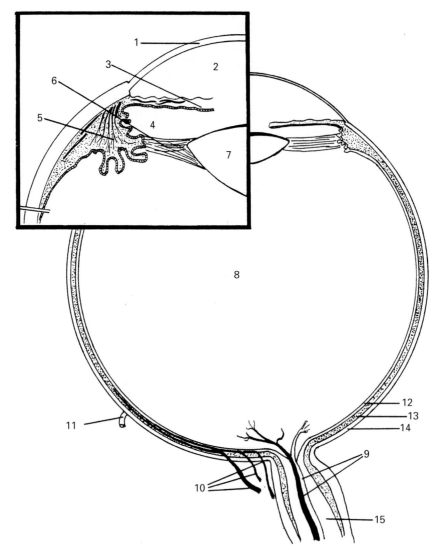

Fig. 12.1 1: cornea; 2: anterior chamber; 3: iris; 4: posterior chamber; 5: ciliary body; 6: zonular fibers; 7: lens; 8: vitreous; 9: central retinal artery and vein; 10: long and short posterior ciliary arteries; 11: vorticose vein; 12: retina; 13: choroid; 14: sclera; 15: optic nerve.

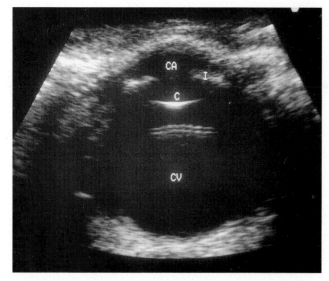

Fig. 12.2 Transverse scan of normal eye. CA: anterior chamber; I: iris diaphragm; C: lens; CV: vitreous body.

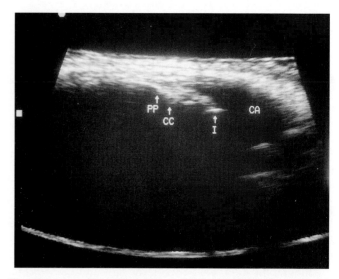

Fig. 12.3 Anterior segment of normal globe (15 MHz transducer). CA: anterior chamber; I: iris diaphragm; CC: ciliary body; PP: pars plana.

The optic nerve

In a transocular axial view, the optic nerve, 3.2–4.4 mm thick, appears as a hypoechoic inverted 'V' with the apex at the level of the papilla and the base posteriorly (Fig. 12.4). According to various reports, it is possible to differentiate the dura mater, the arachnoid space and the nerve only in in vitro studies.

Extraocular motor muscles

The six extraocular motor muscles (four rectus muscles and two oblique) are hypoechoic, slightly inhomogeneous structures (Fig. 12.5) which originate at the orbital apex, run separately toward the orbital globe and join the sclera in front of the global equator. Under normal conditions, the rectus muscles and the belly of the superior oblique muscle are sonographically easily recognizable; the inferior oblique muscle is of very small dimensions and therefore not detectable. The maximum thickness of these muscles should not normally exceed 3.5 mm; the tendinous portion is thinner than the muscular belly.

VASCULAR ANATOMY

Arterial anatomy

The vascularization of the ocular globe is supplied by the ophthalmic artery originating from the internal carotid artery and giving off three branches: the intracranial tract, the intracanalicular tract (running laterally and below the optic nerve), and the intraorbital tract. This last is composed of a posterior segment which follows laterally along the optic nerve, a middle segment which crosses over the optic nerve and an anterior segment which continues medially. However, there are anatomic variations of the course of the ophthalmic artery. The most frequent variation occurs in its middle segment where the vessel can run under rather than over the optic nerve.[10]

The ophthalmic artery is always detectable using color Doppler (Fig. 12.6). The artery is mostly visible in axial scans at the level of the optic nerve.[3,11]

The lateral optical segment of the artery is located posterolaterally while the medial segment is anteromedial. To detect the upper optic segment, the transducer may be angled in a caudocranial direction until the optic nerve is no longer visible.

Spectral analysis presents flow velocity waveforms similar to those of the internal carotid arteries, with a steep maximum peak velocity of approximately 30 cm/s (± 4), often followed by a dicrotic notch. It is noteworthy, however, that flow velocities in the ophthalmic artery may be influenced by the position of the patient: in the supine position velocities are higher than in the sitting or standing position. Furthermore, there is an inverse correlation between velocity and age.

The collateral branches of the ophthalmic artery which originate intraorbitally number 12–14: lacrimal artery, central retinal artery, upper orbital artery, short posterior ciliary arteries (6–8), long posterior ciliary arteries (one medial and one lateral), superior and inferior muscular arteries, anterior and posterior ethmoidal arteries, and superior and inferior palpebral arteries.

The central retinal artery is 0.3 mm thick and runs inside the optic nerve, entering at about 10–15 mm from the sclera.

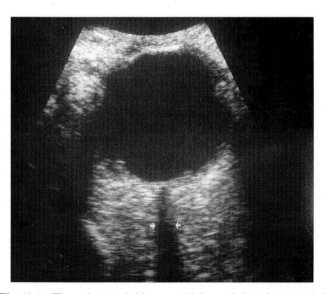

Fig. 12.4 The optic nerve (white arrows) is hypoechoic and surrounded by hyperechoic orbital adipose tissue.

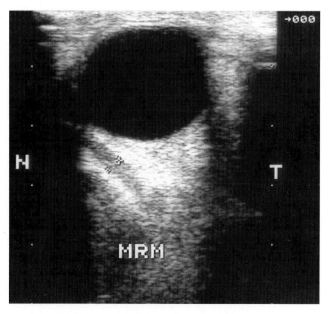

Fig. 12.5 Transverse scan of normal left orbit. The medial rectus muscle (MRM) appears as a band-shaped structure, 2.5 mm thick. N: nasal side of the orbit; T: temporal side.

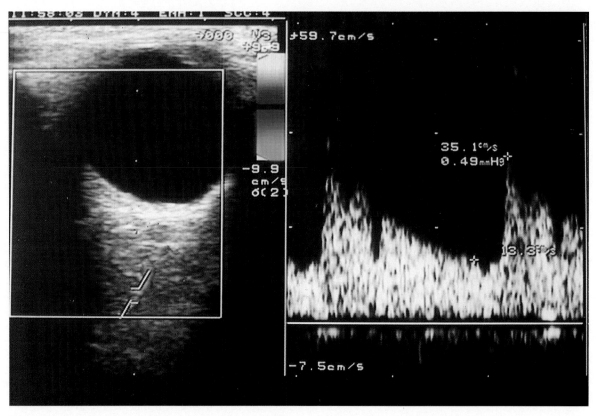

Fig. 12.6   Transverse color Doppler scan showing the ophthalmic artery, color-coded red. Maximum systolic velocity is 35 cm/s.

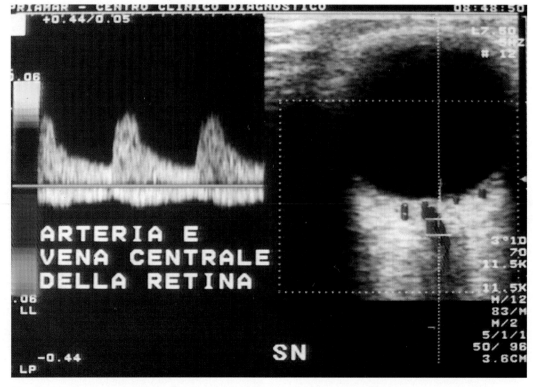

Fig. 12.7   The central retinal artery (red) and vein (blue) are parallel to each other, close to the optic nerve.

In all healthy subjects, in transverse scans color Doppler permits the detection of a 5–10 mm long arterial segment along the optic nerve, with simultaneous observation of both the artery and the vein (Fig. 12.7). Spectral analysis shows an arterial pulsatile flow similar to that of the ophthalmic artery, with a slightly lower systolic peak (12 ± 2 cm/s) and a continuous venous flow. Experimental studies[12] demonstrated that, with increasing intraocular pressure, systolic peak velocities progressively decrease, with disappearance of the telediastolic flow. With an intraocular pressure higher than 80 mmHg, no flow signals are detectable in the central retinal artery with color Doppler.

The posterior ciliary arteries, either long or short (the short being sprinkled throughout the choroid, while the long move more anteriorly up to the ciliary bodies), give rise to the 'choroidal blush' (Fig. 12.8). These arteries are visible on both sides of the optic nerve; their flow patterns are similar to those of the ophthalmic artery, except for a lower systolic velocity peak (10–12 cm/s $\pm$ 4). Distinction of the retinal flow from the choroidal flow is not possible under normal conditions; it can only occur when the two membranes are separated, due to pathologic causes (e.g. retinal detachment).

The lacrimal artery originates from the ophthalmic artery lateral to the optic nerve and goes anterolaterally along the upper surface of the lateral rectus muscle, subsequently dividing into the lacrimal and muscular branches. The terminal segment of the lacrimal artery is visible with color flow Doppler in 75% of normal orbits.[3] The remaining orbital arteries are generally difficult to visualize due to their superior and medial locations.

Venous anatomy

The main veins of the orbit are the superior ophthalmic vein and the inferior ophthalmic vein, both flowing into the cavernous sinus. The superior ophthalmic vein, 1.5 mm in diameter, originates in the internal corner of the palpebral slit and runs above the optic nerve, crossing it in a posterolateral direction.[13] The superior ophthalmic vein is always recognizable with color Doppler in axial caudo-cranially angled scans (Fig. 12.9).

The inferior ophthalmic vein, which runs along the floor of the orbit, is not visible with color Doppler due to its small dimensions.

PATHOLOGIC CONDITIONS OF THE EYE AND ORBIT

Pathology of the anterior chamber and the iris diaphragm

Traumatic injuries can cause hemorrhage in the anterior chamber (hyphema) which is visible as echo 'speckles';

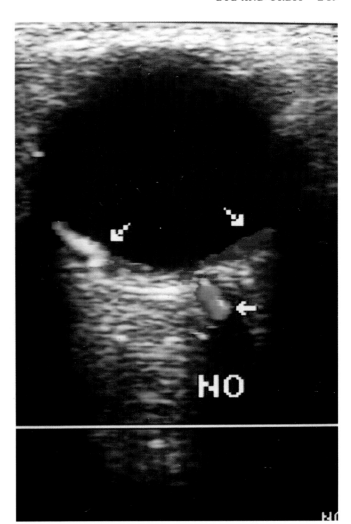

Fig. 12.8 Transverse color Doppler image of the 'choroidal blush' (arrows) produced by the short and long posterior ciliary arteries. NO: optic nerve.

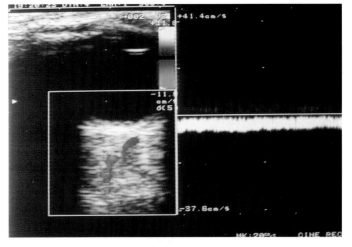

Fig. 12.9 Transverse scan showing a portion of the superior ophthalmic vein, color-coded blue.

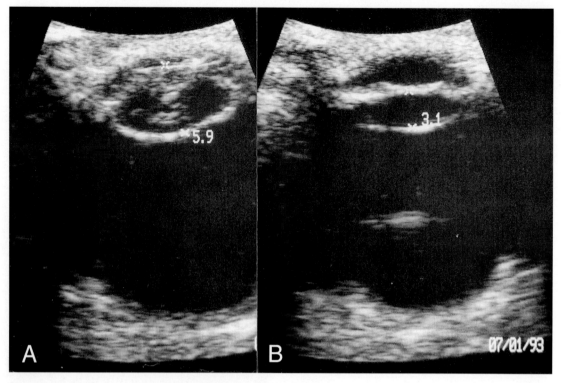

Fig. 12.10 **A** Hyphema caused by penetrating injury. The lesion of the anterior lens capsule causes intumescent cataract with increased diameter (5.9 mm) of the lens. **B** Normal opposite globe.

subsequently the chamber may collapse, becoming unrecognizable with ultrasound (Fig. 12.10). As a result the cornea comes in contact with the iris diaphragm. Increase in size of the anterior chamber, however, may indicate acute congenital glaucoma.[14]

Penetrating injuries to the anterior lens surface cause swelling of the lens with severe thickening and the subsequent occurrence of intumescent cataract. This is sonographically visible as a progressive increase in the echogenicity of the lens.[15] When the capsule and nucleus are also involved, they are displayed as a 'double concentric circle' (Fig. 12.11). Calcifications of the lens may occur in inveterate cataracts, mimicking foreign bodies.

In the case of cataract, the aim of ultrasound is to measure the anteroposterior diameter of the ocular globe in order to determine the strength of the corrective substitute lens, and to exclude the possibility of related pathologies such as retinal detachment which would preclude the replacement of the lens.

Following a traumatic injury, it is possible to demonstrate a subluxation or, more commonly, a posterior luxation of the lens – indicated by the absence of the lens in its physiologic location and its presence in the vitreous chamber.

Traumatic injuries, inflammatory and neoplastic diseases may cause an increase in the volume of the ciliary bodies which, as a result, may become visible with ultrasound; however, there are no specific elements to assist in the differential diagnosis.

Pathology of the vitreous chamber

The most common pathologies of the vitreous chamber which cause opacity of the chamber are the following:

1. vitreous hemorrhage
2. asteroid hyalosis
3. synchysis scintillans

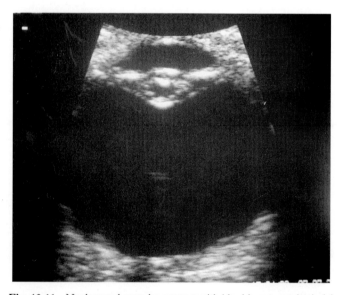

Fig. 12.11 Nuclear and capsular cataract with 'double concentric circle' appearance.

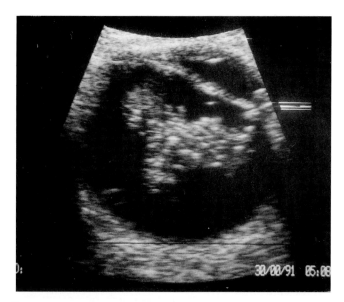

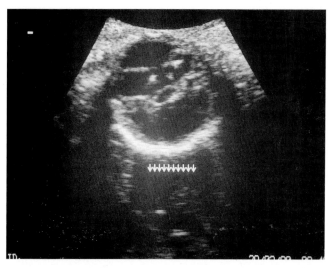

Fig. 12.12 Vitreous hemorrhage. Recent bleeding increases the acoustic reflectivity of the vitreous cavity.

Fig. 12.13 Phthisis bulbi. Severe atrophy with thickening of the ocular wall. Note the presence of vitreal membranes and calcifications of the wall, with typical acoustic shadow (arrows).

4. foreign bodies
5. air bubbles.

The most common cause of opacity of the vitreous is hemorrhage; this may be traumatic, degenerative (diabetic retinopathy) or neoplastic (choroidal melanoma) in nature, or can occur in hematopoietic diseases (leukemia, purpura, hemoglobinopathy).

Vitreous hemorrhage is characterized sonographically by the appearance of 'speckled' echoes which may be either localized or dispersed throughout the entire vitreous chambers (Fig. 12.12). The echoes' mobility is pathognomonic of hemorrhage. Traumatic hemorrhages may be reabsorbed over a period of time, or may persist, forming permanent vitreous membranes.

Atrophy (phthisis bulbi) may follow serious trauma to the ocular globe. The sonographic pattern includes size reduction of the globe, the presence of thick vitreous membranes, and thickening of the chorio-retina with subsequent calcifications (Fig. 12.13).

Asteroid hyalosis is a rare degenerative pathology, usually monolateral, which tends to develop in male, elderly (70–80 years) patients.[16] It is characterized by the presence of palmitate crystals and calcium stearates in the vitreous chamber. These substances are sonographically visible as coarse, slightly moving echoes whose arrangement may mimic a 'starry night'. A band of echo-free vitreous is typically present and, if localized peripherally, may stimulate vitreous detachment (Fig. 12.14).

Synchysis scintillans, which is even rarer than asteroid hyalosis, is usually bilateral and affects rather younger subjects; crystals are composed of cholesterol.[16] Both asteroid hyalosis and synchysis scintillans are asymptomatic.

Intraocular foreign bodies, whether radio-opaque or radio-transparent, appear sonographically as highly-reflective echoes of variable shape and size, usually free-floating within the vitreous in close proximity to the wall, and at times within the lens itself (Fig. 12.15). A particular characteristic of foreign bodies of regular morphology ('ball bearings') is the phenomenon of a posterior chain of multiple signals ('ringing') which greatly facilitates their differentiation from the often closely associated vitreous echoes.[15]

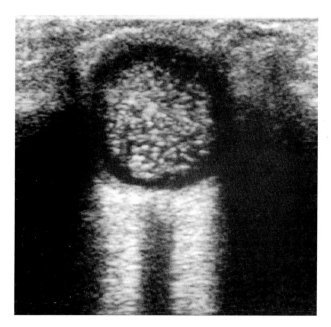

Fig. 12.14 Asteroid hyalosis. Calcium crystals are extremely dense. An anechoic retrovitreal space is still present close to the ocular wall.

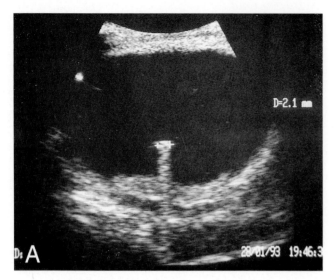 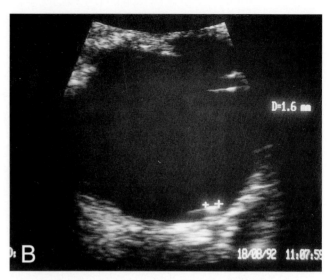

Fig. 12.15 **A** Round foreign body in the center of the vitreous cavity with posterior 'ringing artifacts'. **B** Foreign body (calipers) close to the ocular wall.

Sonography is essential to determine the location of foreign bodies and hence the viability of the magnetization test[17] which can be carried out only when foreign bodies are free within the vitreous and are sufficiently distant from the wall. Otherwise, the movement of the electromagnetically stimulated foreign bodies may cause retinal traction detachment.[18] Foreign bodies of magnetic nature are removed either through the injury path or the pars plana. In the case of foreign bodies with no magnetic properties, vitrectomy is routinely carried out.

Foreign bodies located in the retro-ocular space are hard to visualize with ultrasound, being masked by highly-reflective fatty tissue. Only the posterior acoustic shadow may enable their detection.

Perforating injuries may cause air bubbles to enter the ocular globe. The sonographic differentiation of bubbles from foreign bodies is based upon the larger amount of high level echoes produced by air bubbles as well as their antigravitational movement during head position changes. In doubtful cases additional sonograms should be obtained a few days later since air bubbles are quickly reabsorbed.

Pathology of the ocular global wall

Retinal detachment

Retinal detachment is the separation of the neurosensorial retina from the pigmented epithelium. It can be either idiopathic or secondary to trauma (detachment by traction) or neoplasm (choroidal melanomas).[19]

Detachment may be either partial or total. The sonographic diagnosis of total detachment is generally easy since the retina remains anchored to its two fixation sites (optic nerve posteriorly and ora serrata anteriorly) and sono-

graphically takes a 'V' shape (Fig. 12.16). Epiretinal cysts appear in inveterate detachments. Partial detachments are scarcely distinguishable from the vitreous membranes with the use of a conventional ultrasound system, as their echo-

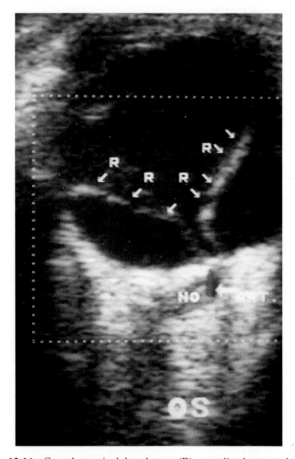

Fig. 12.16 Complete retinal detachment (R) extending between the optic nerve head and the ora serrata. NO: optic nerve.

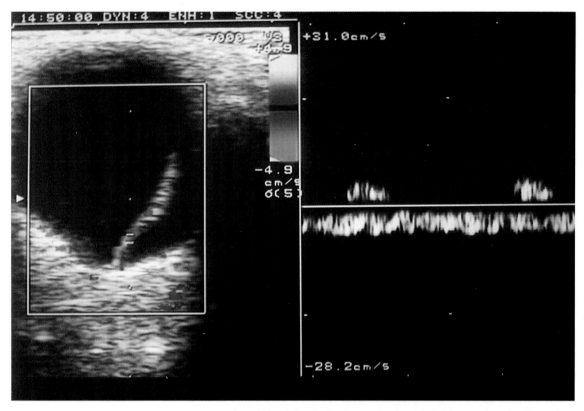

Fig. 12.17 Partial retinal detachment. Visualization of blood flow in the detached retina is helpful to confirm the diagnosis.

genicity is identical. With color Doppler the diagnosis is greatly facilitated[20] because the retina is vascular while the vitreous membranes are avascular (Fig. 12.17).[20] These differential criteria cannot, however, be applied to diabetic patients in whom intense neovascularization of the vitreous membranes may spontaneously occur. Detachments may become more complex in the case of subretinal hemorrhages, which have the characteristic pattern of mobile 'speckle' echoes.

Choroidal detachment

Choroidal detachment is most frequently caused by hypotonia of the ocular globe resulting from surgical therapies or perforating traumas. It is easily distinguished from retinal detachment by its location as well as by its morphology and kinetics (Table 12.1). It is situated between the ciliary body and the origin of the vorticose veins at the level of the ocular equator, never reaching the papilla. Choroidal detachment has a globular form, with slight mobility of the echoes (Fig. 12.18), and may also be associated with retinal detachment (Figs 12.19, 12.20).

Diabetic retinopathy

Ultrasound plays an important role in monitoring diabetic patients with proliferative retinopathy. In its initial stages

this consists of minor hemorrhages of the vitreous, or, more frequently, of the subvitreous space with subsequent posterior vitreous detachment (Fig. 12.21). On ultrasound scans low level 'speckle'-like echoes representing blood are visible. In its advanced stages, thick vitreous membranes with a polycystic shape and vitreo-retinal adhesions occur. These are the first sonographic signs of vitreo-retinal disease in diabetic patients. Subsequently vitreous retraction causes retinal detachments with primary prepapillary localization and, in the later stages, with a tent shape or flat shape. Sonographic monitoring therefore plays a decisive role in planning vitrectomy, and in identifying precisely the introduction site of the vitreotome.

Table 12.1 Choroidal detachment and retinal detachment – differential diagnosis.

	Choroidal detachment	Retinal detachment
Shape	Convex toward the vitreous, posterior pole not involved	Varies
Borders	Does not reach the optic nerve's head/iris; lens diaphragm may be reached	Optic nerve head/ora serrata
Aftermovements	Absent	Present

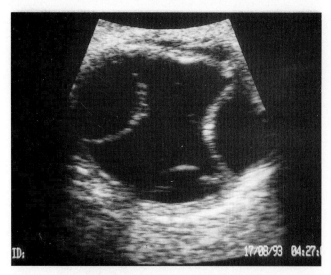

Fig. 12.18 Choroidal detachment. It differs from retinal detachment in that it does not extend to the optic nerve head. The two parts of the detached choroid approximate along the optical axis ('kissing choroidals').

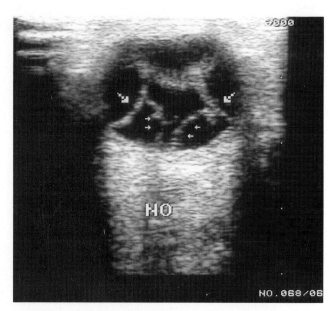

Fig. 12.19 Traumatic retinal detachment (small arrows) associated with choroidal detachment (large arrows). Note the different arrangements of the two membranes. NO: optic nerve.

Inflammatory diseases

Endophthalmitis

Endophthalmitis is an inflammatory condition caused by perforating injuries or endo-ocular surgery and involves the vitreous chamber and the ocular walls. The clinical symptoms are pain and inflammation. Ultrasonically, coarse and high level echoes partially or completely occupy the vitreous; the choroid and the retina appear thickened. Posterior vitreous detachment is also possible. If adhesions between the vitreous and the walls occur, traction retinal detachment may develop.

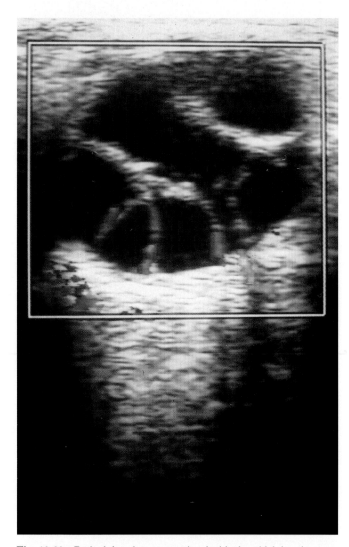

Fig. 12.20 Retinal detachment associated with choroidal detachment. With color Doppler the presence of blood flow is demonstrated.

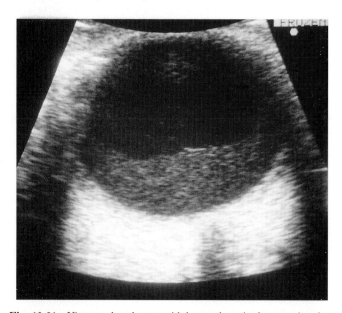

Fig. 12.21 Vitreous detachment with hemorrhage in the retrovitreal space.

Neoplastic pathology

Choroidal melanoma

Clinical aspects. Choroidal melanoma accounts for 2–4% of all orbital tumors[6] and frequently becomes symptomatic in elderly people. Histologically, it originates from choroid melanoblasts, which are thickly packed in combination with vascular lakes. The most common locations are the juxtapapillary region and the posterior pole of the globe.

Clinical symptoms are related to the site and volume of the tumor. When the posterior pole is involved, premature reduction of vision usually occurs, while more peripherally located tumors may be completely asymptomatic. Ocular hypertension may be present; the occurrence of necrotic changes may simulate uveitis.

Sonographic pattern. Small melanomas are vault-shaped,[21] with a solid homogeneous structure (Fig. 12.22) and a large base. Partial replacement of the choroid by neoplastic tissue ('choroidal excavation') is characteristic.

Larger melanomas grow toward the vitreous chamber, and the vitreous Bruch's membrane (the innermost layer of the choroid consisting of collagenous and elastic fibers) may be infiltrated. As a result, tumors herniate toward the vitreous chamber with a mushroom shape and a well-defined collar.[9] The echo pattern of large melanomas is more inhomogeneous since necrotic changes and rich vascularization can create hypoechoic areas. Calcifications are found rarely and only on the surface of melanomas.

Invasion of the retro-ocular space may conceal the highly reflective sclera, or, if extending out of the sclera, appear as a nodular lesion adjacent to the base of the tumor. Ultrasound is particularly useful in tumors with major extraocular growth; in such cases an ophthalmoscopic examination underestimates tumor dimensions. Retinal detachments may be detected with ultrasound; these generally occur along the boundaries of melanomas (Fig. 12.23), but may also occur at the apex of the tumors or in other sites. Furthermore, either vitreous or subretinal hemorrhages may develop; when they are very intense, melanomas can be 'obscured'.

Differential diagnosis. Small melanomas should be sonographically distinguished from other ocular nodular lesions, e.g. metastases, hemangiomas and choroidal nevi. In comparison with melanomas, both metastases and hemangiomas have a flatter surface and a more echogenic structure. Metastases are also more inhomogeneous. The lack of growth on follow-up examinations is the only diagnostic feature of nevi.

Color Doppler patterns. The degree of vascularization of choroidal melanomas is extremely useful in planning therapy. More highly vascularized melanomas are more

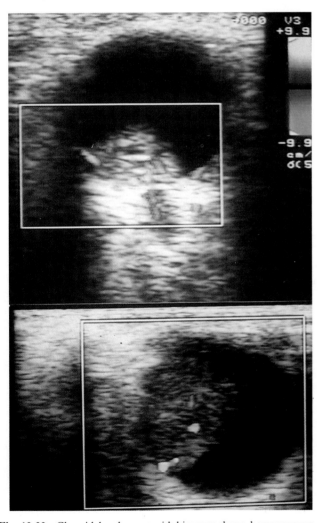

Fig. 12.22 Choroidal melanoma with biconvex shape, homogeneous structure and intense flow signals.

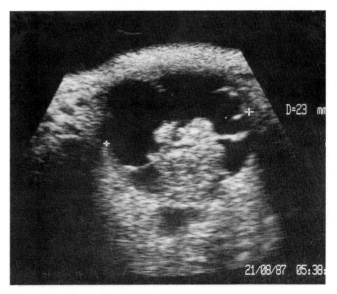

Fig. 12.23 Choroidal melanoma. The tumor has broken through Bruch's membrane and displays a 'mushroom' shape. There is associated retinal detachment.

radiosensitive,[22] while, on the other hand, less well vascularized tumors are more sensitive to hyperthermic treatment.

With color Doppler the presence of vascularization can be detected in a high percentage of melanomas (Fig. 12.22), allowing easy differentiation from subretinal hemorrhages and hematomas which are avascular.

Mean peak systolic frequency of melanoma vessels is 1 kHz (range 0.3–2.7 kHz) and the mean frequency is 0.6 kHz. The mean pulsatility index (PI) is 0.7, indicating a low impedance flow. In a study of 41 melanomas[23] the average maximum systolic velocity was 18.8 cm/s (± 2.6 cm/s).

Velocity parameters are useful in follow-up evaluation of tumor treatment. Currently conservative treatment is preferred; on follow-up studies of patients treated with surgery a higher mortality rate due to dissemination of neoplastic emboli was observed.[24]

Color Doppler is also useful in evaluating the results of radiotherapy, whether using [106]Ru plaques or a proton accelerator. In some cases, melanomas remain morphologically unchanged following treatment; only color Doppler can demonstrate the success of treatment, confirming the disappearance of vascularization (mummified melanoma). In a study of 18 melanomas[25] which underwent radiotherapy, the mean peak frequency progressively decreased from 1 to 0.34 kHz after four months and to 0.18 kHz after six months; complete flow disappearance was observed on eight-month follow-up.

When melanomas are associated with glaucoma flow studies are not meaningful since the high intraocular pressure caused by glaucoma severely reduces blood flow in the ocular globe.

Retinoblastoma

Retinoblastoma is a rare tumor, either mono- or bilateral, uni- or multifocal, affecting mostly children in the first 10 years of life. It is highly malignant with a high incidence of early recurrences and metastases. Retinoblastoma can grow either towards the vitreous or the choroid, involving the sclera and the retro-ocular space. Crossing the subarachnoid space, it may extend to the sellar region.

On sonographic scans retinoblastomas show irregularities of both morphology and contour, but the possibility of sonographic diagnosis relies substantially on the presence of calcifications, either coarse or tiny, always with acoustic shadows (Fig. 12.24).

Pathology of the retro-ocular space

Retro-ocular space pathologies have a variety of etiologies:

1. endocrine
2. vascular
3. neoplastic
4. inflammatory.

Endocrine pathology

Thyroid ophthalmopathy (in autoimmune Graves' disease) is responsible for 20% of all exophthalmos. It is caused by infiltration of lymphocytes and mucopolysaccharides into the recto-ocular muscles. Exophthalmos is associated with impaired venous flow and subsequent congestion in the orbit, leading to motor disturbances.[6]

On ultrasound scans the posterior extraocular muscles appear typically thickened (Fig. 12.25), either mono- or bilaterally, symmetrically or asymmetrically. The ten-

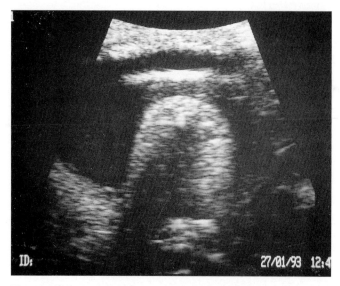

Fig. 12.24 Large retinoblastoma. The appearance of the tumor is inhomogeneous due to the presence of calcifications casting an acoustic shadow.

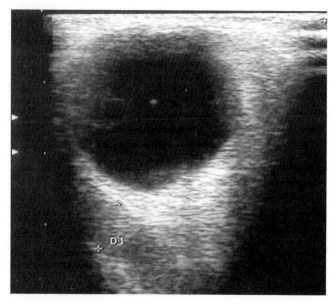

Fig. 12.25 Orbital involvement in Graves' disease. The medial rectus muscle (calipers) is enlarged.

dineous portions of the muscles remain unaffected. Muscle echogenicity may be normal or slightly increased. The medial and inferior rectus muscles are primarily involved. Less frequently, the optic nerve may also be affected, exhibiting an increased diameter.

Lacrimal glands may also be affected, becoming visible with ultrasound as homogeneously solid, oval and regularly marginated masses in the external temporal quadrant of the orbit.

The above mentioned sonographic signs are detectable in the early stages of hyperthyroidism and may precede any clinical and laboratory findings. In Graves' disease orbital scans are useful:

1. to exclude the presence of orbital masses, especially in monolateral exophthalmos
2. to demonstrate muscle thickening
3. to assess the involvement of the optic nerve and/or the lacrimal gland.

The differentiation of thyroid ophthalmopathy from acute or chronic ocular myositis or muscular tumors is important. In myositis, which may involve one or more muscles mono- or bilaterally, simultaneous involvement of the belly and tendineous portions of the muscles and remarkable hypoechogenicity are the clues for diagnosis.

Tumors of the extraocular muscles may be classified into primary (lymphomas, sarcomas) or secondary (originating from carcinomas or melanomas). Generally only one muscle is involved, appearing thickened and hypoechoic.

Vascular pathology

Carotid cavernous sinus fistulas originate from carotid wall ruptures, with subsequent direct passage between the internal carotid artery and the cavernous sinus. Fistulas can be classified as:

1. spontaneous, following intracavernous aneurysm ruptures or wall impairments caused by dysplastic diseases of the connective tissue
2. post-traumatic, occasionally bilateral
3. iatrogenic, due to incorrect endovascular treatment or surgical damage.

Dural arteriovenous malformations are predominantly localized at the transverse sinus and sigmoid level and, less frequently, at the cavernous sinus. According to Djindjian & Merland's classification,[26] drainage may occur in four different ways:

1. Type 1: into a dural sinus or meningeal vein without flow inversion
2. Type 2: into a venous sinus with backflow in the deep venous system
3. Type 3: directly into the cortical veins which appear dilated
4. Type 4: into a venous lake, typically during infancy.

With color Doppler,[27] clinical suspicions of a carotid cavernous sinus fistula, traumatic or spontaneous, responsible for pulsating exophthalmos can be confirmed. Color Doppler shows dilatation of the ophthalmic vein with inverse arterialized and biphasic flow and increased velocity (Fig. 12.26). A bidirectional flow (retrograde in systole, anterograde in diastole) may appear in the vorticose veins. Color Doppler can demonstrate flow normalization following embolization treatment of the fistula.[28]

Orbital varices of the superior ophthalmic vein are clinically evident as intermittent exophthalmos accentuated by the Valsalva maneuver causing a possible transitory

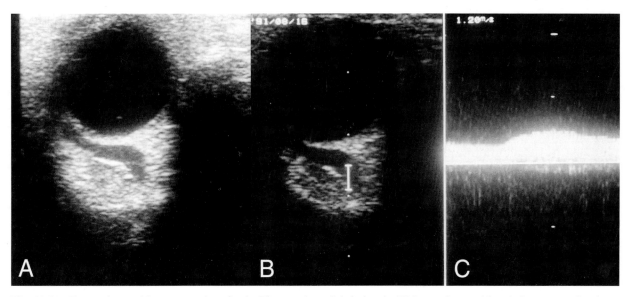

Fig. 12.26 Traumatic carotid cavernous sinus fistula. The superior ophthalmic vein (**A**) is prominent, with turbulent, reversed and arterialized flow (**B**).

inversion of flow.[29] With color Doppler, varices appear as venous lakes at the level of the root of the orbit with intra- or extraconic localization. During the Valsalva maneuver a transitory flow inversion can be seen.

Neoplastic pathology

Meningioma. Meningioma is a rare tumor of the optic nerve which originates from the arachnoid's endothelial cells, and, starting from the orbit, may involve the middle cerebral fossa across the optic canal or the superior orbital tissue. Meningioma affects mainly adults (30–50 years of age) and causes early visual reduction as the first clinical symptom.

On ultrasound scans meningiomas present as hypoechoic, cylindrical masses surrounding the optic nerve, with possible calcifications.[30–32]

Glioma. Glioma primarily affects children and young adults and is frequently associated with systemic neurofibromatosis.[33] It originates from the optic nerve and may extend to the chiasm, enlarging the optical canal.[34] Fusiform, hypoechoic thickening of the nerve, either localized or diffuse, represents the characteristic sonographic presentation (Fig. 12.27). CT and MRI are mandatory for delineating the precise extent of both meningiomas and gliomas in the periorbital space.

Metastases. Metastases, predominantly originating from carcinomas of the lung and breast, appear as solid lesions, hypoechoic in comparison with the surrounding fatty tissue. The margins of small metastases are clearly identifiable, but those of large masses are irregular and ill-defined. There are no ultrasound criteria which can suggest the location of the primary tumor.

Neoplasms of the paranasal sinuses. Primary tumors of the paranasal sinuses, mostly carcinomas and sarcomas, may invade the orbit. With ultrasound they appear as intraorbital, solid, hypoechoic masses in an extraconical location. CT is mandatory to obtain an accurate staging of these tumors.

Rhabdomyomas, rhabdomyosarcomas and lymphomas. These neoplasms affect the extraocular muscles which undergo aspecific thickening, differential diagnosis being impossible either with ultrasound, CT, or MRI. In suspected malignancies characterized by irreducible monolateral exophthalmos, sonography can define the morphology, structure, and intra- or extraconical location, but cannot determine the nature of the lesions.

Inflammatory pathology

Pseudotumors. Pseudotumors (or inflammatory masses) represent a frequent cause of monolateral exophthalmos, a condition characterized by pain and reduced ocular motility, generally affecting patients between 10 and 40 years of age.

Pseudotumors are considered 'idiopathic' and are likely to be caused by autoimmune diseases frequently associated with systemic pathologies, like Wegener's granulomatosis. The symptoms can mimic malignancies.[35]

Two types of pseudotumor are pathologically classified:

1. acute disease characterized by vasculitis
2. chronic disease characterized by infiltration of lymphocytes, plasmacytes, and macrophages.

The sonographic pattern is characteristic, even though non-specific: hypoechoic masses with ill-defined margins, located in the retro-ocular adipose tissue and often associated with myositis and thickening of extraocular muscles. Typically these lesions are highly sensitive to cortisone treatment; the healing process can be easily followed up with ultrasound until recovery is complete.

Optic neuritis. Optic neuritis is an inflammatory condition of the optic nerve which manifests as reduced vision, typically in the central area. An aspecific thickening of the optic nerve is demonstrated on ultrasound.

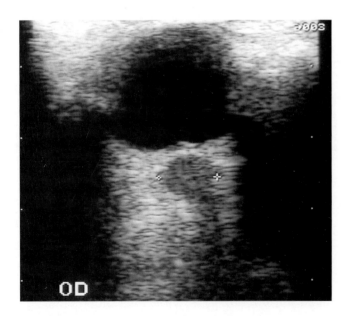

Fig. 12.27 Transverse scan of fusiform optic glioma (calipers), with a homogeneous and hypoechoic structure.

REFERENCES

1. De Albertis P, Quadri P, Serafini G, Cavallo A 1991 Ecografia dell'orbita. Spirito, Savona
2. Cavallo A, Serafini G, Quadri P 1993 Occhio. In: SIUMB (ed) Trattato Italiano di Ecografia, Poletto, Milan, vol 1, pp 70–79
3. Erickson S J, Hendrix L E, Massaro B M et al 1989 Color Doppler flow imaging of the normal and abnormal orbit. Radiology 173: 511–516
4. Lieb W E, Cohen S M, Merton D A et al 1991 Color Doppler imaging of the eye and orbit. Arch Ophthalmol 109: 527–531
5. Giovagnorio F, Quaranta L, Bucci M G 1993 Color Doppler assessment of normal ocular blood flow. J Ultrasound Med 12: 473–477
6. Miglior M 1989 Oftalmologia clinica. Monduzzi, Bologna
7. Coleman D J, Lizzi F L, Jack R L 1977 Ultrasonography of the eye and orbit. Lea and Febiger, Philadelphia
8. Shammas H J 1984 Atlas of ophthalmic ultrasonography and biometry. Mosby, St Louis
9. Mazzeo V 1987 Ecografia dell'apparato oculare. Fogliazza, Bologna
10. Hayreh S S, Dass R 1962 The ophthalmic artery, second intra-orbital course. Br J Ophthalmol 46: 165–185
11. Canning C R, Restori M 1988 Doppler ultrasound studies of the ophthalmic artery. Eye 2: 92–95
12. Guthoff R, Berger R W, Winkler P et al 1991 Doppler ultrasonography of the ophthalmic and central retinal vessels. Arch Ophthalmol 109: 532–536
13. Montanara A 1976 Elementi di radiodiagnostica oftalmologica. Minerva Medica, Turin
14. François J, Goes F 1981 Ocular biometry: introductory lecture. Doc Ophthalmol Proc Ser 29–135
15. Cavallo A, Polizzi A, De Albertis P 1991 Ruolo della ecotomografia nella traumatologia del bulbo oculare. G Ital Ultrasonol 2: 98
16. McLeod D, Restori M 1977 Real time B-scanning of the vitreous. Trans Ophthalmol Soc UK 97: 547
17. Machemer R 1972 A new concept for vitreous surgery. Am J Ophthalmol 74: 1022–1033
18. Puttman W, Reuter R, Trier N G 1977 Change of orientation and intensity of a magnetic field as an aid for ultrasonic foreign body localization. In: White D, Brown R E (eds) Ultrasound in medicine. Plenum, New York, pp 1011–1018
19. Munk P L, Vellet A D, Levin M, Lin D T C, Collyer R T 1991 Sonography of the eye. AJR 157: 1079–1086
20. Wong A D, Cooperberg P L, Ross W H et al 1991 Differentiation of detached retina and vitreous membrane with color flow Doppler. Radiology 178: 429–431
21. Poujol J 1986 L'ecografia in oftalmologia. Masson, Milan
22. Coleman D J, Silverman R H, Iwamoto T et al 1988 Histopathologic effects of ultrasonically induced hyperthermia in intraocular malignant melanoma. Ophthalmology 95: 970–981
23. Guthoff R, Berger R W, Winkler P et al 1991 Doppler ultrasonography of malignant melanomas of the uvea. Arch Ophthalmol 109: 537–541
24. Guthoff R, Berger R W, Helmke K et al 1989 Doppler sonographische befunde bei intraokularen tumoren. Fortschr Ophthalmol 86: 239–241
25. Wolff-Kormann P G, Kormann B A, Riedel K G et al 1992 Quantitative duplex and color Doppler ultrasound in the follow up of β-irradiated (^{106}Ru/^{106}Rh) choroidal melanomas. German J Ophthalmol 1: 151–155
26. Djindjian R, Merland J J 1978 Superselective arteriography of the external carotid artery. Springer Verlag, Berlin
27. Ferro C, Perona F, Cavallo A 1992 Diagnosi eco Doppler e trattamento embolizzante di malformazione arterovenosa durale. Radiol Med 83: 464–467
28. Scialfa G, Vaghi A, Valsecchi F et al 1982 Neuroradiological treatment of carotid and vertebral fistulas and intracavernous aneurysms. Technical problems and results. Neuroradiology 24: 13–25
29. Lieb W E, Merto D A, Shields J A et al 1990 Color Doppler imaging in the demonstration of orbital varix. Br J Ophthalmol 74: 305–308
30. Byrne S F, Green R L 1992 Ultrasound of the eye and orbit. Mosby, St Louis
31. Guthoff R 1991 Ultrasound in ophthalmologic diagnosis. Thieme, New York
32. Lloyd G 1982 Primary orbital meningioma: review of 41 patients investigated radiologicaly. Clin Radiol 33: 181–184
33. Cavallo A, Polizzi A, De Albertis P 1990 Reperti ecografici in patologia neoplastica orbitaria. G Ital Ultrasonol 1: 231
34. Stern J, Jakobiel F A, Housepian E M 1980 The architecture of optic nerve gliomas with and without neurofibromatosis. Arch Ophthalmol 98: 505–511
35. Goes F 1987 Ultrasonographic and clinical characteristics of orbital pseudotumors. In: Ossoinig K C (ed) Ophthalmic echography. Nijhoff/Junk, Dordrecht, p 499

13

Skin and subcutaneous tissues

S. Baldassarre   A. M. Offidani   L. Solbiati

The use of ultrasonography in dermatology is not very widespread, despite the fact that the first papers appeared in the literature more than 20 years ago.[1] Initially US was utilized to depict normal skin in a rapid and non-invasive way as cross-section images, especially for the measurement of skin thickness.[2,3] It was only later, at the beginning of the 80s, that the use of US was extended to cutaneous pathologies, with particular regard to neoplasms.[4-6]

The rationale for this relatively recent application may be found in the characteristics of echographic examination which provides quickly and harmlessly repeated cross-section images of the skin and underlying tissues. This examination has recently become even more accurate because of the availability of high-frequency probes, which allow high axial and lateral resolution.

Three types of sonographic equipment are currently employed for skin studies:

- 10–20 MHz mechanical sector transducers with water bath, in some instances associated with a thin layer of gel mattress which allows optimal focalization of the US beam in the near field. Thanks to its moderate size, this particular type of transducer is suitable for the study of irregular surfaces, especially of the face, and for lesions situated in large cutaneous plicae or folds.

- 7.5–10 MHz linear electronic probes, currently available also with color Doppler facilities, in most cases coupled with thin blocks of synthetic spacer. These probes are particularly suitable for lesions which are found on smooth areas, such as the skin of the limbs, back and hypogastrium, or on areas away from articular or irregular surfaces. Compared with sector transducers, linear probes have the clear advantage of a wider near field of view.

- Quite recently a new generation of US equipment dedicated to the study of the dermatologic pathologies has been introduced, consisting of a translating, 20 MHz transducer in a built-in water chamber. This equipment has a very limited field of view (1.2–2.5 cm) and minimal depth of penetration (2 cm), but provides a theoretic axial resolution of 80 μm and theoretic lateral resolution of 200 μm.[7] Furthermore, it has a slow frame rate; Doppler facilities are not available. In its representation of the skin this equipment employs a false color coding system, where light colors correspond to hyperechoic tissues.

In all dermatologic US applications the use of large amounts of gel is essential in order to produce a continuous, homogeneous and uniform contact between probe and skin or between spacer and skin, thus avoiding the formation of small air bubbles which may also be caused by the presence of hair, skin folds, or irregularities resulting from the lesion itself.

The examination should always include the study of the homologous, contralateral region for comparison and technical calibration of the equipment. Hair removal is advisable only in the case of hypertrichosis. Correct pressure should be applied on the skin to avoid the formation of small air bubbles and to stabilize the contact between transducer, spacer and skin.

GENERAL CHARACTERISTICS OF THE SKIN

Skin is composed of two mutually interdependent major layers, the epidermis and the dermis, connected to the underlying muscular structures by the subcutaneous, adipose layer (hypoderm) whose thickness varies greatly from region to region, ranging from 0.5 mm (eyelids) to 4 mm (plantar areas). The external cutaneous surface is not uniform: there are punctiform depressions (pilosebaceous units), superficial and deep sulci and raised folds.

The epidermis is the most superficial layer of the skin; it is a scaly, stratified epithelium which is composed of four types of cells: keratinocytes, melanocytes, Langerhans cells and Merkel cells. Its thickness ranges from 0.06–0.6 mm; it has no blood or lymphatic vessels but there are free nerve endings. Keratinocytes constitute about 90–96% of epidermic cells; they originate from the cells of the basal layer and as they move toward the surface, they form the following layers from the bottom upward: basal, prickle-cell, granular, clear and corneous. The latter is not present in mucosa.

The cutaneous layer beneath the epidermis is called the dermis; it represents the stroma of the skin. It is a layer of fibroelastic, connective tissue immersed in a ground substance, creating a supporting structure where the glands, appendages, vessels and nerves of the skin are found. The thickness of the dermis ranges from 1 mm, as on the scalp, to 4 mm, as on the back.

The hypoderm, beneath the dermis, forms a fibro-adipous layer between skin and aponeurotic fascia. Its thickness varies according to race, age, sex and even nutritional and endocrine factors.

US PATTERNS OF NORMAL SKIN

Thorough knowledge of the sonographic features of normal skin is essential for the study of skin pathology. Some aspects are constant, but others vary according to region of the body, age, race, sex and exposure to different factors.

Sonographically, the normal skin is composed of multiple layers with differing echo structures, starting from the surface and moving down[3,6-8] (Figs 13.1, 13.2).

The first layer, which is highly reflective, corresponds to the entry echo; it appears as an intensely echoic, continuous line whose thickness varies in relation to the part being examined and to skin elasticity. Generally, it does not exceed 2 mm. It is produced by the interface between gel and epidermis, reinforced by the corneous layer. This hyperechoic, continuous line may be interrupted, either by

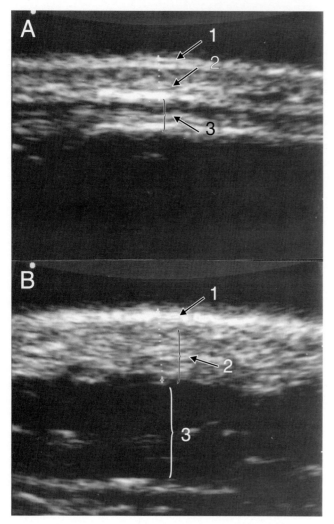

Fig. 13.1   Normal skin imaged with a 20 MHz mechanical sector transducer. **A** Dorsum of the hand (thickness 0.8 mm). **B** Chin region (thickness 2.2 mm). 1: entry echo; 2: dermis; 3: subcutaneous adipose tissue.

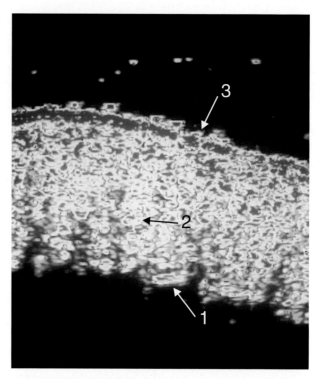

Fig. 13.2   Normal skin imaged with a 20 MHz dedicated translating transducer. Volar side of the forearm. 1: entry echo; 2: dermis; 3: subcutaneous adipose tissue.

air contained within the scales (especially in psoriasis) or by keratinous material in seborrheic verrucas, which may create strong reflections with acoustic shadows.

The next layer is the dermis; the demarcation between this and the epidermis above is not clear. Observations of psoriatic and acanthotic skin show that the ultrasonic interface between epidermis and dermis is mainly determined by the edges of the dermic papillae.[9,10]

The dermis is clearly echogenic (Figs 13.1, 13.2) because of its well-organized fibers, but is less echogenic than the transducer–epidermis interface. Its homogeneity is interrupted by small hypoechoic areas which correspond to hair follicles.

Conditions which cause edema typically result in a reduction in reflectiveness. In some areas however, such as palms and soles, face and scalp, dermic echoes are faint because of the variability in the direction of dermic fibers.[11]

The regular fibrous web of the dermis provides optimal contrast resolution with pathologic lesions, which are generally hypoechoic. Its thickness varies according to the areas of the body and patient age; this also affects the reflectiveness of the dermis. As a matter of fact, in neonates the dermis is hyporeflective; after a few months, it becomes progressively more echogenic. The level of skin relaxation may also affect the reflectiveness of the dermis.[11–13]

The next layer (hypoderm) is normally hypoechoic due to its mainly adipose nature, but there may be hyperechoic bands representing connective septa. Its thickness is greatly variable, ranging from 5–20 mm.

Below this layer, the superficial fascia is visualized as a hyperechoic line that divides subcutaneous from muscular tissue.

US not only depicts the structure of normal skin as described but also allows accurate measurement of its thickness; data obtained are reproducible and comparable even after some time, as long as the same technical and methodologic conditions are applied. Sonographically measured skin thickness is higher in the upper portion of the forearm and on the dorsum of the hand, where the dermo–hypodermic delimitation is clearer, and lower in the lumbar region and around the nape and chin[12] where the dermo–hypodermic delimitation is generally less clear. Usually skin is thicker in women than in men.

Apart from the measurement of skin thickness described above, the main indications for US in dermatology at present may be summarized as follows:

- measurement of thickness and invasion depth of skin tumors prior to cryosurgery, laser surgery or radiotherapy
- determination of therapeutic effects in chronic inflammatory dermatoses (e.g. psoriasis)
- assessment of the size of cutaneous metastases during the course of chemotherapy treatment
- studies on the effects of steroids on the skin (Fig. 13.3).

The outstanding application of US in dermatology is in the study of malignant melanomas. Sonography can also usefully be employed in the follow-up of psoriasis during treatment and in the assessment of the extent of other benign and malignant skin pathologies.

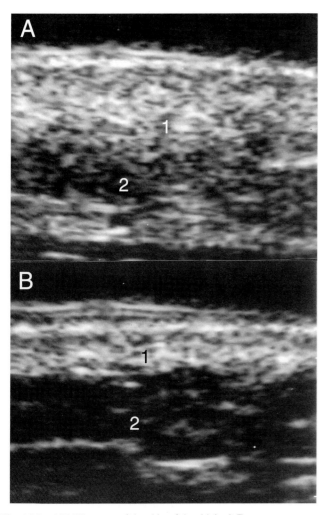

Fig. 13.3 20 MHz scans of the skin of the thigh. **A** Eczematous dermatitis with severe thickening of the dermis (1) which extends toward the subcutaneous fatty tissue (2). **B** Following steroid therapy, complete remission with normal morphology of the skin.

MELANOMA

Malignant melanoma is a highly invasive cutaneous tumor which metastasizes via the lymphatics and blood vessels. It is likely to start in the melanocytes of the epidermal–dermal junction, from a pre-existing nevus or in normal-appearing skin.

It is the most malignant but least common (3%) of skin tumors. Its natural history is extremely variable: it may metastasize rapidly and diffusely or not until 10 or 20 years after the diagnosis. This varying behavior also depends on the site affected.

Unfortunately, the incidence of melanomas has dramatically increased worldwide in the last 20 years: 27 new cases annually per 100 000 inhabitants have been reported in Arizona, and 12/100 000 in Connecticut. In Scandinavian countries the rate doubles every decade.

As regards Italy, in the last 30 years the incidence has almost doubled, from 2–3 cases per 100 000 inhabitants, to 5 cases at the current time. However, the highest incidence is in Australia, with a rate of 32.7 cases per 100 000 inhabitants, and where the number of cases doubles every decade.[14,15]

The death rate has increased in parallel with the number of cases but statistics demonstrate that there is a general improvement in prognosis, linked to early diagnosis, as a consequence of better understanding of histogenesis and risk factors.

Melanoma may develop at any age, but is rare before puberty; the peak incidence is between 40 and 60 years, while the lentigo type usually affects people between 60 and 80 years.

Common sites include the lower limbs in women, the trunk in men and the depigmented areas (e.g. plantar region) in black people.

From a strictly morphologic point of view, melanomas are classified as flat, cupped or flat-cupped. The flat melanoma is an irregularly-shaped pigmented lesion growing centrifugally (horizontal growth). This is the most common form (80%) and may arise in any part of the skin or mucosa. The cupped melanoma (18%) is less common and generally appears on healthy skin, tending to grow vertically.

The progression of melanoma can occur in two ways:

A. superficial spread, characterized by a phase of radial growth of variable duration and a subsequent invasive phase of the dermis in which metastases may occur;
B. nodular growth, which is vertically invasive and metastasizes more quickly.

The presence and type of intradermal tumor adjacent to the invasive component allowed the categorization of different kinds of melanomas with differing prognoses: nodular melanoma, superficial spreading melanoma, lentigo-type melanoma, and lentiginous acral melanoma.

Nodular melanoma accounts for 15–30% of cases[15] and is characterized by vertical progression. It is the most aggressive and invasive type; its prognosis, which is the poorest, is related to tumor thickness.

Superficial spreading melanoma is the most common type and accounts for 70% of cases.[15] Its early recognition and moderate thickness make its prognosis more favourable compared with the nodular type. It can arise in healthy skin or in a small, acquired or congenital nevus. Initially it appears as a spotted lesion, then becomes slightly elevated and spreads progressively and irregularly. During its growth, areas of spontaneous regression can be seen, characterized by a strong, infiltrating, lymphocytic response.[15]

The lentigo-type melanoma typically affects the elderly, especially women. In most cases it occurs on the face. It is characterized by slow progression; local or lymphatic metastases may occur.[15]

As described above, the prognosis of melanoma is assessable by means of morphologic parameters which define the various stages of tumor progression. These stages consist of the phase in situ, the phase of radial and/or vertical growth, characterized by deep invasion, and finally metastatic spread. Thus, assessment of the level of dermic invasion according to Clark and measurement of tumor thickness according to Breslow,[16] share importance in prognosis with the histologic identification. The prognostic value of both methods is widely acknowledged; as a matter of fact, a strict correlation between these parameters and patient survival exists (Tables 13.1, 13.2).

In addition, there are other morphologic parameters of lesser prognostic relevance such as ulceration, sublesional inflammatory infiltration, mitotic activity, cell type and vascular invasion.

It is therefore necessary to assess precisely the thickness of the lesion in order to formulate a prognostic hypothesis and to apply the appropriate treatment. Sonography can be very helpful in this assessment.

The high survival ratio of patients with thin melanomas (thickness less than 0.75 mm according to Breslow, or 0.85 mm as suggested by Day et al)[16,17] caused a radical change in surgical approach: simple excision has been proposed as an alternative to wide exeresis. The same therapeutic strategy may be adopted even for tumors up to 2 mm thick. Thus an accurate preoperative determination of tumor thickness is mandatory in order to plan precisely the extent of excision, the type of anesthesia and, last but not least, the correct information for the patient.

Previous descriptions[4,18–23] demonstrate that precise, quantitative information concerning the morphovolumetric characteristics and the thickness of cutaneous melanomas can be obtained by the use of high-resolution ultrasonography, and that these data are virtually comparable to those provided by histologic examination (Figs 13.4–13.6).

Sonographically, melanomas appear as hypoechoic lesions, clearly distinguishable from the surrounding dermis because of the higher echogenicity of the latter. The lateral borders are irregular in 75% of cases, whereas the basal demarcation is generally well-defined. Interruption of the entry echo with ill-defined posterior contours can be found in the ulcerated or warty type (Fig. 13.7)

It has already been reported[4,19,22,23] that sonographic determination of melanoma thickness is comparable to the histologic assessment. Sonographic errors are generally

Table 13.1 Melanoma: Clark's levels versus prognosis (5-year survival).

Levels	Invasion	5-year survival
I	epidermis (melanoma in situ)	100%
II	subtotal papillary dermis	80–90%
III	total papillary dermis	65–75%
IV	reticular dermis	50–55%
V	subcutaneous tissue	30–38%

Table 13.2 Classification of cutaneous melanomas by thickness (Breslow) versus prognosis (5-year survival).

thickness (mm)	5-year survival
< 0.75	88–100%
0.76–1.50	74–83%
1.51–3.00	60–70%
> 3.01	22–47%

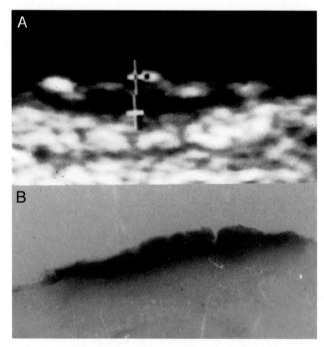

Fig. 13.4 Clark's level II melanoma. Scan with a 13 MHz probe. **A** Sonogram shows a serpiginous, 0.70 mm thick, nearly anechoic lesion with a small irregularity of the dermis. **B** Pathologic specimen.

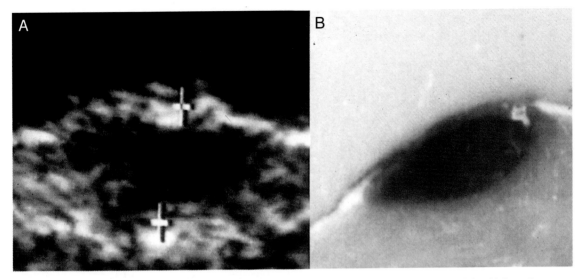

Fig. 13.5 Clark's level III melanoma. Scan with a 13 MHz probe. **A** Hypoechoic, 2.4 mm thick nodule with irregular margins and dermic invasion. **B** Pathologic specimen.

more frequent in the case of thin lesions, whereas the error rate is significantly lower for Clark's level IV melanomas or for lesions more than 3 mm thick, according to Breslow's classification. Errors are related to a variety of factors; paradoxically some of them have greater impact when higher frequency probes are used. With 13–20 MHz transducers a larger number of anatomic structures (e.g. hair follicles, sweat glands) can be visualized close to the tumor and may be misinterpreted as part of the lesion itself, thus overestimating the tumor stage. Overestimation can also be related to the presence of perilesional inflammatory infiltration: sonographic measurement of tumor thickness will include the inflammatory area as well, because of its tumor-like echo structure (Fig. 13.8). In Clark's level II–III melanomas, it is sometimes possible to detect inflammatory supratumoral infiltration, also producing overestimation of the stage of the lesion. Such errors are less frequent in the evaluation of advanced stage melanomas, when peritumoral infiltration is generally less important.

The causes of sonographic underestimation of melanoma stages are not very clear. Inaccurate setting of the US equipment gain can lead to defective measurements in ulcerative melanomas. Further causes may be incorrect pressure of the transducer on the skin or the presence of tumor islands which escape sonographic scanning.

In order to obtain better contrast resolution between the melanoma and surrounding tissues it is advisable gently to stretch the skin surrounding the lesion, which, particularly if it is affected by elastosis, will show an increased echo response whilst the echo structure of the neoplasm remains unchanged.

More recently, color Doppler sonography has been employed to increase the informative potential of the examination, enabling the identification of major blood flow signals in melanomas compared to normal skin (Fig. 13.9).

The sensitivity of US in detecting regional metastatic lymph nodes and distant metastases in patients with melanoma is well established. The sonographic patterns of metastatic nodes in melanoma do not differ from the characteristics described in Chapter 14 for all neoplastic superficial lymph nodes.

In the follow-up of patients who have undergone surgery for melanoma (or any other skin malignancy) sonography affords accurate study of recurrences, scarring and inflammatory sequelae.

PSORIASIS

Psorias is an erythematous scaly dermatosis of unknown etiology; there is genetic predisposition. It is characterized by a chronic course, with frequent exacerbations occurring at variable time intervals. Psorias affects 1–2% of the population, and onset can occur at any age.

The basic lesion is an erythematous scaly patch of varying shape and dimensions (punctate, lenticular, nummular and plaque lesions) with sharp edges and a color varying from bright red to pale pink, partially hidden by scales. The scales appear dry and stratified, and are easily removable; their color varies from whitish to silver. Size and thickness are variable; they may be small and thin with a pityriasic appearance, or large and thick. The number of patches is also highly variable: lesions may be single or, more commonly, multiple, but the disease may involve the whole tegument (universal psoriasis).

Common sites of onset are the extensor surfaces of the extremities (elbows, knees), the scalp, the lumbosacral and periumbilical regions, but any cutaneous zone may be affected.

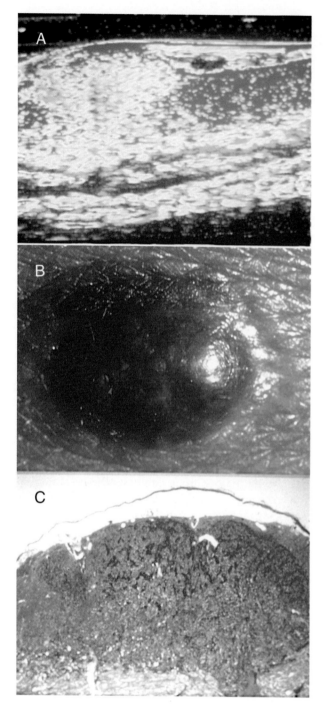

Fig. 13.6 Clark's level IV melanoma. **A** 20 MHz scan showing an oval hypoechoic mass (arrow), 4 mm thick, localized in the dermis, with poor deep demarcation. **B** Physical examination: nodular melanoma of the back. **C** Histopathologic features (×40). (Courtesy of G Borroni, MD, Institute of Dermatology, University of Pavia, Italy.)

Histologically, psoriasis is characterized by epidermal as well as dermal lesions: lamellar stratified hyperkeratosis associated with parakeratosis; lack of the granular layer; acanthosis with lengthened interpapillary crests; and Munro–Sabouraud's microabscesses consisting of sub-

corneal polymorphonuclear cells. Infiltrates mainly composed of mononuclear cells are present in the dermis. Papillae are edematous, and the capillaries are dilated and tortuous. Increased proliferative activity originates the psoriatic process, accompanied by anomalies in the differentiation process (keratinization), resulting in parakeratotic desquamation.

Trials of the therapeutic effectiveness of antipsoriatic drugs have always been based mostly on clinical observations and therefore are highly subjective. This kind of evaluation, even when carefully standardized, does not allow for reproducible data or, in particular, for comparison of data from different centers.

Histologic evaluation, on the other hand, certainly yields data which are precise, objective, reproducible and comparable with those from different centers, but it is also minimally invasive and consequently not suitable for time-serial protocols. In the search for other non-invasive methods[24] several parameters for evaluation were considered: erythema (spectrophotometry in remission and colorimetry),[25,26] microcirculation (laser Doppler flowmetering,[27,28] mechanical properties of the skin (elastometry),[29] trans-epidermic evaporation of water (evaporimetry),[30] hydration (impedance and capacitance)[31,32] and, finally, thickness of the skin (A-mode US).[5,9]

The last approach is certainly more reliable and direct than the others; nowadays high-frequency B-mode sonography has replaced A-mode, fulfilling the need for precise quantification, repeatability and reproducibility.

Sonographically, the psoriatic plaque is characterized by a varying increase in the width of the entry echo. Under this echo a hypoechoic band related to inflammatory and vascular changes is detectable and is more evident in the acute stages. The dermis appears thicker and inhomogeneous and is not always clearly differentiable from the epidermis (Fig. 13.10A). Air retained under cutaneous scales may produce small parallel acoustic shadows. Using extremely high frequencies, richly keratinized plaques may show a marked absorption of the acoustic beam, making visualization of dermis and hypodermis impossible (Fig. 13.11).

If clinical improvement occurs, a typical sonographic finding is decrease in the thickness of the skin and, more particularly, of the subepidermal hypoechoic band, or even its disappearance (Fig. 13.10B). The dermis and the entry echo also return to their normal thickness, and posterior shadows due to air microbubbles on the surface disappear.

The subepidermal hypoechoic band is probably related to inflammatory infiltrate with vasodilation; the more active the disease, the more marked and evident is the band. Moreover, its modification in response to therapy correlates well with the clinical course. While normalization of skin thickness occurs immediately after the start of therapy, disappearance of the subepidermal hypoechoic band takes

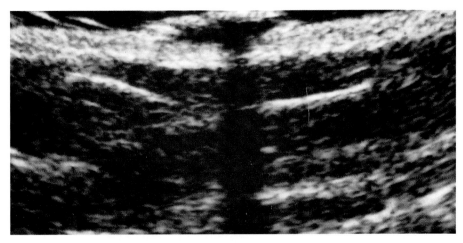

Fig. 13.7   Melanoma with a posterior shadow due to its warty form. 13 MHz scan.

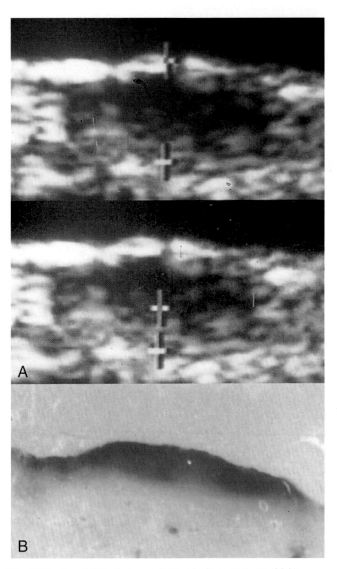

Fig. 13.8   **A** and **B** Posterior perilesional edema (0.8 mm thick) increasing the thickness of the melanoma (1.3 mm). Total thickness: 2.1 mm. **C** (*overleaf*) Pathologic specimen.

place in a more gradual and uniform way, according to clinical outcome.

OTHER PATHOLOGIC CONDITIONS OF THE SKIN

Sonographic differentiation of the various histologic types of skin tumors, either benign or malignant, is not at present feasible, even though strong correlations have been recently demonstrated for echogenicity versus spacing and size of collagen bundles and echogenicity versus cellularity.[33]

The bullous lesions of pemphigoid appear as subepidermal, oval anechoic lesions (Fig. 13.12) with well-defined posterior and lateral edges.

Purely epidermoid cysts of the skin contain only keratinized stratified epithelium; sonographically they appear as roundish, homogeneously solid nodules, with 'parenchymal-like' echogenicity and regular smooth borders (Fig. 13.13A). The keratinous debris completely filling their lumen is responsible for their fine homogeneous echo texture. This pattern is similar to the sonographic appearance of sebaceous cysts (Fig. 13.13B), even though the latter may exhibit a more inhomogeneous echo texture.

Hemangiomas of the skin and subcutaneous tissue generally develop in the dermis and subsequently may involve the epidermis. They usually appear as hypo- or anechoic lesions, but may contain hyperechoic septa (Fig. 13.14). Margins are always regular and well-defined, and sound transmission is mostly good, except in thrombosed angiomas which may cause posterior sound attenuation. The main indication for US is the assessment of the thickness and deep extension of subcutaneous and mucosal hemangiomas in order to define accurately the kind of treatment required.

Dermatofibromas usually display a parenchymal, homogeneous echo texture, with a medium to high level of echoes and clearly defined outlines (Fig. 13.15).[7,34]

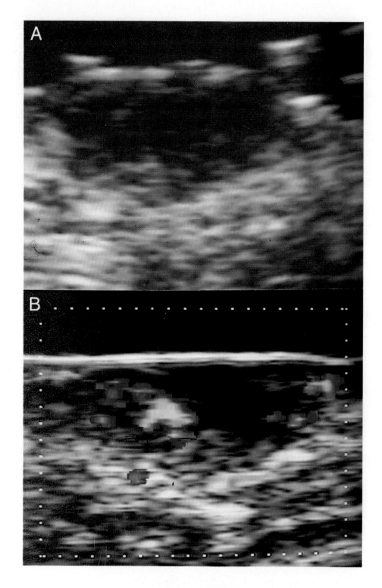

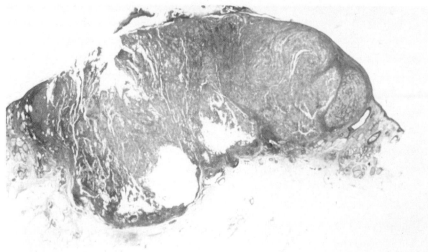

Fig. 13.9   3 mm thick melanoma of the cheek (**A**). The intense flow signals detected by color Doppler in the posterolateral portions of the lesion (**B**) correspond to the wide vascular lakes seen in the pathologic specimen (**C**).

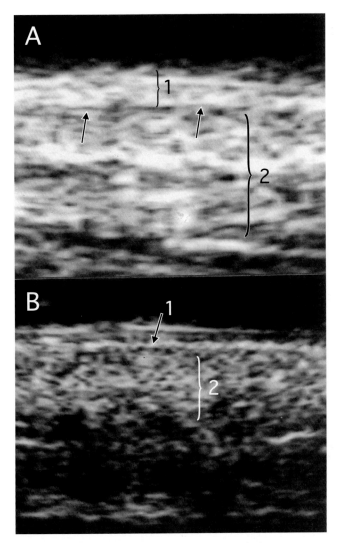

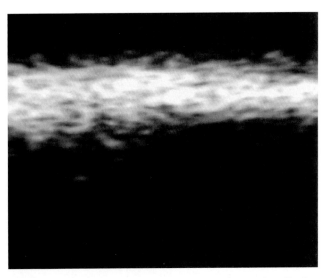

Fig. 13.11 Highly keratinized psoriatic plaque with complete distal attenuation of the ultrasound beam.

Fig. 13.10 Psoriatic patch of the elbow region: marked hyperechogenicity and thickening of epidermis (1) and dermis (2); note the presence of the subepidermal hypoechoic band (arrow). **B** Sonographic control after calcipotriolium therapy: the thicknesses of the epidermis (1) and dermis (2) are greatly reduced and the subepidermal band has disappeared.

Nevus cell nevi are roundish nodules with low-level, inhomogeneously distributed internal echoes and sharp demarcation (Fig. 13.16); benign nevi, dysplastic nevi and melanomas are not distinguishable on the basis of the sonographic appearance. Pigmented nevi can cast acoustic shadows.

The sonographic findings in cutaneous fibrolipomas are described in Chapter 7, whereas the rare subcutaneous pure lipomas may occasionally show a homogeneously hypoechoic pattern (Fig. 13.17).

Histiocytomas (Fig. 13.18) and cutaneous lymphomas may exhibit a wide variety of echo patterns, from low to high levels of echoes, and from homogeneous to mixed echo texture. With currently available high-sensibility color Doppler equipment, intense flow signals may be detected in histiocytomas. Diffuse cutaneous lymphomas may present as hyperechoic, ill-defined areas, with thickening of the dermis and hypodermis; nodular lymphomas, on the contrary, appear predominantly as hypoechoic, inhomogeneous nodules with irregular outlines.

Unlike other skin malignancies, basal cell carcinomas (hypoechoic, homogeneous lesions) usually display smooth borders, the typical hypoechoic projections of most malignancies (Fig. 13.19) being extremely rare in this condition. US can be helpful in measuring the tumor volume, mainly in the sclerodermic forms, but, as in melanomas, the often coexisting basal inflammatory infiltrate may be difficult to differentiate from neoplastic tissue.

Kaposi's sarcoma, often associated with AIDS and with a multicentric presentation, does not have a peculiar echo pattern; it is hypoechoic, with occasional high level echoes, poor lateral demarcation, and well-defined posterior margins. The main purpose of US is precise size assessment before treatment, laser therapy being possible only if the upper dermis is not infiltrated. When interferon therapy is given, US can be used to monitor change in lesion size.

Finally, modern high-frequency sonography can be employed for the accurate evaluation of other cutaneous pathologies, such as fistulas in neonates (Fig. 13.20), foreign body granulomas (Fig. 13.21), serous or inflammatory fluid collections in subcutaneous spaces (Fig. 13.22) and also inflammatory complications of peritoneal catheters in uremic patients (Fig. 13.23).

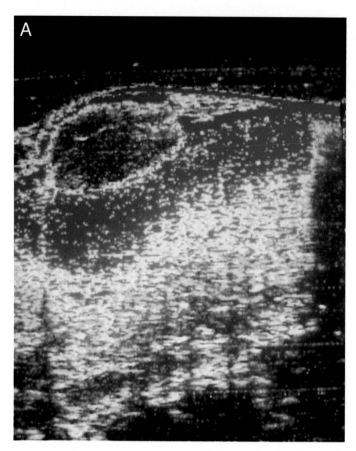

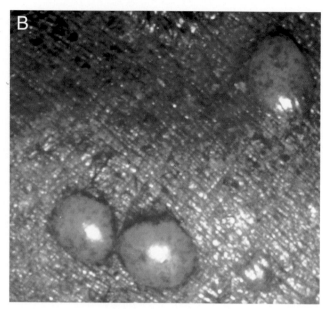

Fig. 13.12 20 MHz scan featuring a subepidermal, oval, anechoic nodule (arrow) corresponding to a subepidermal bulla of pemphigoid (**B**). (Courtesy of G Borroni, MD, Institute of Dermatology, University of Pavia, Italy.)

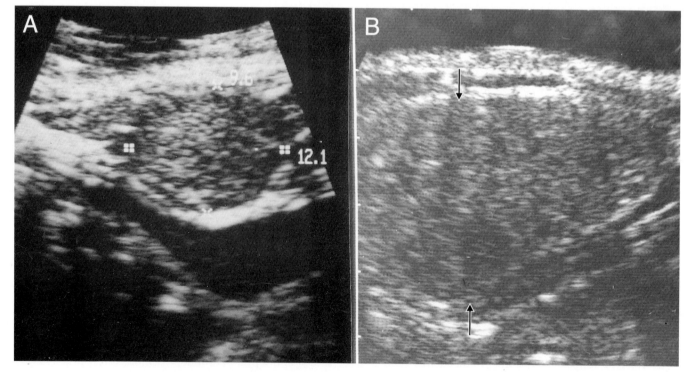

Fig. 13.13 **A** Epidermoid cyst of the neck in the midline region. **B** Sebaceous cyst (arrow), slightly more inhomogeneous than the lesion in **A**.

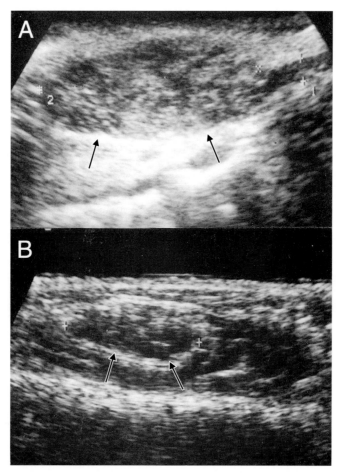

Fig. 13.14 **A** Cutaneous hemangioma (arrow). **B** Hemangioma in an intramuscular location (arrow).

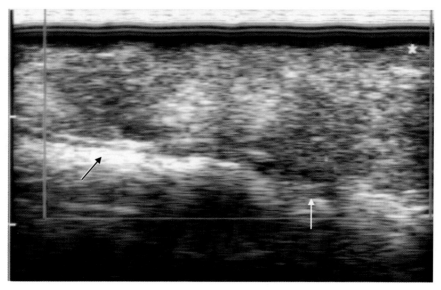

Fig. 13.15 Dermatofibroma (arrow) with a medium to high level of echoes.

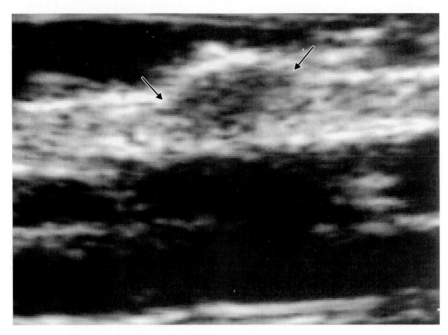

Fig. 13.16   Small (3 mm) nevus (arrow) of the thoracic skin.

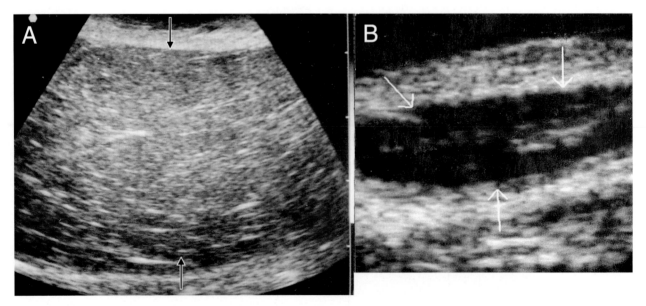

Fig. 13.17   Typical superficial fibrolipoma (arrow). **B** Fat deposit in subcutaneous tissue, markedly hypoechoic (arrows).

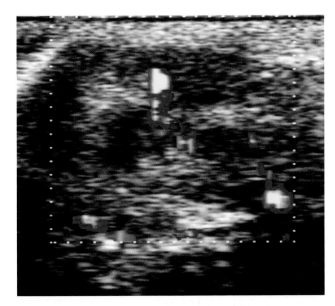

Fig. 13.18   A 15 mm histiocytoma with hypervascularity.

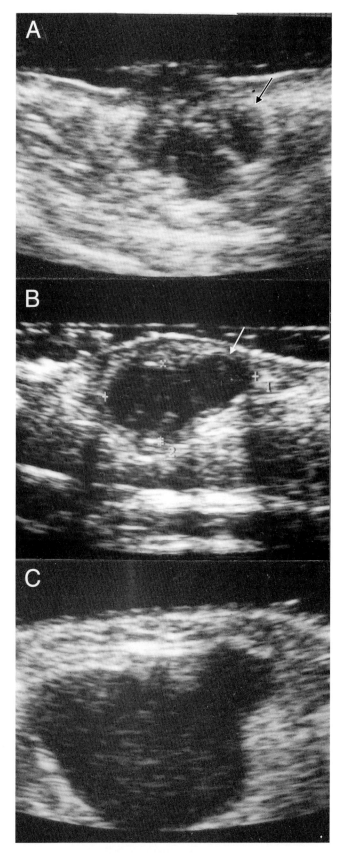

Fig. 13.19   Three markedly hypoechoic nodules with irregular margins: Merkel's neuroendocrine tumor (**A**), squamous cell carcinoma (**B**) and cutaneous metastasis from adenocarcinoma (**C**).

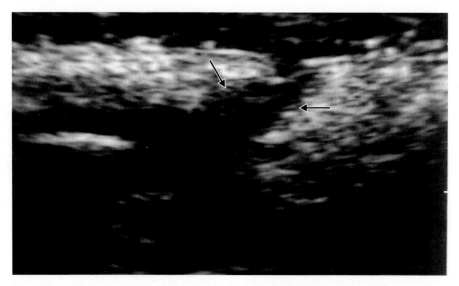

Fig. 13.20 A 2 mm cutaneous fistula (arrow) in the coccygeal region in a neonate.

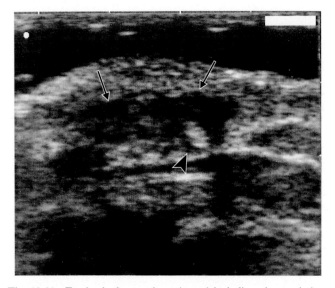

Fig. 13.21 Foreign body granuloma (arrow) including a hyperechoic core (arrowhead) consisting of the foreign body.

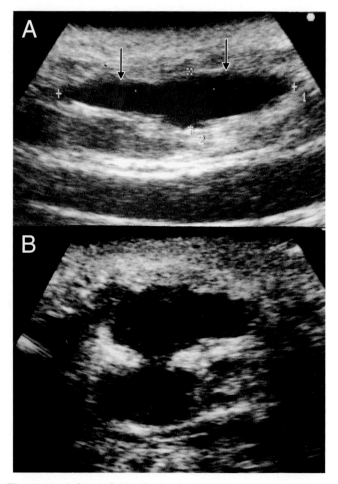

Fig. 13.22 **A** Serous fluid collection in the subcutaneous tissue (arrow) following trauma. **B** Biloculated abscess of the subcutaneous spaces.

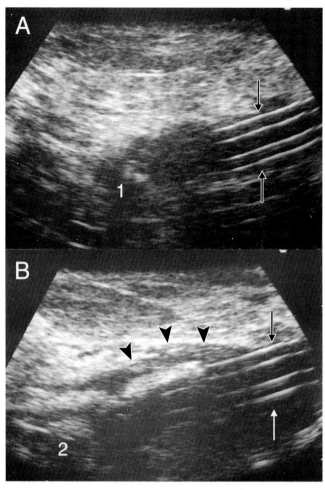

Fig. 13.23 15 MHz sonographic studies of peritoneal catheters in uremic patients (arrow) **A** Normal pattern. **B** Inflammatory changes (arrowhead) at the internal catheter cuff, close to the peritoneum (1).

REFERENCES

1. Daly C H, Wheeler J B 1971 The use of ultrasonic thickness measurement in the clinical evaluation of the oral soft tissues. Int Dent J 21: 418–429
2. Rukavina B, Mohar N 1979 An approach of ultrasound diagnostic techniques of the skin and subcutaneous tissue. Dermatologica 158: 81–92
3. Alexander H, Miller D L 1979 Determining skin thickness with pulsed ultrasound. J Invest Dermatol 72: 17–19
4. Shafir R, Itzchak Y, Heyman Z 1984 Preoperative ultrasonic measurements of thickness of cutaneous malignant melanoma. J Ultrasound Med 3: 205–208
5. Sondergaard J, Serup J, Tikjob G 1985 Ultrasonic A- and B-scanning in clinical and experimental dermatology. Acta Derm Venereol (Stockh) 120 (suppl): pp 76–82
6. Fornage B D, Deshayes J L 1986 Ultrasound of normal skin. JCU 14: 619–622
7. Fornage B D, McGavran M H, Duvic M 1993 Imaging of the skin with 20 MHz US. Radiology 189: 69–76
8. Miyauchi S A, Miki Y 1983 Normal human skin echogram. Arch Dermatol Res 275: 345–349
9. Serup J 1984 Non invasive quantification of psoriasis plaques: measurement of skin thickness with 15 MHz pulsed ultrasound. Clin Exp Dermatol 9: 502–508
10. Serup J 1990 Ultrasound patterns of the papillary dermis. 8th Int Symp on Bioengineering and the Skin, Stresa, Italy, p 31
11. Seidenari S, Di Nardo A, Giannetti A 1990 L'indagine ultrasonografica in dermatologia. G Ital Dermatol Venereol 125: 295–300
12. Bossi Fusco M C, Cammarota T 1993 Cute e sottocute. In: SIUMB (ed) Trattato italiano di ecografia. Poletto Edizione, Milan, vol II, pp 593–605
13. De Rigal J, Escoffier C, Pharm M et al 1989 Assessment of aging of the human skin by in vivo ultrasonic imaging. J Invest Dermatol 93: 621–625
14. Balch C M, Soong S J, Milton G W 1983 Changing trends in cutaneous melanoma over a quarter century in Alabama USA and New South Wales, Australia. Cancer 52: 1748–1753
15. De Vita V T, Hellman S, Rosenberg S A 1989 Cancer principles and practice of oncology, 3rd edn. Lippincott, Philadelphia
16. Breslow A 1970 Thickness, cross sectional areas and depth of invasion in the prognosis of cutaneous melanoma. Ann Surg 172: 902–908
17. Day C L, Lew R A, Mihm M O 1981 The natural breakpoints for primary tumor thickness in clinical stage I melanoma. N Engl J Med 305: 1155–1159
18. Bagley F H, Cady B, Lee A 1981 Changes in clinical presentation and management of malignant melanoma. Cancer 47: 2126–2131
19. Hoffmann K, Jung J, El Gammal S, Altmeyer P 1992 Malignant melanoma in 20 MHz B scan sonography. Dermatology 185: 49–55

20. Nessi R, Betti R, Bencini P L 1990 Ultrasonography of nodular and infiltrative lesions of the skin and subcutaneous tissues. JCU 18: 103–109

21. Hughes B R, Black D, Srivastava A 1987 Comparison of techniques for the non-invasive assessment of skin tumors. Clin Exp Dermat 12: 108–111

22. Reali U M, Santucci M, Paoli G 1989 The use of high resolution ultrasound in preoperative evaluation of cutaneous malignant melanoma thickness. Tumori 75: 452–455

23. Murakami S, Miki Y 1989 Human skin histology using high-resolution echography. JCU 17: 77–82

24. Di Nardo A, Seidenari S, Giannetti A 1991 Valutazione ecografica della risposta al trattamento con ditranolo della psoriasi in placche. G Ital Dermatol Venereol 126: 611–617

25. Ryatt K S, Feather J W, Dawson J B 1983 The usefulness of reflectance spectrophotometric measurements during psoralens and ultraviolet therapy for psoriasis. J Am Acad Dermatol 9: 558–562

26. Broby J V 1990 Ranking of the antipsoriatic effect of various topical corticosteroids applied under a hydrocolloid dressing. Skin-thickness, blood-flow and colour measurements compared to clinical assessment. Clin Exp Dermatol 15: 343–348

27. Klemp P, Staberg B 1983 Cutaneous blood flow in psoriasis. J Invest Dermatol 81: 503–506

28. Khan A, Schall L M, Tur E 1987 Blood flow in psoriatic skin lesions: the effect of treatment. Br J Dermatol 193–201

29. Serup J, Northeved A 1985 Skin elasticity in psoriasis. In vivo measurement of tensile distensibility, hysteresis and resilient distension with a new method. Comparison with skin thickness as measured with high frequency ultrasound. J Dermatol 12: 318–324

30. Frodin T, Skogh M, Molin L 1988 The importance of the coal tar bath in the Ingram treatment of psoriasis. Evaluation by evaporimetry and laser Doppler flowmetry. Br J Dermatol 118: 429–434

31. Clar E J, Cambrai M, Heid E 1976 Le parametres electrophysiologiques dans le psoriasis. Ann Dermatol Syphiligr 83: 291–295

32. Tagami H, Yoshikuni K 1985 Interrelationship between water barrier and reservoir function of pathologic stratum corneum. Arch Dermatol 121: 642–645

33. Harland C C, Bamber J C, Gusterson B A, Mortimer P S 1993 High frequency, high resolution B-scan ultrasound in the assessment of skin tumours. Br J Dermatol 128: 525–532

34. Gropper C A, Stiller M J, Shupack J L, Driller J, Rorke M, Lizzi F 1993 Diagnostic high-resolution in dermatology. Int J Dermatol 32: 243–250

14

Lymph nodes

J. N. Bruneton   *L. Rubaltelli*   *L. Solbiati*

Palpation has always been the mainstay in the diagnostic work-up of the neck, the axilla and the inguinal region. Since most lymph nodes are located superficially, enlarged nodes may be easily identified. However, small nodes may escape attention, even when palpation is performed by an experienced oncologist. Moreover, when large lymph nodes are present, clinical examination is insufficient to determine nodal size, extracapsular growth and vascular connections. In some cases, other structures may be incorrectly identified as lymph nodes clinically, and a more accurate test is needed.

Several exploratory techniques, including lymphography and lymphoscintigraphy, have been proposed to reduce the false negative rate.[1,2] Likewise, carotid angiography has been suggested as a means of investigating venous return. In practice CT and MRI provide the solution to both problems: in addition to their capacity to investigate the tumor itself, CT and MRI can detect lymph nodes and their vascular connections with a high sensitivity.

Since 1984, the use of ultrasonography has been proposed in the search for lymph node diseases in the neck, breast and inguinal regions.[3-9]

ANATOMIC DATA AND EXAMINATION TECHNIQUE

Neck

Anatomic data

The lymph nodes of the head and neck regions lie between the deep cervical fascia and the prevertebral fascia. Rouviere classed them into 10 main groups, which can be divided into three main chains: the pericervical collar, the deep cervical nodes, and the accessory chains.

The pericervical collar consists of nodal groups located at the junction of the head with the neck. These groups include:

- the occipital nodes (draining the regions of the nape and scalp)
- the retroauricular (mastoid) nodes (parietal scalp, part of the auricle of the ear, and external auditory canal)
- the parotid nodes (parotid gland, middle and external ear, and part of the face and scalp)
- the submandibular nodes including preglandular and retroglandular nodes (located at the anterior and posterior poles of the gland), prevascular nodes (the most constant group, which runs along the facial artery), and intracapsular nodes (lips, cheeks, upper and lower gums, tongue, soft palate, and floor of the mouth)
- the submental nodes (chin, part of the lower lip, floor of the mouth, and tip of the tongue).

Most of the nodes of the pericervical collar drain into the internal jugular chain; only the occipital lymph nodes drain into the spinal accessory chain.

According to Rouviere, **the deep cervical lymph nodes** include three different chains:

- The internal jugular chain, subdivided into anterior and lateral groups. The anterior nodes lie in front of the internal jugular vein, predominantly in the upper neck, between the digastric muscle and the omohyoid muscle. Three divisions can be distinguished: a superior subdigastric group, often limited to a single large node (principal node of Kuttner, or jugulodigastric node) (Fig. 14.1), which is the most frequent relay of upper respiratory and digestive tract cancers, a middle division (midjugular nodes) lying anterior to the thyro-linguofacial venous trunk, and an inferior division (low jugular nodes) located in the supraomohyoid region.

The lateral group consists of smaller nodes. The internal jugular chain receives lymph either directly from the tissues or indirectly, after passage through outlying nodes, from the nasal fossa, tonsils, tongue, hard palate, thyroid gland, ear, submandibular gland, and sublingual glands.

- The spinal accessory chain consists of 8–10 nodes; it lies obliquely along the general course of the spinal accessory nerve, and is divided into two groups: the upper group blends with the superior internal jugular vein nodes while the lower group becomes continuous with the transverse cervical chain.
- The transverse cervical chain (supraclavicular chain) also follows an oblique course, behind the clavicle. The transverse nodes prolong the lower end of the spinal accessory chain up to the thoracic duct on the left and the lymphatic duct on the right. This chain comprises 8–10 nodes; the most medial on the left is connected to the subdiaphragmatic lymph pathways by the thoracic duct.

The accessory chains include both superficial chains and deep juxtavisceral chains:

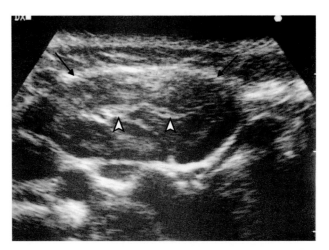

Fig. 14.1 Large (2.7 × 1 cm), non-pathologic jugulodigastric (Kuttner) lymph node (arrow) with oval shape and hyperechoic central hilum (arrowhead).

- The superficial chains are satellites of the anterior jugular vein and the external jugular vein.
- The deep juxtavisceral chains are scarcely accessible either on physical examination or on ultrasonography. They include the lateral retropharyngeal nodes, one or two prelaryngeal (cricothyroid) nodes, the pretracheal nodes, and the nodes of the recurrent chain (Fig. 14.2). The latter mostly drain the thyroid region.

Examination technique

US examination is performed with 7.5–13 MHz probes, either linear-array or sector mechanical; very superficial nodes are better assessed with the interposition of thin layers of gel mattress or with higher frequency transducers (15–20 MHz) (Fig. 14.3).

The superficial cervical nodes are examined after determination of the positions of the common carotid artery and the internal jugular vein. Transverse scans between these two important landmarks, starting from the lower neck, allow accurate evaluation of the relationship of a nodal mass to the carotid artery or internal jugular vein at any point. US can generally visualize the jugular chain nodes lying anterior to the carotid artery and the internal jugular vein (Fig. 14.4) and the spinal chain nodes posterior to these two landmarks. Despite their limited diagnostic value, sagittal scans are useful from an iconographic standpoint.

US detection of the recurrent nodes, lying deeply and caudally to the lower pole of the thyroid gland, is often possible only on dynamic scans during swallowing: the cranial displacement of the thyroid gland permits the exploration of deep neck spaces (see Fig. 14.2).

Reporting sonographic data

In agreement with surgeons and histopathologists, it is practical to divide the lateral neck into eight different zones. As it is easier to localize vessels, and particularly the carotid bifurcation, than cervical muscles, nodes anterior to the major neurovascular bundle (common carotid artery, deep jugular vein, vagus nerve) can be termed jugular nodes, while nodes lying behind this bundle can be considered spinal nodes. Using height in the neck as a criterion, nodes situated at the level of the carotid bifurcation or above can be termed superior nodes, those lying 3 cm below the carotid bifurcation can be considered middle jugular or spinal nodes, and those located between the clavicle and the middle region can be referred to as inferior nodes.[3] Along with a written report on the sonographic findings, the sonographer should indicate the exact site and maximum diameter of any abnormal nodes detected by US on a surgical map (Fig. 14.5).

Axilla

Anatomic data

The axilla is a pyramidal space between the arm and the chest wall. Its base, formed by the axillary fascia, extends

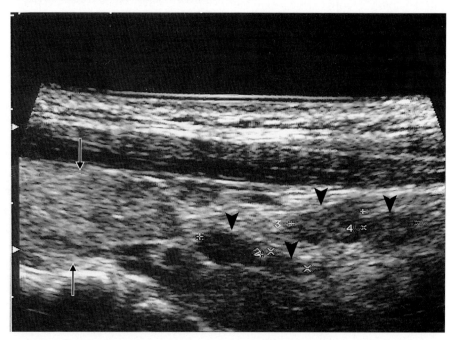

Fig. 14.2 Sagittal scan of the lower neck. Four small metastatic nodes from medullary thyroid cancer (arrowhead) are shown caudal to the lower pole of the thyroid lobe (arrow) along the recurrent nodal chain.

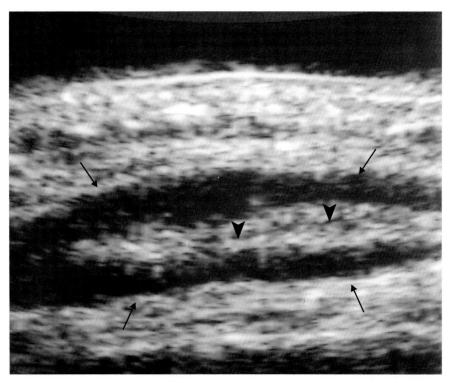

Fig. 14.3 Normal, elongated (L:S ratio = 5) subcutaneous lymph node (arrow) of the inguinal region, detected with a 20 MHz mechanical sector transducer. The wide hyperechoic hilum contains thin hypoechoic bands (arrowhead) consisting of blood vessels.

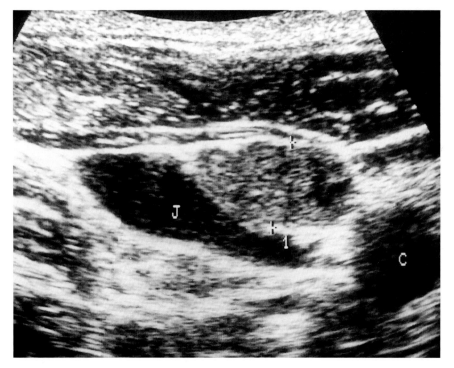

Fig. 14.4 Metastatic, 12 mm thick lymph node (+) of the jugular chain, lying anterior to the common carotid artery (C) and internal jugular vein (J).

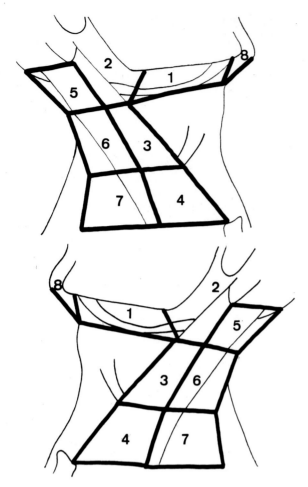

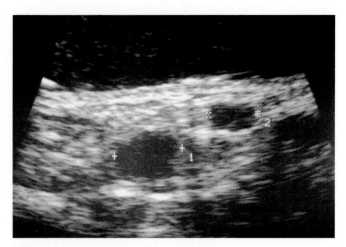

Fig. 14.6   Two small metastatic nodes (+) of the axilla from breast cancer. The nodes are located between the subcutaneous tissue and the smaller pectoral muscle (first level).

Fig. 14.5   Schematic map used to indicate the exact location of abnormal nodes detected with US.

between the inferolateral margins of the pectoralis major and latissimus dorsi muscles. Its apex is the interval between the posterior border of the clavicle, the superior border of the scapula, and the external border of the first rib. The anterior wall of the axilla is formed by the pectoralis major and minor. The axilla contains the axillary artery and vein, several nerves, and the axillary lymph nodes.

The axillary nodes act as a series of filters between the breast and the venous circulation. Carcinoma cells that enter a lymphatic vessel usually have to pass through two or three groups of nodes before reaching the venous circulation.

Examination technique

US examination is performed in real time with a 7.5–13 MHz transducer, selected according to the thickness of the pectoral wall of each patient.[3] Adenopathies are searched for essentially on transverse scans, following the axillary vessels and then the subclavicular vessels using a

transpectoral approach. Nodes are searched for in front of the greater pectoral muscle; the smaller pectoral muscle is used to delineate the different levels (first level, outside the smaller pectoral muscle – Fig. 14.6; second level, behind the smaller pectoral muscle; third level, within the pectoral muscle).

Internal mammary region

Anatomic data

The internal mammary artery passes downward through the thorax, behind the upper six costal cartilages and the intervening internal intercostal muscles, just lateral to the sternum. It is accompanied by two venae comitantes and by lymphatic vessels.

Collecting vessels from the central and medial parts of the breast follow the perforating blood vessels through the pectoralis major and end in the parasternal (internal thoracic) nodes behind the internal intercostal muscles and in front of the endothoracic fascia. These nodes, commonly only 1 or 2 mm in diameter, are about three to five in number on each side. Lymphatic routes across the median plane, either in the skin or in the pectoral fascia, are sometimes present.

Examination technique

Once the median line is noted, a bilateral US study is performed through the intercostal spaces, from the first to the fifth interspace. The following parameters are investigated: depth of the anterior wall of the internal mammary artery and position of the inner border of the internal mammary artery with respect to the median line. All these data are useful prior to radiotherapy of the internal mammary chain for the treatment of breast cancer.[10]

Inguinal region

Anatomic data

The uppermost parts of the femoral artery and vein lie behind the inguinal ligament in the vascular compartment situated in the groove between the iliopsoas and the pectineus muscles.

The femoral triangle is located in the upper third of the front of the thigh. It contains femoral vessels, nerves and lymph nodes and is bounded laterally by the medial border of the sartorius muscle, medially by the medial border of the adductor longus, and superiorly by the inguinal ligament.

Examination technique

It is possible to explore an area of about 10 cm, with the probe held perpendicular to the femoral vessels.

Fine-needle aspiration biopsy (FNAB) under US guidance

Conventional FNAB of superficial, palpable nodal masses has been used for more than 30 years and provides an alternative to surgery. The percentage of unsatisfactory aspirates does not exceed 14%.

When small, non-palpable nodes are detected with US, aspiration under ultrasound guidance is required and may be accurately performed with 10–13 MHz small-parts transducers with lateral adaptors for needle placement (Fig. 14.7).

This diagnostic procedure is useful in the clinical management of patients, having a high sensitivity and a high specificity.[6,11–13] There are no major complications related to aspiration.

Some specific difficulties relate to cytopathology: keratinizing cancers are readily identifiable, whereas non-keratin-forming cancers are more difficult to diagnose. Another pitfall is the smear showing necrosis only (resulting from inflammatory or neoplastic disorders). Finally, immunocytologic techniques are required to differentiate lymphoma from metastases of poorly differentiated carcinoma.

OTHER IMAGING TECHNIQUES

CT

Contrast-enhanced CT is of unquestionable value for cervical node exploration as it can determine both the number and position of enlarged nodes and their relations to neck vessels. With CT, extracapsular nodal spread is diagnosed when enhancement of the nodal capsule and poorly defined nodal margins (without prior surgery or radiotherapy) are detected.

CT criteria for assessing nodal metastases include nodal size and shape, and the presence of central necrosis and

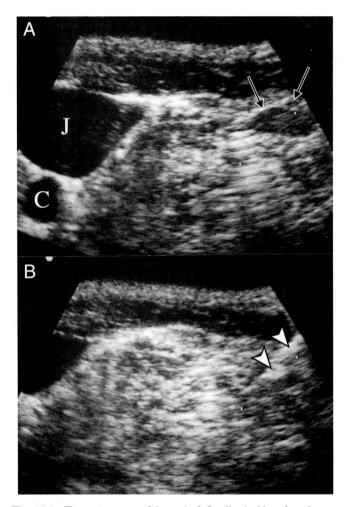

Fig. 14.7 Transverse scans of the neck. **A** Small spinal lymph node (arrow) in a patient with squamous cell carcinoma. **B** In order to assess its nature, US-guided FNAB is performed with a 13 MHz sector mechanical probe with lateral biopsy adaptor. The needle tip (arrowhead) is clearly visualized into the target. C: carotid artery; J: internal jugular vein.

of multiple localized nodes. On CT scans the generally accepted upper limit of normal lymph node diameter is 1 cm, except in the case of the jugulodigastric and submandibular nodes (1.5 cm).[14,15]

CT cannot differentiate between inflammatory and tumoral nodes and, in addition, is unable to demonstrate extracapsular extension of small nodes. By contrast, compared with US, CT allows more thorough topographic investigation of ENT tumors and nodal metastases, particularly of large masses (Fig. 14.8) and the exploration of anatomic sites inaccessible to US (retropharyngeal space, upper mediastinum) (Fig. 14.9).[16,17] CT is also indicated for the detection of the subclinical lymphomatous lesions frequently found in Waldeyer's ring. According to March et al,[18] considering axillary lymph nodes measuring greater than or equal to 1 cm to be abnormal, CT has a sensitivity of 50% and a specificity of 75%.

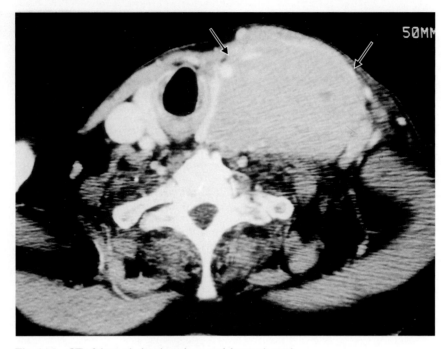

Fig. 14.8 CT of the neck showing a large nodal mass (arrow).

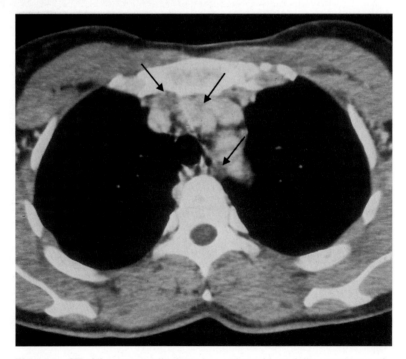

Fig. 14.9 CT of the upper mediastinum in a patient with medullary carcinoma of the thyroid gland. Several metastatic nodes (arrows) are detectable behind the sternum.

MRI

Enlarged cervical lymph nodes can be identified on various MRI sequences. The fat which surrounds the lymph nodes and helps their identification by CT decreases their detectability on MRI. Differential diagnosis between hyperplastic and metastatic lymph nodes is not easy: most hyperplastic nodes have a homogeneous low signal intensity on T_1-weighted images and a high signal intensity on T_2-weighted images, but this same pattern is found in non-necrotic metastatic nodes.[19]

The same size and shape criteria used for CT are applied to the MRI evaluation of cervical lymph nodes.[14,20]

Using MRI contrast media, as on CT scans, nodes with necrotic changes show a central region of lower signal intensity and a periphery with enhancing higher signal on T_1-weighted images. However, according to Yousem et al,[21] CT actually seems to be more sensitive than MRI for the detection of central nodal necrosis and extracapsular nodal spread.

Lymphomatous lymph nodes are hypointense to fat and slightly hyperintense to muscle in T_1-weighted images but isointense to fat and hyperintense to muscle in T_2-weighted images.[22]

SONOGRAPHIC PATTERNS OF LYMPH NODES AND PATHOLOGIC CORRELATIONS

In 1984, we claimed that normal lymph nodes were not visualizable sonographically and that even large lipomatous nodes were not visible with US because their fatty component was indistinguishable from the subcutaneous tissue.[5] Since this report, various authors have described the echostructural–pathologic correlations of superficial nodes, both in vitro and in vivo, especially with the development of very high-frequency transducers (10–13 MHz) capable of visualizing fine structural details.[6–8,23–30]

The assessment of the structural patterns of superficial lymph nodes is extremely important, considering the high rate of detection of lymph nodes in the neck, axilla and inguinal regions. In a recent study[31] one or more normal cervical lymph nodes (weakly echoic oval structures with an echoic central hilum) were detected in 67.6% of 1000 healthy volunteers. This occurrence was not related to recent ENT infections, sex or age.

Six parameters have to be evaluated in the assessment of the benign or malignant nature of superficial lymph nodes:

- shape (rounded or oval)
- presence/absence and thickness of nodal hilum
- thickness of nodal cortex
- structural patterns of the cortex
- blood flow patterns (with color Doppler)
- presence/absence of extracapsular nodal spread.

The parameter of minimal transverse diameter seems to have limited value, even though, according to Van Den Breckel et al,[9] nodes of 8 mm minimal diameter in the digastric area and of at least 7 mm in other areas of the neck should be considered malignant when ENT cancer is suspected. As for lymphomatous nodes, no anatomic correlations have ever been published in the literature; 10 mm seems to be the minimal transverse diameter suggesting multiple enlarged nodes indicative of lymphoma and requiring cytologic assessment.

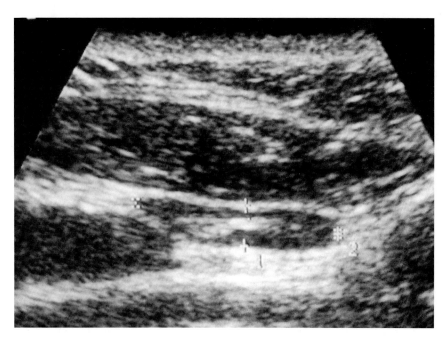

Fig. 14.10 Typical normal lymph node (+) with L:S (or Solbiati ratio) of 4.5 and a wide hyperechoic hilum.

The six parameters mentioned above should be considered separately and correlated with the histologic patterns.

Normal lymph nodes are formed by an outer cortex with lymphoid follicles and an inner medulla with lymphatic sinuses, connective tissue and blood vessels. Reactive (or hyperplastic) nodes, usually the sequelae of inflammatory processes and sonographically indistinguishable from normal nodes, increase in size because of enlargement of both lymphoid follicles and sinusoids, with the possible development of hilar lymphoid germinal centers.[28] Most inflammatory diseases (except for granulomatous infections, like tuberculosis)[30] involve lymph nodes diffusely and homogeneously, generally preserving their oval shape. Malignant involvement (metastatic or lymphomatous),

however, occurs primarily in the cortex, mostly with a multifocal arrangement, resulting in rounded, asymmetric morphology of the nodes.

These morphologic data are sonographically represented by the long:short (L:S) axis ratio (longitudinal:transverse diameter ratio, Solbiati ratio, or roundness index) which can be obtained on long-axis scans of the lymph nodes, measuring the largest and smallest diameter.[7,8,24,26–29,31] Sonography is the only imaging technique enabling easy assessment of nodal diameters in all directions. If the threshold value of the L:S ratio employed is low (1.5)[24] the accuracy of US in differentiating normal/reactive nodes (oval shape) (Figs 14.3, 14.10) from pathologic nodes (rounded shape) (Fig. 14.4) is relatively low (sensitivity 71%, specificity 65%). If the ratio used is 2.0, sensitivity increases to 81–95% and specificity to 67–96%.[7,8,26–29]

The second parameter to be assessed is the hyperechoic central line of lymph nodes (the hilum). With sonographic-pathologic related studies[23,25,26,28] the hilum has been defi-

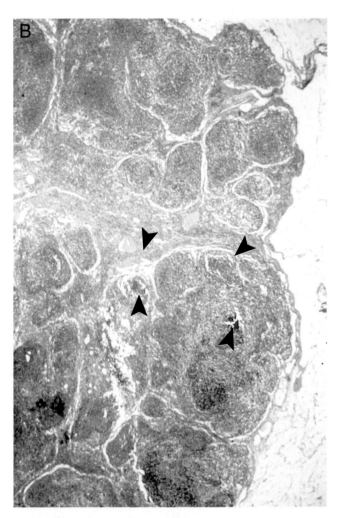

Fig. 14.11 **A** In vitro sonographic scan of normal lymph node with a thin hyperechoic hilum (arrowhead) (top). The gross specimen (bottom) confirms the oval shape and the regular margins. **B** The histologic examination demonstrates that the sonographic hyperechoic hilum corresponds to the lymphatic sinuses converging on the medulla together with connective tissue (arrowhead).

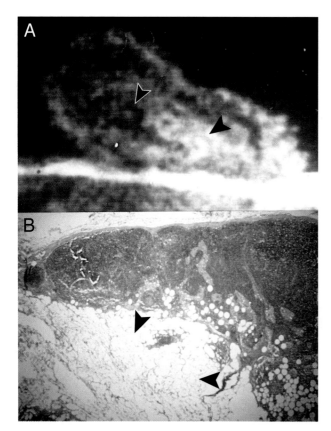

Fig. 14.12 **A** In vitro scan of a normal lymph node with a markedly thickened hyperechoic hilum (arrowhead) which is histologically shown (**B**) to be due to massive fatty infiltration (arrowhead).

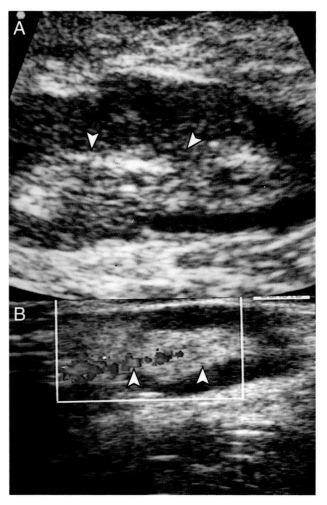

Fig. 14.13 Two large, normal lymph nodes of the inguinal region with thickened hila (arrowheads) owing to abundant fat deposition. In (**B**) the vascular hilum of the node is clearly shown by color Doppler.

nitely demonstrated to correspond to the dense network (with lots of sonographic interfaces) of lymphatic sinuses converging on the internal part of the medulla and supported by loose connective tissue (Fig. 14.11). Fatty infiltration does not seem to play a role in the formation of the hyperechoic hilum when it is of normal thickness, compared with the whole thickness of the lymph node.[29] However, principally in in vitro studies, when fatty changes are abundant they can make the central echogenic line much thicker[25] (Fig. 14.12).

In contrast, the main cause of in vivo 'thickened hilum' could be the increasing number of lymphatic sinuses and vessels, which proliferate as a consequence of chronic inflammatory stimuli.[29] In benign lymph nodes in the inguinal and pelvic region fat deposition is frequent, with development of a broad, echogenic medulla[23] (Fig. 14.13).

The sonographic detection of the hyperechoic hilum has always been related to probable benign nature of the lymph node, since infiltration of the nodal cortex, inflammatory

active diseases and malignancies cause progressive thinning of the hilum ('slit-like hilum'), which is often also eccentric[28] (Fig. 14.14) and finally its complete disappearance (Fig. 14.15). In fact, in reports in the literature 85–90% of lymph nodes with a wide, elliptical hilum, conforming with the shape of the lymph node, turned out to be benign at pathologic examination, whereas slit-like hilum and absence of hilum were detected respectively in 67% and 76–92% of malignant nodes.[8,25,28,29] Only in the group of cases studied by Evans et al[23] was the echogenic hilum present in as many as 58% of pathologically malignant nodes. Since in this study group most of the nodes were of small size, the possible explanation of this discrepancy could be that 'in early malignancies the converging sinuses within the medulla have not been sufficiently disrupted to eradicate the hilus sign'.[23]

In a few cases the presence of diffuse, massive adipose infiltration (which mostly occurs in elderly or immunosuppressed patients or following chemotherapy or

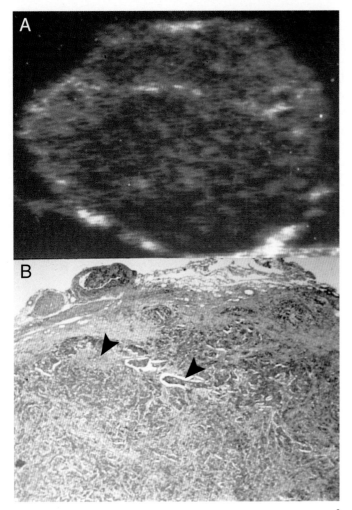

Fig. 14.14   A In vitro sonographic scan of a rounded lymph node including a hypoechoic area in the lower portion, causing displacement and thinning of the hilum (arrowhead). Histologically (**B**), the sonographically hypoechoic area corresponds to a metastatic deposit from adenocarcinoma.

radiotherapy) makes the nodes totally hyperechoic; thus the sonographic detection of the hilum becomes impossible even in benign nodes[23,25] (Fig. 14.16).

In a limited number of cases (4–6%) the hilum may not be visible in completely normal lymph nodes (Fig. 14.17), whilst it may be falsely observed in 3–8% of pathologic nodes owing to the presence of hyperechoic structures mimicking the hilum: metastatic hyperechoic deposits involving the medulla (mostly from highly keratinizing squamous cell carcinomas), fibrotic changes of the medulla, or coagulation necrosis.[9,23,25,28] This latter condition, due to ischemic degeneration of the lymph node, may occur both in infectious and in malignant diseases. It can result in an echogenic appearance of the medulla, more rounded and less echogenic than the hilum, usually associated with cystic areas and sometimes involving the whole node[23] (Fig. 14.18).

The thickness of nodal cortex, studied in particular by Vassallo et al,[28,29] is sonographically assessable only in the presence of a hilum, which serves as a reference structure.

A narrow cortex (thickness less than half the transverse diameter of the hilum) is mostly seen in benign nodes; only in 9% of malignant nodes (always with extensive hilar hyperechoic metastases) has a narrow cortex been detected.

Concentric cortical widening (Fig. 14.19) has been reported in multifocal/diffuse cortical malignant involvement of lymph nodes (70% of cases), but also in benign nodes with hypertrophied peripheral lymphatic follicles (30%). Eccentric cortical widening (Fig. 14.20) may be due to focal cortical malignant involvement (70% of cases), but also to cortical non-caseating granulomas or focal cortical follicular hyperplasia.[28]

According to Vassallo et al[28] evaluating L:S ratio, hilum and cortical thickness, 82% of nodes with L:S < 2, 81% with no hilum and 70% with eccentric cortical widening were malignant, whereas 72% with L:S > 2, 86% with wide hilum and 91% with narrow cortex were benign.

The internal echo texture of normal/reactive nodes is constant, with hypoechoic cortex and hyperechoic hilum (see Fig. 14.3). Diseased nodes may have varying structural patterns:

- markedly hypoechoic (even pseudocystic) in lymphomas (Fig. 14.21), due to the homogeneous arrangement of cellular sheets; their echogenicity increases following chemotherapy owing to fibrotic changes
- with a 'parenchymal' level of echoes or even hyperechoic (Fig. 14.22) in large metastatic nodes in which tumoral areas are adjacent to normal nodal zones
- anechoic because of liquefaction necrosis in metastatic deposits from squamous cell carcinomas or because of cystic changes in metastatic nodes from cystic papillary cancer of the thyroid gland (Fig. 14.23) or from carcinomas of the rhinopharynx
- with patchy hyperechoic areas (due to coagulative necrosis) associated with cystic degeneration in tuberculous nodes (polymorphous pattern)[23] (Fig. 14.24)
- with large cortical calcifications in granulomatous diseases or in metastatic nodes following radiotherapy or chemotherapy
- with microcalcifications in metastases from papillary or medullary carcinomas of the thyroid gland (Fig. 14.25).

Only recently have color Doppler and power Doppler been employed in the study of superficial lymph nodes; to date only preliminary observations are available. In normal/reactive nodes, even with instrumentation which is highly sensitive to slow flows, flow signals are either completely lacking[31] or limited to the hilar region (Fig. 14.26).

In most non-necrotic metastatic nodes from carcinomas diffuse hypervascularization with a wide range of velocities and uneven distribution (but mainly concentrated in the

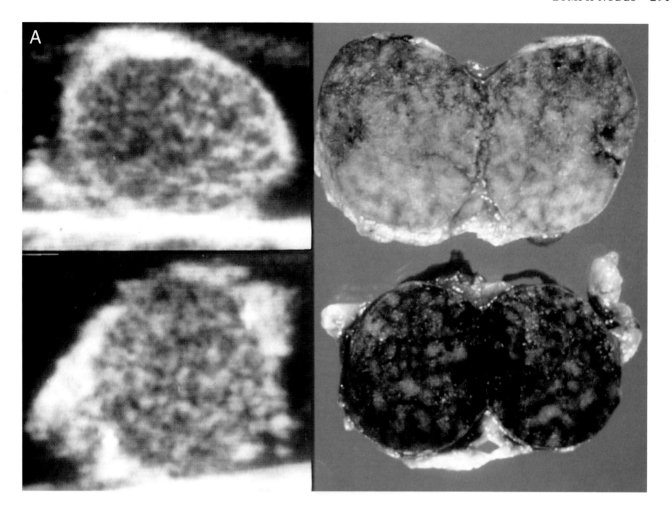

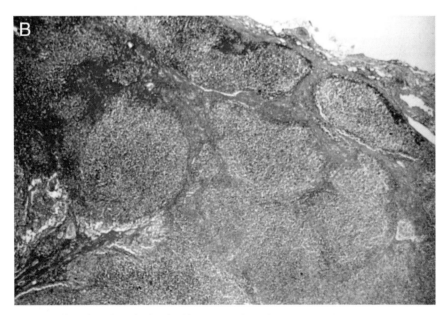

Fig. 14.15   In vitro sonograms of two lymph nodes involved by non-Hodgkin follicular-type lymphoma: the hyperechoic hilum is absent and the echo texture is inhomogeneous with a micronodular appearance. The surface of the gross specimen shows micronodular diffuse infiltration, and histology (**B**) demonstrates large, hypertrophied follicles suggesting the diagnosis of follicular lymphoma.

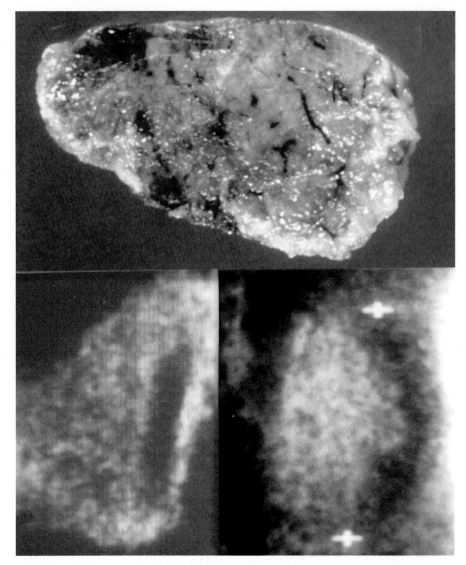

Fig. 14.16   Two sonograms of the same lymph node (on the right) featuring a wide hyperechoic component and small, eccentric hypoechoic bands. The gross specimen demonstrates that the hyperechoic zone corresponds to fatty replacement and hypoechoic bands to normal lymphatic tissue.

cortex, as showed by power Doppler) is generally detected (Fig. 14.27).

In low grade non-Hodgkin lymphomas a root-like distribution of flow signals with a large central vessel and small departing branches has been reported (Fig. 14.28A).[32] In high grade non-Hodgkin lymphomas short and small tortuous vessels with irregular distribution are seen from the color flow pattern, whereas in Hodgkin lymphomas a short vascular pole formed by a small artery and vein has been described (Fig. 14.28B).[32]

In inflammatory adenopathies a hilar distribution of vascularity may be seen, albeit inconstantly; general experience in inflammatory diseases is even more limited, because the widespread administration of antibiotics and anti-inflammatory drugs at an early stage quickly modifies the pathologic pattern and halts the enlargement of lymph nodes.

As for spectral analysis, a high resistive index seems to be quite frequently measured in reactive nodes, whereas a low resistive index related to a high diastolic component seems to be rather characteristic of malignant nodes.

Extracapsular nodal spread

This problem essentially involves the cervical lymph nodes, because it is mainly assessable through the relationship between adenopathies and the internal jugular vein. In our experience, jugular vein thrombosis (Fig. 14.29) suggests a diagnosis of metastasis (regardless of node size), as we have observed it in 75 cases of metastasis and only 3 cases

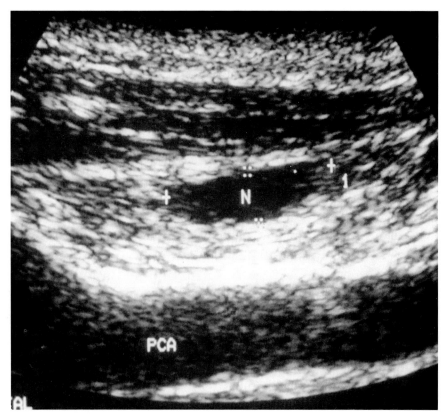

Fig. 14.17   Small, normal cervical lymph node (N) with a L:S ratio of more than 2 but without a hyperechoic hilum. PCA: common carotid artery.

of lymphoma; jugular vein compression without thrombosis can be observed in both metastasis and lymphoma. Inflammatory pathologies do not cause jugular vein thrombosis unless an endoluminal venous process is responsible for inflammation of the lateral neck.[33]

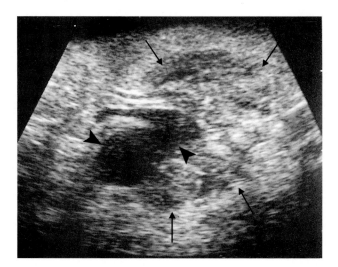

Fig. 14.18   Large inguinal node (arrow), diffusely hyperechoic because of coagulative necrosis, associated with a cystic area (arrowhead).

Carotid artery invasion is a preterminal event and is most likely to affect the external carotid artery (direct local invasion). Carotid invasion produces a focal hypoechoic lesion of the carotid wall.[34]

Differential diagnosis

The differential diagnosis of enlarged cervical nodes depends on whether only one or several lesions are present. Except in cases of neurofibromatosis (where there are cutaneous symptoms), multinodular lesions involve no diagnostic problems. The major difficulty is the obtaining of accurate topographic data rather than the identification of such masses as enlarged nodes.

In the neck, the possibility that a solitary, non-thyroid, non-salivary, non-vascular cervical mass is an enlarged lymph node can only be considered if there is a neoplastic or lymphomatous context. From a purely sonographic standpoint, an anechoic nodule in the mid-jugulocarotid region, along the anterior belly of the sternocleidomastoid muscle, may be a branchial or lymphoepithelial cyst. By contrast, thyroglossal duct cysts usually occupy a midline infrahyoid or prehyoid position. Vascular tumefaction (aneurysm, phlebectasia) is readily identified by US. Solid solitary nodules may have a rare etiology such as a neuro-

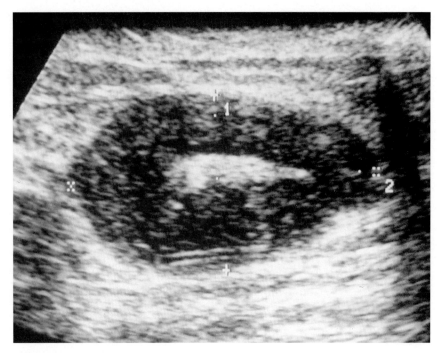

Fig. 14.19 Lymphomatous inguinal node with concentric cortical widening and hyperechoic central hilum.

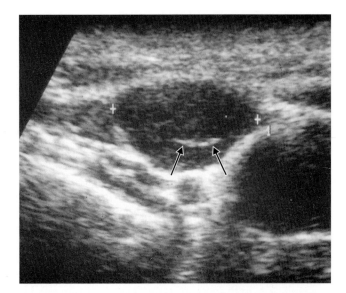

Fig. 14.20 Superficial enlarged lymph node (Hodgkin lymphoma) with eccentric cortical widening and thin, posteriorly displaced hilum (arrow).

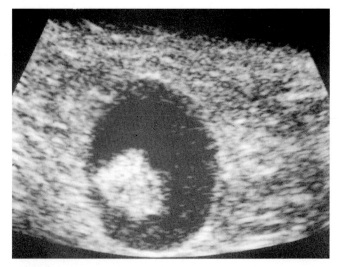

Fig. 14.21 Lymphomatous lymph node; apart from the hyperechoic hilum (arrow) the whole cortex is markedly hypoechoic, almost anechoic.

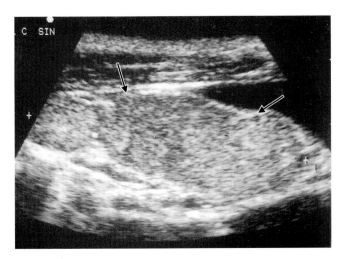

Fig. 14.22 Large, conglomerating cervical nodes (arrows) with homogeneously hyperechoic echo texture: metastases from renal carcinoma.

genic tumor. Solitary sarcomatous lesions tend to be larger in diameter than nodal lesions.

INDICATIONS FOR US OF SUPERFICIAL LYMPH NODES

ENT cancer

Numerous studies have emphasized the failure of physical examination to detect lymph node metastases in patients with ENT cancer. Depending on the series, the incidence of false-negative errors varies between 27.6% and 38.1%.

Moreover, when a nodal mass in the lateral neck occurs concomitantly with a primary ENT tumor, physical examination cannot determine whether or not the jugular vein is truly thrombosed.

CT and MR imaging have been used to upgrade a lesion in a large percentage (38–67%) of examinations of lateral necks which had given false-negative results at palpation. Consequently, 33–62% of these occult lymph node metastases have not been detected.[17, 20]

US and pretherapeutic work-up of metastatic nodes

The accuracy of US alone never exceeds 70%, as any rise in sensitivity is always accompanied by a decrease in specificity. According to Van Den Breckel et al,[9] FNAB under US guidance has an accuracy of 89%, a sensitivity of 76% and a specificity of 100%, and must play an important role in directing treatment of ENT cancers.

Pretherapy work-ups must obviously determine whether there is any venous thrombosis and/or bilateral nodal involvement. Jugular vein thrombosis precludes a modified neck dissection; in addition to node exeresis, the mandatory radical procedure involves removal of the internal jugular vein, the spinal nerve, and the sternocleidomastoid muscle. The value of US in the work-up of superficial nodes in ENT cancers is heightened by its topographic accuracy:

- Detection of subclinical ipsilateral nodes: this can be achieved by US, which is more sensitive than physical examination, especially in patients with thick necks.
- Accurate analysis of the size of palpable nodes: as US can accurately determine lesion size, the sonogram con-

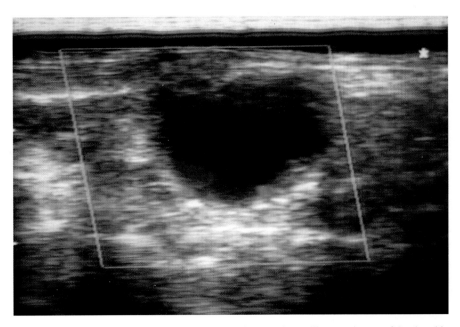

Fig. 14.23   Entirely cystic metastatic lymph node from cystic papillary carcinoma of the thyroid gland.

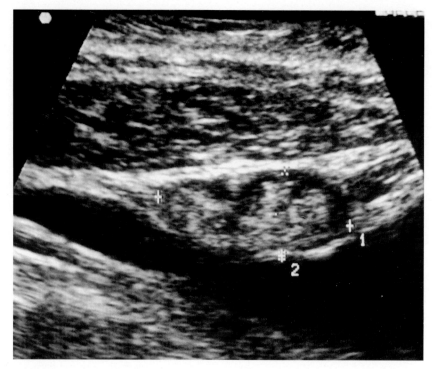

Fig. 14.24 Patchy hyperechoic areas in a tuberculous node (+) in front of the internal jugular vein.

stitutes an invaluable reference document for the surveillance of patients treated non-surgically. This is increasingly the case because of the present trend for the use of induction (neoadjuvant) chemotherapy. Precise volumetric data on superficial nodes are extremely helpful for monitoring response to therapy in such cases.

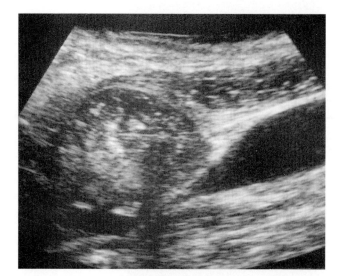

Fig. 14.25 Cervical adenopathy with hyperechoic spots (arrowheads) representing microcalcifications: metastasis from thyroid papillary carcinoma.

However, neither US nor any other imaging technique can currently detect extracapsular extension for lesions smaller than 1 cm in transverse diameter.

● Analysis of vascular relations: as mentioned earlier, US is sufficiently sensitive to detect thrombosis.

● Analysis of the contralateral cervical node regions: disease spread to the contralateral neck is not uncommon and modifies the therapeutic protocol (up-stage to N2c). Pathologic contralateral nodes are usually small, and the discrepancy in sensitivity between US and physical examination is at a maximum in these cases.[11]

However, there will remain patients in whom ultrasound with FNAB fails to demonstrate metastatic neck disease; microscopic disease in non-enlarged nodes will continue to evade recognition.

Ultrasonography and monitoring of non-surgical treatment

Along with its determinant role in the staging of ENT cancers, US is an ideal method for monitoring the course of patients who do not undergo surgery. Being less invasive than CT, ultrasonography is particularly indicated for follow-up studies aimed at assessing the efficacy of chemotherapy or radiotherapy. This is especially true for patients with radiation-induced cutaneous thickening of the neck. Even though a primary ENT tumor may be well controlled,

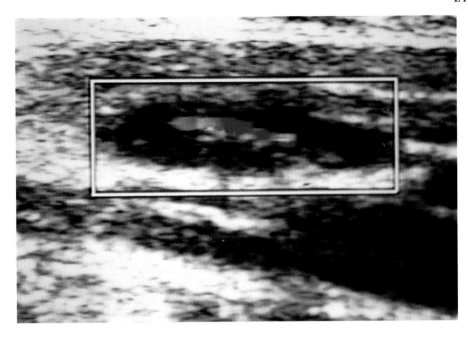

Fig. 14.26 Color Doppler study of normal lymph node: flow signals are present only in the hilar region.

the prognosis often depends on the status of the cervical nodes. Our analysis of patients followed up for cervical node involvement which was not treated by surgery confirmed these classic data. Of the 33 patients in whom sonograms demonstrated stable or progressive disease, only 2 were still alive at 1 year. By contrast, only 9 of 67 patients with a sonographically demonstrated improvement in node status died in less than 12 months.[5] These findings emphasize the importance of regular, effective monitoring of node size during therapy. Whereas chemotherapy does not alter the nature of the skin of the neck, irradiation generally causes cutaneous thickening which reduces the value of physical examination still further. Even though its sensitivity remains markedly superior to that of physical examination, US can also be hampered by postirradiation induration. In our experience CT and MRI are more sensitive than US in such cases.

Lymphomas

Superficial adenopathies are the most frequent manifestation of lymphomatous involvement during both initial staging work-up and follow-up in cases of disease recurrence.[35,36] Although usually larger in diameter than metastatic nodes, lymphomatous adenopathies have a 'soft' consistency that can make physical examination difficult.

Precise information on possible superficial nodal involvement, regardless of the disease form, is extremely important. In patients with supradiaphragmatic Hodgkin disease, for example, US findings of inguinal nodal involvement reflect subdiaphragmatic spread and result in modification

of the staging. The number of nodal sites involved also has prognostic significance in Hodgkin disease. In non-Hodgkin lymphoma, for which the prognosis depends more on histologic disease type, detection and accurate evaluation of the extent of superficial nodal involvement enable additional targets to be defined for evaluating the response to therapy.

In Hodgkin disease, relapses tend to occur during the first 3 years. Recurrence in a superficial node, whether or not it is associated with a deep site of involvement, occurs in 89–95% of relapses.[35] In non-Hodgkin lymphoma 69% of relapses affect the lymph nodes.[36]

Regardless of the type of lymphoma, superficial nodes are the most common sites for disease recurrence. The frequency of such relapses is difficult to determine at this time because of progressive improvements in the response rates to chemotherapy.

In order to reduce the potential number of false-positive findings without increasing the risk of false-negatives, we require a minimum transverse node diameter of 1 cm and the presence of multiple lesions.

In our experience with 120 patients, US revealed clinically impalpable lesions in an average of 10.8% of cases for the cervicosupraclavicular region, 17.9% for the axillary region, and 4.1% for the inguinal region. 8 of the 29 relapses were not detected at physical examination, and 3 were demonstrated solely with US.[4]

Not all superficial nodes affected by lymphoma require puncture biopsy, but histologic proof is required in the work-up of patients with supradiaphragmatic Hodgkin disease when sonograms show subclinical inguinal aden-

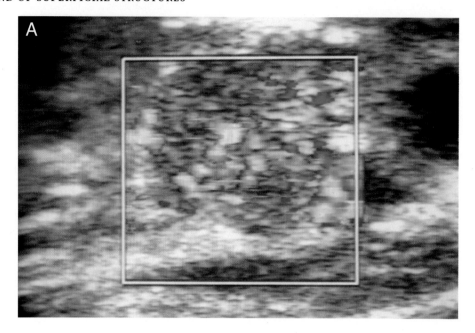

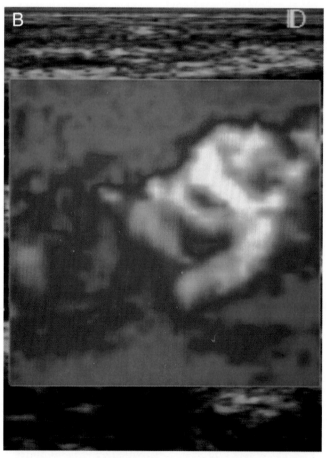

Fig. 14.27   Color (**A**) and power Doppler (**B**) studies of metastatic nodes from adenocarcinoma: hypervascularization with uneven flow distribution in **A** and evidence of predominantly cortical ('parenchymal') blood flow in **B**.

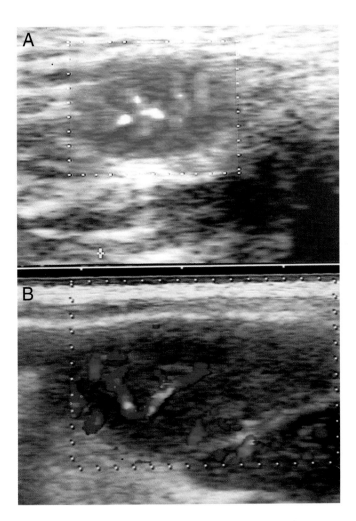

Fig. 14.28 Color flow signals in lymphomatous nodes: rootlike distribution with thin branches in low grade non-Hodgkin lymphoma (**A**) (power Doppler image) and single vascular pole in Hodgkin lymphoma (**B**).

opathies and whenever US findings raise a suspicion of recurrence, regardless of the type of lymphoma. Although puncture biopsy does not yield as much diagnostic information as examination of a surgically excised node, it can enable identification of non-lymphomatous nodal masses. In some instances, transformation of a lymphoma from a less aggressive to a more aggressive type can be evaluated by means of puncture biopsy. As such adverse evolution occurs in 20–40% of all cases of non-Hodgkin disease, repeated histologic analysis of nodes is particularly important; if needle biopsy is insufficient, surgical node dissection may be necessary. Finally, because of the importance of the superficial nodal status in lymphomas and the limited value of physical examination, systematic real-time sonographic examination of the superficial lymph node regions with a high-frequency transducer has become indispensable for both staging and follow-up.

Breast cancer

The importance of nodal status for the prognosis of breast cancer has led to the development of numerous methods for the detection of axillary lymph nodes, which can occur from levels one to three (subclavicular region within the smaller pectoral muscle). Clinical examination, axillary mammography, and lymphography are all insufficiently sensitive. US depicts lymph node enlargement but provides no information on the histology. In our experience, sensitivity of clinical examination was 45.4%, versus 72.7% for US.[3] However, in practice, for patients with breast cancer, US is no better suited than other methods as a replacement for axillary dissection for teams who perform this procedure.

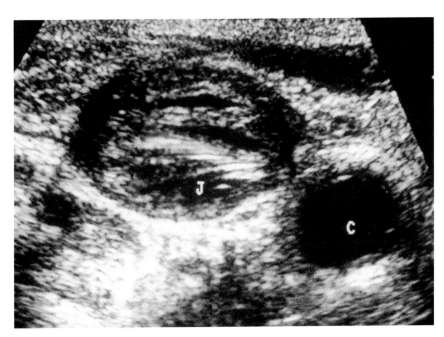

Fig. 14.29 Jugular thrombosis. J: jugular vein; C: common carotid artery.

Presently, color Doppler appears to be of little value in determining whether a primary tumor of the breast is malignant or benign. It does appear to be useful, however, in the follow-up of cancers during initial chemotherapy (partial regression of the signal and of tumor volume), and in the diagnosis of metastatic lymph nodes, with a sensitivity of 63% and a specificity of 100% in our initial results.[28]

If there is a risk of involvement of the internal mammary chain, precise localization of the internal mammary vessels by US allows optimization of radiotherapy.[10]

Apart from the problem of color Doppler (which needs more studies) and of internal mammary irradiation, US possesses real advantages in some instances, including (a) cancers treated solely by irradiation; (b) insufficient axillary dissection, with less than seven negative nodes (the predictive value of axillary sampling in such cases is insufficient); and (c) large tumors not amenable to primary surgery (chemotherapy). The use of US in these cases allows better evaluation of the nodal factor for prognosis and optimizes the follow-up of adenopathies under chemotherapy. For stage I patients treated by surgery and/or irradiation (nodal recurrence in only 1%), monitoring with US appears unnecessary. By contrast, when the axillary region is not treated, the recurrence rate rises to 16% and US remains justified.[37]

REFERENCES

1. Ege G N 1978 Internal mammary lymphoscintigraphy: a rational adjunct to the staging and management of breast carcinoma. Clin Radiol 29: 453–456
2. Sanda K, Sasaki T 1980 Scintigram of the cervical lymph nodes. Jpn J Clin Radiol 25: 413–414
3. Bruneton J N, Caramella E, Hery M, Aubanel D, Manzino J J, Picard J L 1986 Axillary lymph node metastases in breast cancer: preoperative detection with US. Radiology 158: 325–326
4. Bruneton J N, Normand F, Balu-Maestro C et al 1987 Lymphomatous syperficial lymph nodes: US detection. Radiology 165: 233–235
5. Bruneton J N, Roux P, Caramella E, Demard F, Vallicioni J, Chauvel P 1984 Ear, nose, and throat cancer: ultrasound diagnosis of metastasis to cervical lymph nodes. Radiology 152: 771–773
6. Eichhorn T, Schroeder H G 1993 Ultrasound in metastatic neck disease. ORL J Otorhinolaryngol Relat Spec 55: 258–262
7. Shozushima M, Suzuki M, Nakasima Y et al 1990 Ultrasound diagnosis of lymph node metastasis in head and neck cancer. Dentomaxillofac Radiol 19: 165–170
8. Solbiati L, Rizzatto G, Bellotti E et al 1988 High-resolution sonography of cervical lymph nodes in head and neck cancers: criteria for differentiation of reactive versus malignant nodes Radiology 169 (P): 113 (Abstract)
9. Van den Brekel M W M, Castelijns J A, Stel H V et al 1991 Occult metastatic neck disease: detection with US and US-guided fine-needle aspiration cytology. Radiology 180: 457–461
10. Bruneton J N, Dalfin F Y, Caramella E, Roux P, Hery M 1986 Value of ultrasound in localizing the internal mammary vessels. Eur J Radiol 6: 142–144
11. Baatenburg de Jong R J, Knegt P, Verwoerd C D A 1993 Assessment of cervical metastatic disease. ORL J Otorhinolaryngol Relat Spec 55: 273–280
12. Boland G W, Lee M J, Mueller P R, Mayo-Smith W, Dawson S L, Simeone J F 1993 Efficacy of sonographically guided biopsy of thyroid masses and cervical lymph nodes. AJR 161: 1053–1056
13. Sutton R T, Reading C C, Charboneau J W, James E M, Grant C S, Hay I D 1988 US-guided biopsy of neck masses in postoperative management of patients with thyroid cancer. Radiology 168: 769–772
14. Som P M 1992 Detection of metastasis in cervical lymph nodes: CT and MR criteria and differential diagnosis. AJR 158: 961–969
15. Van den Brekel M W M, Stel H V, Castelijns J A et al 1990 Cervical lymph node metastasis: assessment of radiologic criteria. Radiology 177: 379–384
16. Carvalho P, Baldwin D, Carter R, Parsons C 1991 Accuracy of CT in detecting squamous carcinoma metastases in cervical lymph nodes. Clin Radiol 44: 79–81
17. Stern W B P, Silver C E, Zeifer B A, Persky M S, Heller K S 1990 Computed tomography of the clinically negative neck. Head Neck 12: 109–113
18. March D E, Wechsler R J, Kurtz A B, Rosenberg A L, Needleman L 1991 CT pathologic correlation of axillary lymph nodes in breast carcinoma. J Comput Assist Tomogr 15: 440–444
19. Lee A S, Weissleder R, Brady T J, Wittenberg J 1991 Lymph nodes: microstructural anatomy at MR imaging. Radiology 178: 519–522
20. Van den Brekel M W M, Castelijns J A, Croll G A et al 1991 Magnetic resonance versus palpation of cervical lymph node metastasis. Arch Otolaryngol Head Neck Surg 117: 667–673
21. Yousem D M, Som P M, Hakney D B, Schwaibold F, Hendrix R A 1992 Central nodal necrosis and intracapsular neoplastic spread in cervical lymph nodes: MR imaging versus CT. Radiology 182: 753–759
22. Negendank W G, Al-Katib A M, Karanes C, Smith M R 1990 Lymphomas: MR imaging contrast characteristics with clinico-pathologic correlations. Radiology 177: 209–216
23. Evans R M, Ahuja A, Metreweli C 1993 The linear echogenic hilus in cervical lymphoadenopathy – a sign of benignity or malignancy? Clin Radiol 47: 262–264
24. Ischii J, Amagasa T, Tachibana T et al 1989 Ultrasonic evaluation of cervical lymph node metastasis of squamous cell carcinoma in the oral cavity. Bull Tokyo Med Dent Univ 36: 63–67
25. Rubaltelli L, Proto E, Salmaso R, Bortoletto P, Candiani F, Cagol P 1990 Sonography of abnormal lymph nodes in vitro: correlation of sonographic and histologic findings. AJR 155: 1241–1244
26. Sakai F, Kiyono K, Sone S et al 1988 Ultrasonic evaluation of cervical metastatic lymphadenopathy. J Ultrasound Med 7: 305–310
27. Steinkamp H J, Hosten N, Langer R, Mathe F, Ehritt C, Felix R 1992 Cervical node metastases: sonographic evidence of malignancy. Fortschr Geb Rontgenstr Nuklearmed Erganzungsbd 156: 135–141
28. Vassallo P, Edel G, Roos N, Naguib A, Peters P E 1993 In-vitro high-resolution ultrasonography of benign and malignant lymph nodes. A sonographic-pathologic correlation. Invest Radiol 28: 698–705
29. Vassallo P, Wernecke K, Roos N, Peters P E 1992 Differentiation of benign from malignant superficial lymphadenopathy: the role of high-resolution US. Radiology 183: 215–220
30. Winkelbauer F, Denk D M, Ammann M, Karnel F 1993 Sonographische Diagnostik der Halslymphknotentuberkulose. Ultraschall Med 14: 28–31
31. Bruneton J N, Balu-Maestro C, Marcy P Y, Melia P, Mourou M Y 1994 Very high frequency (13 MHz) ultrasonographic examination of the normal neck: detection of normal lymph nodes and thyroid nodules. J Ultrasound Med 13: 87–90
32. Calliada F, Raieli G, Corsi G, Campani R, Bottinelli O, Carnevale G 1992 Color Doppler US of pathologically enlarged neck lymph nodes in differential diagnosis of Hodgkin and non-Hodgkin lymphoma. Radiology 185(P): 280
33. Bruneton J N, Balu-Maestro C, Merran D et al 1990 Rapports veineux des adénopathies cervicales. Revue d'une série de 300 cas. J Radiol 71: 57–60
34. Gooding G A W 1993 Malignant carotid invasion: sonographic diagnosis. ORL J Otorhinolaryngol Relat Spec 55: 263–272

35. Bayle-Weisgerber C, Lemercier N, Teillet F et al 1984 Hodgkin's disease in children: results of therapy in a mixed group of 178 clinical and pathologically staged patients over 13 years. Cancer 54: 215–222

36. Schein P S, Chabner B A, Canellos G P et al 1975 Non Hodgkin's lymphoma: patterns of relapse from complete remission after combination chemotherapy. Cancer 35: 354–357

37. Balu-Maestro C, Bruneton J N, Giudicelli T, Chauvel C, Hery M D 1991 Doppler couleur en pathologie tumorale mammaire. J Radiol 72: 579–583

15

Peripheral nerves

L. De Pra   L. E. Derchi   G. Balconi

ANATOMIC CONSIDERATIONS

Peripheral nerves are strong whitish cords with a complex internal structure resembling that of a cable. They are made up of many basic units, the nerve fibers, running along their course. Each nerve fiber consists of an axon, a myelin sheath (only in myelinated fibers) and a neuro-lemmal sheath. Both the neurolemma and the myelin sheath are surrounded by Schwann cells. The fibers of all but the smallest peripheral nerves run along the course of the nerve arranged in small fasciculi.

The nerve fibers are protected and strengthened by connective tissue coverings. The whole nerve is surrounded by a thick membranous sheath containing fatty tissue, blood vessels and lymphatics, called epineurium. A more delicate membrane encloses each fasciculus and provides a barrier to penetration of substances in and out of the nerve fibers. Individual fibers are embedded within a delicate connective tissue called endoneurium.[1-3]

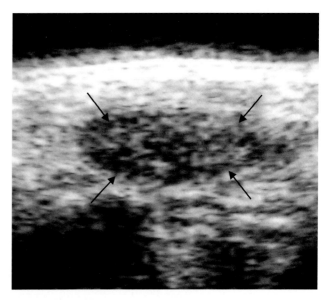

Fig. 15.1   20 MHz transverse scan of normal, 2.5 mm thick median nerve (arrows) in the wrist, with the typical coarsely dotted pattern.

EXAMINATION TECHNIQUE

US evaluation of peripheral nerves is not an easy task; knowledge of the course and anatomic relationships of the nerves to be examined and careful correlation with clinical findings and, if available, with the results of other imaging tests are of greatest importance in obtaining clinically useful and accurate information.

The choice of the transducer is based on the depth of the nerve to be studied: high-frequency small-parts probes have to be used for superficial nerves; evaluation of sciatic nerves in the gluteal or in the posterior thigh regions, where penetrative capabilities are needed, can be obtained with 5 or even 3.5 MHz probes.[4]

Examination should be performed bilaterally, usually starting from the normal side and then evaluating the region where pathologic changes are suspected. In order to obtain comparable images, the same scan planes have to be followed on both sides. When needed, dynamic maneuvers can be performed in order to evaluate better the relationships of muscles and tendons with nerves.

US ANATOMY

On US images, the normal peripheral nerve has an elongated or oval or rounded shape, depending on the scan plane used to image it, and presents with high reflectivity, directly related to the angle of incidence of the US beam: it is hyperechoic when the beam strikes it at 90°, but it has lower reflectivity at lower angles of incidence. When high-frequency small-parts probes are used, its structure reveals, in cross section, a coarsely dotted pattern (Fig. 15.1) and, on longitudinal images, elongated hypoechoic lines running along its course, more irregularly arranged than tendon fibers (Fig. 15.2).[5-7] In vitro studies have shown that such images correlate well to the small fasciculi of which nerves are composed (Fig. 15.3).[8]

Careful analysis of this structural pattern can help differentiate nerves from adjacent hyperechoic tendons, ligaments and muscular aponeuroses. This can be helpful in difficult anatomic sites, such as in the volar aspect of the wrist, where many structures with similar echogenicity can be present within the same image, and differentiation based on anatomic relationships alone can be difficult.

Nerves in the neck have been described as hypoechoic images surrounded by high-level echoes[9] (Fig. 15.4). The peripheral hyperechogenicity is due to the presence of fatty tissue surrounding the nerve; the hypoechoic structure may be explained by difficulties in obtaining a good scanning angle in a complicated anatomic region such as the neck.

NERVOUS DISEASES

Peripheral nerves may undergo pathologic changes from either extrinsic or intrinsic causes.

Extrinsic lesions

Such pathologic changes may occur anywhere in the body, but are more common where the nerve passes within unextensible osteofibrous canals and can undergo compression by adjacent structures.

Nerves have relatively high resistance to mechanical stress due to the presence of their outer connective covering. However, nerve fibers are altered when compression forces overcome such resistance, and functional changes develop. Longstanding compression leads to gross changes of the nervous morphology, with either diffuse flattening

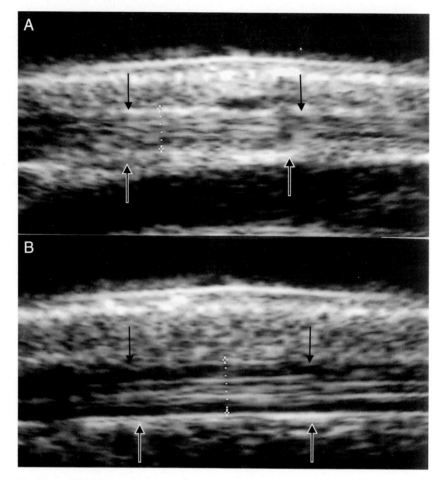

Fig. 15.2 Different sonographic appearances of a peripheral nerve (median nerve) (arrows) (**A**) and a tendon (arrows) (**B**) on longitudinal 20 MHz scans. Both of them are 1.5–1.8 mm thick. The nerve fibers are more irregularly arranged than the tendon fibers.

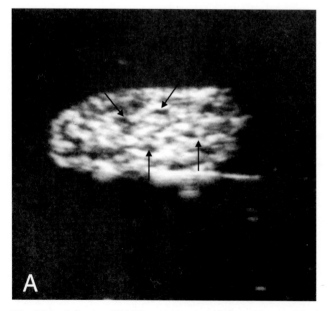

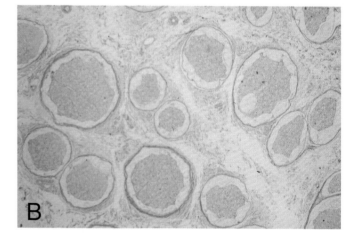

Fig. 15.3 **A** In vitro 15 MHz transverse scan of normal nerve. The hypoechoic small dots (arrows) correspond to the fasciculi visible in the histologic section (**B**).

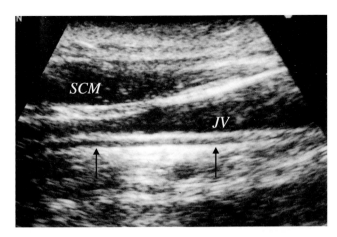

Fig. 15.4 13 MHz longitudinal scan of normal vagus nerve (arrows) appearing as a hypoechoic line surrounded by hyperechoic tissue. JV: jugular vein; SCM: sternocleidomastoid muscle.

or localized constrictions and, in many cases, associated swelling of the proximal portion of the nerve (Fig. 15.5). These are the only changes which can be detected by ultrasound; at present, in fact, structural alterations of the nerve cannot be detected.[2,5]

Compression syndromes are characterized by burning pain, numbness and paresthesia in the territory of the involved nerve. In advanced cases muscle weakness and atrophy can develop. The diagnosis is made by a combination of clinical symptoms, electromyography and nerve conduction studies. However, symptoms may be nonspecific in the early stages of the disease, and the results of conduction tests can be equivocal. In fact, focal compressions of nerves may cause slowing of conduction, but if even a few fibers are not compressed test results may be normal.[4]

Detecting the presence of a lesion which may be the cause of compression symptoms on the nerve and determining its

exact location are of great importance for both proper diagnosis and treatment planning.

A large number of pathologic conditions may cause compression syndromes.

In patients with trauma, symptoms may be due to hematoma, fractured or dislocated bony fragments, or even scar tissue located in close proximity to the nerve.

Any condition that increases the volume of structures within an unextensible osteofibrous canal may cause a compression syndrome on the nerve passing through it. The most common of such conditions is tenosynovitis, in which symptoms are produced by compression on adjacent nerves by the thickened synovial tendinous sheaths (see Ch. 17).

Both solid and fluid-filled space-occupying lesions may be encountered. Ganglion cysts develop from an adjacent joint, with which they communicate; they have a lobulated appearance and the thin connection with the joint is usually detected (Fig. 15.6).

Compression may be due also to congenital anomalies; anomalous location of the flexor muscles of the fingers whose bellies protrude in the carpal tunnel has been described as a cause of carpal tunnel syndrome (Fig. 15.7).

The carpal tunnel syndrome is a relatively frequent complication of chronic hemodialysis. Both thickening of the flexor retinaculum and development of collections of amyloid deep to the flexor tendons have been suggested as possible causes of this condition in these patients (Fig. 15.8).

In longstanding compression syndromes, especially when due to ligament fibrosis or calcification, the nerve can be impossible to demonstrate, and only indirect signs can be detected by US. However, direct imaging of the nerve and its changes is quite important: determining the degree of thinning (see Fig. 15.5A) and measuring the length of involvement is quite helpful in planning accurately the best therapeutic approach in each case.[5,7]

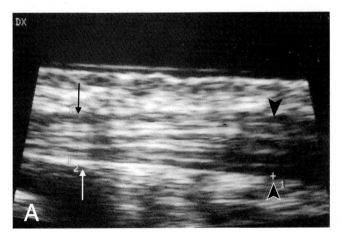
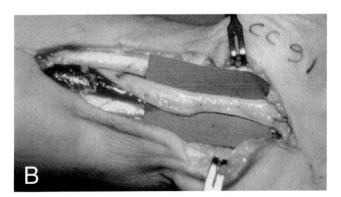

Fig. 15.5 **A** 15 MHz longitudinal scan of the median nerve showing marked distal flattening (arrows) due to longstanding compression. Proximally the nerve is moderately swollen (arrowheads). **B** At surgical exploration both compression and proximal swelling of the nerve are evident.

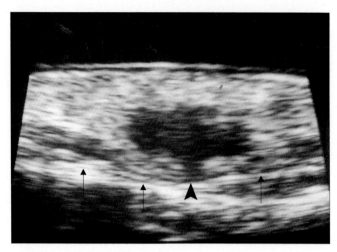

Fig. 15.6 12 mm ganglion cyst of the wrist with posterior connection (arrowhead) with the joint and compression on the posteriorly located nerve (arrows).

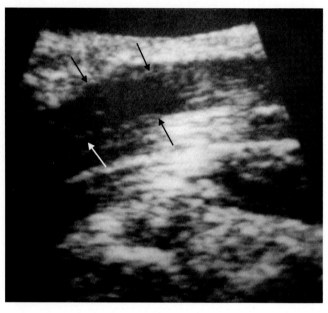

Fig. 15.7 Longitudinal scan of the wrist showing anomalous protrusion of flexor muscle bellies (arrows) into the carpal tunnel.

Intrinsic lesions

Primary lesions present as focal enlargements of nerves which are not always easy to detect; in fact, only superficially located nodules can be palpated, and clinical problems ensue only when lesions cause either sensory or motor disturbances. In most cases either clinical or functional tests may be normal.

Benign tumors of the nerves (schwannomas or neurinomas, and neurofibromas) originate from the Schwann cells and cause progressive compression on the axons of the nerve cells running within the nerve; they deform the nervous architecture but do not destroy its fascicular arrangement.

Solitary schwannomas are a typical example of this kind of slow and constant growth pattern. They are encapsulated

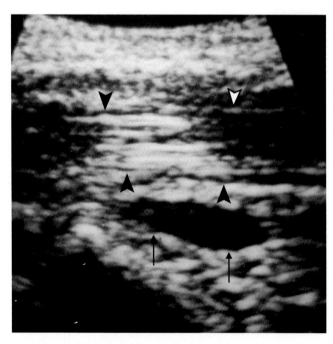

Fig. 15.8 Small ovoid collection of amyloid substance (arrows) compressing a superficially located peripheral nerve (arrowheads).

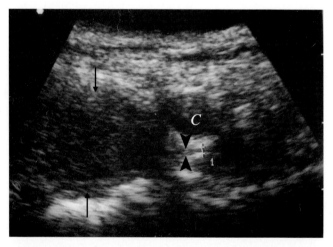

Fig. 15.9 Neck schwannoma (arrows) with homogeneous hypoechoic pattern. The visualization of the junction with the nerve of origin (arrowheads) is essential for the sonographic diagnosis of nerve tumor. C: carotid artery.

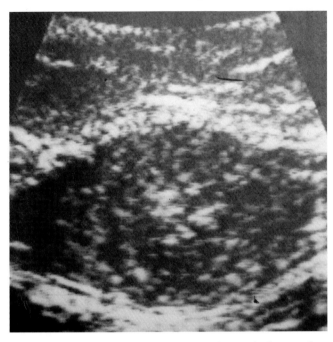

Fig. 15.10   2.5 cm schwannoma with echogenic areas in the central portion.

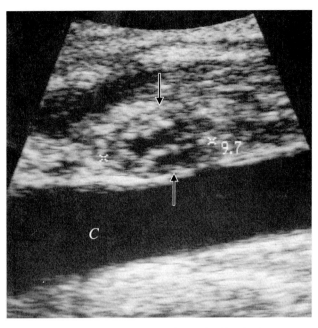

Fig. 15.11   0.9 cm neck schwannoma (arrows) with mixed structure due to small cystic areas. C: carotid artery.

tumors, which develop at the periphery of the nerve and grow eccentrically.[1,5,10,11] Schwannomas have significant vascularization and often internal cystic changes.[1] On physical examination they can be mobilized only transversely and not along the nerve axis.[10] Sonographically most schwannomas have a hypoechoic solid and homogeneous structure, well-defined margins, and posterior acoustic enhancement (Fig. 15.9).[10,12,13] However, albeit rarely, slightly echogenic (Fig. 15.10) and heterogeneous (Fig. 15.11)[14] schwannomas have been described. Since multiple lesions (schwannomatosis) can be exceptionally encountered[15] (Fig. 15.12), or the same nodule can extend for a variable length, it is always necessary to explore the whole course of the involved nerve and to extend the study also to the contralateral side.

Solitary neurofibromas develop in the endoneurium and grow concentrically in an elongated shape along the nerve axis (not encapsulated, plexiform pattern); surgical excision can therefore be very difficult.[5,10,11] Plexiform neurofibromas present with diffuse alteration of the nerve structure, but do not interrupt the nerve fibers. These tumours occur usually in young people, mostly in subcutaneous nerves, and their growth speed may increase at puberty or during pregnancy.[10] On US studies they are mostly hyperechoic, with coarse internal echoes and lobulated margins (Fig. 15.13).[5,10,12,13,16]

Non-plexiform neurofibromas and tumors in von Recklinghausen's neurofibromatosis (hereditary phakomatosis) appear as asymptomatic nodules with fusiform shape and hypoechoic structure on US scans. Although they do not

have a histologic capsule, they present with relatively regular and well-defined margins (Fig. 15.14). When sudden increases in size are detected, the possibility of malignant transformation should be considered.[10] Small intratumoral cystic changes (usually a clue to the diagnosis of schwannoma) may be present due to foci of myxoid degeneration.[11]

The sonographic diagnosis of a nerve sheath tumor relies on the detection of a mass along the presumed course of a peripheral nerve, in association with neurologic signs. However, sonography can be completely reliable only when the junction between a tumor and the nerve of origin can be demonstrated[10] (see Fig. 15.9). Fine-needle aspiration biopsy can be performed in doubtful lesions; the excruciating pain triggered by the needle insertion is also a clue for the diagnosis of nerve tumor.[10]

Glomus tumors originate from sympathetic nervous fibers; they are highly vascular, mostly of small size, and often located at the extremities of the fingers.[11,17] They appear as hypoechoic small lesions with well-defined margins, and slight posterior acoustic enhancement (Fig. 15.15).[17]

Ultrasonography plays an important role in patients with Morton neuromas. Such lesions are focal masses of perineural fibrosis, with connective tissue, vascular thrombosis and ischemic nervous changes, involving plantar nerves of the foot, which cause pain and/or numbness in the forefoot exacerbated by walking and relieved by rest.[18] They are located in the intermetatarsal spaces, most frequently in the 3–4 and the 2–3 ones. Ultrasonography can detect the

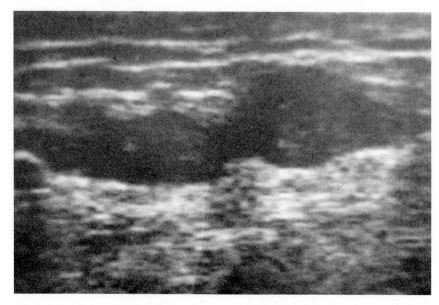

Fig. 15.12 Schwannomatosis. Two small adjacent hypoechoic schwannomas along the course of the same nerve.

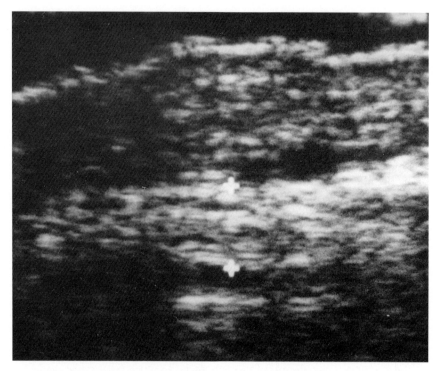

Fig. 15.13 Focal enlargement of a peripheral nerve (calipers) with coarse hyperechoic structure: plexiform neurofibroma.

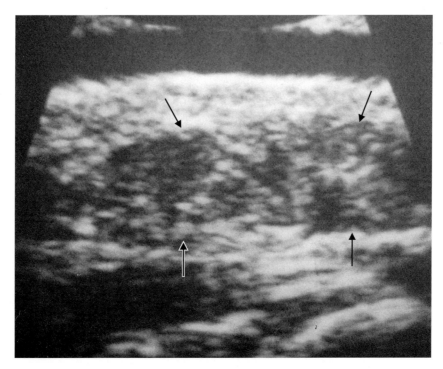

Fig. 15.14   Solitary non-plexiform neurofibroma (arrows) with fusiform shape and hypoechoic structure.

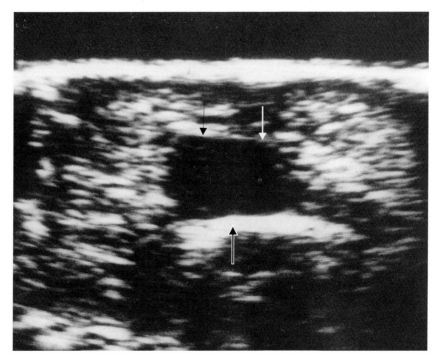

Fig. 15.15   4 mm homogeneously hypoechoic glomus tumor (arrows) of a finger extremity.

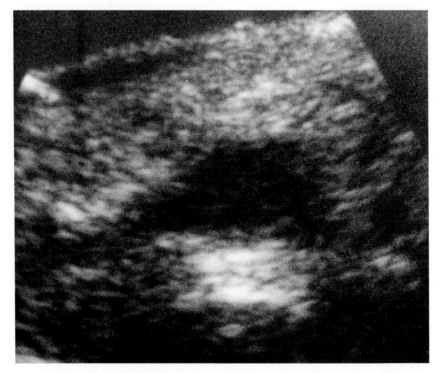

Fig. 15.16 9 mm oval hypoechoic Morton neuroma in the 3–4 intermetatarsal space (longitudinal scan).

presence of Morton neuromas and localize them accurately, thus directing surgery to the appropriate intermetatarsal space and avoiding exploration of adjacent regions. Lesions appear as ovoid hypoechoic masses oriented along the major axis of the metatarsals[11,19] (Fig. 15.16). Only a few false-negative results have been reported for lesions which are smaller than 5 mm.

Traumatic neuromas can also be identified by ultrasound. They are painful, nodular lesions formed by the random proliferation of regenerating axonal sprouts, Schwann cells and scar tissue at the site of trauma or amputation of a peripheral nerve. They can grow rapidly soon after the trauma and may infiltrate the surrounding soft tissues.[10] On US scans they present as elongated

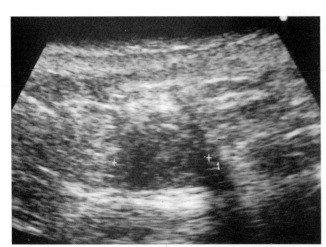

Fig. 15.17 Traumatic neuroma of the thigh: 10 mm hypoechoic mass with irregular margins.

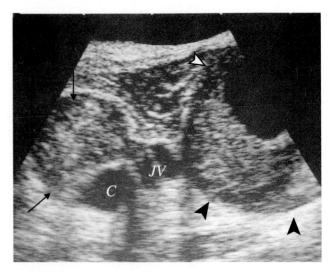

Fig. 15.18 Transverse scan of the left laterocervical region. Malignant schwannoma of the neck (arrows) anterior to the carotid artery (C) and jugular vein (JV). Laterally a large metastatic node with wide cystic change is evident (arrowheads).

hypoechoic masses (Fig. 15.17); well-defined margins and posterior enhancement are not always present.[5,6,11]

Malignant schwannomas (neurofibrosarcomas) are the most frequent malignant nerve tumors. They are poorly differentiated spindle-cell sarcomas, approximately 50% of which occur in patients with neurofibromatosis. Neurofibrosarcomas can reach large dimensions; regional lymphatic spread is not common, even if possible. Sonographically they appear as hypoechoic masses causing enlargement of the nerve with internal complete disorganization and interruption of nerve fibers. Necrotic or hemorrhagic changes may be present. These tumors cannot be differentiated from other benign lesions on the basis of echogenicity; the only sonographic findings which may make the examiner suspect malignancy are the presence of irregular margins and adhesions with surrounding tissues and the detection of associated cervical metastatic lymph nodes (Fig. 15.18).[5,11]

REFERENCES

1. Harkin J C, Reed R J 1969 Tumors of the peripheral nervous system. In: Firminger H I (ed) Atlas of tumor pathology. AFIP, Washington DC, pp 29–59
2. Lundborg G 1988 Nerve injury and repair. Churchill Livingstone, Edinburgh
3. Moore K L 1985 Clinically oriented anatomy, 2nd edn. Williams and Wilkins, Baltimore, p 45
4. Graif M, Seton A, Nerubai J, Horoszowski H, Itzchak Y 1991 Sciatic nerve: sonographic evaluation and anatomic–pathologic considerations. Radiology 181: 405–408
5. De Pra L, Petrolati M, Gandellini S, Del Bene M, Solbiati L 1987 L'ecografia nella patologia nervosa dell'arto superiore. Solei, Milan
6. Fornage B D 1988 Peripheral nerves of the extremities: imaging with US. Radiology 167: 179–182
7. Solbiati L, De Pra L, Gandellini S et al 1992 High-resolution sonography of the carpal tunnel syndrome: J Echograph Med Ultrasons 13: 48–54
8. Silvestri E, Derchi L E, Bertolotto M et al 1993 High-resolution US of peripheral nerves. Radiology 189 (P): 210
9. Solbiati L, De Pra L, Ierace T, Bellotti E, Derchi L E 1985 High-resolution sonography of the recurrent laryngeal nerve: anatomic and pathologic considerations. AJR 145: 989–993
10. Fornage B D 1993 Sonography of peripheral nerves of the extremities. Radiol Med 85: 162–167
11. Enzinger F M, Weiss S W 1983 Soft tissue tumors. Mosby, St Louis
12. Hoddick W K, Callen P W, Filly R A, Mahony B S, Edwards M B 1984 Ultrasound evaluation of benign sciatic nerve sheath tumors. J Ultrasound Med 3: 505–507
13. Hughes D G, Wilson D J 1986 Ultrasound appearances of peripheral nerve tumors. Br J Radiol 59: 1041–1043
14. Chinn D H, Filly R A, Callen P W 1982 Unusual ultrasonographic appearance of a solid schwannoma. JCU 10: 243–245
15. Purcell S M, Dixon S L 1989 Schwannomatosis: an unusual variant of neurofibromatosis or a distinct clinical entity? Arch Dermatol 125: 390–393
16. Reuter K L, Raptopoulos V, De Girolami U et al 1982 Ultrasonography of a plexiform neurofibroma of the popliteal fossa. J Ultrasound Med 1: 209–211
17. Fornage B D Schernberg F L 1984 Sonographic diagnosis of glomous tumour of the finger. J Ultrasound Med 3: 523–524
18. Mulder J D 1951 The causative mechanism in Morton's metatarsalgia. J Bone Joint Surg 33: 94–95
19. Redd R A, Peters V J, Emery S F, Branch H M, Rifkin M D 1989 Morton neuroma: sonographic evaluation. Radiology 171: 415–417

16

Muscles

G. Balconi   G. Monetti   L. De Pra

In the human body there are 327 matched and 2 unmatched skeletal muscles, i.e. the dynamic organs of the locomotor system, made up of a fleshy central portion, the muscle belly, generally connected to a fibrous element, the tendon. Their morphology allows muscles to be divided into two large groups: the long muscles are so described because they develop their maximum dimension primarily along their longitudinal axis; they feature a bulky central portion and are often composed of several bellies (e.g. biceps, triceps and quadriceps) with a single distal tendon insertion and multiple proximal insertions. The long muscles have a great ability to extend and shorten themselves. The wide muscles generally have a flatter belly and are less able to extend and shorten themselves: they serve primarily to supply power.

The different morphologic relationships existing between muscle bellies and tendons allow muscles to be classified as pennate, semipennate and orbicular. The muscles are generally enclosed in fibrous bands of connective tissue, which separate them from adjacent structures and often unite them in groups or bundles. The muscle bundles enclose blood vessels and nerves. The dynamics of a muscle may be altered or obstructed by factors intrinsic to the muscle belly or by alterations in adjacent structures, i.e. other muscles, muscle bands, epidermis, or osseous borders. Given the anatomic and functional characteristics of muscles, any study of them requires a morphologic evaluation of the belly and musculotendinous junction, and of their dynamic capability. In the study of muscles, the close anatomic relations between muscles and adjacent structures and the possible functional interferences that may develop also call for a careful evaluation of all perimuscular structures.

The study of periskeletal soft tissue is performed utilizing the different imaging methods currently available. Conventional radiology, including the 'soft-ray' technique, often provides only poor results in the study of superficial structures, due to its weak inherent contrast. Ultrasonography, computed tomography and magnetic resonance imaging provide a better 'panoramic' view of specific structures than ultrasound and a better characterization of all structural focal and diffuse alterations of the muscle. Ultrasonography is the only examination which permits the dynamic phase of muscles to be studied. The choice among such techniques will be based upon their availability and accessibility, as well as on an appropriate indication; if possible, the integration of various methods may prove helpful. Other imaging techniques currently available are scintigraphy, a technique which can be useful in some types of pathological conditions, and thermography, which can on occasion be highly sensitive, but which is too poorly specific for detecting functional, inflammatory or vascular alterations.

The ultrasonographic evaluation of muscles must also include an assessment of the structures contained within and those lying adjacent to them.

TECHNOLOGICAL OPTIONS AND EXAMINATION METHODOLOGY

In order to perform an ultrasound study of muscle, it is essential to use real-time equipment: this is the only way to carry out a dynamic study. To study larger muscle structures, it is necessary to use medium- to high-frequency probes (7.5 MHz), while the study of small muscle structures requires the use of high-frequency probes (10–13 MHz). The high-frequency probes can also be valuable for studying the surface details of bulky muscles. This type of study may employ linear, sector or convex probes. However, linear probes are to be preferred, since they reduce artifacts and provide a more panoramic view. Convex probes, and especially sector probes, can easily produce artifacts due to probe placement on the surface being examined; the muscle is a 'soft' structure that can easily be compressed and 'altered' even by the light pressure of a probe being placed on the skin. Linear probes have a larger contact surface, thus reducing the likelihood of such artifacts. The angle of incidence of the ultrasound beam on the lamellar structures of a muscle can modify their echogenicity. With convex and sector probes, the angle of incidence of the ultrasound beam on the muscle bundles in the central section of the image can differ with respect to the peripheral parts, while linear probes have the same angle of incidence across the entire field. The use of a spacer between the probe and the skin may be useful in reducing artifacts produced by the pressure of the probe on the skin, and, especially on a highly curved surface, can improve contact between probe and skin, thus facilitating the dynamic phase study.

The examination technique should consist of three steps which must be fully integrated: the clinical evaluation, the ultrasound evaluation and the patient report.

The clinical evaluation must identify the most commonly used muscle activity or athletic movement causing the symptoms, and the mode of onset of the lesion. Clinical examination should detect any macroscopic muscle or tendon abnormalities, and any sites of spontaneous or provoked pain, in addition to noting the absence or presence of functional limitations. The clinical-anamnestic details are essential to enable the physician to interpret correctly all ultrasound findings; for instance, the 'trained' muscle of an athlete looks quite unlike an 'un-trained' muscle on ultrasound, with differences in both size and echogenicity. Such findings may also be common to certain pathological conditions. An accurate clinical evaluation permits the prompt identification of muscle pathologies and should also provide some valuable guidance regarding the dynamic movements to be performed during the US examination to detect and describe more accurately any lesions present.

The ultrasound examination needs to include sagittal scans along the longest axis of the muscle or tendon being examined, in addition to axial and oblique scans. The scan must be performed during both active and passive dynamic phases. The dynamic examination, performed during isometric and isotonic contractions and during passive stretching, facilitates the identification of various muscles, and the recognition of several abnormalities as well as any artifacts. Adhesions, which tend to prevent muscles from sliding smoothly with respect to adjacent structures, can also be detected easily. During dynamic phase studies, the operator must look for movements producing contractions, stretching or shortening in the smallest number of muscles, so that a highly selective evaluation can be made. Comparisons with the contralateral tendon or muscle may be useful, beginning always with the healthy side. Comparative examinations permit the evaluation of muscle trophism, and can speed up the detection of pathologies. However, it should not be forgotten that certain pathological conditions may be bilateral and even symmetrical.

When performing an ultrasound examination, the operator must remember to look at all the other structures closely connected with the muscles, such as blood vessels, nerves, bone margins, bursae and ligaments, which may be present in the area.[1] A good ultrasound study on skeletal muscle should always take into account the results of other imaging techniques, without disregarding the valuable contributions that may be made by conventional radiology (standard X-ray, arthrography, tenography and bursography, xerography). Several more recent methods also have great potential, including infra-red telethermography, CT and MRI. The ultrasound examination must endeavor to identify, quantify and visualize anatomic alterations; when these are interpreted in the light of the clinical findings, it should be possible to identify correctly any existing pathology. The examination must also include the patient report, which constitutes the only information truly accessible to the attending physician, and may be of critical medico-legal importance. The report must specify the region examined, describe the lesion detected (site, extension, US features) and provide an interpretation of the injury; there should also be an evaluation of the adjacent structures, helpful suggestions based on comparative examination methods, and any other recommendations, such as monitoring. The report must be accompanied by photographic documentation (even video recordings), in support of the findings presented, and which will also be critical for later comparisons.[1]

ULTRASONOGRAPHIC ANATOMY

The anatomo-ultrasonographic study of muscles must include an identification of the involved muscles and an evaluation of the relevant muscle structure.[2–4]

Large muscles or muscles surrounded by thick fascia or bone margins are very easy to recognize on ultrasound. It is, however, rather more difficult to detect accurately certain small muscles, delimited by a thin sheath and lying adjacent to other muscles, particularly if they are synergic. In synergic muscles, even the dynamic phase examination may not be able to discriminate between one muscle and another. Hence, sonography may more easily detect anatomic variants, such as the presence of an accessory soleus muscle, or agenesis of the pectoralis major muscle, such as in Poland syndrome. However, at other times it may be very difficult, if not impossible, to distinguish sonographically between muscle hypotrophy and agenesia.

All muscles present the same structural characteristics. They are enclosed by a band of connective tissue, the epimysium. Ultrasound shows the epimysium to be a thin hyperechoic stria, with regular edges, surrounding the muscles and separating them from adjacent structures (Fig. 16.1). The integrity of the epimysium must be evaluated at rest and during active contraction. As well as surrounding and delimiting muscles, the epimysium, lying in close contact with the adjacent structures, also enables the muscles to slide smoothly during the various dynamic phases.

The cleavage plane between two contiguous muscles can generally be recognized as a thin hypoechoic line defined by the epimysium of the two adjacent muscles (see Fig. 16.1). The dynamic phase study enables the operator to check that there are no adhesions between the two planes.

From the epimysium arise several thin connective tissue septa called perimysia, which subdivide the muscle into smaller segments, the tertiary bundles. These are subdivided, in turn, into secondary bundles, which include small groups of functional units – the muscle cells. The

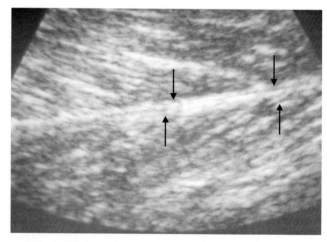

Fig. 16.1 Ultrasound anatomy. Study with a 10 MHz probe shows the comb-like structure of muscle. Hypoechoic cleavage plane between hyperechoic epimysium of two adjacent muscles (arrows).

connective tissue surrounding the muscle cells is called the endomysium.[5] The tertiary bundles are responsible for the typical ultrasound image of muscles. In scans taken along the functional axis of a muscle, the hypoechoic muscle fibers are divided by hyperechoic perimysial connective septa, resulting in the typical 'comb-like' effect (see Fig. 16.1). The echogenicity of a muscle is determined by the alternating pattern of muscle fibers and connective tissue fibers, and by their thickness. The increase in intramuscular fat occurring with advancing age, in certain pathological conditions, or simply resulting from reduced physical activity or weight gain, is very important in determining the enhanced diffuse echogenicity of muscle.[1] The overall echogenicity of muscle partly depends on the angle of incidence of the US beam with respect to the direction of the muscle fibers. This technical detail must be kept clearly in mind during the examination, to avoid incorrect evaluation of muscle echogenicity. The muscle bellies may be divided, or crossed, by well-circumscribed hyperechoic fibrous septa. These must not be confused with the sequelae of trauma which are generally coarser and less regular.

The intrinsic vascularity of muscle is derived from one or more vascular pedicles. The principal arteries run longitudinally through the connective tissue of the perimysium. Only the largest vascular pedicles can be recognized on ultrasound. Similarly, only the largest longitudinal arteries can be seen on ultrasound, particularly those with an adequately long intramuscular portion (Fig. 16.2). Color flow Doppler may facilitate the recognition of intramuscular arteries, even those with a meandering course (Figs 16.3, 16.4).

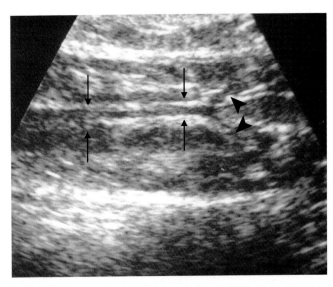

Fig. 16.2 Ultrasound anatomy. Study with a 10 MHz probe. Arteriole with longitudinal intramuscular pathway (arrows). Bifurcation into branches running transversely (arrowheads).

The arteries running through the perimysium give rise to arterioles which penetrate the endomysium and subsequently branch out into capillaries supplying the muscle fibers. Other branches originating from the main arteries run in a transverse direction and remain within the epimysium or perimysium. These vessels anastomose with other arterial branches or shunt directly into veins. They do not supply blood, but permit blood drainage during

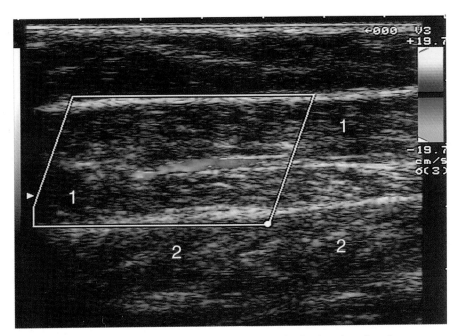

Fig. 16.3 Ultrasound anatomy. Colour flow Doppler permits the detection of small intramuscular arteries. Longitudinal scan. 1: median gemellus muscle; 2: soleus muscle.

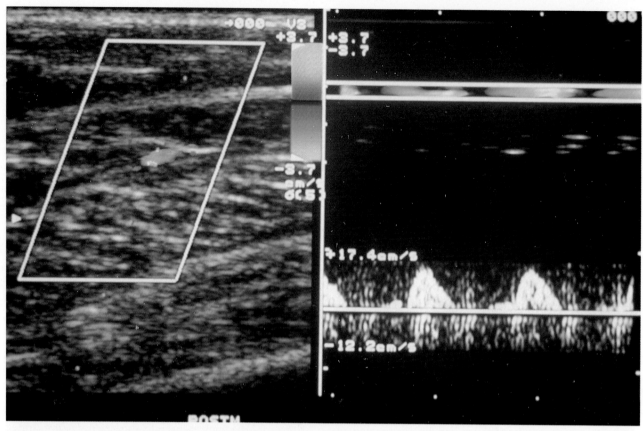

Fig. 16.4 Doppler image of intramuscular artery. Muscle during rest phase.

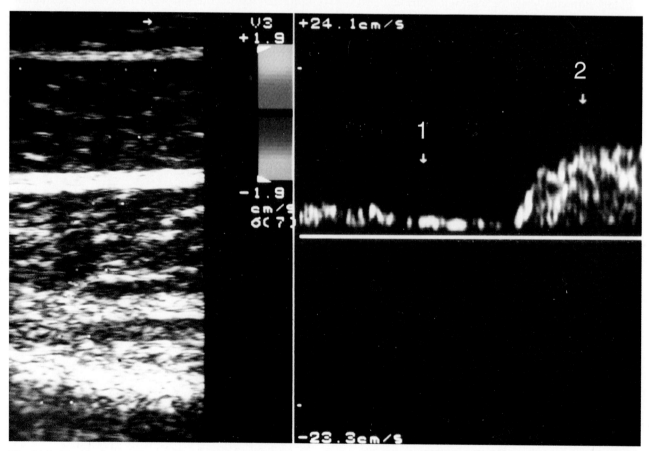

Fig. 16.5 Doppler image of intramuscular artery. Cessation of blood flow during muscle contraction phase (1). Restoration of flow during muscle relaxation phase (2).

contraction, when the trophic circulation is compressed and may become obstructed[5] (Fig. 16.5).

The intramuscular venous vascular tree follows the same course as the arterial system. On ultrasound, veins are even more difficult to detect than arteries; even the light pressure of the probe can cause them to collapse. A tourniquet placed upstream of the examination site will often allow adequate dilation of the intramuscular veins. If this precaution is taken, and the muscle is observed during relaxation, ensuring that the pressure exerted by the probe is minimal, the intramuscular veins can be accurately identified, particularly in certain difficult areas (e.g. the gemellus muscles in the leg) (Fig. 16.6).

The muscle belly is joined to the tendon by means of the connective tissue present in both structures. The muscle cells do not penetrate into the tendon collagen fibers. Some tendons extend for quite a long distance before attaching to the bone margin; others are considerably shorter. The musculotendinous junction is clearly identifiable sonographically when the tendon is a long one. In such cases, the gradual narrowing of the muscle belly and the myotendinal junction are unmistakable. The epimysium appears as a continuation of the outer edge of the tendon. When the tendon is very short, it may be difficult to discern on ultrasound; the muscle fibers appear to attach directly to the bone margin (Fig. 16.7).

The ultrasound examination of muscles must also include a study of all neighboring structures: bone margins, skin, vessels, nerves, bursae and joints.

TRAUMA

Acute muscle trauma

Traumatic muscle damage may be caused by external agents, the mechanism being that of contusion (direct trauma); however, at times no external agent is present (indirect trauma). In indirect trauma, injuries occur due to the excessive contraction or passive extension of muscle. Trauma to muscle is generally described as either 'minor' or 'major', depending on the degree of anatomic damage present. The extent and type of injury affects the prognosis and dictates the treatment options. In minor trauma, there is no macroscopic anatomic damage; such damage is, however, present in major trauma. The clinical symptoms are not always proportional to the degree of anatomic damage. The diagnostic reliability of clinical semeiotics in assessing and quantifying superficial (palpable) muscle injuries is very good, but it cannot document them. The clinical evaluation of deep (non-palpable) muscles must be functional in almost all cases, and therefore is relatively less accurate. The reliability of sonography in detecting and documenting traumatic muscle damage is extremely high and relates closely to the size of the anatomic lesion present.

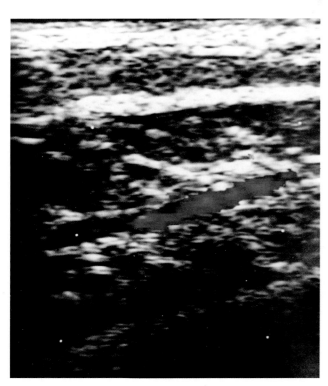

Fig. 16.6 Colour flow Doppler image of intramuscular vein. Muscle relaxed.

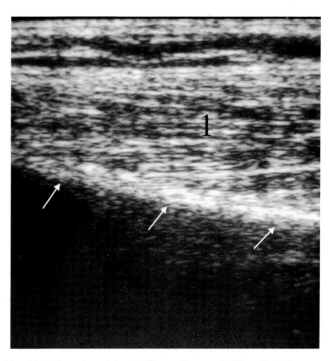

Fig. 16.7 Insertion of the tibialis anterior muscle (1) to the tibia (arrow).

Ultrasound is therefore of great, and acknowledged, help in identifying, quantifying and documenting traumatic lesions, thus permitting appropriate rehabilitative treatment to be embarked upon; this is particularly important for athletes.[6,7]

Minor traumas include slight contusions, contractions and cramps, the 'aching muscles' felt by unfit individuals after strenuous activity, and elongations. No macroscopic anatomic alterations are present, thus there are no significant sonographic findings. More serious contusions or elongations, verging on a partial fracture, may show moderate echographic signs, which usually correspond to the elective pain felt as the probe is passed over the injured area. The lesions that are detectable sonographically may appear weakly echogenic, due to edema, or may present as small hyperechogenic spots produced by recent minimal extravasations (Fig. 16.8), generally associated with slight swelling. The term 'distraction' often generates confusion. Some authors use the term to indicate partial tears caused by indirect trauma (i.e. distractive trauma); others use it to describe an indirect injury to a minimal number of muscle fibers, intermediate between an elongation and a minimal partial rupture.

Major traumas include muscle tears, musculotendinous detachments, and hematomas. Ruptures or detachments may involve only part of the muscle (partial tears) or the whole muscle (total ruptures). Ultrasonography detects any discontinuity in muscle fibers, whether total or partial, and can detect the presence of hematoma at the tear site. Immediately following the trauma, the blood effusion appears strongly echogenic, with ill-defined margins. Several hours later, the appearance of the hematoma is hypo-anechoic due to the development of fluid (partially organized due to the presence of clots), and well defined, with distal wall enhancement. In total or subtotal ruptures, the muscle stumps penetrate the hematoma (Fig. 16.9). In partial tears, sonography can not only detect the site of the injury, but should also endeavor to estimate the percentage of broken fibers: injury to more than two thirds of the muscle can be an indication for surgical repair. This evidence is easy to obtain using axial scans of the muscle. Small partial tears may be more easily detected during contraction or passive extension of the muscle: these movements separate the muscle stumps or broken fibers. There are many particular forms of partial rupture, such as small tears in the intramuscular fibrotic septa or in the vascular hilum of the muscle, where the clinical symptoms are generally severe, apparently far in excess of the anatomic injury detected on ultrasound. In indirect traumas, the muscle stumps are generally well circumscribed, with no evidence of intrinsic abnormalities. In ruptures caused by contusion, not only are there tears in the muscle fibers, but also lesions caused by crushing. On ultrasound the muscle stump fibers appear to be irregular and inhomogeneous. Occasionally evidence is found of irregular muscle fibers that have migrated into the hematoma.

Special attention must be devoted to the US evaluation of muscle injuries following trauma, particularly direct trauma. The hyperechogenicity of the bruise area may easily lead to overestimation of the extent of a contusion, but may also camouflage a partial tear. Therefore, the ultrasound examination must be repeated several days later, in order to make a reliable assessment of the degree and extent of the injury.[1]

In the case of muscle trauma caused by external agents that have also caused skin lesions, the muscle belly may be penetrated by foreign bodies, such as metal or glass fragments, etc. The appearance of foreign bodies that have penetrated muscle has been widely described in the literature,[8] and also in 'in vitro' studies.[9] Depending on their specific nature, foreign bodies appear as echogenic images with reverberations, posterior acoustic shadows and comet tail artifacts. If the examination is performed a long time after the trauma, the strongly echogenic foreign body may be encircled by a hypoechoic rim due to the surrounding granulomatous reaction.

Another form of muscle rupture is the detachment of the muscle belly from the tendon. The US image is identical to that of a muscle belly tear, with broken fibers and hematoma, into which the muscle and tendon stumps penetrate (Fig. 16.10). The muscles most prone to musculotendinous detachments are the median gemellus of the

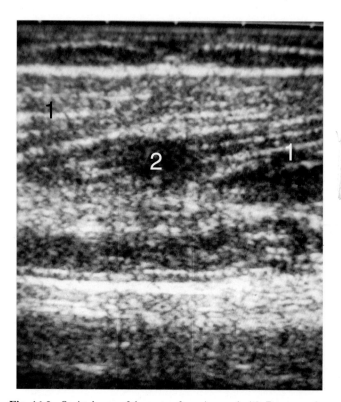

Fig. 16.8 Sagittal scan of the rectus femoris muscle (1). Presence of small lesion (2) caused by contusion.

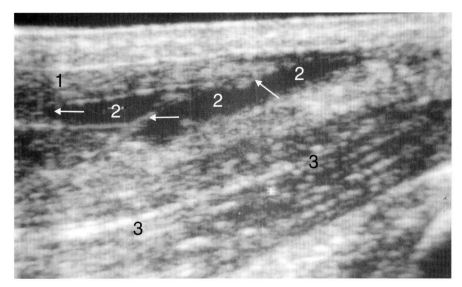

Fig. 16.9 Partial rupture of the distal portion of the vastus lateralis muscle (1). Presence of hematoma (2) with breakage of several muscle fibers (arrows). 3: internal vastus muscle.

lower limb and the biceps brachialis muscle. This type of rupture must be promptly recognized, as it is associated with a distinctly poorer prognosis than a muscle belly tear. Musculotendinous ruptures take longer to heal and also frequently develop serosanguineous cysts and, subsequently, extensive areas of permanent fibrosis.[1]

Intra- or inter-muscular hematomas are classed as major muscle pathologies. They generally occur following muscle tears or musculotendinous detachments. Hematomas may rarely develop between one muscle and another following a traumatic blood vessel rupture. The US appearance of this condition is, in part, identical to that of a muscle tear. After an initial phase, featuring the formation of a hyperechoic hematoma, the area becomes well defined and displays coagulation. The hematoma is more easily detected on ultrasound, its echogenicity weakens, and distal wall enhancement occurs. Several days later, unless it is rapidly absorbed by the healing process, internal lysis tends to transform the hematoma into a serosanguineous cyst. A fluid-filled sac forms, surrounded by its own wall. When the clots have 'dissolved' but before any actual cyst wall has formed, the cyst may be effectively drained.[10] Otherwise, shortly thereafter, the serohematic cyst wall may become consolidated and delay healing even after the cyst has been drained. Ultrasonography can determine exactly when to perform the drainage procedure, i.e. when

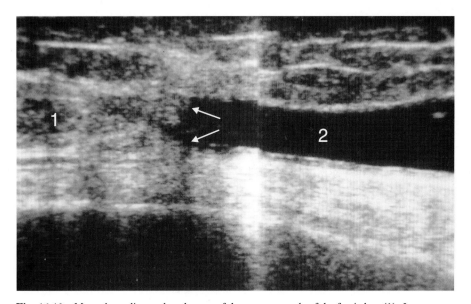

Fig. 16.10 Musculotendinous detachment of the tensor muscle of the fascia lata (1). 2: haematoma.

the contents become anechoic. At this point, the cyst can be drained using a fine needle and the procedure is totally atraumatic. Ultrasound guidance enables the needle to be centered safely and accurately (Fig. 16.11). In trauma due to contusion, and occasionally also to distraction, the structures neighboring the injured muscle are also generally affected, i.e. nerves, blood vessels, bursae and ligaments. The lesser intra- or inter-muscular vessels may be broken or thrombosed and may display wall irregularities. Vessel involvement causes the formation of extensive hematoma. The presence of any sonographically detectable vessel injuries must be very carefully reported and assessed, particularly in the presence of thrombosis, as such findings will have a bearing on treatment. Blood vessels can be examined more easily by color flow Doppler, which is also able to detect any internal thrombi. Artery or vein involvement may lead to the development of an arteriovenous fistula, surrounded by fibrotic tissue originating from a scar reaction or an organized hematoma.[11]

Trauma outcomes

Muscle trauma may heal with complete *restitutio ad integrum*. In such cases, the hematoma is gradually reabsorbed and the partially undifferentiated syncytial cells restore the continuity of the muscle fibers. A partial muscle tear takes about three weeks to heal. A good correlation exists between the ultrasound findings and the progressive anatomo-pathologic recovery.[12] The healing process generally results in complete recovery of muscle integrity, for smaller lesions. Painful sequelae may remain even after the US examination no longer reveals evidence of alterations in echo structure.

When injuries are more extensive, a *fibrous scar* forms. Small areas of fibrosis, initially hypoechoic and subsequently hyperechoic, may form within the muscle belly (Fig. 16.11C), or may spread throughout the muscle, especially after extensive contusive ruptures followed by a long period of inactivity. Special attention should be paid to a particular form of muscle fibrosis – that of the sternocleidomastoid muscle, which causes congenital myogenic torticollis. In this case, the onset of the fibrosis may occur during the intrauterine development of the fetus, or in the early postnatal period as a result of muscle trauma during delivery. It is difficult to distinguish the two forms clinically during the first few days after birth. A US examination during the early neonatal period may detect an injury caused by perinatal trauma and guide treatment to prevent the onset of fibrosis. Fibrous, poorly elastic areas reduce muscle function and may generate further ruptures some time later and in different sites. Scarring fibrous tissue may be present between muscles, and between muscle and subcutaneous tissue or bone. In such cases the muscle does not slide correctly in relation to the structure which it is adhering to by fibrosis. Sonography not only documents the fibrosis, but, during dynamic phase studies, can also detect functional damage caused by the adhesions.

Complications associated with the evolution of muscle trauma include organized hematomas, serohematic cysts, calcifications and ossifications, and muscle hernias. An incorrectly treated or overlooked hematoma may become organized or evolve into a serosanguineous cyst. *Organized hematomas* appear on ultrasound as solid, inhomogeneous and generally well-defined masses. The US finding of an organized hematoma may simulate a neoplasm. Anamnestic data generally enable an accurate interpretation to be made.

Serohematic cysts have thin, generally regular walls, and contain serous fluid. Ultrasound can easily recognize them as anechoic formations with fairly distinct walls, occasionally containing thin strands of fibrin.

Calcium salts are commonly deposited in injured muscles, often within days of the trauma. Small *calcifications* are generally reabsorbed during healing. However, if there are permanent fibrous areas that have been inadequately treated, or the patients have predisposing factors such as young age, metabolic disorders or longstanding inactivity, the calcium salt deposits may develop into intramuscular calcifications. Ultrasonography identifies these as hyperechoic areas with posterior acoustic shadows. The US examination cannot distinguish between calcification and *muscular ossification*, which may also develop following an injury (circumscribed myositis ossificans), particularly in younger patients and when the injury site is close to the bone margins. The US findings are similar in both cases. Occasionally, the position of the periosteum may arouse suspicion of ossification; however, only an X-ray can detect newly formed bone tissue and differentiate it from a calcification. Although sonographically indistinguishable, calcifications and ossifications are two histologically different entities: calcifications are caused when calcium salts are deposited in fibrous tissue, while ossification takes place when muscle tissue undergoes osseous metaplasia.

Under certain conditions muscle tissue can even differentiate into bone tissue.[13] Ossifications are disabling for athletes, restricting muscle movement and elasticity. Eventually, post-traumatic ossifications tend to be reabsorbed, whilst calcifications tend to become permanent.

Unless properly treated, muscle fascia injuries may give rise to muscle belly hernias. On ultrasound, the lesion appears as a gap in the epimysium with muscle tissue protruding through it (Fig. 16.12).

INFLAMMATORY CONDITIONS

Rhabdomyolysis

Rhabdomyolysis is a rare condition. Its etiology seems to have no common denominator. The condition may develop

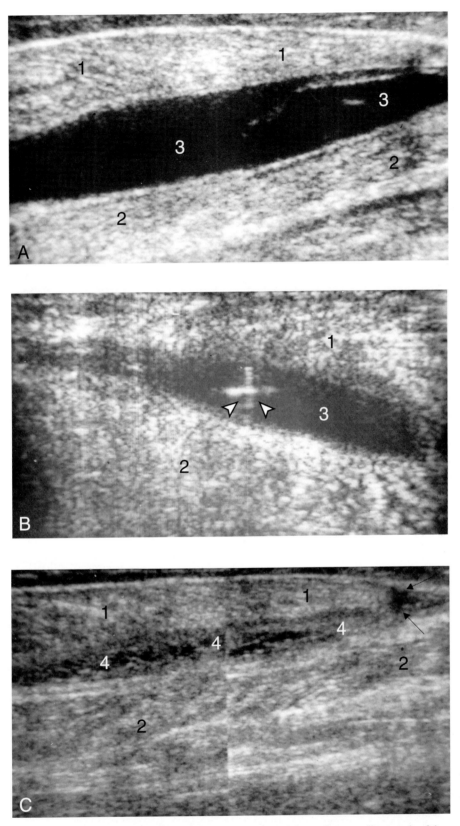

Fig. 16.11   Partial musculotendinous detachment (arrow) of the median gemellus muscle of the leg (1). 2: soleus muscle. **A** Sagittal scan. Presence of haematoma (3) undergoing lysis (10 days following trauma). **B** Axial scan. US-guided fine-needle aspiration of the hematoma. Arrowhead: needle tip. **C** Sagittal scan. After emptying of the hematoma the gemellus and soleus muscles appear closer together, separated only by several clots and by early-forming scar tissue (4).

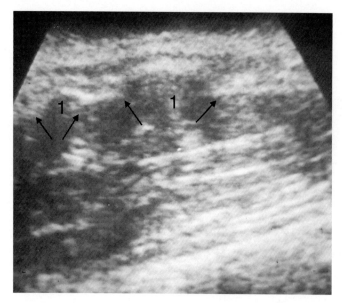

Fig. 16.12 Two small muscle hernias (1) with evident rupture of the epimysium (arrow).

following trauma (surgery possibly due to the prolonged compression of several muscles) and also intoxication. Frequently no apparent cause can be identified. The diagnosis is made primarily on the basis of clinical findings (i.e. pain) and laboratory findings (myohemoglobinuria, CPK elevation, LDH, aldolase). Ultrasound reveals increased muscle volume, elective pain on placing the US probe on the affected area, hypoechoic zones with diffuse and irregular internal echoes, and disruption of the normal muscle architecture, without formation of pus[14] (Fig. 16.13). After approximately two weeks, the US follow-up reveals a gradual reappearance of the normal muscle structure, which is complete within three or four weeks.

Myositis

The term myositis is used to describe all muscle lesions of inflammatory etiology, including acute, chronic, exudative, suppurative and granulomatous forms. The etiology may be viral (Coxsackie B), bacterial (Staphylococcus, Streptococcus, Clostridium, BK), or parasitic (cysticercosis, hydatidosis).

Diffuse muscle pain appears and may last for several days, often accompanying a wide range of viral, bacterial and parasitic infections, and even chronic rheumatic disorders. These forms of myalgia doubtless have an inflammatory origin, but do not produce sonographically detectable signs.

Acute suppurative forms are often associated with injuries featuring skin lesions and direct contamination of the muscle, and include iatrogenic abscesses developing after muscle surgery. The clinical manifestations are typical of acute infection, featuring pain, burning sensation, reddening of the overlying skin, and functional limitation. During the onset of the abscess, ultrasound reveals a slightly hypoechoic area with irregular and ill-defined margins; the typical 'comb' structure of the muscle gradually disappears. During the pus-forming phase, a central hypo-anechoic area appears, containing some fluctuating echoes, with posterior enhancement; the margins of the lesion become more distinct (Fig. 16.14). If gas-producing anaerobes are present, it is possible to recognize bubbles in the pus collection (Fig. 16.15).

Abscesses can generally be diagnosed on the basis of clinical findings. Ultrasonography can be useful for detecting the extent of the abscess, particularly if it is very deep, and for recognizing the colliquative phase, when drainage is required. When the abscess is deep, sonography can effectively guide the placement of a drainage needle or catheter. It should be stressed that both primary and metastatic soft tissue malignancies may develop abscesses; these should not be misdiagnosed as simple suppurative forms. In such cases, a painless swelling generally precedes the first signs of inflammation. Moreover, the ultrasound examination can detect the suppurative area of the lesion, but a solid, infiltrating border is also evident.

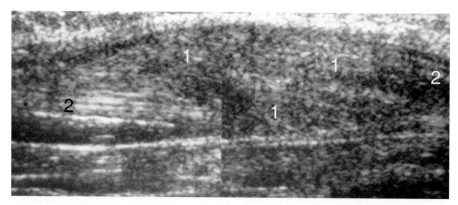

Fig. 16.13 Sagittal scan. Rhabdomyolysis with evidence of hypoechoic area (1) showing disruption of normal muscle architecture. 2: brachial triceps muscle.

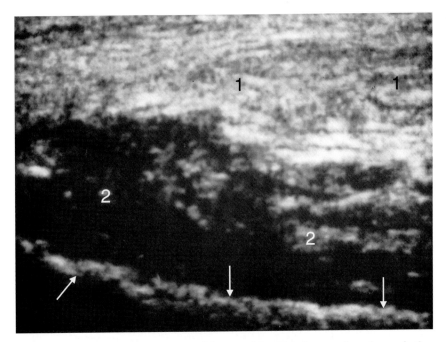

Fig. 16.14 Longitudinal anterior scan of the root of the thigh. 1: rectus femoris muscle. 2: colliquative abscess of the internal vastus muscle. Arrows: anterior margin of the femur.

Chronic exudative-suppurative forms are generally associated with osteomyelitis, or with infected bone prostheses, and are characterized by a collection of fluid with minimal pain in the soft tissues adjoining the infection site. The fluid sac tends to form a fistula with the skin by means of a thin passage that is recognizable on the US image as a hypoechoic line with a diameter of 0.5–1 cm. No fluid can be visualized in the fistula once it has been drained, since the walls collapse. The fistula may be quite long and run from the site of the infection to sloping parts. Ultrasound is valuable in recognizing the entire length of the fistula and in ascertaining its reabsorption once the opening on to the skin has closed.

Parasitic infections due to Echinococcus tapeworms are identified by the typical formation of hydatid cysts; they have the same ultrasound characteristics as in the more typical abdominal localization.

In cysticercosis the parasitic lesions appear as hyper-

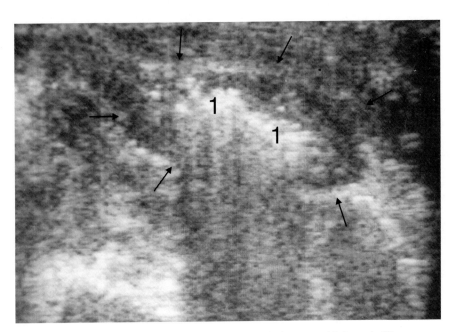

Fig. 16.15 Muscle abscess (arrows) caused by gas-producing anaerobic bacteria (1).

echoic nodular lesions with posterior acoustic shadows. Generally multiple, and measuring up to 1 cm in diameter, these lesions must be distinguished from post-traumatic calcifications. In doubtful cases, the X-ray pattern is usually decisive.

Myositis may also be of immunologic etiology, and it is commonly diagnosed in patients affected by diffuse connective tissue disorders: schleroderma, dermatomyositis, periarteritis nodosa, rheumatoid polyarthritis, diffuse lupus erythematosus, and AIDS. Sonography provides little significant evidence, detecting only moderate increases in muscle volume at the affected site, and a slight reduction in its echogenicity.

DEGENERATIVE DISORDERS

The term 'degenerative' is applied to a group of diseases of unrelated etiology and pathogenesis, with no evidence of inflammatory, traumatic or neoplastic origin, involving the gradual destruction of muscle tissue and its progressive replacement with fibroadipose tissue. The muscle loses its elasticity and its ability to contract, i.e. it loses its function.

Progressive or malignant progressive myositis ossificans is a hereditary syndrome, encountered more frequently in males, which appears at around 10 years of age, and is characterized by inflammation of the muscle tissues followed immediately by ossification of the muscles themselves. The ossification gradually spreads to the tendons and fasciae. No ultrasound findings have been described of this rare disorder, which must, however, be kept in mind when making a differential diagnosis of post-traumatic ossi-

fication, since the ultrasound image of early stage progressive myositis ossificans is very likely to resemble closely that of the benign post-traumatic form.

In amyotrophic disorders, the muscle cells gradually shrink in volume and, later, in number. The muscle becomes increasingly smaller, more fibrous and less elastic. Sonography reveals the muscle to be smaller than normal, and smaller than the contralateral muscle. It should be noted, however, that some forms are bilateral, therefore US findings based on a comparison between two sides may be misleading. The muscles are also hyperechoic and show a reduction in the thickness and number of hypoechoic lines corresponding to muscle fibers (Fig. 16.16). The causes may be myogenic (myopathy, Steinert's disease, dermatopolymyositis, concomitance with metabolic and endocrine disorders) or neurogenic (central or peripheral denervation). In any case, US findings are not diagnostic in the early stages and may be helpful only in monitoring the course of the disease, i.e. providing documentation of the progressive onset of muscle fibrosis.

Muscular dystrophies are characterized by the progressive destruction of muscle fibers. Genetic diseases and disorders classified into a wide variety of forms, based on the age of onset and the different muscles involved (Duchenne's, limb-girdle, Landouzy–Dejerine's facioscapulohumeral, Erb-type scapulohumeral, Gowers' distal limb muscular dystrophy), all lead to the same type of muscle damage. In the early stages, there is minimal fiber destruction, with relative hypertrophy of the healthy fibers, producing a finding of pseudohypertrophy. During this phase the muscle is normal in size or slightly enlarged, but with poor contractile capability, supported only by a few

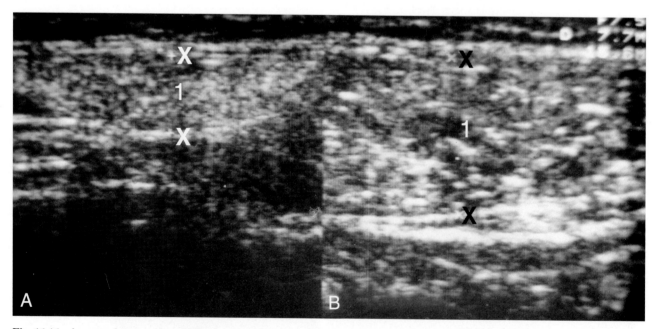

Fig. 16.16 Amyotrophy caused by peripheral denervation of the right rectus abdominis muscle (1). **A** Axial scan of the right rectus abdominis muscle. **B** Axial scan of the left rectus abdominis muscle.

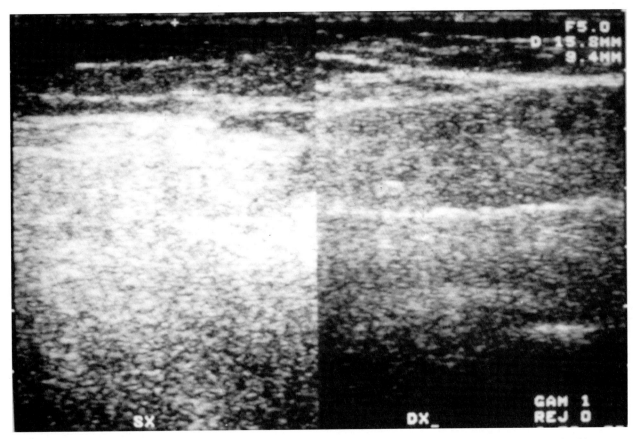

Fig. 16.17 Muscular dystrophy (Becker's type), grade 7 (according to Vignos scale) on the left side and grade 5 on the right side.

hypertrophic fibers. More and more fibers progressively degenerate, until eventually all muscle function is lost. The muscle becomes smaller and the muscle fibers are gradually replaced by fibrous tissue and fat. The ultrasound findings are identical in all forms, displaying the anatomic alterations described above. During the pseudohypertrophic phase, the dimensions of the muscle may be unchanged; the hypoechoic spaces may increase, with hyperechoic areas separating them. The muscle later develops a patchy appearance, with ill-defined hyper- and hypo-echoic areas. In the more advanced stages, the muscle has a hyperechoic, finely inhomogeneous structure, with no evidence of the typical 'comb' pattern (Fig. 16.17) and marked attenuation of the ultrasound beam. The subcutaneous fat layer remains generally unaffected. The typical US pattern reported in the literature appears:[15–17] reversal in the normal thickness ratio of muscle to fat, increase in the echogenicity of the muscle, and disappearance of the underlying bone margin (Fig. 16.18). Sonography is of little or no help for diagnostic purposes: evidence of macroscopic anatomic muscle alterations can be achieved, but only once the clinical symptoms have become quite marked. Ultrasound may accurately document the distribution of the disease, monitor its progression, and help to locate the best site for a biopsy,[18] which is essential for a reliable diagnosis.

SOFT TISSUE NEOPLASMS

Muscle neoplasms include a wide range of histologic forms. This is because muscle contains many different tissues, e.g. muscle cells, blood vessels, nerves, fasciae. Each may give rise to benign or malignant neoplasms.

Although many ultrasound studies on muscle tumors have been reported in the literature,[19] in reality ultrasound is an unreliable method for histologic typing of such tumors. Ultrasound's ability to detect muscle tumors has always been considered to be excellent, if not absolute, even with now obsolete US equipment.[20,21] However, it should be kept in mind that by the time the patient undergoes sonographic examination, the neoplasm, be it benign or malignant, is generally already clearly palpable.

The various histologic types of *benign muscle tumors* are indicated in Table 16.1. The commonest among these are the lipoma, fibroid, neurinoma and angioma. Fibroids generally develop in the fasciae, and therefore are extramuscular; they are frequently multiple (fibromatosis). Lipomas and angiomas may be intrafascial, but extramuscular or intramuscular; in other words, they may be enclosed by muscle fascia without involving the muscle itself, or develop within the muscle, between the muscle fasciae. The sonographic pattern of both lipomas[22] and

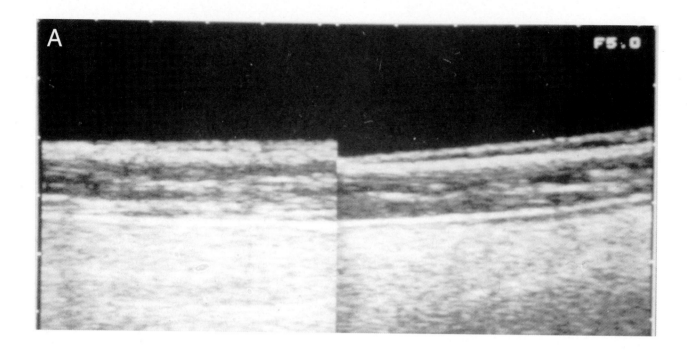

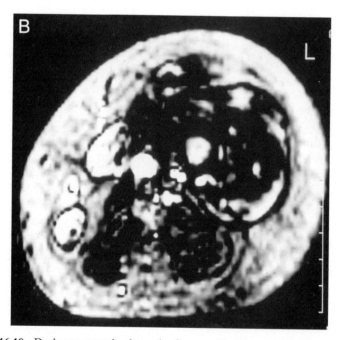

Fig. 16.18 Duchenne muscular dystrophy. Sonographic (**A**) and MRI (**B**) appearance.

Table 16.1 Histologic classification of soft tissue tumors

Original tissue	Benign	Malignant
Osseous	Myositis ossificans	Extraosseous osteosarcoma
Cartilaginous	Chondroma	Chondrosarcoma
Fibrous	Fibroid tumor	Fibrosarcoma Malignant histiocytoma
Synovial membrane	Pigmented synovitis Synovial cysts	Synovial sarcoma
Adipose	Lipoma	Liposarcoma
Muscular	Myoma	Myosarcoma
Vascular	Angioma	Angiosarcoma
Nervous	Neurofibroma	Neurofibrosarcoma

angiomas[23] may be hyper- or hypoechoic with respect to the surrounding muscle tissue (Figs 16.19, 16.20), with neither form prevailing over the other to any statistically significant extent. Growth is not always intracapsular, and the appearance of the margins is strongly influenced by the structure in which the tumor is located, i.e. a lipoma enveloped by muscle fascia will show irregular margins on ultrasound. Ultrasonography is thus very reliable in detecting benign tumors, and can be helpful in locating the exact position of the neoplasm and describing its relationship with neighboring elements, thus facilitating the planning of any surgical procedure that may be required.

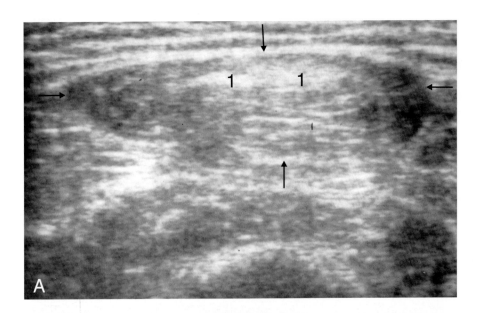

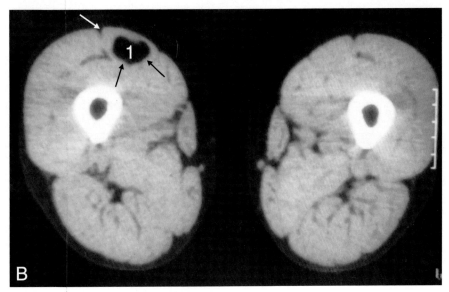

Fig. 16.19 Lipoma (1) of the rectus femoris muscle (arrow).
A Ultrasound axial scan. **B** CT scan.

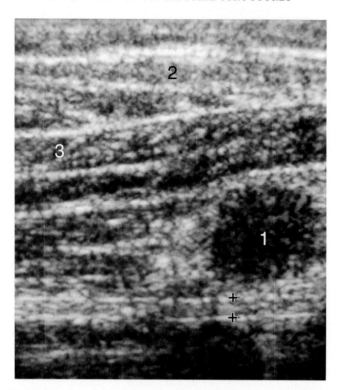

Fig. 16.20 Posterior sagittal scan of the leg. Angioma (1) immediately adjacent to the posterior tibial nerve (+ ... +). 2: gemellus muscle; 3: soleus muscle.

Sonography is, however, less reliable in the histologic typing of benign tumors. There are no pathognomonic ultrasound criteria for determining the benign nature of a neoplasm, only orientative criteria, such as small size, regular margins, hyperechoic structure, location in a single anatomic compartment, and absence of necrotic areas. A very distinctive form of soft tissue benign neoplasm is the desmoid tumor. This tumor is cytologically benign, but tends to infiltrate the surrounding tissues, thus displaying histologic malignancy. Recurrences are common after surgical removal, but distant metastases are infrequent. Desmoid tumors initially develop in fibrous tissue, generally in the muscle fasciae or musculotendinous junctions. They occur most frequently in women, during or following pregnancy, and are located predominantly in the anterior abdominal wall. The tumor may thus be mistaken, both clinically and on ultrasound, for an organized hematoma of the abdominal wall following trauma during delivery. The desmoid tumor appears on ultrasound as a hypoechoic mass, well-defined from outside the fascia of origin, and occasionally presenting recognizable signs of infiltration into the adjacent tissues, but always remaining within the fascia. When US-guided biopsy of a desmoid tumor is performed, the histologic sample must be taken from the periphery of the neoplasm; samples taken from the central portion of the neoplasm are not significant, and only show evidence of mesenchymal tissue with no cellular abnormalities.

Malignant muscle tumors are all described as sarcomas, regardless of their histologic tissue of origin. These neoplasms are often very difficult to dissociate from the other tissues in which they are embedded or which they have invaded. Often, indeed in up to 38% of the cases reported in the literature, such sarcomas are undifferentiated; in other words, the tissue of origin cannot be identified. Sarcomas account for 1.5% of all malignant neoplasms.[24] The most widely used staging method for soft tissue sarcomas is based primarily on clinical and surgical considerations,[25] i.e. on assessment of local tumor dissemination (T), degree of aggressiveness (G) and metastatic spread (M) (Table 16.2). The extent of local dissemination (T) allows the primary localization to be classified as intracapsular (T0), extracapsular but intracompartmental (T1), or extracompartmental (T2). The compartment represents an area well defined by anatomic structures such as fasciae or periosteum. The tumor may be classed as extracompartmental if it spreads beyond the limits of its compartment of origin, or develops in areas not entirely enclosed by fasciae (e.g. hamstrings, armpits, groin).[26] Ultrasonography is 90% accurate in diagnosing such tumors, distinguishing between a compartmental or extracompartmental site, and determining whether the tumor is benign or malignant. The same considerations made in relation to benign tumors also apply here: by the time the patient undergoes the US examination, the neoplasm is generally already clinically detectable and is thus visible on ultrasound. Any invasion of bone can easily be documented by ultrasound, which immediately identifies discontinuities in the regular hyperechoic lines corresponding to the bone margins. Even major vessel involvement can generally be well documented by color Doppler, either in the case of the neoplasm spreading from the vessel wall[27] or due to extrinsic neoplastic invasion. Ultrasonography is of limited value in the case of initial bone and vessel invasion, and must therefore be augmented with X-rays, CT scan and, if necessary, angiography. MRI provides a good 'panoramic' view of the extension of the sarcoma and surrounding structures, but the technique is still not widely available and its costs are extremely high; as a result MRI cannot yet be recommended as the method of choice and first approach in the study of soft tissue

Table 16.2 Anatomo-surgical staging in malignant musculoskeletal tumors

Stage	Grade	Site	Metastasis
IA	G1	T1	M0
IB	G1	T2	M0
IIA	G2	T1	M0
IIB	G2	T2	M0
IIIA	G1/2	T1	M1
IIIB	G1/2	T2	M1

G1: low grade of malignancy; G2: high grade of malignancy; T1: intracompartmental; T2: extracompartmental; M0: absence of metastasis; M1: presence of metastasis.

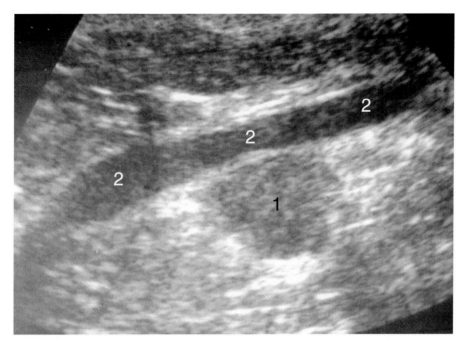

Fig. 16.21 Sagittal scan of the elbow. Sarcoma (1) of the brachialis muscle, very close to the cephalic vein (2).

swellings. The method is therefore still being treated as a second-level examination, to be used in selected cases.[28] Sarcomas commonly appear on ultrasound as hypoechoic, inhomogeneous masses containing extensive hypo-anechoic necrotic changes. The margins are, by definition, irregular (Fig. 16.21), but such characteristics may be masked by the presence of reactive pseudocapsules in the smaller neoplasms, or of anatomic structures such as fasciae or bone margins, which may partly but only transiently obstruct the spread of the tumor and thus simulate an apparently sharp border. Colour Doppler has been used in the study of soft tissue sarcomas,[29] but the results so far have not been significant. Several reports have described generic parameters such as increased vascularity and reduced resistance, however the method is still being developed and more extensive experience will be required before its true value can be judged.

Muscle infiltration by an adjacent sarcoma causes irregular muscle sliding, and this can be detected effortlessly during dynamic phase ultrasound testing, even when the degree of infiltration is only moderate.

The aggressiveness of the tumor is assessed according to its histologic characteristics and clinical behavior. Ultrasonography does not provide a valuable contribution in this regard, but it can effectively guide biopsies. Histologic assessment obviously requires a sample to be collected from the neoplasm; biopsy may comprise an open incision or excision, or may involve percutaneous fine-needle aspiration, for cytologic or histologic examination. When performing an ultrasound-guided percutaneous biopsy, the shortest route should always be chosen, through the smallest possible number of organs, and avoiding any large bundles of vessels and nerves. The pathway of the needle must be surgically removed en bloc with the tumor, therefore the needle entrance must be located on the surgical incision line; alternatively, the needle pathway must be accurately reported to the surgeon (by tattooing it on the skin). It is essential for biopsies to be taken from soft tissue tumors not only to ascertain the degree of aggressiveness of the growth, but also to determine origin, as metastases often spread to soft tissues from tumors of other organs (lung, breast, thyroid). Ultrasonography does not possess reliable diagnostic criteria for differentiating a primary tumor from a metastatic one, although some guidelines are reported in the literature for secondary forms (smaller size, better defined margins, more homogeneous echo structure, multifocal (Fig. 16.22). In general, fine-needle biopsy for cytologic testing can differentiate between a primary and a secondary tumor, but this method is rarely sufficient for staging the histotype or aggressiveness of a primary sarcoma. For such evaluations, a histologic sample is mandatory. When the neoplasm affects both the muscle and the neighboring bone tissue, both sonography and X-rays are seldom able to determine its origin, and only histologic sampling can clarify the situation. In such cases, X-rays and ultrasound are complementary in detecting the intra- and extraosseous spread of the tumor, respectively (Fig. 16.23).

When both methods are integrated, it is generally possible to diagnose even rare forms of circumscribed non-

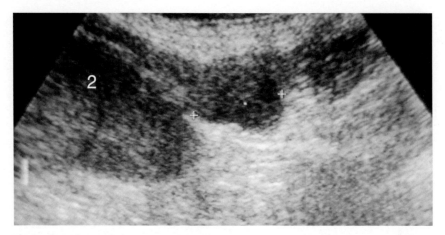

Fig. 16.22   Metastasis (+ ... +) originating from carcinoma of the kidney, in the muscle wall of the abdomen. 2: spleen.

traumatic myositis ossificans. This disease, affecting mainly young people, involves the proximal portions of the limbs; the tumor grows quite quickly and painlessly in the muscle tissue, and is clinically hard and fixed. These factors guide the clinical diagnosis toward a sarcomatous form. Sonography detects an intramuscular mass, highly inhomogeneous due to the presence of bone tissue, and hyperechoic, with posterior acoustic shadow. These findings cannot permit distinction from an extraosseous osteosarcoma. X-rays may detect regular bone margins and thus lead to an accurate diagnosis. If suspicions persist, a biopsy is required.

It should be noted that biopsy punctures, when performed in neurinomas, may be extremely painful and generate clinically significant vagal reactions, even if a fine needle is employed.

Ultrasonography is unquestionably the method of choice for evaluating *neoplastic relapses* deriving from soft tissue sarcomas following treatment. The method is highly reliable in recognizing recurrences and differentiating them from scar tissue, and outperforms CT, even when contrast medium is employed.[30] Ultrasonography can, in fact, identify minimal alterations which would otherwise require high-resolution CT for their detection. Sutures and metal staples can create interference in the CT examination, but they do not generate artifacts on ultrasound. Relapses examined on ultrasound appear as hypoechoic, homogeneous masses (Fig. 16.24), generally well defined by the surrounding scarring fibrous tissue; conversely, recurrences studied by CT show enhancement and this tends to produce overstaging, generating the appearance of irregular margins. This is particularly problematic shortly after surgery, when

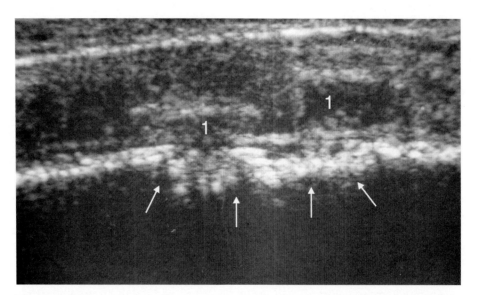

Fig. 16.23   Extraosseous Ewing's sarcoma (1), originating from the fibula (arrows) and displaying irregular margins.

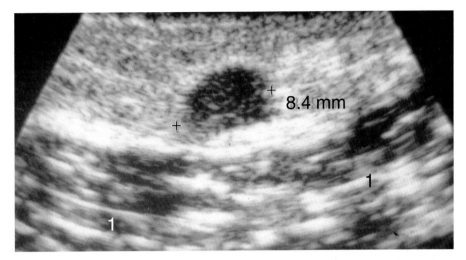

Fig. 16.24   Sagittal scan of the thigh. Relapse of sarcoma (+ ... +). 1: vastus medialis muscle.

the fibrous granulation tissue is highly vascularized. Even MRI, which is a highly sensitive technique for detecting sarcoma recurrences in soft tissues in the presence of stabilized scars, shares the same drawbacks indicated earlier for CT in the evaluation of early relapses, even if para-

magnetic contrast medium is used (gadolinium).[31] However, this early period is also the most crucial for detecting recurrences, since at this stage they can still be surgically removed.

REFERENCES

1. Laurac J, Felix F 1989 Echographie en pathologie musculaire et tendineuse. Vigot, Paris
2. Fornage B D 1987 Echographie du systeme musculo tendineux des membres. Vigot, Paris
3. Lefebvre E, Pourcelot L 1991 Echographie musculo-tendineuse. Masson, Paris
4. Harcke T H, Grisson L E, Finkelstein M S 1988 Evaluation of the musculoskeletal system with sonography. AJR 150: 1253–1261
5. Netter F H 1988 Musculoskeletal system: anatomy, physiology, and metabolic disorders. Ciba-Geigy, Varese
6. Leonardi M, Ulivi M, Balconi G 1983 L'esame ecotomografico in patologia dello sport. Ital J Sports Traumatol 5: 49–58
7. Pfister A 1987 Experimental and clinic results of ultrasound imaging in sports orthopedic soft tissue diseases. Sportverlets Sportschaden 1: 130–141
8. Fornage B D, Schernberg F L 1986 Sonographic diagnosis of foreign bodies of the distal extremities. AJR 147: 567–569
9. De Flaviis L, Scaglione P, Del Bò P 1988 Detection of foreign bodies in soft tissues: experimental comparison of ultrasonography and xeroradiography. J Trauma 28: 400–404
10. Christensen R A, Van Sonnenberg E, Casola G et al 1988 Interventional ultrasound in the musculoskeletal system. Radiol Clin North Am 26: 145–156
11. Helvie M A, Rubin J M 1989 Evaluation of traumatic groin arteriovenous fistulas with duplex doppler sonography. J Ultrasound Med 8: 21–24
12. Letho M, Alanen A 1987 Healing of a muscle trauma. Correlation of sonographical and histological findings in an experimental study in rats. J Ultrasound Med 6: 425–429
13. Khouri K R, Koudsi B, Reddi H 1991 Tissue transformation into bone: in vivo potential practical application. JAMA 266: 1953–1955
14. Kaplan G N 1980 Ultrasonic appearance of rhabdomyolysis. AJR 134: 375–377
15. Kamala D, Suresh S, Githa K 1985 Real-time ultrasonography in neuromuscular problems of children. JCU 13: 465–468
16. Heckmatt J Z, Pier N, Dubowitz A 1988 Assessment of quadriceps femoris muscle atrophy and hypertrophy in neuromuscular disease in children. JCU 16: 177–181
17. Forst R, Casser H R 1985 7-MHz real-time sonographie der skelettmuskulatur bei Duchenne muskeldystrophie. Ultraschall 6: 336–340
18. Heckmatt J Z, Dubowitz V 1985 Diagnostic advantage of needle muscle biopsy and ultrasound imaging in the detection of focal pathology in a girl with limb-girdle dystrophy. Muscle Nerve 8: 705–709
19. Peetrons P, Stienon M, Carrier L et al 1984 Ultrasonographie des sarcomes des tissues musculaires. JEMU: J Echograph Med Ultrasons 5: 305–310
20. Bernardino M E, Jing B S, Thomas J L 1981 The extremity soft tissue lesions: a comparative study of ultrasound, computed tomography, and xeroradiography. Radiology 139: 53–59
21. Braunstein E M, Silver T M, Martel W et al 1981 Ultrasonographic diagnosis of extremity masses. Skeletal Radiol 6:157
22. Fornage B D, Tassin G B 1991 Sonographic appearances of superficial soft tissue lipomas. JCU 19: 215–220
23. Derchi L E, Balconi G, De Flaviis L, Oliva A, Rosso F 1989 Sonographic appearances of hemangiomas of skeletal muscle. J Ultrasound Med 8: 263–267
24. Enzinger F M, Weiss S W 1983 Soft-tissue tumours. Mosby, St Louis
25. Enneking W F 1985 Staging of musculo skeletal neoplasm. Skeletal Radiol 13: 183–184
26. Netter F H 1991 Musculoskeletal system: developmental disorders, tumors, rheumatic diseases, and joint replacement. Ciba-Geigy, Varese
27. Gramith F, Smith L 1989 Ultrasound demonstration of a superficial femoral artery leiomyosarcoma. J Ultrasound Med 1988 5: 269–272
28. Demas B, Heelen R, Lane J et al 1988 Soft-tissue sarcomas of the extremities: comparison of MR and CT in determining the extent of disease. AJR 150: 615–620
29. Mitchell D G, Merton D A, Liu J B, Goldberg B B 1991 Superficial masses with color flow doppler imaging. JCU 19: 555

30. Tregnaghi A, Bidoli L, De Candia A et al 1992 Confronto tra ecografia e Tomografia Computerizzata nella valutazione delle recidive neoplastiche dei tessuti molli superficiali. Radiol Med 84: 204–207

31. Erlemann R, Reiser M F, Peters P E et al 1989 Musculoskeletal neoplasms: static and dynamic Gd-DTPA-enhanced MR imaging. Radiology 171: 767–773

17

Tendons

L. De Pra   G. Monetti   L. E. Derchi

ANATOMIC CONSIDERATIONS

Tendons are white fibrous cords of variable length and thickness, with either a round or flattened shape, which have the function of connecting the muscle bellies to movable structures such as bones and cartilages. Transmission of the force created in the muscles is made possible by the considerable strength and lack of elasticity of tendons. Tendons are composed of collagen fibres oriented in different planes, but preponderantly along the longitudinal axis. The fibres are united and bound together in a three-dimensional network of endotendineum septa originating from a fine connective tissue sheath, called epitenon, which surrounds the whole tendon. In large tendons, blood vessels, nerves and lymphatics run within these septa, while small tendons are almost avascular.

Tendons are of varying lengths and may run within specialized sheaths which allow them to move freely with respect to surrounding structures.

Long tendons running in osteofibrous canals are surrounded by a fluid-filled synovial sheath which facilitates free tendon movement and variably extends both upwards and downwards the canal. Long tendons which are not surrounded by synovia lie within a highly vascularized, loose areolar and adipose tissue, called paratenon.

ULTRASOUND ANATOMY

All normal long tendons are highly echogenic structures, with either an elongated or rounded shape, according to

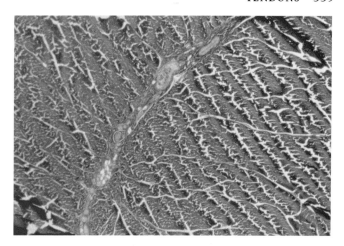

Fig. 17.2 Histologic specimen of a tendon displaying the arrangement of the fibrils surrounded by the endotendineum septa.

the scan plane used to image them; they exhibit an echo texture made up of many fine, parallel and longitudinally specular echoes resembling fibrils (Fig. 17.1). Fibrils are more numerous and thin and easy to distinguish one from another as the frequency used to image the tendon is increased[1] Fibrils are aligned along both the longitudinal and transverse axes of the tendon and their appearance thus represents superimposed planes rather than superimposed lines.[2] Histologic correlation has shown that the echoes correspond to the endotendineum septa running within the tendon[3] (Fig. 17.2).

The hyperechoic appearance of tendons can be dem-

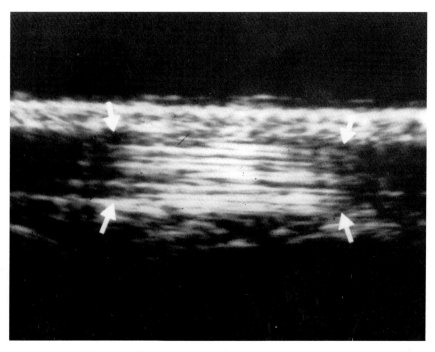

Fig. 17.1 15 MHz longitudinal scan of a superficial tendon (arrows), obtained in vivo. The typical fibrillar structure of the tendon is clearly visible.

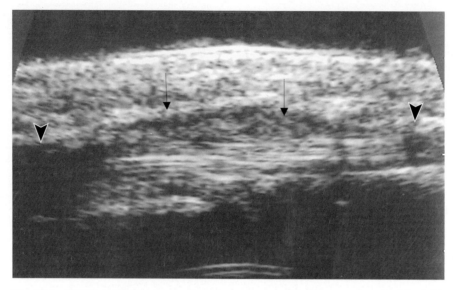

Fig. 17.3 20 MHz longitudinal scan of an extensor tendon of the fingers at the wrist. The fluid-filled synovial sheath (arrow) in the central portion of the tendon and the thin paratenon (arrowhead) proximally and distally are visible.

onstrated only when the US beam has a 90° angle of incidence on fibrils running within them. Even slight obliquity of the angle of incidence results in a hypoechoic appearance which obscures textural details and may even mimic tendinous disease.[4] This artifact is well demonstrated when tendons are examined with sector probes: the hyperechoic pattern is visible only in the center of the image and a false hypoechoic structure appears on both lateral portions.

The small amount of fluid which is normally contained within the synovial membrane is visible, on US images, as a thin hypoechoic rim, surrounding the hyperechoic tendon. In a sagittal scan of the dorsal region of the wrist, along the course of an extensor tendon of the fingers, the difference between the part of the tendon surrounded by the synovial sheath and that surrounded only by the paratenon can be easily appreciated (Fig. 17.3). Tendons without synovial sheaths, like the Achilles tendon, are sur-

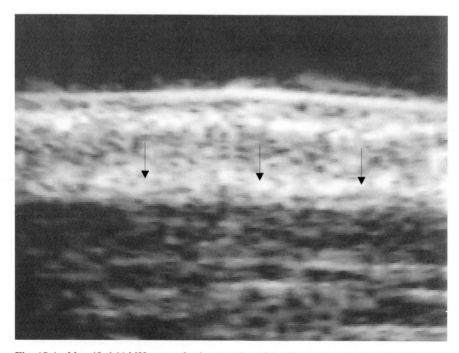

Fig. 17.4 Magnified 20 MHz scan of a short portion of Achilles tendon showing the thin hyperechoic paratenon (arrow).

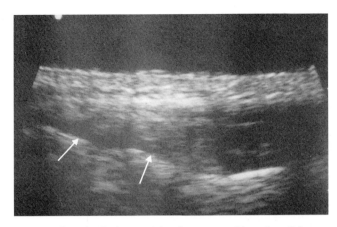

Fig. 17.5 Longitudinal scan of the elbow: normal insertion of short tendons to the humeral epicondyle (arrow).

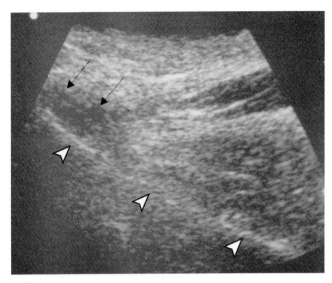

Fig. 17.6 Normal insertion (arrow) of the short tendon of adductor longus to the ischiopubic bone (arrowhead). The tendon is hypoechoic with respect to the muscle belly.

rounded by homogeneous hyperechoic tissue within which they can be seen to move freely[3,5-7] (Fig. 17.4). Synovial bursae are often interposed between tendons and adjacent osseous surfaces: they can be appreciated as hypoechoic elongated areas which are rarely thicker than 2–3 mm.

The attachment of short tendons to their muscles appears either as a crowding of the muscular fibers, with rapid reduction in the volume of the muscle itself (Fig. 17.5), or as an irregularly triangular, hypoechoic and homogeneous area with a well-defined margin with respect to the muscle (Fig. 17.6).

TENDINOUS DISEASES

The most frequent lesions encountered in tendons are due to trauma, either acute or chronic. Other common lesions are of degenerative origin, but their etiology is not well known; repeated microtrauma and/or functional stress seem to play a role in their production.

Trauma

Traumatic ruptures of tendons can occur either in the middle of the tendon body or as a result of avulsion from the osseous insertion. Clinically, the patient describes a sensation of 'rupture', pain and functional impairment. Retraction of the muscle produces a subcutaneous mass, and a cutaneous bruise is often present. It must be remembered that, in most cases, pre-existing degenerative changes and/or small recurrent microtraumas predispose tendons to rupture; damaged tendons may then undergo rupture as a result of relatively minor trauma.[7]

Tendon fracture may occur without associated rupture

of the tendon sheath. In such cases, a small hypoechoic hematoma develops at the site of fracture, with retraction of both fragments[7-10] (Fig. 17.7). When the sheath is also ruptured the hematoma is larger, with irregular and indistinct margins (Fig. 17.8); fresh hemorrhagic lesions may be either hyperechoic or heterogeneous, and this can be an additional cause of difficulty in distinguishing their margins. Movement causes further separation of the fragments with better delineation of the fracture site.

When the lesion is not complete, the intact portion of tendon, the hematoma, and the retracted ruptured parts can be demonstrated[11] (Fig. 17.9). Careful analysis of the structure of both the intact and fractured parts of tendon

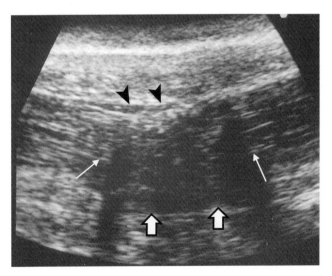

Fig. 17.7 Traumatic rupture of the Achilles tendon with retraction of the fragments (arrows) and large hematoma (open arrows). The tendon sheath is not involved (arrowhead).

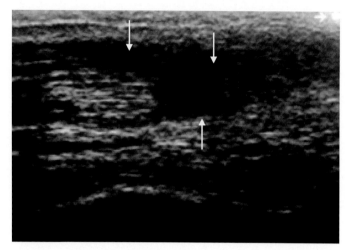

Fig. 17.8 Complete traumatic rupture of the Achilles tendon and its sheath, with a large hematoma (arrow).

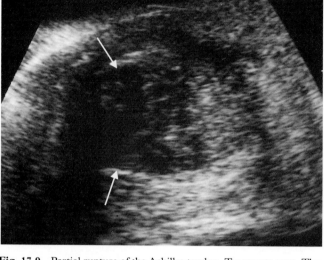

Fig. 17.9 Partial rupture of the Achilles tendon. Transverse scan. The left half of the tendon (arrow) is ruptured, while the right portion is preserved.

is important before submitting the patient to surgery, since the presence of textural abnormalities can predict a difficult recovery after therapy (Fig. 17.10). Tendons are structures of considerable strength which undergo rupture only as a consequence of significant trauma. It is usually considered that only tendons with pre-existing pathologic changes, be they of inflammatory, traumatic or degenerative origin, undergo 'spontaneous' rupture or rupture after minor traumatic insult. US can play a role in detecting minor changes of tendon echo texture which predispose tendons to rupture;[8–10] these can be recognized as focal enlargements of the involved tendon, and as either diffuse or focal disappearance of the normal hyperechoic fibrillar texture (Figs 17.10, 17.11).

Following treatment, be it medical or surgical, US can provide information both about the internal structure and integrity of the tendon, and evaluation of its movement with respect to surrounding tissues. The postoperative texture of the tendon is non-homogeneously hypoechoic, with internal sutures visible as hyperechoic spots with a thin acoustic shadow. This pattern can be difficult to differentiate from tendinitis or partial recurrent rupture. Following rupture of the peritenon or after the development of adhesions between the peri- and paratenon, tendon movements can be hampered, and this can be easily evaluated with real-time US.[7,10,12]

Avulsion of the tendon from its bony insertion can detach bony fragments, or even cause small cortical fractures (Fig. 17.12). The osteotendinous insertion is the weakest point of the musculo-tendinous-skeletal system in the adult; in

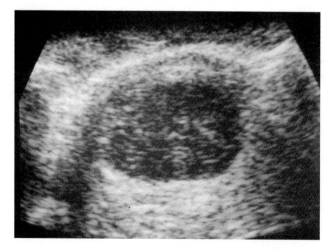

Fig. 17.10 Transverse scan of the cranial portion of the ruptured Achilles tendon shown in Fig. 17.9. The texture is irregular and hypoechoic, suggesting pre-existing tendinosis.

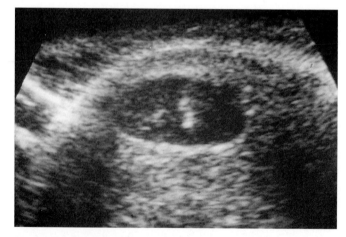

Fig. 17.11 Transverse scan of an Achilles tendon affected with tendinosis: it is not enlarged but is markedly hypoechoic, with small calcifications.

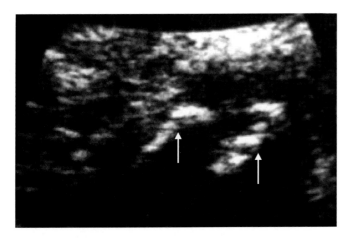

Fig. 17.12 Oblique scan of iliac crest. Two detached bony fragments (arrows) are evident, sequelae of partial traumatic avulsion of the sartorius muscle from its insertion.

Inflammatory conditions

US can be used for diagnosing tendinitis and peritendinitis; a variety of findings can be observed in these cases, depending on both the site of involvement of the tendon and associated involvement of synovial bursae or sheaths.

When inflammatory changes develop at the osteotendinous or musculotendinous junction (insertional diseases), mostly due to longstanding microtraumas, there is thickening of the involved tendon, whose structure can become heterogeneous, with both hyper- and hypoechoic alternating areas, due to either fibrotic or degenerative changes[7–9,13] (Figs 17.13, 17.14). Erosions of the cortical surface of bone can be demonstrated (Fig. 17.15) and, when present, small associated cortical detachments are easily visible (Fig. 17.16).

When long tendons are involved, marked thickening of the insertion can develop, with both micro- and macrocalcifications (Fig. 17.17). When a synovial bursa is present, the presence of internal fluid indicating inflammatory involvement is often observed (Fig. 17.18).

Inflammatory changes which develop in tendons surrounded by synovial sheaths are called tenosynovitis. Histologically, this is due to infiltration of inflammatory cells, associated with fibrosis and myxoid changes. US shows a collection of hypoechoic fluid within the synovial sheath surrounding the hyperechoic normal-appearing tendon. The fluid may be corpusculated. When axial images are obtained, a target pattern, with the hypoechoic dilated synovial sheath and the hyperechoic central tendon, is

children the weakest point is the metaphysis. The lesion is usually due to a pull-up force applied to the insertion of the tendon; it typically involves the tibial and ischial tuberosities, and the iliac crests. Clinical symptoms include sudden pain with local swelling and loss of function. Pain is increased by movement and pressure on the involved insertion. Conservative treatment is usually preferred. US can play a role in the follow-up of such lesions by monitoring the development of the scarring process.[12] When the avulsion is not complete, US can demonstrate a 'V-shaped' image at the site of the lesion, with slight irregularities of the adjacent bony surfaces.

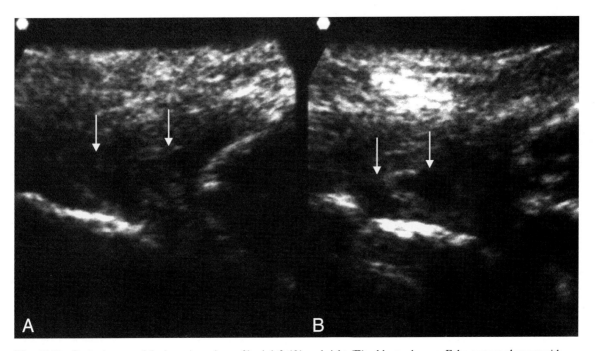

Fig. 17.13 Sagittal scans of the bony insertions of both left (**A**) and right (**B**) adductor longus. Echo texture changes with hypoechoic areas (arrows) are visible on both sides, due to inflammatory insertional disease.

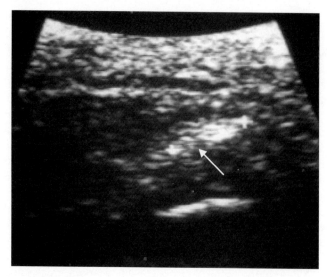

Fig. 17.14 Oblique scan of the tendinous insertion of the adductor longus with a hyperechoic band (arrow) representing fibrotic degenerative change.

observed (Fig. 17.19). The amount of fluid is usually directly related to the degree of inflammation.

In tendons surrounded by paratenon, inflammation causes thickening of peritendinous tissues and adhesions between them and the outer tendinous surface, fibrosis being the main histologic alteration. This creates pain during movement, leading to functional impairment. Peritendinous regions, which normally are of regular thickness

and hyperechoic, become thickened and irregular, with blurred outer margins and heterogeneous structure; their outer surface often has a nodular appearance (Fig. 17.20).

Degenerative changes

Degenerative changes involving tendons can be the result of metabolic diseases (such as familial hypercholesterolosis), repeated microtrauma, or chronic tendinitis. Pain and tenderness are absent in most cases, and patients are usually asymptomatic; enlargement of the involved tendons is the only sign of disease.[8–12] US can show tendinous enlargement and irregularities of the textural appearance, with small hypoechoic areas within the tendon body and associated microcalcifications (see Figs 17.10, 17.11). Histologically, fibrosis with mucoid degeneration is the main pathologic event, with complete absence of inflammatory changes.

Tendinous xanthomas occurring in familial hypercholesterolosis appear as focal hypoechoic areas causing disruption of the normal tendinous structure.

Degenerative changes can reduce the resistance of tendons to stress and predispose them to rupture. In many cases, in fact, an episode of rupture following minor trauma is the presenting symptom of a previously unsuspected degenerative tendinous disease. As mentioned above high-resolution US can be used to identify tendinous textural changes which may predispose to rupture in patients at high risk of developing degenerative diseases.

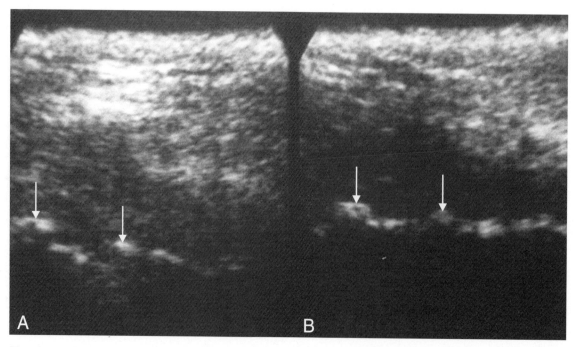

Fig. 17.15 Tendinous insertions of right (**A**) and left (**B**) adductor longus. Multiple, fine erosions (arrows) of the bone surface are detected.

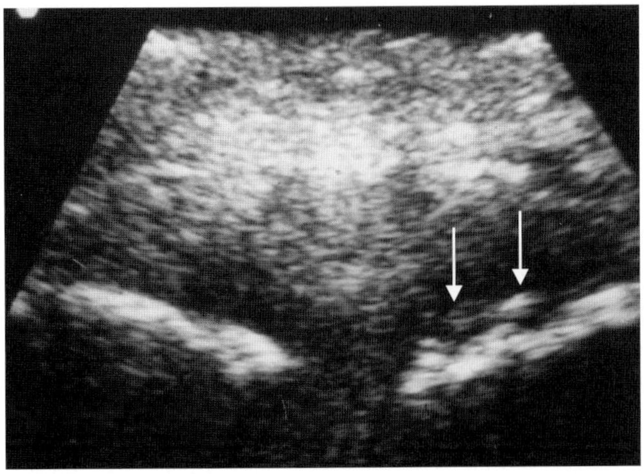

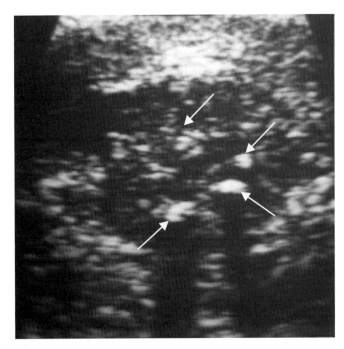

Fig. 17.16 Transverse scan of pubic symphysis: there is a small cortical detachment (arrow) on the left side.

Fig. 17.17 Transverse scan of the patellar insertion of the quadriceps tendon with multiple calcifications due to degenerative changes (arrows).

Other diseases

Tendinous involvement can occur in systemic diseases such as rheumatoid and psoriatic arthritis, lupus, gout, and scleroderma. The findings cannot be differentiated from those observed in other inflammatory lesions, and only correlation with clinical findings can allow a specific diagnosis to be made. Gout tophi are echogenic, with posterior acoustic shadow. In patients with rheumatoid arthritis, US evaluation of tendons can be used to differentiate between functional impairment due to primary joint changes and ankylosis caused by tendinous rupture.

Primary neoplasms of tendons are rare. Lesions arising from the tendinous sheaths, such as the giant cell tumor and synovial sarcoma, are relatively more common. Secondary lesions may also be encountered.

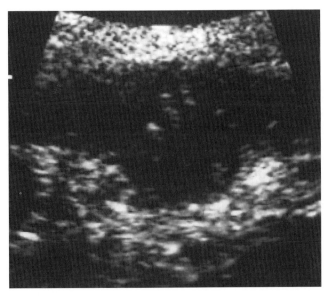

Fig. 17.18 Transverse scan. Median portion of the patellar insertion of the quadriceps tendon showing marked hypoechogenicity due to inflammatory involvement.

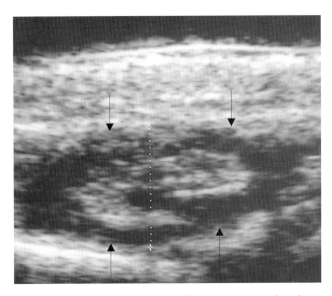

Fig. 17.19 Tenosynovitis. Axial view of hyperechoic normal tendon surrounded by hypoechoic dilated synovial sheath (arrow).

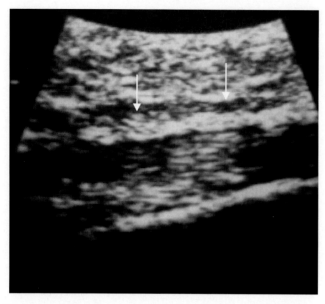

Fig. 17.20 Sagittal scan of quadriceps tendon. Severe thickening of hyperechoic peritenon (arrow) with nodular margins.

REFERENCES

1. Bagnolesi P, Cilotti A, Lencioni R, Campassi C, Tessa C, Bartolozzi C 1993 Tendine di Achille: ecografia con diverse frequenze. Radiol Med 35: 741–747
2. Jozsa L, Kannus P, Balint J B, Reffy A 1991 Three dimensional ultrastructure of human tendons. Acta Anat 142: 306–312
3. Martinoli C, Derchi L E, Pastorino C, Bertolotto M, Silvestri E 1993 Analysis of echotexture of tendons with US. Radiology 186: 839–843
4. Fornage B D 1987 The hypoechoic normal tendon. A pitfall. J Ultrasound Med 6: 19–22
5. Balconi G 1987 Muscoli e tendini. In: Rizzatto G, Solbiati L (eds) Anatomia ecografica. Masson, Milan, pp 303–311
6. Fornage B D 1986 Achilles tendon: US examination. Radiology 159: 759–764
7. Fornage B D, Rifkin M D 1988 Ultrasound examination of tendon. Radiol Clin North Am 26: 87–107
8. Balconi G, Miraglia A 1991 L'ecografia in traumatologia ortopedica: muscoli e tendini. In: Rizzatto G, Solbiati L, Derchi L, Busilacchi P (eds) Imaging – US. Avanzamenti '90. Masson, Milan, pp 177–188
9. Campani R, Bottinelli O, Genovese E et al 1990 Ruolo dell'ecotomografia nella traumatologia da sport dell'arto inferiore. Radiol Med 79: 151–162
10. Kainberger F M, Engel A, Barton P et al 1990 Injury of the Achilles tendon: diagnosis with sonography. AJR 155: 1031–1036
11. Leekam R N, Salsberg B B, Bogoch E et al 1986 Sonographic diagnosis of partial Achilles tendon rupture and healing. J Ultrasound Med 5: 115–119
12. Fornage B D 1992 Musculoskeletal evaluation. In: Mittelstaedt C A (ed) General ultrasound. Churchill Livingstone, New York, pp 1–57
13 Benazzo F, Barnabei G, Jelmoni G P et al 1990 L'ecografia nella traumatologia da sport: indicazioni e limiti. J Sports Traumatol Rel Res 12: 13–23

18

Joints

G. Monetti   L. De Pra   G. Balconi

In this chapter only the anatomic and pathologic elements of the joints which can be examined with high-frequency ultrasound are included. The hip joint is not described as in adults it is adequately visualized with lower frequencies.

Benign and malignant neoplasms have similar patterns in all the joints and will be described in the final section of the chapter.

As for examination technique, each joint must be studied both in static and dynamic phases, always comparing with the contralateral unaffected side and employing probes of as high a frequency as possible.

KNEE

The knee is the most complex joint of the human body; it includes the tendons of the extensor and flexor apparatus, ligaments, menisci, capsule, cartilage and the structures forming the synovial membrane.

Standard X-rays are still fundamental in the diagnostic assessment of the skeletal apparatus of the knee, but the study of knee disorders is currently mostly based on computed tomography (CT) and magnetic resonance imaging (MRI) which allow visualization of all the anatomic components.[1-3] US investigation has some limitations, due to the complexity of the knee and to the fact that its main structures are predominantly intra-articular.

Tendons

The tendons which can be assessed with sonography are the quadriceps (Fig. 18.1) and the patellar (Fig. 18.2) tendons, the biceps femoris tendon and, less easily, the popliteus tendon.[4-6]

The quadriceps tendon attaches to the base of the patella. The patellar tendon extends from the patella to the tibial tuberosity: it is normally 4–5 mm thick and 20–25 mm wide, with a convex anterior shape. Both are adequately displayed with high frequencies. The deep infrapatellar bursa is always visible as a flattened, 2–3 mm thick anechoic structure. The prepatellar and superficial infrapatellar bursae are not commonly visualized with US. Along the medial portion of the joint the insertions of the three tendons – semitendinosus, gracilis and sartorius – forming the so-called 'pes anserinus' can be seen (Fig. 18.3).

The echo patterns of these tendons and their disorders are quite similar to those of tendons elsewhere in the body (see Ch. 17). However, due to functional overloading, tendinous diseases peculiar to the knee may occur, such as the insertional tendinopathies of the patellar tendon, either of its proximal end (Sinding-Larsen–Johnson disease) (Fig. 18.4) or of its distal end (Osgood–Schlatter disease or anterior tibial apophysitis) (Fig. 18.5).[8]

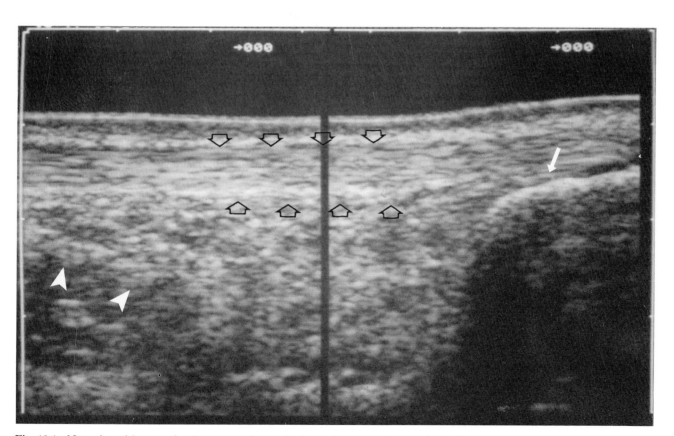

Fig. 18.1 Normal quadriceps tendon (open arrows) on sagittal scan. Arrow: patella; arrowheads: femur.

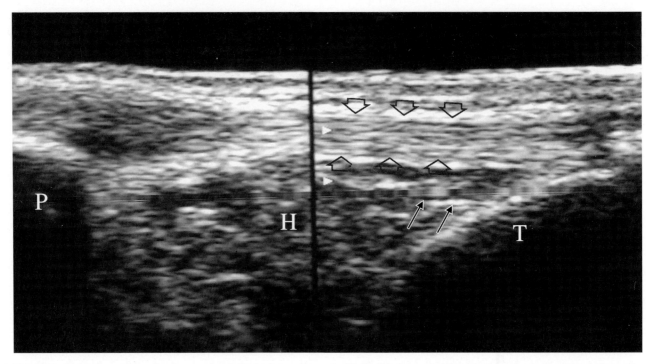

Fig. 18.2   Normal patellar tendon (open arrows). Sagittal scan. P: patella; H: Hoffa's fatty pad; T: tibial tuberosity; arrows: deep infrapatellar bursa.

Tendinous diseases are frequently associated with inflammatory involvement of the serous bursae (reactive bursitis) which can be acute in character or undergo chronic evolution with internal organization and occasionally microcalcifications (Fig. 18.6).[9,10]

The most common bursitis involves the semi-membranosus-gastrocnemius bursa in the popliteal fossa and is improperly termed a 'Baker cyst'. When it is widely distended, its short, thin articular pedicle is easily seen with US (Fig. 18.7).[11,12] During inflammatory episodes, Baker cysts frequently show parietal thickenings, internal septa, echogenic debris, fibrin clots and widespread micro-calcifications, often due to cortisone. Baker cysts should be differentiated from other disorders of the popliteal fossa, such as popliteal aneurysms or deep popliteal thrombosis. The popliteus tendon can be subject to both peritendinitic

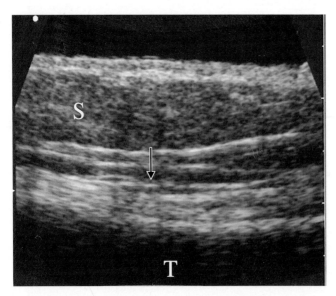

Fig. 18.3   Sagittal scan showing the insertion of the tendon of the semitendinosus muscle (arrow) to the tibia (T). S: subcutaneous tissue.

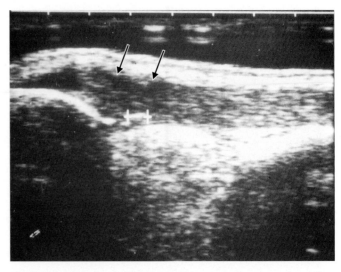

Fig. 18.4   Degenerative changes of the patellar tendon (arrow) at its proximal insertion, with a calcification (+).

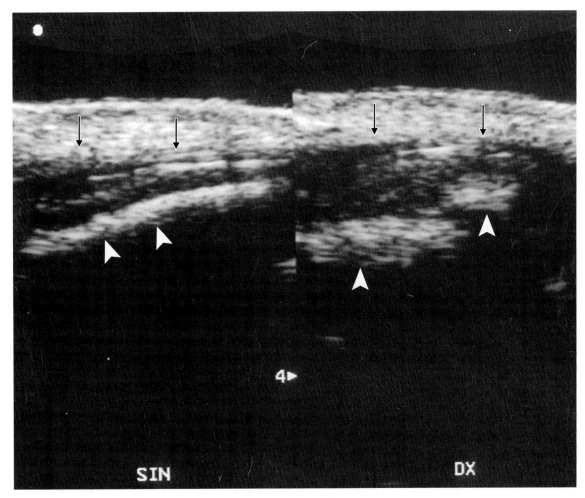

Fig. 18.5 Osgood–Schlatter disease. Sagittal scans of the patellar tendons (arrows) of the same patient at their tibial insertions. On the left side the tibial tuberosity (arrowhead) is normal, while on the right side it is fragmented (apophysitis).

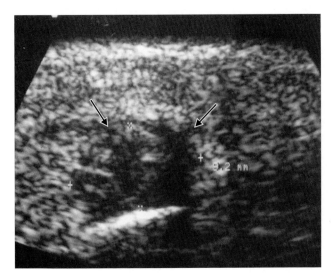

Fig. 18.6 Longstanding infrapatellar bursitis (arrow) with fibrotic changes.

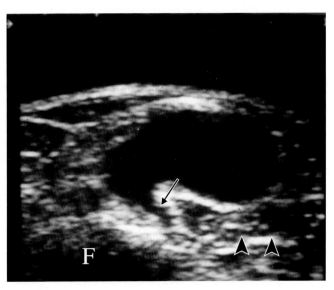

Fig. 18.7 Transverse scan at the level of the proximal end of the tendon of the gastrocnemius (arrowhead). Typical Baker cyst with thin posterior pedicle (arrow). F: medial condyle of the femur.

disorders and tenosynovitis, as it is provided with a synovial sheath.

Ligaments

The ligaments of the knee (anterior and posterior cruciate ligaments, lateral and medial collateral ligaments) are currently best visualized with CT and MRI. Only the collateral ligaments can be completely displayed by US.

In the case of traumatic lesions, three different degrees of tears of the collateral ligaments can be listed. The first degree consists of hyperextension of the ligament, with overstretching of the fibers and edema. Ultrasound shows uninterrupted ligament, with hypoechogenicity and homogeneous widening due to edema, which can also involve the adjacent subcutaneous tissues (Fig. 18.8).

The second degree is consistent with an incomplete tear of the ligament with concomitant edema and extravasation of blood into surrounding tissues. The capsule is generally not involved. Sonographically, in the early phase, the ligament appears markedly widened and shows a sharp internal hypoechoic defect, corresponding to the fresh partial rupture, associated with peripheral hematoma. After appropriate therapy, progressive healing of the ligament can be assessed[13] (Fig. 18.9).

The third degree corresponds to the complete rupture of the ligament, associated with a large hematoma and, in most cases, with a capsular lesion. US shows full thickness discontinuity of the ligament with a large hematoma filling the space between the torn fragments. A capsular tear with endoarticular blood effusion is a frequent association.

In ligament tears, US investigation is useful primarily during the acute stage, since edema and blood effusion create an ideal contrast. In subacute or chronic conditions the main purpose of US is to quantify the lesions.

At present, the US study of cruciate ligaments is usually

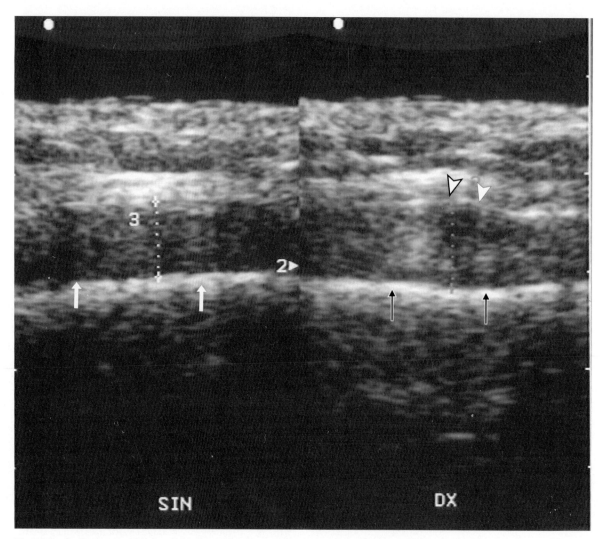

Fig. 18.8   Sagittal scans of the medial collateral ligaments (arrows) of both sides in the same patient, close to the femoral insertion. Normal ligament on the left, first degree tear on the right, with moderate enlargement due to edema (arrowhead).

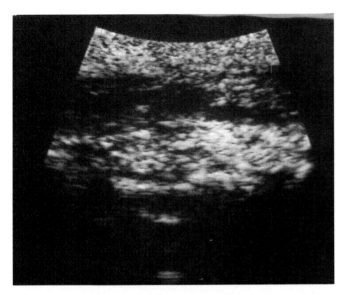

Fig. 18.9 Sagittal scan of the middle third of the external collateral ligament featuring slight enlargement (arrow) and irregular echo texture due to healing of traumatic injury.

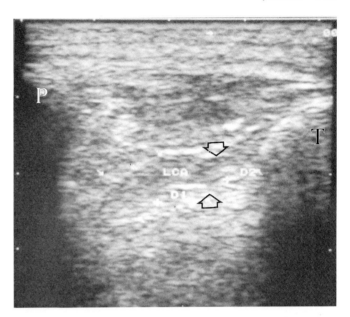

Fig. 18.10 Sagittal scan of the articular space of the knee. Tibial insertion of the anterior cruciate ligament (open arrows). P: patella; T: tibia.

inadequate as they have an intra-articular course and are masked by the bony structures. US investigation allows visualization only of the distal insertions of both anterior and posterior cruciate ligaments (Fig. 18.10). It is well known that posterior or anterior ligament tears are usually associated with fractures of the spongiosa, Segond fractures, capsular detachments or meniscal tears; thus only the global imaging provided by CT or MRI can provide an accurate and complete diagnosis (Figs 18.11, 18.12).

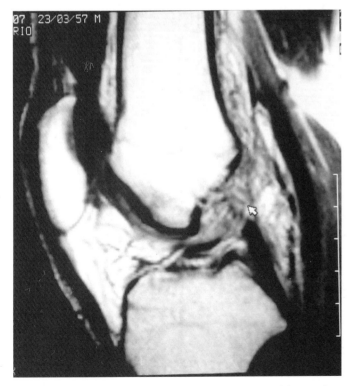

Fig. 18.11 MR image (sagittal) featuring complete tear of the anterior cruciate ligament (arrow).

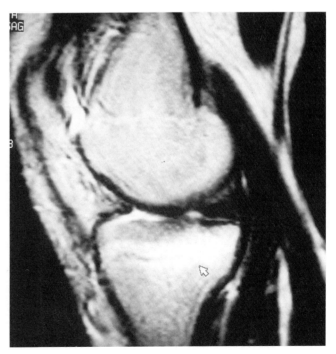

Fig. 18.12 MR sagittal scan. Fracture of the tibial plate (arrow) following complete rupture of the anterior cruciate ligament.

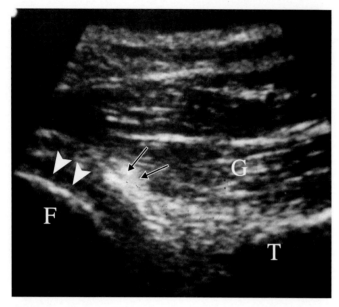

Fig. 18.13 Sagittal-oblique view of the popliteal fossa at the level of the posterior horn of the medial meniscus (arrow). F: femur condyle; T: posterior margin of tibial epiphysis; arrowhead: articular space; G: medial head of gastrocnemius.

Menisci

Menisci are fibrocartilaginous triangular structures easily detected on anatomic investigations but hard to examine with US. Ultrasound coronal scans performed anteriorly display the medial and lateral portions of the anterior horns of the menisci. With posterior sagittal planes adjacent to

the popliteal fossa the posterior horns of the lateral and medial menisci can be visualized. Sonographically, menisci appear as wedge-shaped, relatively hyperechoic structures, clearly defined only in their outer portions[14] (Fig. 18.13). The inner portions, which more frequently undergo traumatic injuries (due to their poor vascularization), are not visible with US.[15]

Only large meniscal tears (at least 2 mm and 5 mm wide for vertical and horizontal defects, respectively)[15] can be diagnosed with US, and appear as hyperechoic lines. Unfortunately the diagnostic sensitivity of US is also affected by the angle of incidence of the US beam, causing structural inhomogeneities which can be interpreted only with difficulty (Fig. 18.14). Arthroscopy, arthrography, CT and MRI remain the preferred investigations,[7] even though they too can provide wrong diagnoses both in meniscal tears and in other pathological conditions such as discoid dysplasias and degenerative changes (Fig. 18.15).

US is, however, excellent for displaying parameniscal or meniscal cysts, which mostly occur laterally and present as firm swellings on the knee margins. Sonographically they appear as either hyperechoic or hypoechoic masses, single or septate (pseudocyst-like), arising from the lateral border of the meniscus and extending cranially or caudally, adjacent to the bone (Fig. 18.16). This pattern may be hardly distinguishable from that of other diseases, such as bursitis of collateral ligaments, synovial extroflexions, or post-traumatic hematomas. MRI is currently the method of choice for imaging meniscal cysts; it also assists in excluding associated injuries of the ligaments.

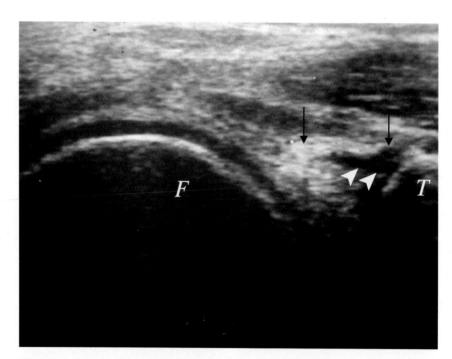

Fig. 18.14 Sagittal-oblique scan of the popliteal fossa. Posterior horn of medial meniscus (arrow) with fracture (arrowhead) featured as a hypoechoic line. F: medial femoral condyle; T: tibia.

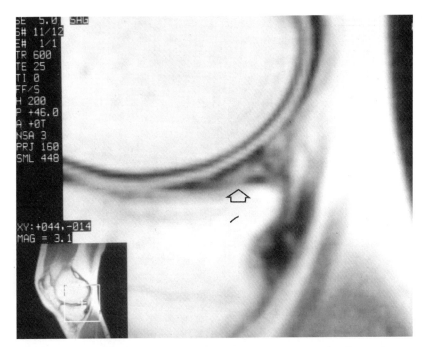

Fig. 18.15 MR image of knee articular space. High grade degenerative changes (open arrow) of the posterior horn of the medial meniscus.

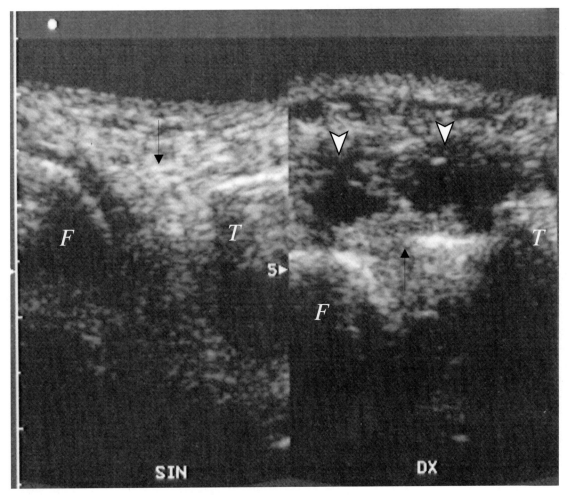

Fig. 18.16 Sagittal-oblique scans between the body and anterior horn of the lateral meniscus (arrow). Comparative views of both sides in the same subject. On the right side a large parameniscal cyst (arrowhead) is featured. F: lateral condyle of femur; T: tibia.

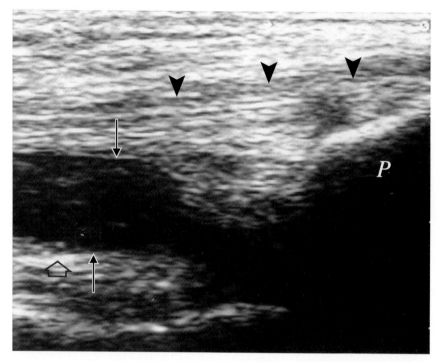

Fig. 18.17 Sagittal suprapatellar scan. Fluid effusion in the suprapatellar pouch (arrow). P: patella; arrowhead: quadriceps tendon.

Another sonographic diagnosis which can be made, even though it is seldom necessary, is the capsulo-meniscal detachment of the posterior horns of the medial menisci.

Synovia

The accuracy of US in the assessment of synovial alterations is very poor, whereas the sonographic detection of

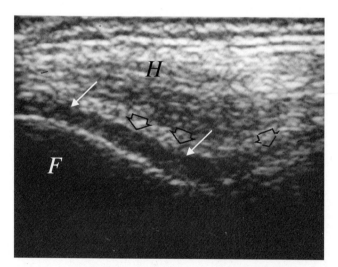

Fig. 18.18 Rheumatic disease. Transverse scan on 90° flexed knee. Synovial thickening (arrow) in front of the femoral condyle (F). H: Hoffa's fatty pad.

even small effusions in the anterior infrapatellar space is highly accurate. Effusions of the suprapatellar pouch are also visible, mostly after compression of the sides of the joint (Fig. 18.17).

In rheumatic diseases synovial thickenings (pannus) can be observed predominantly along the femoral condyles, through axial scans performed on 90° flexed knees (Fig. 18.18).[16]

In many sites, such as the suprapatellar pouch, Hoffa's fat pad, and popliteal fossa, nodular or villonodular synovial thickenings can be displayed by US as hyperechoic, roundish and ovoid nodules, adherent to the synovial surface or joined to it by a hyperechoic pedicle[17] (Fig. 18.19). The nodules of synovitis may mimic fibrin clots: if, on exerting local compression with the probe, a thorough scattering of hyperechoic spots in the synovial fluid is observed, the diagnosis of simple clots is easily obtained. In villonodular synovitis the villi remain tightly packed close to the synovia because of pedicles.

In reactive synovitis, a marked and inhomogeneous hyper- or hypoechoic thickening of the fibrous septa of Hoffa's fat pad is often detected with US.

Cartilage

The articular cartilage is assessable with US only in a few areas of the knee, mostly along the surface of the femoral condyles, appearing as a hypoechoic thin line. The normal thickness of the cartilage should not be less than 1 mm in

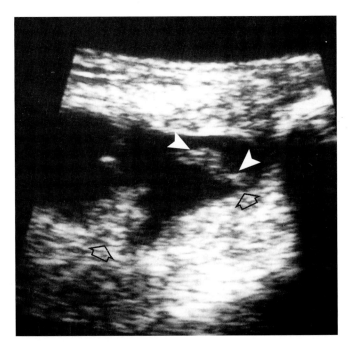

Fig. 18.19 Villonodular synovial thickening (open arrow) in the patellar pouch, with solid projections (arrowheads).

adults and 2 mm in adolescents.[7,18] Defects as small as 1 mm may be detected by US.

In rheumatic diseases the cartilage appears markedly irregular, with hyperechoic defects and diffuse thinning due to erosion (Fig. 18.20). Double contrast arthrography and gadolinium–DTPA enhanced MRI are the most accurate imaging methods for studying the knee cartilage.[20]

Capsule

The normal knee capsule is difficult to visualize with any imaging technique. Capsular tears involving limited areas can be sonographically suspected in some instances through indirect signs, such as the disinsertion of the posterior horns of the medial menisci at the level of the capsule.

More of the capsule can be seen with US if a large endoarticular effusion is present.

Blood vessels

The popliteal artery is the largest arterial vessel of the knee. It may undergo either degenerative changes in rheumatic disease or traumatic lesions, as in sports injuries.

The presence of aneurysms in the medial tract of the popliteal artery, associated with saccular dilatation and calcified ring thrombus, is a very frequent occurrence. Popliteal aneurysms need to be differentiated from large multiloculated cysts at the level of the semimembranosus-gastrocnemius bursa and from post-traumatic pseudo-aneurysms, easily evaluated by color Doppler.

The pathology of the popliteal veins can also be accurately studied with US, both thrombophlebitic processes involving deep venous vessels, and variceal disease of superficial branches.[21]

The most frequent cause of 'entrapment' of the popliteal artery, a well-known clinical condition, is the compression of the vessel by either the medial or the lateral head of gastrocnemius (often hypertrophic), resulting in ischemia. US and color Doppler can easily demonstrate this occurrence.

ANKLE AND FOOT

The ankle joint includes four bony structures, a capsule, and some ligaments and tendons.

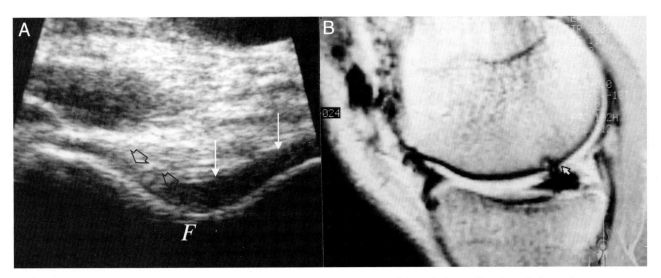

Fig. 18.20 Rheumatic disease. **A** Hyperechoic defects and erosions (open arrows) of the articular cartilage (arrow), featured even more clearly by MRI (**B**). F: femur condyle.

Ligaments

In the medial compartment of the ankle is located the large deltoid ligament, which is composed of three bundles – the anterior and posterior tibiotalar ligaments and the tibiocalcanean ligament. In the outer compartment of the ankle three main ligaments are located: the anterior and posterior talofibular ligaments and the calcaneofibular ligament. Sonographically these ligaments appear as hyperechoic, band-like structures, whilst the deltoid ligament has a triangular shape (Fig. 18.21).

The sonographic study of ligaments should always be performed under stress conditions, either varus or valgus, in order to achieve the best resolution of ligament echo texture. In the outer compartment of the ankle all the ligaments are easily investigated with US (Fig. 18.22), apart from the posterior talofibular ligament which can be examined only with MRI. In the inner compartment the deltoid ligament is clearly visible with US, but its three main bundles are not individually distinguishable.

Tendons

A considerable number of tendons are located in the ankle, mainly extensor tendons dorsally and flexor tendons ventrally. All of them are provided with a synovial sheath. The Achilles tendon is the largest tendon of the human body; it has a peritenon, but not a sheath. Around the Achilles tendon the subcalcaneal deep (flattened, 2–3 mm thick, visible with high-frequency US) and superficial subcutaneous (undetectable with US) bursae are located, allowing a regular sliding plane between the tendon and periosteum. Below the Achilles tendon, in addition to the bursa, lies a fat triangular, hypoechoic tissue, the so-called Kager's fatty triangle; this has a pad-like function (Fig. 18.23).

On sagittal scans the Achilles tendon appears as an echogenic, homogeneous band-like structure (Fig. 18.23), surrounded by the thin peritenon (see Ch. 17). It is examinable from the calcaneal insertion to its junction with the gastrocnemius. In its medal portion the normal tendon is 5–6 mm thick and 8–10 mm wide.[5,10,21]

Flexor and extensor tendons have the same pattern of echo structure described in Chapter 17. The principal tendons which can be evaluated ultrasonically are those of the peroneus longus and peroneus brevis muscles laterally, the tendon of the tibialis posterior muscle medially and the tendon of the tibialis anterior muscle anteriorly. All these tendons are wrapped in synovial sheaths,[7] but have the same echo pattern as the Achilles tendon which is only provided with peritenon.

The dynamic study of tendons is helpful for differentiating the mobile tendons from the fixed nerves of the ankle region (tibial nerve, superficial peroneal nerve); the latter appear as hyperechoic ribbon-like bands, as described in Chapter 15.[9]

Tarsal tunnel and sinus

In the central subtalar portion of the foot is located the tarsal sinus, characterized by the bifurcated ligament (or 'Y' ligament) with its medial (calcaneonavicular) and lateral bundles. The tarsal sinus can not be assessed with US, but can with MRI (Fig. 18.24). Close to the sinus the tarsal tunnel is visible, crossed by the neurovascular bundles and the flexor tendons, here provided with sheaths. The last clinically relevant structure in this area is the transverse ligament at the intermetatarsal level, where the neurovascular bundles and the interdigital nerves are found.

The tendons of the extensor muscles course over the dorsal aspect of the foot, provided with sheaths in the middle of their tracts.

Finally, the normally hypoechoic, ribbon-like plantar

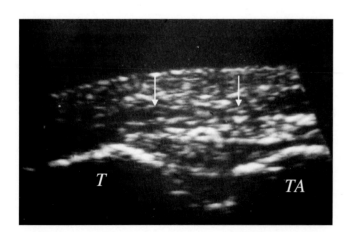

Fig. 18.21 Sagittal scan of the triangular-shaped, hyperechoic deltoid ligament (arrow). T: tibia; TA: talus.

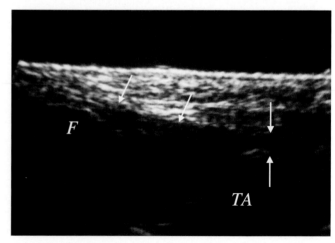

Fig. 18.22 Sagittal scan of the anterior talofibular ligament (arrow). F: fibula; Ta: talus.

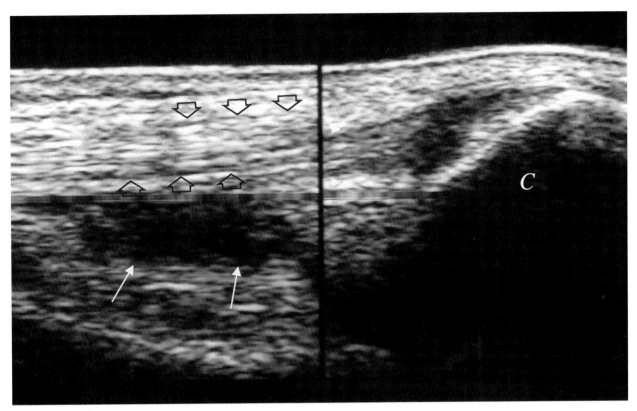

Fig. 18.23 Sagittal scan of a normal Achilles tendon (open arrows). (Arrow): Kager's fatty triangle; C: calcaneus.

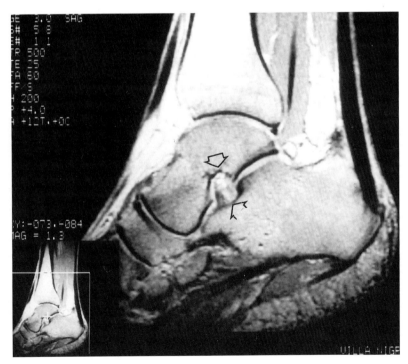

Fig. 18.24 MR image of normal tarsal sinus with spring ligament (open arrows).

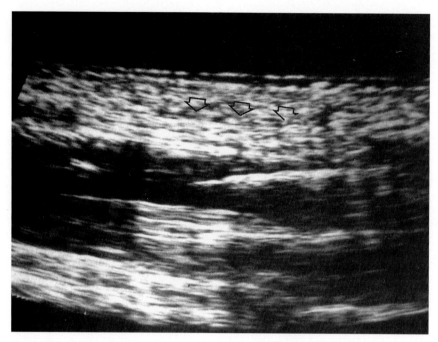

Fig. 18.25 Normal plantar aponeurotic fascia (open arrows). Sagittal scan.

fascia with its aponeurosis is detectable (Fig. 18.25); this is of considerable relevance in inflammatory diseases of the foot. In the intermetatarsal area MRI provides more complete and detailed information than US.[21]

Pathological conditions of the ankle and foot

The sonographic patterns of the different tendinous pathologies (insertional diseases, tenosynovitis, partial tears, complete ruptures, etc.) have been already described in Chapter 17. As regards the Achilles tendon, its only peculiar aspect is that its peritenon is highly vascularized, while its fibers have very poor vascularization. As a consequence, most inflammatory diseases of this tendon involve only its peritenon, with thickening and marked hyperechogenicity. Inflammatory changes may extend to the deep retro-calcanean bursa and to Kager's fatty pad, which becomes hyperechoic.[5,21]

Xanthomatosis

Xanthomatosis occurs mostly in women after the fourth decade of life; it is associated with familial hyper-cholesterolemia. The tendons undergo myxoid changes with a vacuolar arrangement, appearing as tiny hypoechoic areas mixed with widespread microcalcifications (Fig. 18.26). The tendons appear markedly thickened and thoroughly degenerated.

Tendons in patients who have undergone LDL apheresis therapy show an almost complete normalization of the structural pattern.

Surgical repair of the Achilles tendon

US studies achieve extremely useful results in the post-surgical evaluation of the Achilles tendon.

A variety of repair techniques are employed nowadays, from the simplest, i.e. biologic reconstruction through the plantar gracilis, to prosthetic repairs using biologically absorbable materials like Teflon[R], Dacron[R], Goretex[R] and Kennedy-Lad[R] (Fig. 18.27). US examinations must be performed at least one month after surgery, due to the presence of the acoustic shadow from the scar. The tendon always appears markedly thickened (as wide as 15–16 mm), with an inhomogeneous pattern. In some instances the

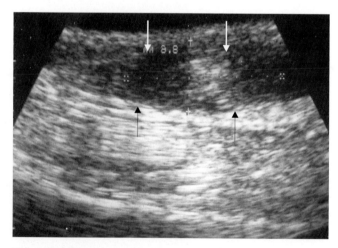

Fig. 18.26 Sagittal scan. Markedly thickened Achilles tendon (arrow) due to xanthomatosis.

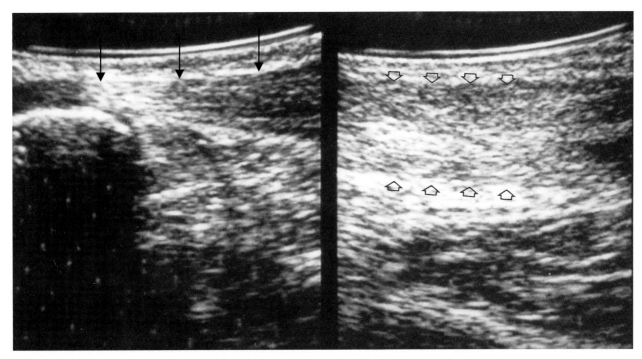

Fig. 18.27 Sagittal scans of both Achilles tendons in the same patient. The tendon on the right side (arrow) is normal, the tendon on the left is thickened and hyperechoic (open arrows) following injury and reconstruction by means of Kennedy-Lad[R].

stitches can be visualized as hyperechoic stripes together with post-surgical microcalcifications.

The purpose of US examination is to detect possible post-surgical tears due to recurrences. In our group of cases, tendons repaired by Kennedy-Lad[R] presented a more homogeneous echo texture.[21]

Ligament pathology

When traumatic lesions of ligaments occur, it is essential to perform the sonographic examination in the acute phase, since the contrast resolution created by the presence of hematoma, edema and blood effusion from capsular tear allows an adequate assessment of the degree of ligament tear. The completely or partially torn ligament appears highly hyperechoic within the hypoechoic hematoma ('bell clapper' image) (Fig. 18.28). In addition, in the acute stage US investigation should be carried out in varus and valgus stress conditions: the diastasis of the stumps of the ligaments allows a more accurate interpretation of the type of tear.

Sonographic monitoring following the acute traumatic event is helpful since, 15–20 days after a partial tear, increased thickness of the ligament, due to scar tissue, and a hyperechoic repaired area can be demonstrated.

Tarsal tunnel pathology

High-frequency sonography is currently able to assess most of the various pathological conditions of the tarsal tunnel.

The tarsal tunnel can appear severely narrowed as a result of sheath thickening in tenosynovitis, or be involved by venous varicosities or arterial aneurysms, easily assessable with color Doppler.

Space-occupying lesions of the tarsal tunnel do not differ from those of any other joint and are described on page 371.

Pathologies of the tarsal sinus, especially of the bifurcated ligament, can be studied only by MRI.[23]

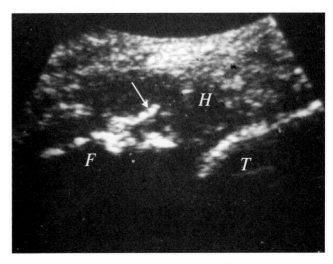

Fig. 18.28 Transverse scan of the anterior tibiofibular ligament (arrow) following complete rupture. H: hematoma; F: fibula; T: tibia.

Foot pathology

A wide variety of painful syndromes have been described in the foot, most of which are localized at the calcanear and metatarsal regions. The best known etiology of inter-metatarsal pain is Morton's neuroma, described in Chapter 15. Other causes include plantar inflammatory diseases, gout, chondrocalcinosis, nerve compression, bursitis, bone malformations or dysplasias, etc.

A typical pathology of the foot is Ledderhose disease, consisting of the development of longitudinally oriented fibrous cords in the plantar aponeurosis, with subsequent formation of nodules and adhesions to the subcutis. As a result, progressive retraction of the aponeurosis occurs. The sonographic detection of hypoechoic, oval nodules with lobulated margins in the fascial planes of the plantar region is relatively easy with US, using high frequencies.

SHOULDER

The shoulder region includes the acromioclavicular and glenohumeral joints, various ligaments (superior, middle and inferior glenohumeral ligaments, coracoacromial and coracohumeral ligaments), and the tendons forming the rotator cuff. These structures provide stability to the shoulder joint at the level of the glenoid fossa and its fibro-cartilaginous ring. The rotator cuff consists of the tendons of the supraspinatus, infraspinatus and teres minor muscles, but the tendons of subscapularis and the long head of the humeral biceps also have a role in formation of the cuff.

Due to biomechanical considerations, shoulder path-ology is currently subdivided into two main categories, i.e. the impingement syndrome, and shoulder instability (anterior, posterior or multidirectional).[25–28]

Examination technique

The echographic examination of the shoulder is usually performed using either 7.5–13 MHz linear electronic probes or 7.5–15 MHz mechanical sector transducers. Synthetic pads are useful to improve resolution of more superficial structures and to facilitate dynamic maneuvers in intra- and extrarotation.

The first, basic scan to be carried out is a transverse scan crossing the tendon of the long head of the biceps, lying over the transverse ligament in the intertubercular groove[29] (Fig. 18.29). The same tendon is detected in a longitudinal scan along its major axis, either in its intra- or extra-articular course (Fig. 18.30); in the intra-articular location the tendon is covered by synovial sheath. Moving the transducer medially, the insertion of the subscapularis tendon to the humeral lesser tuberosity is visible (Fig. 18.31). Moving the transducer externally and laterally, a general coronal view of the rotator cuff is achieved. The most anterior bundle is the attachment of the supraspinatus tendon to the greater tuberosity, the most medial bundle is the insertion of the infraspinatus tendon, and the most posterior is the teres minor tendon (Fig. 18.32).

Moving posteriorly with transverse scans along the courses of the tendons, the insertions of the infraspinatus and teres minor tendons can be assessed (Fig. 18.33).

The most important scan plane is at the level of the attachment of the supraspinatus tendon to the humeral greater tuberosity: this area is referred to as 'critical', due

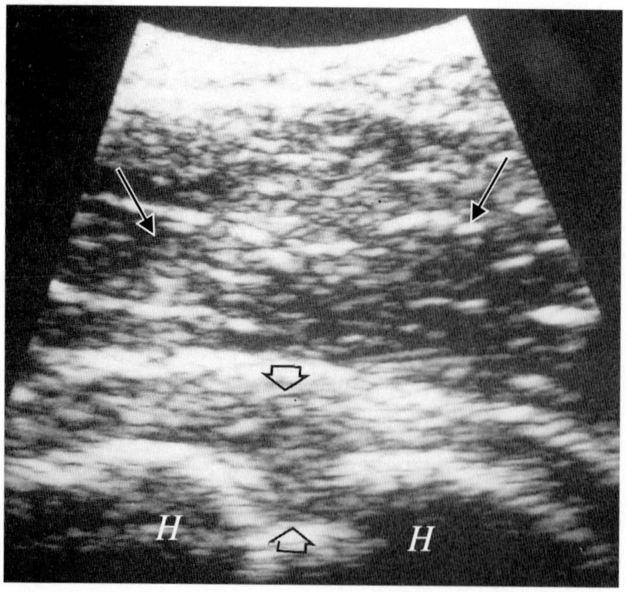

Fig. 18.29 Transverse scan through the tendon of the long head of the humeral biceps (open arrows). Arrow: rotator cuff; H: humeral sulcus.

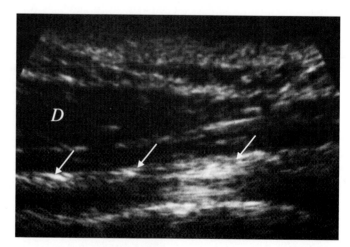

Fig. 18.30 Sagittal scan. Normal tendon of the long head of the biceps (arrow). D: deltoid muscle.

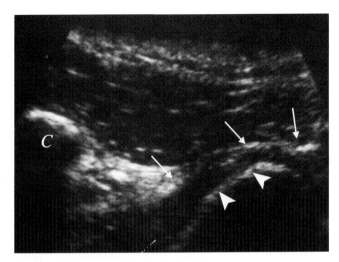

Fig. 18.31 Transverse anterior scan. Insertion of the subscapularis tendon (arrow) to the humerus (lesser tuberosity) (arrowhead). C: coracoid process.

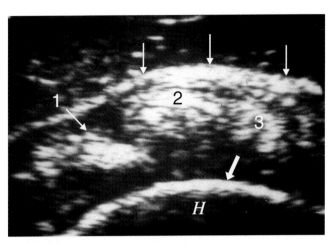

Fig. 18.32 Anterolateral transverse scan with posteriorly intrarotated arm. Normal rotator cuff. 1: supraspinatus tendon; 2: infraspinatus tendon; 3: teres minor tendon; arrow: articular capsule; H: humerus.

to its physiologic hypovascularization (Fig. 18.34). The maximum normal thickness of the supraspinatus tendon is 5–7 mm. The rotator cuff is thicker anteriorly (6 mm) than posteriorly (4 mm); its length, measured on longitudinal scans between its humeral attachment and the shadow cast by the acromion, is about 25 mm.

An essential maneuver, if the patient's discomfort will allow it, consists in moving the arm posteriorly in extra-rotation, in order to achieve better visualization of the supraspinatus tendon in the subacromial site where the acromion can cause visualization problems due to its acoustic shadow.

The articular cartilage is seen as a thin hypoechoic line overlying the humeral head. At the superior margin of the rotator cuff a hyperechoic line is visible, representing the barely separated walls of the subacromial-deltoid bursa,

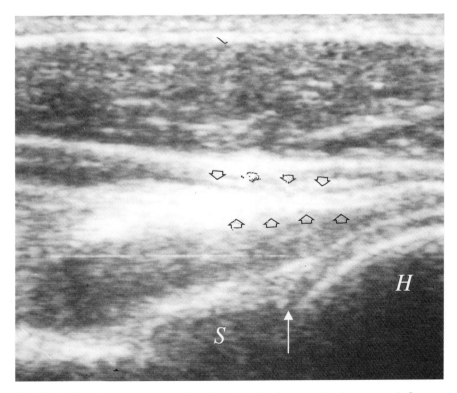

Fig. 18.33 Posterior transverse scan featuring the infraspinatus tendon (open arrows). S: scapula; H: humerus; arrow: glenoidal labrum.

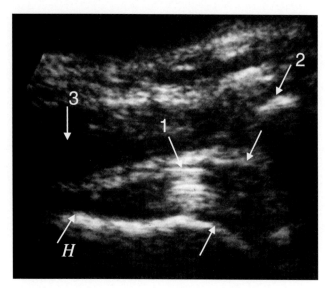

Fig. 18.34 Attachment of the supraspinatus tendon (arrow) to the humeral greater tuberosity (H). 1: critical area of the tendon; 2: acromion; 3: acromial bundle of deltoid muscle.

and a fatty cleavage plane: both structures separate the rotator cuff from the deltoid muscle.[9,30,31]

Most of the shoulder ligaments are poorly displayed by US, as are the glenoid fibrocartilaginous ring and the articular capsule.

The impingement syndrome

The impingement syndrome (or acromio-coraco-humeral syndrome) is a 'conflict pathology' taking place between the humeral head and acromion on one side and the coraco-acromial ligament on the other. Deep to this ligament are located the rotator cuff tendons, the subacromial-deltoid bursa and the biceps tendon.[32]

The pathologic classification of this syndrome into three stages has been described by Neer et al.[26] In the first stage limited blood effusion and thickening of the subacromial-deltoid bursa associated with edema of the rotator cuff occur. On US scans the cuff appears inhomogeneous and hypoechoic, compared with the unaffected side, while the subacromial-deltoid bursa is hyperechoic and markedly thickened, with reduced mobility during extrarotation movements[33,34] (Fig. 18.35).

The second stage is represented by initial fibrotic retraction of the deltoid bursa ('adhesive capsulitis') followed by initial degeneration of the rotator cuff tendons. The latter affects chiefly the attachment of the supraspinatus tendon to the greater tuberosity in the 'critical' area and the intra-articular tract of the biceps tendon (tenosynovitis). On US scans all these pathologic changes can be visualized.

With progression of the disease, increasing friction between acromion and rotator cuff occurs, with subsequent partial tear of the cuff and calcium deposition into the cuff and the deltoid bursa. These pathologic changes can also be visualized on US. Subacromial-deltoid bursitis appears as a fluid-filled mass, either anechoic or hypoechoic due to fibrin clots and possible microcalcifications. Initial rotator cuff lesions are seen in the critical area of the supraspinatus tendon as hypoechoic focal defects (with possible microcalcifications) originating from the marginal portions and causing loss of the regular convexity of the tendon (Fig. 18.36). Due to the tenosynovitic process, the biceps tendon in the intra-articular tract appears to be 'floating' within the fluid-filled sheath (Figs 18.37, 18.38).

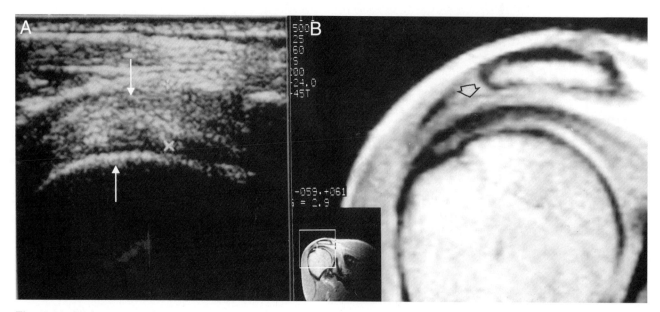

Fig. 18.35 Impingement syndrome – first stage. **A** The supraspinatus tendon (arrows) is thickened due to edema. **B** The same lesion (open arrow) imaged by MRI.

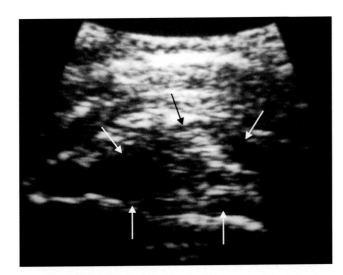

Fig. 18.36 Structural changes of the supraspinatus tendon (arrow) at the critical area.

cuff with retraction of the tendons and communication between the subacromial-deltoid bursa and the articular cavity. According to Neer et al[26] this is caused by hypertrophic sclerosis of the acromion, reducing the distance between the humeral head and the acromion, and hypertrophic sclerosis of the acromioclavicular joint and of the coracoacromial ligament.

Neer's third stage is easily assessable with US, both in the acute phase and in the chronic condition. In acute third stage impingement a complete tear of the rotator cuff is detected, with interposition of a large hematoma among the torn fibers. The complete rupture of the fibers can be better evaluated during the extrarotation stress maneuver, allowing visualization of the retracted fibers. In addition, a direct sign of high-grade impingement is the relevant fluid distension of the subacromial-deltoid bursa, communicating through a wide aperture with the articular cavity. An indirect sign is the concave appearance of the superior margin of the rotator cuff, due to loss of substance.

In the chronic phase the sonographic diagnosis is easier; due to the complete tear of the cuff with retraction of the fibers, the deltoid muscle and the subacromial-deltoid bursa move in contact with the humeral cortex. Comparative examination demonstrates the different thickness of the rotator cuff on the two sides (Fig. 18.41).

The accuracy of US in the diagnosis of tears of the rotator cuff is currently very high, even though it mostly relies on operator experience, particularly in the assessment of fissurative partial tears during the early post-traumatic stages.[36-38] If it is true that CT, MRI and arthrography may

Furthermore, lesions of the proximal attachment of the supraspinatus and infrascapular tendons may occur (Fig. 18.39), in some instances associated with fluid collections in the infrascapular pouch (Fig. 18.40).[35]

In chronic second stage impingement hyperechoic foci representing scars and calcifications can be detected in the cuff; it is important to define the exact location of the calcifications (intratendinous or in the subacromial bursa) since the subsequent therapeutic approach may be different in each case.

The third stage consists of complete tear of the rotator

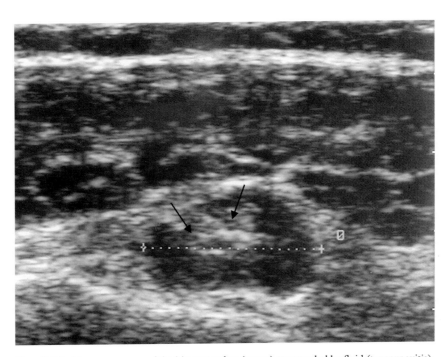

Fig. 18.37 Transverse scan of the biceps tendon (arrow) surrounded by fluid (tenosynovitis).

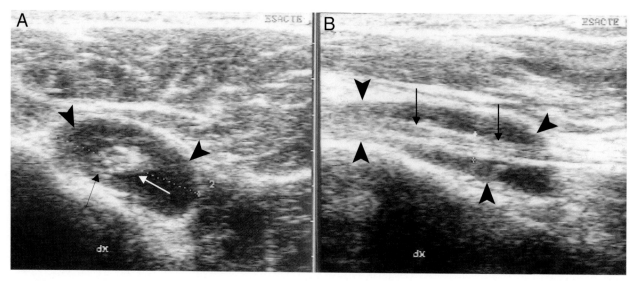

Fig. 18.38 Transverse (**A**) and sagittal (**B**) scans of the biceps tendon (arrow) 'floating' in the fluid-filled sheath (arrowhead), due to severe tenosynovitis.

not visualize small tears detected with US, it is also true that sonography may have other limitations. The impingement syndrome caused by contact of the coracoacromial ligament (partially assessable with US) (Fig. 18.42) and the attachment of the supraspinatus tendon may be poorly diagnosed by sonography, but can be clearly demonstrated by MRI (Fig. 18.43). In conclusion, whenever surgery is scheduled as therapy for impingement syndrome, gadolinium-DTPA MRI is to be considered the imaging modality of choice. When medical treatment is suggested, sonography is definitely the most useful diagnostic test.

Shoulder instability

Shoulder instability is mostly due to traumatic lesions of the superior, middle or inferior glenohumeral ligaments (Fig. 18.44), of the articular capsule, or of the humeral bony surface, involving the glenoid pad. Shoulder instability can be anterior, posterior or multidirectional. In all these instances US has important limitations for diagnosis.

First of all, the superior, middle and inferior glenohumeral ligaments can not be visualized at all. However, the transverse ligament lying below the long head of the humeral biceps at the interosseous groove level is easily

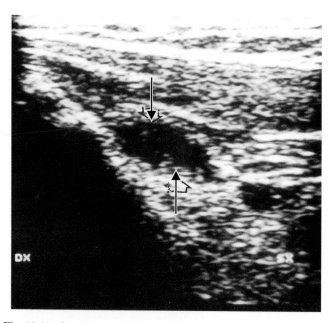

Fig. 18.39 Partial rupture of the supraspinatus tendon (arrow) with degenerative changes (arrowhead) and small hematoma (open arrows).

Fig. 18.40 Impingement syndrome. Fluid collection in the infrascapular pouch (arrow).

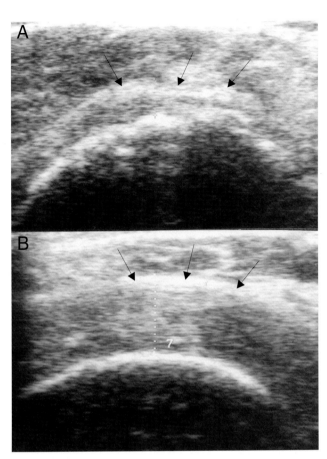

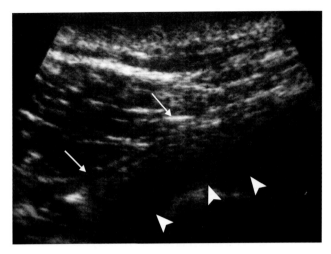

Fig. 18.42 Transverse-oblique scan featuring the normal coracoacromial ligament (arrow). Arrowhead: rotator cuff.

Fig. 18.41 Impingement syndrome. Complete rupture of the supraspinatus tendon (arrow) (**A**), compared with the normal contralateral supraspinatus tendon (**B**).

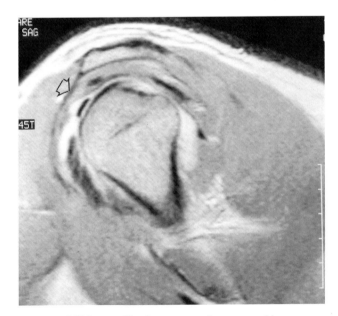

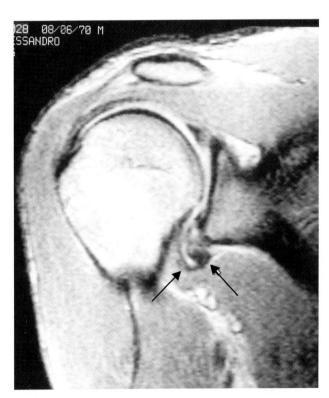

Fig. 18.43 MR image of impingement syndrome caused by contact (open arrow) of the coracoacromial ligament with the supraspinatus tendon.

Fig. 18.44 MR scan featuring a traumatic lesion of the inferior glenohumeral ligament (arrow) causing shoulder instability. The lesion was not detected with US.

seen. The function of this ligament is related to the stability of the long head tendon itself. In the case of subluxation of the long head, high-frequency sonography may therefore demonstrate partial or complete tears, whereas visualization of possible tears of the anterior or posterior glenoid pads is extremely poor.[39]

The only point in favor of US is the possibility of assessing cortical osseous tears at the posterosuperior aspect of the humeral head.[40] This lesion, caused by anterior luxation of the shoulder, is named 'Hill-Sachs' disease.

ELBOW AND WRIST

The elbow joint is enveloped by a single capsule, reinforced by two collateral ligaments whose function is to stabilize the articular complex formed by the distal end of the humerus and the proximal ends of the ulna and radius. In functional terms there are three articular components: humero-ulnar, humeroradial and proximal radio-ulnar. Articular movement, dictated mainly by the humero-ulnar joint, is complex, being flexor-extensor with associated pronato-supinator movements. The latter are possible in any position, with simultaneous involvement not only of the elbow joint, but also of the distal radio-ulnar joint.[41]

Ultrasound studies serve to quantify the changes present and are performed in sequelae of trauma and in the presence of inflammation or space-occupying lesion.

Sequelae of trauma and inflammatory disease

The most common acute post-traumatic changes are bursitis, muscular disinsertions and inflammatory processes due to functional overloading.[42]

Normal synovial bursae are not detectable with US. Bursitis, clearly appreciable clinically, looks like a well-demarcated tumor whose texture ranges from echofree to structured (Fig. 18.45).

After muscle disinsertion or rupture of a tendon the hematoma is always imaged at the point of rupture and retraction, complete or partial, of the fibers involved in the lesion, together with perilesional edema (Fig. 18.46). In stabilized conditions, especially when appropriate treatment has been given, the sequelae may not be very clear, in which case identification and assessment are not simple. In untreated cases, scars with calcifications and/or serous-hemorrhagic collections may be found (Fig. 18.47).

Inflammation due to overloading has characteristic features which may affect the cortical tissue of the epicondyle and of the epitrochlea and always involve the insertions of the extensor muscles on the epicondyle and of the flexors on the epitrochlea. Cortical changes, if present, take the form of small spurs and/or microerosions (Fig. 18.48). The insertions of the muscles show an increase in overall volume, a convexity at the insertion (Fig. 18.49) and a coarse irregular structure with accentuation of the fibrous component and occasional calcifications.[7,21,25] If an acute event is superimposed on chronic damage, areas of degeneration may be present (Fig. 18.50).

The normal joint compartment is always well demarcated by the capsulo-ligamentous system and presents an echofree or hypoechoic texture. In the case of arthrosynovitis, post-traumatic or inflammatory, the articular compartment is increased in volume, the capsulo-ligamentous system is convex, and the texture of the articular compartment may be regular, hypoechoic or hyperechoic, but more irregular than the unaffected contralateral joint

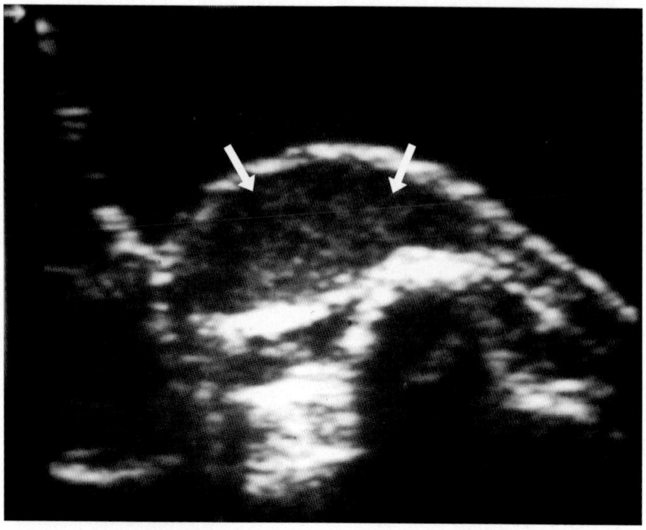

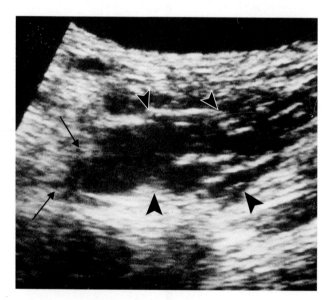

Fig. 18.45 Well-demarcated, hypoechoic mass with posterior enhancement (arrow) in the olecranon fossa: post-traumatic bursitis.

Fig. 18.46 Sagittal scan of the distal tendon of the humeral biceps: partial rupture with fresh hematoma (arrowhead) and retraction of the injured proximal fibers (arrow).

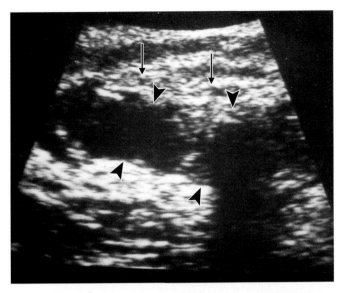

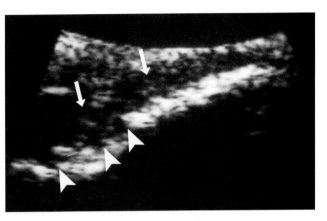

Fig. 18.48 Epicondylitis. Sagittal scan of the epicondyle showing erosions (arrowheads) of the bone cortex at the site of insertion of the extensor muscles (arrows).

Fig. 18.47 Sagittal scan of the distal brachialis tendon (arrow) showing a large, partially calcified post-traumatic pseudocyst (arrowhead).

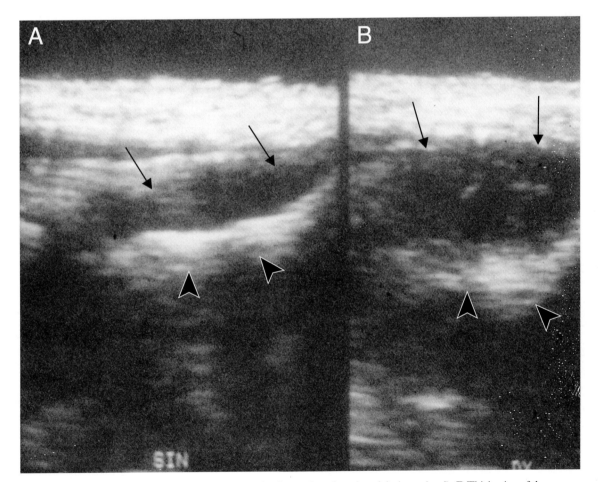

Fig. 18.49 **A** Normal insertion of the extensor muscles (arrows) to the epicondyle (arrowhead). **B** Thickening of the muscles, with convex margins due to inflammatory changes.

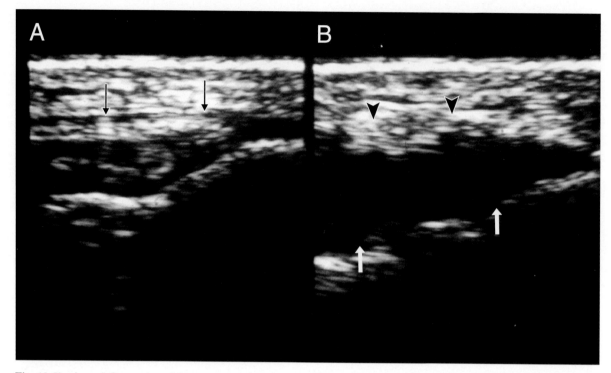

Fig. 18.50 Acute inflammation of the extensor tendons (arrows) (**B**) superimposed on pre-existing degenerative changes. The tendons are markedly hypoechoic with intense fibrosis of the superficial layers (arrowheads). Normal appearance of the contralateral side (**A**).

(Fig. 18.51). The change may be diffuse or localized. Intra-articular calcifications may also be present.

WRIST AND HAND

The principal structure of the wrist is the carpal tunnel, consisting dorsally of the two rows of carpal bones which form a groove with a volar concavity that is converted into an osteofibrous canal by the anterior annular ligament of the carpus. From its depth rises a fibrous septum which is fixed to the volar surface of the scaphoid bone: thus two

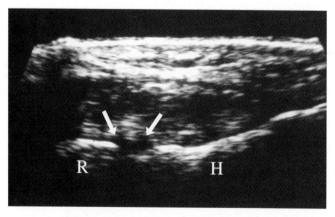

Fig. 18.51 Sagittal scan of the joint between the head of the radius (R) and the humeral condyle (H). The articular compartment has a convex morphology due to low-grade synovitis (arrow).

osteofibrous canals of different width are created. In the radial groove runs the tendon of the radial flexor muscle of the carpus. In the medial groove, which is the wider, run the tendons of the superficial and deep flexors of the fingers, the tendon of the long flexor of the thumb and the median nerve. On the ulnar side of the carpal tunnel lies Guyon's compartment, occupied by the ulnar artery and nerve. On the dorsal side lies the posterior annular ligament of the carpus which divides the space into six compartments, in which run the tendons of the extrinsic extensor muscles.

The movements of the hand are governed by the intrinsic and extrinsic muscles. The intrinsic muscles are all short muscles. The extrinsic muscles have their proximal insertions in the elbow and forearm and their distal insertions in the metacarpals and phalanges and are divided into two main groups – extensor and flexor extrinsic muscles. Synovial sheaths enclose the flexor tendons almost completely from the distal metaphysis of the radius and ulna to the distal insertion of the tendons. The metacarpal portions of the flexor tendons of the second, third and fourth fingers have no sheaths. The extensor tendons have synovial sheaths only in the dorsal osteofibrous canal of the wrist.

In the presence of sequelae of trauma, inflammatory processes and tumors, sonography permits an assessment of the damage and a determination of how it affects the neighboring structures.

The normal joint compartments are well delineated and

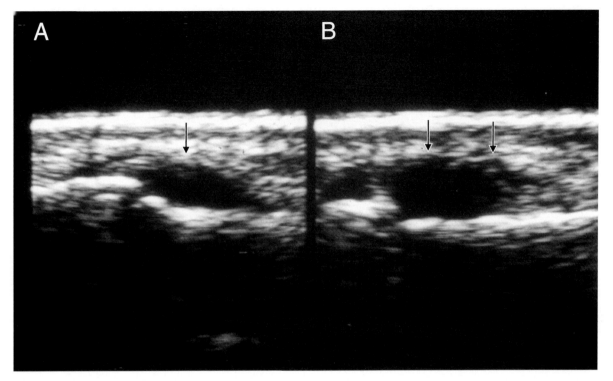

Fig. 18.52 Sagittal view of the proximal interphalangeal joint of the middle finger. On the right side (**B**) the joint compartment is enlarged (arrow), compared with the contralateral normal side (**A**).

their texture is anechoic or hypoechoic. In sequelae of trauma or in inflammatory or metabolic disease there is often an increase in volume, diffuse or localized, of the joint space, which may present a fine internal echogenicity (Fig. 18.52).[21,25] Following joint lesions it is possible to demonstrate and quantify the sequelae in the form of hypoechoic lumps which interrupt the hyperechoic linear image of the capsulo-ligamentous system. In sequelae of injury the metacarpophalangeal joint of the first finger is important, especially the ulnar ligament (Fig. 18.53).

The pathologic and sonographic aspects of tendon lesions have been described in Chapter 17, whereas glomus tumors of the fingers have been dealt with in Chapter 15.

The commonest tumors of the hand are hygromas (Fig. 18.54). Trochlear cysts appear as well-defined anechoic areas with posterior enhancement. As a rule, they lie volar to the tendon and appear immobile on dynamic examination (Fig. 18.55). Foreign body granulomas are easily diagnosed; they usually present as well-defined hypoechoic nodules with a hyperechoic core (Fig. 18.56).

SPACE-OCCUPYING LESIONS

Space-occupying lesions may affect any of the joints and may arise from any of the anatomic components, from bone to skin.

Lipomas usually present as well-defined solid masses with a hypoechoic structure mixed with hyperechoic streaks (Fig. 18.57), mostly located in the subcutaneous tissue. On dynamic examination and under targeted pressure the tumor (unless large) usually slides over both superficial and deep planes.

Fibromyolipomas are generally large and lack cleavage planes with the surrounding tissues.

Hygroma (see Fig. 18.54) always presents as a well-defined tumor, with regular, often multilobate margins and

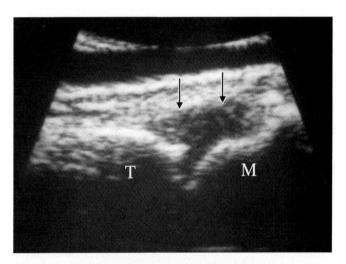

Fig. 18.53 Sagittal scan of the metacarpophalangeal joint of the thumb (ulnar side). The joint compartment (arrow) is enlarged and ill-defined due to sequelae of rupture of the collateral ulnar ligament. T: base of the proximal phalanx of the thumb; M: first metacarpal bone.

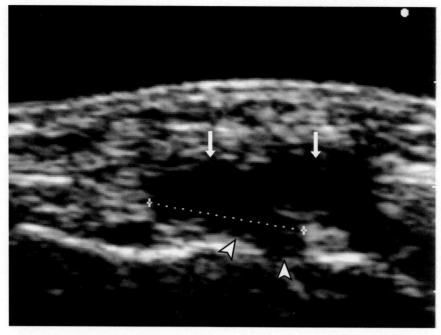

Fig. 18.54 Transverse scan of the wrist (radial volar view). Well-demarcated, oval hygroma (arrow), with posterior peduncle (arrowhead).

peduncle. It may be anechoic (if recent) or septate or echogenic (if of longer standing or treated with local infiltrations).

Echinococcal cysts of the musculoskeletal system have the same structural variability as hydatid cysts of any other body region (Fig. 18.58) and preferentially develop in the muscles of the shoulder.

Hemangiomas are solid lesions which are not always well delimited, with a coarse pattern and small anechoic, posteriorly enhancing areas. Signs of hypervascularization may be detected with color Doppler.

Scar tissue is often clearly visible. Its morphology and texture depend on the anatomic structure of the damaged part and on the time that has elapsed between the trauma and US examination. The texture ranges from anechoic to hyperechoic.

Benign tumors differ in appearance according to the tissues of origin and usually have regular margins.

Malignant tumors are generally hypoechoic (or mixed, due to necrotic changes) and frequently do not show signs of local infiltration. In most cases further diagnostic investigations (CT, MRI and X-rays) are mandatory.

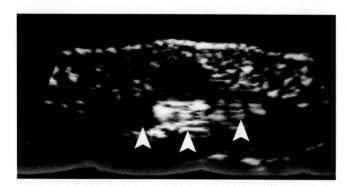

Fig. 18.55 Sagittal scan of the middle phalanx of the forefinger (volar side). Small trochear cyst in front of the flexor digitorum profundus tendon (arrowhead).

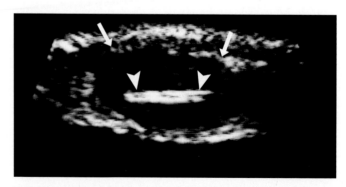

Fig. 18.56 Foreign body granuloma (arrow) with hyperechoic core (arrowhead). Sagittal scan of the palm of the hand.

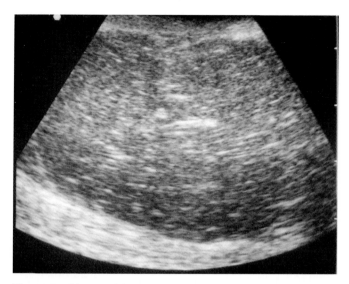

Fig. 18.57 Lipoma of the elbow joint.

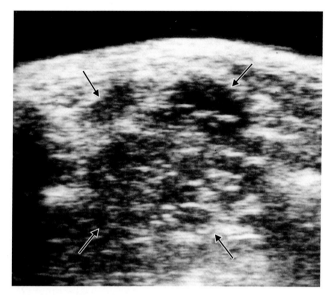

Fig. 18.58 Echinococcal cyst (arrow) of the deltoid muscle.

REFERENCES

1. Bloem S L, Sartoris D J 1992 MRI and CT of musculoskeletal system. Williams & Wilkins, Baltimore
2. Helenon O, Roger B, Laval C, Jeantet M 1991 IRM du genou. Masson, Paris
3. Mink J H, Reicher M A 1993 MRI of the knee. Raven Press, New York
4. De Flaviis L 1987 L'Ecografia dinamica del ginocchio varo-valgo: tecnica, indicazioni, risultati. US Med 8: 39–44
5. Fornage B D 1987 Echographie du systeme musculo-tendineux des membres. Vigot, Paris
6. Fornage B D, Rifkin M D 1989 Ultrasound examination of tendons. Radiol Clin North Am 26: 27–107
7. Wilson D J, Fornage B D, Bossi M C, Nessi R 1993 Musculoskeletal system and skin. In: Cosgrove D, Meire M, Dewbury K (eds) Abdominal and general ultrasound. Churchill Livingstone, London, pp 795–832
8. De Flaviis L 1989 Ultrasonic diagnosis of Osgood-Schlatter and Sinding-Larsen-Johnson diseases of the knee. Skeletal Radiol 18: 193–197
9. Laurac J, Felix F 1991 Echographie en pathologie musculaire et tendineuse. Vigot, Paris
10. Monetti G 1989 Ecografia muscolo-tendinea e dei tessuti molli. Solei Ed, Milan
11. Laine H R, Harjula A, Peltokallio P 1987 Ultrasound in the evaluation of the knee and patellar regions. J Ultrasound Med 6: 33–36
12. Richardson M L, Selby B, Montana M A, Mack L A 1988 Ultrasonography of the knee. Radiol Clin North Am 26: 63–75
13. De Flaviis L, Nessi R, Leonardi M, Ulivi M 1988 Dynamic ultrasonography of capsulo-ligamentous knee joint traumas. J Clin Ultrasound 16: 487–498
14. Selby B, Richardson M L, Montana M A, Teitz C C, Larson R V, Mack L A 1986 High resolution sonography of the menisci of the knee. Invest Radiol 21: 332–335
15. Selby B, Richardson M L, Nelson B D, Graney D O, Mack L A 1987 Sonography in the detection of meniscal injuries of the knee: evaluation in cadavers. AJR 149: 549–553
16. Van Holsbeeck M, Van Holsbeeck K, Gevers G et al 1988 Staging and follow-up of the arthritis of the knee. Comparison of sonography, thermography, and clinical assessment. J Ultrasound Med 7: 561–566
17. Gagnerie F, Taillan B, Bruneton J N et al 1986 Three cases of pigmented villonodular synovitis of the knee. Ultrasound and computed tomographic findings. ROFO 145: 227–228
18. Helzel M V, Schindler G, Gay B 1987 Sonographische messung des gelenkknorpels uber den femurkondylen. Fortschr Rontgenstr 147: 10–14
19. Aisen A M, McCune W J, MacGuire A et al 1984 Sonographic evaluation of the cartilage of the knee. Radiology 153: 781–784
20. Sintzoff S 1989 Imagerie du genou. Masson, Paris
21. Van Holsbeeck M, Introcaso J H 1991 Musculoskeletal ultrasound. Mosby, St Louis
22. De Flaviis L, Musso M C 1993 Arto inferiore. In: SIUMB (ed) Trattato Italiano di ecografia. Poletto Edizioni, Milan
23. Deutsch L, Mink J H, Kerr R 1992 MRI of the foot and ankle. Raven Press, New York
24. Basset R W, Cofield R H 1983 Acute tears of the rotator cuff: the timing of surgical repair. Clin Orthoped Relate Res 175: 1824–1827
25. Monetti G, Santoli G, Monteduro F 1993 Arto superiore. In: SIUMB (ed) Trattato Italiano di ecografia. Poletto Edizioni, Milan
26. Neer C S II, Craig E V, Fakuda H 1983 Cuff tear arthropathy. J Bone Joint Surg (Am) 65A: 1232–1244
27. Patten R M, Mack L A, Wang K Y, Lingel J 1994 Nondisplaced fractures of the greater tuberosity of the humerus: sonographic detection. (in press)
28. Seeger L, Leanne J 1992 Diagnostic imaging of the shoulder. Williams and Wilkins, Baltimore
29. Brandt T D, Cardone B W, Grant T H, Post M, Weiss C A 1989 Rotator cuff sonography: a reassessment. Radiology 173: 323–327
30. Mack L A, Matsen F A, Kilcoyne J F, Davies P K, Sickle M E 1985 Ultrasound evaluation of the rotator cuff. Radiology 157: 205–209
31. Miller C L, Karasick D, Kurtz A B, Fenlin J M 1989 Limited sensitivity of ultrasound for the detection of rotator cuff tear. Skeletal Radiol 18: 179–183
32. Crass J R, Craig E V, Feinberg S B 1988 Ultrasonography of rotator cuff tear: a review of 500 diagnostic studies. J Clin Ultrasound 16: 313–327
33. Harryman D D T II, Mack L A, Wang K Y, Jackins S E, Richardson M L, Matsen F A III 1991 Rotator cuff repair: correlation of functional results with cuff integrity. J Bone Joint Surg 73A: 982–989
34. Hodler J, Fretz C J, Terrier F, Gerber C 1988 Rotator cuff tears: correlation of sonography and surgical findings. Radiology 167: 791–793
35. Mack L A, Nyberg D A, Matsen F A III 1988 Sonographic evaluation of the rotator cuff. Radiol Clin North Am 26: 161–177
36. Masten F A, Arntz C T 1990 Subacromial impingement. In: Rockwood C A, Matsen F A (eds) The shoulder, vol II. W B Saunders, Philadelphia

37. Middleton W D 1989 Status of rotator cuff sonography. Radiology 173: 307–309

38. Monetti G 1989 L'ecografia nella patologia traumatica della spalla. Aulo Gaggi Editore, Bologna

39. Calvert P T, Packer W P, Stoker D J, Bayley J K, Kressel B L 1986 Arthrography of the shoulder after operative repair at the torn rotator cuff. J Bone Joint Surg (Br) 68B: 147–150

40. Crass J R, Craig E V, Feinberg S B 1986 Sonography of postoperative rotator cuff. AJR 146: 561–564

41. Barr L L, Babcock D S 1991 Sonography of the normal elbow. AJR 157: 793–798

42. Koski J M 1990 Ultrasonography of the elbow joint. Rheumatol Int 10: 91–94

19

Bone and callus

G. Rizzatto   M. Abbona   G. Mininel

Bone cannot be completely visualized because of the almost complete attenuation or reflection of sound at its interface. Nevertheless, the evaluation of its outer margin adds significant information to the diagnosis of several changes involving joints and muscles (see Chs 16–18). Some pathological conditions cause interruption of the cortical bone and open a window on the inner components of the spongiosa (Fig. 19.1). However, these cases are unusual.

Ultrasound studies are generally applied to the assessment of bone characteristics and to the evaluation of fracture healing.

BONE ASSESSMENT

Sound transmission and absorption in bone have long been considered to have potential diagnostic value. Many studies have established that sound transmission velocity is influenced both by mass density and by the architectural and material properties along the transmission path.[1] When the frequency of ultrasound waves varies between 200 and 600 kHz, the gradient of attenuation provides accurate information on the bone density.[2] Two of the most commonly used ultrasound measures are the speed of sound (SOS) and the broad-band ultrasound attenuation (BUA). SOS represents the velocity of ultrasound transmission through the bone. It is influenced by the elasticity and the density of the bone measured; generally, SOS is higher for relatively dense materials.[3] BUA represents the loss of energy resulting from the interaction of the ultrasound waves with the medium through which they pass. In trabecular bone BUA reflects not only the absorption of ultrasound, but also its scattering by the trabeculae;[2] they act as successive filters which selectively reduce the frequency components across the transmission band. There is indirect evidence that BUA is related to density as well as to architecture, i.e. trabecular quantity, spacing and orientation.[4] The strength of bone, and consequently the risk of fracture, is related to the amount of bone and to its structure.[5] Because of high turnover, cancellous bone is an ideal site for detection of early bone loss and monitoring of response to therapy. Commercially available scanners have been developed, some of which measure the ultrasonic properties of the patella; most of them work on the os calcis. The os calcis is subcutaneous, easily accessible even in obese patients, and has virtually flat and parallel surfaces. It is mainly composed of cancellous bone, with 90–95% of cancellous bone by volume. Moreover, the trabecular pattern of os calcis, a weight-bearing bone, closely parallels that in the upper end of the femur; its decrement in bone mass is similar to those of the femur and radius.[6]

The Achilles system (Lunar Corporation, Madison, WI, USA) consists of two large transducers, mounted coaxially; one transducer acts as the transmitter and the other as the receiver. Acoustic coupling is accomplished by submerging the transducer pair and the heel in a water bath (Fig. 19.2). The waveform collection time is very short, which minimizes motion artifacts. SOS value is obtained measuring the transit time; this procedure eliminates the need to measure skin thickness.[7] BUA value is obtained through the discrete Fourier analysis of a broad spectrum of frequencies.

The Achilles instrument combines BUA and SOS measurements to derive a third value, the stiffness, which represents an attempt to define a clinical index of bone quality. Stiffness is expressed as a percentage deviation from expected young normal, and in Z-score, which is the difference divided by intrapopulation standard deviation (Fig. 19.3).

Many reports[6–8] have demonstrated that SOS and BUA measurements have clinical significance because they are

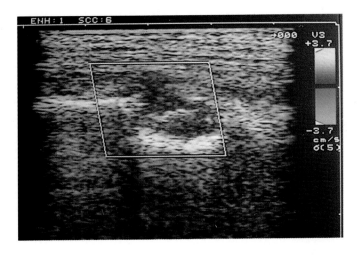

Fig. 19.1 Secondary involvement of the left tibia from lung carcinoma. The cortical bone is interrupted; the spongiosa is partially occupied by a highly vascularized tissue that also invades the adjacent muscles.

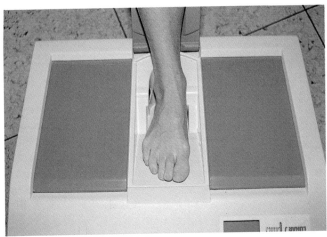

Fig. 19.2 The control box and the heel bath of the Achilles bone densitometer. The control box houses the Achilles electronics; it preprocesses the signals from the transducers in the heel bath before sending them to the computer for storage and analysis.

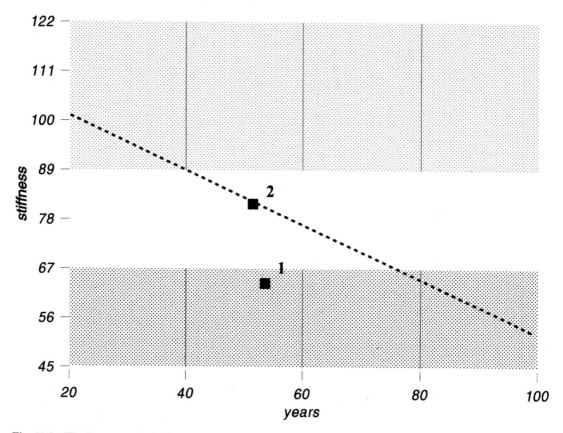

Fig. 19.3 The %-age-matched value compares the patient's stiffness value with the expected stiffness values of a reference group of the same age and sex. In this graph the value for Patient 2 clearly deviates from the normal regression line. (Patient 1: SOS 1555, BUA 116, Stiffness 82; Patient 2: SOS 1501, BUA 102, Stiffness 63.)

significantly different between normal and osteopenic women. The values of SOS, BUA, and bone mineral density (BMD) measured with dual energy X-ray absorptiometry (DXA) correlate moderately well (from $p < 0.05$ to $p < 0.0001$), especially if they are related to the femoral neck BMD measurements. Stiffness values correlate slightly better, also with BMD measurements found in the spine and in the distal radius.[7] To date, there is no reliable explanation for the cases in which DXA and ultrasound measurements do not correlate; in most of these patients, DXA values fall within a group with higher risk of osteoporosis. Given that X-ray and ultrasound examine different aspects of bone, a strong correlation is not so important. Long-term prospective studies will establish the predominant importance of density or structure in predicting a risk of fracture; probably they are complementary. Apart from screening for osteoporosis, the ultrasound evaluation of os calcis may add significant information in some diffuse metabolic diseases and in the follow-up of patients with severe fractures of the lower limb.

FRACTURE HEALING

Multiple factors affect fracture healing, including the severity of injury to bone and soft tissue, the age of the patient and his or her nutritional status, and the local nutrition at the fracture site. There is also an inherent metabolic controlling mechanism. The treatment method, which markedly influences the mechanical conditions prevailing at the fracture site, is also an important factor.[9]

Fractures that are surgically stabilized tend to undergo *primary healing*, in which the fragments are joined by direct, angiogenic bone formation. On the other hand, the imperfect immobilization produced by external fixators mostly gives rise to *secondary fracture healing*. In this process the fracture hematoma is enclosed by a tension-resistant envelope of soft tissues; this hematoma may be absent in the case of surgery for an exposed fracture. Connective tissue cells and subsequently cartilage cells develop within the hematoma. The intercellular component calcifies and forms stable masses that are invaded by blood vessels; osteons are formed along these vessels. A successive progression from connective tissue to cartilage and thence to calcification is characteristic of secondary healing. First, it gives rise to an irritation callus, which gradually converts to a hard fixation callus. A few weeks after treatment, this callus stabilizes the fracture and the frame can be removed. The fixation callus is followed by a remodeling process;

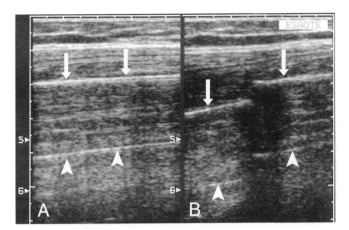

Fig. 19.4 Normal (**A**) and fractured tibia (**B**). Arrows indicate the strong reflection due to the cortical bone; arrowheads indicate the artifactual inner surface caused by the reverberation.

there is a significant reduction of its size and a bony cicatrix represents complete recovery.

If the bone fragments have a good blood supply, there are good conditions for osteogenesis, resulting in a *vascular non-union* in which the mechanical pathogenesis is predominant. If the fragments have little or no blood supply, or if a significant osseous defect is present, the result is an *avascular union*. Its pathogenesis is mainly biological and the fragments have a characteristic radiographic appearance: absence of visible callus and sclerosis of the bone ends.

In patients with external fixators, ultrasound can be used in the follow-up of the fracture healing process, to augment X-ray and clinical information.[10] The scanning area is partially limited by the design of the external frame; the use of small intraoperative probes with a frequency of 5–7.5 MHz gives the best results. The diaphyseal cortical bone gives rise to very strong linear reflections; these cause marked reverberations that are responsible for deeper artifactual echoes that simulate a second, parallel bone surface (Fig. 19.4). The area between the probe–skin interface and the bone is occupied by muscles, vessels and soft tissues. Their

characteristics differ according to the anatomic site.

In the *first phase* (4–15 days after the fracture and the application of the external fixators), ultrasound shows the gap between the cortical ends; the deeper reverberation artifact exhibits the same pattern (Fig. 19.4B). In 90% of closed fractures, a hypoechoic area, consisting of hematoma, fragments and tissue, alters the adjacent muscles and fills the osseous defects (Fig.19.5); this hypoechoic area may be small or absent in the case of exposed fracture created by surgical reduction. Normally, color Doppler shows vessels proximal to and within the fracture site (Fig. 19.6).

In the *second phase* (15–30 days after the fracture) the fragments show smoother ends. The hypoechoic area reduces in size and becomes more echogenic, mainly at its periphery. Small linear echoes suggest the formation of periosteal collars (Fig. 19.7). In the case of correct dynamization the outer margin of the hypoechoic area is convex; excessive dynamization often gives rise to angular, spire-like morphologies.

In the *third phase* (20–40 days after the fracture) the hypoechoic area becomes more echogenic; the outer rim often reflects linear echoes due to calcification (Fig. 19.8). Ultrasound still penetrates the deeper portion of the callus, showing vessels and small highly echogenic spots due to calcification. In this phase radiography shows initial periosteal apposition.

Abnormal healing processes often show very poor vascularity. However, subjective evaluation of vascularity alone seems to be insufficient to predict the final outcome. Spectral analysis suggests that vessels showing a low resistance flow may predict a good final outcome.[11] Near the end of the healing process, these vessels exhibit a characteristic telesystolic indentation due to the formation of a muscular tunica (Fig. 19.9). By contrast, a high resistance flow is typical of altered or delayed healing processes (Fig. 19.10).

In the *fourth phase* (40–90 days after the fracture) there is a progressive increase in the echogenicity of the periosteal callus, resulting in different degrees of posterior acoustic shadowing (Fig. 19.11). In this phase, radiography clearly

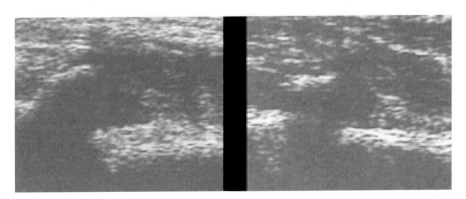

Fig. 19.5 Different aspects of the acute phase: fracture gaps, hypoechoic hematomas and bony fragments.

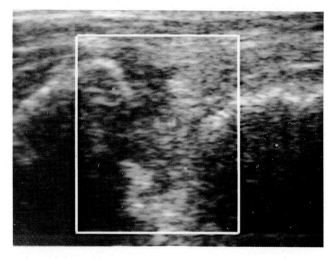

Fig. 19.6 The osseous defect is filled by an area of low echogenicity caused by hematoma and residual tissues; vascularity is observed inside and proximal to this area.

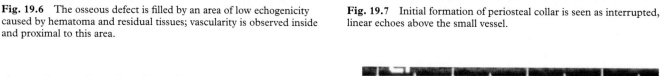

Fig. 19.7 Initial formation of periosteal collar is seen as interrupted, linear echoes above the small vessel.

shows the periosteal callus; the radiographic image is smaller because sonography also shows the fibrous and cartilagineous portions. The final, positive outcome is reconstruction of cortical bone and restoration of its deeper reverberation artifact. The subsequent remodeling process gives rise to a regular bony cicatrix that represents complete recovery (Fig. 19.12).

Good correlation has been demonstrated between the ultrasound image and the mechanical status of the healing process, evaluated by recording the maximal strain value variations:[10] there is an indirect correlation between the volume of the periosteal callus and its mechanical stability; the appearance of the acoustic shadow coincides with an

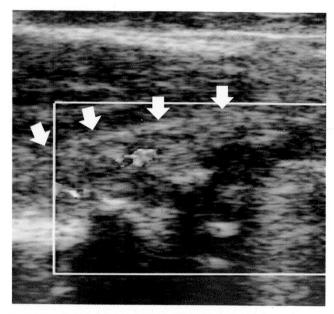

Fig. 19.8 Calcification of the outer margin of the callus gives rise to a continuous echogenic rim (arrows) that well defines the callus morphology.

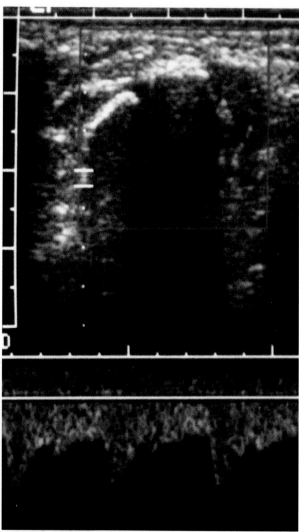

Fig. 19.9 Transverse scan of a fractured patella, 40 days after surgery. Vessels show low resistance index (RI = 48), and a typical indentation is seen on the spectrum at the end of the systole. (By courtesy of F Calliada, Department of Radiology, General Hospital, Lodi, Italy.)

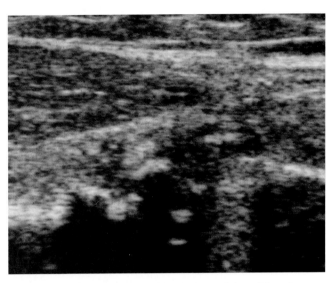

Fig. 19.11 The same case as in Fig. 19.8, 1 week later. There is a significant increase in the echogenicity of the callus components.

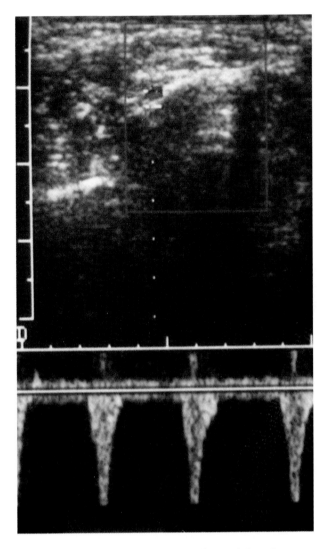

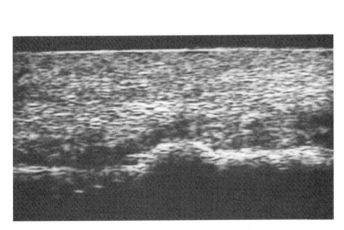

Fig. 19.10 Fractured tibia with altered healing, 110 days after trauma. Vessels show high resistance index (RI = 90). (By courtesy F Calliada, Department of Radiology, General Hospital, Lodi, Italy.)

acceleration of bone apposition and is an index of initial mechanical recovery; the disappearance of the acoustic shadow and the visibility of the deeper reverberation artifact coincide with the final recovery of the bone and the restoration of its mechanical stability.

Ultrasound also shows complications involving the adjacent tissues, like fistulae and abscesses (Fig. 19.13); in these cases ultrasound augments the clinical findings and can enable very precise percutaneous drainage.

Ultrasound also provides information on the rate and quality of new bone formation during distraction osteogenesis for bone lengthening.[12] After osteotomy, the limb is elongated slowly and continuously at a rate of no more than 1–1.5 mm per day. It is very important to determine if the rate of callus formation is equal to the rate of limb lengthening. Poor callus formation is predicted when ultrasound shows areas of decreased echogenicity in the developing bone.

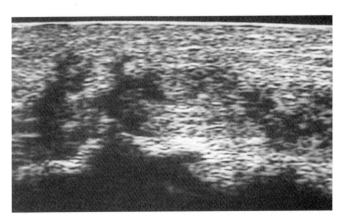

Fig. 19.12 Residual alteration of the cortical profile of a fractured femur after the final remodeling process.

Fig. 19.13 Altered healing process with cuspid-like shape of the callus and inflammatory infiltration of the adjacent muscles.

REFERENCES

1. Abendschein W, Hyatt G W 1970 Ultrasonics and selected physical properties of bone. Clin Orthop 69: 294–301
2. Langton C M, Palmer S B, Porter R W 1984 The measurement of broadband ultrasonic attenuation in cancellous bone. Eng Med 13: 89–91
3. Biot M A 1962 Generalized theory of acoustic propagation in porous dissipative media. J Acoust Soc Am 34: 1254–1264
4. Schott A M, Hans D, Sornay-Rendu E, Delmas P D, Meunier P J 1993 Ultrasound measurement on os calcis: precision and age-related changes in a normal female population. Osteoporosis Int 3: 249–254
5. Mosekilde L 1989 Sex differences in age related loss of vertebral trabecular bone mass and structure–biomechanical consequences. Bone 10: 425–432
6. Laugier P, Giat P, Berger G 1994 New ultrasonic methods of quantitative assessment of bone status. Eur J Ultrasound 1: 23–38
7. Lees B, Stevenson J C 1993 Preliminary evaluation of a new ultrasound bone densitometer. Calcif Tissue Int 53: 149–152
8. Massie A, Reid D M, Porter R W 1993 Screening for osteoporosis: comparison between dual energy x-ray absorptiometry and broadband ultrasound attenuation in 1000 perimenopausal women. Osteoporosis Int 3: 107–110
9. Weber B G, Magerl F 1985 The external fixator. Springer-Verlag, Berlin
10. Ricciardi L, Perissinotto A, Dabalà M 1993 Mechanical monitoring of fracture healing using ultrasound imaging. Clin Orthop 293: 71–76
11. Calliada F, Bottinelli O, Sala G, Raieli G, Corsi G, Conti M P 1993 Color Doppler differential diagnosis between normally and delayed healing bone fractures. Radiology 189 (P): 209
12. Eyres K S, Bell M J, Kanis J A 1993 Methods of assessing new bone formation during limb lengthening. Ultrasonography, dual energy X-ray absorptiometry and radiography compared. J Bone Joint Surg [Br] 75: 358–364

20

Intraoperative ultrasound of the exocrine pancreas

G. Di Candio   A. Pietrabissa   F. Mosca

INTRODUCTION

During the last two decades, ultrasound (US), dynamic CT, MRI, and percutaneous US- and CT-guided biopsies have revolutionized the diagnostic approach to diseases of the exocrine pancreas and reduced the number of diagnostic laparotomies. Preoperative work-up, which also included angiography, abdominal laparoscopy, and ERCP allows us almost always to reach the correct diagnosis and, in the case of pancreatic cancer, to evaluate resectability correctly in 90% of cases.[1] However, at laparotomy, before surgical dissection, difficulties can be encountered in evaluating pancreatic diseases by vision and touch alone because of the deep location of the pancreas, its complex relations with vessels and retroperitoneal connective tissue, and the possibly small dimensions of the nodules (as, for instance, in small endocrine tumors). Hence, sometimes it may be impossible to palpate a nodule, to localize a main pancreatic duct which is slightly dilated, to differentiate pancreatic cancer and chronic pancreatitis, and to detect vascular infiltration.

Operative imaging is usually limited to contrast X-rays, with opacification of biliary and pancreatic ducts, to assess the site and etiology of the obstruction. However, this might not be sufficient to clarify the situation during pancreatic surgery. Intraoperative ultrasonography (IOUS), first introduced in the 1960s for biliary and renal stone location, has been sensibly improved thanks to the real-time and gray-scale facilities and the availability of high-frequency, small, handy probes. IOUS provides a wide and reliable anatomic representation of the abdominal cavity and allows the surgeon easily to localize focal pancreatic lesions, with simultaneous palpation.

The continuous improvement in short- and long-term results obtained in pancreatic surgery has also widened resectability criteria in the case of vascular infiltration and, in selected cases, may justify palliative resection. The new trend to resect what was considered unresectable only a few years ago justifies the use of IOUS for several purposes: localization of occult endocrine tumors (where IOUS is the new 'gold standard' technique), management of chronic pancreatitis, and choice of the surgical approach in a case of pancreatic cancer.

TECHNIQUE AND INSTRUMENTATION

Intraoperative sonographic probes differ from those used in percutaneous sonography in shape, size, and frequency. Three main shapes are available: pen (phased-array or mechanical sector scan), bar, and T-shaped (linear or mini-convex scan). The frequencies range from 5 to 10 MHz. New equipment includes Doppler and color Doppler facilities, increasing the diagnostic capabilities.

The pancreas does not have bare areas as the liver does, therefore it does not require any particular shape of probe for its complete examination. Acoustic coupling is obtained by pouring 200–250 ml of warm saline into the abdominal cavity. A slight tilting of the surgical table to the left increases the capacity of the abdominal cavity, raising the fluid level above the pancreas, particularly when examining the pancreatic body and tail. Some pen-shaped probes have a water-path stand-off in order to increase near-field focalization. With this type of instrument the acoustic coupling can be obtained with a thin layer of saline solution.

The probes are sterilized by either cold-gas sterilization (using ethylene dioxide at normal temperature, under normal pressure), or chemical sterilization (with 2% Hibitane alcohol, 2% glutaraldehyde, or 0.1% sodium hypochlorite), or by plastic sterilized bags filled with sonographic gel. Plastic bags do not damage the probes, which can be used repeatedly during the same day, in emergencies, or in consecutive surgical procedures.

Sonographic scan planes vary according to the area to be examined. Due to the small size of the probes and, consequently, of the field of view, the assessment of the US images is difficult, particularly for inexperienced operators. The traditional vascular landmarks (i.e. the portal trunk and its main branches) may be helpful for orientation in the scanning planes. The pancreatic head and body are better studied using transverse scans, while the tail requires longitudinal and oblique scans.

WHEN TO USE IOUS

During surgery for chronic pancreatitis or cancer the best timing for IOUS is at the opening of the abdominal cavity, before any surgical dissection, when sonography provides significantly more information than inspection and palpation. IOUS can be performed via a transgastric or transduodenal route: slight compression by the probe permits the displacement of gas bubbles and enteric contents in order to obtain clear visualization. The interposition of stomach or duodenum helps when studying the superficial portion of the pancreas, whilst for deeper portions the gastrocolic and gastrohepatic ligaments can be utilized as acoustic windows.

Some authors prefer to approach the pancreas by keeping the probe directly on its surface, after a wide opening of the gastrocolic ligament, carefully preserving the gastroepiploic vessels along the entire length of the greater curvature of the stomach, and after a Kocher maneuver and spleen mobilization.

The first wide survey of the pancreatic region is performed with 5 MHz probes, whilst 7.5 MHz probes are subsequently used for more detailed exploration.

Ultrasound-guided biopsy is usually performed with a 'free-hand' technique, without any puncture adaptor. Cytologic samples can be obtained with 21–22 G Chiba needles, which are safe and effective, whilst histologic material can be obtained by Tru-Cut or Surecut needles, taking care to avoid the use of needles larger than 18 G because of the risk of needle tract tumor implantation and pancreatic fistulas.[2-4]

Usually, after an initial 'learning phase', the complete examination time does not exceed 5–10 minutes.

IOUS AND CHRONIC PANCREATITIS

Most patients with chronic pancreatitis are managed conservatively, but intractable abdominal pain, with or without pancreatic duct dilation, pseudocysts, abscesses, and biliary duct obstruction are indications for surgery.

Palpation of the pancreas is often difficult because of the significant morphologic changes related to fibrosis, intraductal and interstitial calcifications, dilatation of the pancreatic duct and superimposed acute pancreatitis with steatonecrosis. The mobility of the gland may be limited by inflammatory adhesions with periglandular fatty tissue and vessels. IOUS may help the surgeon to overcome this limitation.

The first step should be the identification of the main pancreatic duct (Fig. 20.1): It is generally easy even in normal glands and in fasting patients in whom the duct does not exceed 2 mm in diameter. If the duct is dilated, it can be visualized and palpated on the anterior surface of the pancreas, especially when associated with chronic and atrophic pancreatitis, but in the early stages of the disease and after repeated episodes of superimposed acute pancreatitis it cannot be appreciated by palpation. IOUS allows determination of the site of the main pancreatic duct (usually central and posterior in the pancreatic body), its diameter, the number and location of stenotic tracts and

the presence of intraluminal debris (protein plugs) or stones, with a global accuracy similar to that of ERCP[5] (Fig. 20.1). Furthermore, in selected cases with multiple segmental stenoses, IOUS can guide appropriate surgical section. The immediate assessment of US images allows localization of otherwise undetectable lesions: this cannot be achieved with other image techniques, such as ERCP. IOUS facilitates the safe insertion of thin needles into the pancreatic duct to inject contrast media.

The extrahepatic biliary tree can be studied with longitudinal scans of the pancreatic head; the common bile duct and the cystic duct appear in front of the portal vein. In chronic inflammatory changes the duct undergoes regular and progressive stenosis without pancreatic masses. The pancreatic echo texture is inhomogeneous, with patchy, mainly hypoechoic, areas (Fig. 20.2).

IOUS has high accuracy in detecting common bile duct stones,[6-9] which are not infrequently found in the natural history of chronic pancreatitis. In this situation, sonographic exploration should be performed before any surgical maneuver, particularly intraoperative cholangiography, since false positive results of IOUS may be caused by air microbubbles and intraluminal plugs resulting from physical and chemical reactions between contrast media and bile.

Study of the main venous vessels, mostly with Doppler and color Doppler, has to be performed without any compression, preferably employing stand-off pads to place the probe 1–2 cm away from the pancreatic surface.

When pancreatic pseudocysts (PSC) are found, IOUS is helpful in defining their relationships with the blood vessels, pancreatic duct and biliary tree and in choosing the best

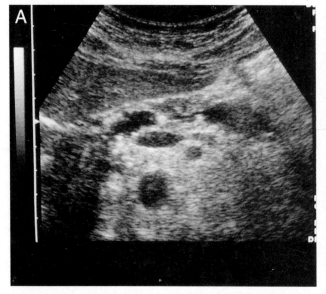
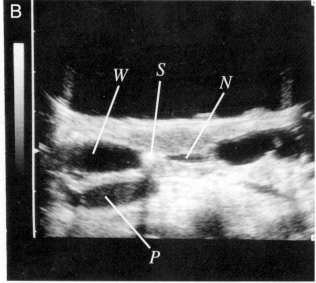

Fig. 20.1 Preoperative (**A**) and intraoperative (**B**) sonography in a patient with chronic pancreatitis and disabling abdominal pain. IOUS shows several irregularities of the pancreatic duct (W), with stenosis, dilatation and a solitary stone (S). P: portal vein; N: narrowing of the pancreatic duct.

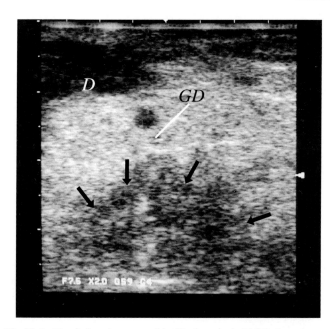

Fig 20.2 Focal chronic pancreatitis (black arrows). IOUS shows a hypoechoic inhomogeneous area of the head of the pancreas. GD: gastroduodenal artery; D: duodenum.

site of drainage, if needed. Small pseudocysts missed in the preoperative imaging work-up can be occasionally detected.[10–12] The sonographic appearance of the walls (thickness, vascularization, calcifications, neoplastic changes) and the content (liquid, solid, mixed, with or without septa) helps in differentiating PSCs from cystic tumors. In doubtful cases either fine-needle aspiration of the fluid with evaluation of amylase, CEA, and Ca 125 content[13] or cytology-histology of the wall irregularities is mandatory.

In the case of pancreatic abscess, IOUS defines the extent of the inflammatory cavity and its vascular relationships (very important during major necronectomy) and allows complete drainage of residual non-communicating sacs.[14]

IOUS AND PANCREATIC CANCER

Palpation and IOUS together are the most accurate diagnostic tools for the detection of small endocrine pancreatic tumors, with better results than those of angiography and transhepatic venous sampling.[15–21] The utilization of IOUS in neoplasms of the exocrine pancreas has recently been reported, mostly for periampullary tumors of the head of the pancreas, whose incidence has increased worldwide in the last 40 years.[22–23] Surgically, in the last ten years the resectability rate of pancreatic pathologies has doubled (from 10 to 20% of cases), still remaining lower in the oncologic field.[24] Several institutions reported a drop in hospital morbidity and mortality after pancreatico-duodenectomy (from 20 to 2%),[25–29] mainly due to better selection of candidates for surgery and improvement of

both surgical technique and postoperative intensive care. Recently, Trede et al reported less than 1% mortality in a series of 118 consecutive resected patients.[30] These results have encouraged more aggressive management of pancreatic cancer, extending resections to cases previously considered inoperable (i.e. cancers with vascular infiltration), or performing, in selected cases, palliative resections instead of simple digestive and biliary by-passes.

The 5-year survival rate has generally improved, being as high as 20% in some reports.[25,26,31] In patients with tumors smaller than 2 cm, with neither vascular invasion nor nodal involvement, the 5-year survival rate can exceed 50%.[32]

Even though preoperative work-up correctly defines unresectability in 90% of cases, with an accuracy of 80%,[33] IOUS is still useful to correct preoperative over- or under-estimations in some particular instances:

- jaundiced patients with cholestasis but without pre- or intraoperatively demonstrated pancreatic masses
- patients with palpable, doubtful pancreatic masses (pancreatitis or cancer)
- patients with associated cancer and pancreatitis (6–10% of cases).[33–34]

IOUS can confirm or exclude the presence of a pancreatic mass in 32% and 4% of patients respectively, according to Plainfosse et al.[35] Additional diagnostic findings (i.e. biliary lithiasis) are provided in 45% of cases.[35–37]

Sonographically, pancreatic cancer appears as a round, hypoechoic and inhomogeneous mass (rarely iso- or hyperechoic)[38] with ill-defined margins. Biliary, ampullary and pancreatic cancers cannot be differentiated on the basis of the sonographic appearance. Differentiation may only be obtained in the early stages by evaluating the relationship of the mass to the biliary tree; final diagnosis is provided only by examination of the surgical specimen.

IOUS allows the safe performance of biopsies, avoiding blood vessels and the pancreatic duct, and reaching any nodule of the pancreatic head via the transduodenal route in order to reduce complications (i.e. pancreatic fistula). The global accuracy of intraoperative biopsy of the pancreas reaches 85–90%.[35–39]

As previously mentioned, the sonographic staging of pancreatic tumors is possible at the very beginning of surgical exploration, with the great advantage of performing 'en bloc' vascular resections with no-touch technique, without the time-consuming and potentially contaminating surgical dissection which sometimes can be complicated by hemorrhage or pancreatic duct injury.

The sonographic evaluation of peripancreatic vessels has a triple aim:

a. detection of vascular anomalies
b. detection of vascular invasion by the tumor
c. detection of invasion by metastatic lymph nodes.

Knowledge of vascular anomalies before surgical dissection influences the operative strategy. The same information can be obtained by preoperative angiography, which demonstrates significant vascular anomalies in 30% of cases: anomalous course of the right hepatic artery (14%) or common hepatic artery (5%)[40–43] (Fig. 20.3), accessory right and/or left hepatic artery, early bifurcation of the hepatic artery, arteriovenous fistulas, aneurysms, thrombosis, etc. Missed identification of these anomalies increases morbidity during surgical preparation for pancreatoduodenectomy, especially when the surgeon's experience is limited.

The study of the relationships between blood vessels (portal vein, mesenteric vein, superior mesenteric artery and celiac axis) and the tumor is the main step in staging pancreatic cancer. Different spatial relationships can occur (Fig. 20.4):

a. vessels distant from the tumor
b. vessels touching the mass without any variation of their courses
c. vessels compressed but with regular margins
d. vessels compressed, with irregular margins (disappearance of the echogenic wall)
e. as in (d), but associated with endoluminal thrombosis (Figs 20.5, 20.6)
f. progressive disappearance of the vascular lumen, completely replaced by neoplastic tissue.

While occurrences (a) and (b) are undoubtedly consistent with non-involved vessels and occurrences (d) to (f) with vessel infiltration, the interpretation of occurrence (c) still remains questionable and requires surgical dissection for its resolution. Feeding vessels of the tumor may be misinterpreted as contiguous infiltrated vessels (false positive diagnosis). These problems may currently be solved by color Doppler. Vascular infiltration can be caused not only by the primary tumor but also by metastatic lymph nodes around the celiac axis, the superior mesenteric artery and, at a later stage, the aorta and vena cava (Figs 20.7, 20.8).

As concerns the condition of the lymph nodes, IOUS has the same limitations as computed tomography and magnetic resonance, in that it is always difficult to define the nature of any enlarged lymph node. Oval shape, regular margins, the presence of a hyperechoic hilum and homogeneous echogenicity are all landmarks of benignity, while large size (more than 15–20 mm), irregular shape, ill-defined margins, and inhomogeneous, hypoechoic structure can raise the suspicion of neoplastic involvement. False negative results can be due to microscopic neoplastic invasion. When the common bile duct is involved by the cancer, it appears dilated with an abrupt and irregular end at the level of the neoplastic mass.

CONCLUSIONS

Several reports relating a significant drop in mortality rate and prolonged survival times have led to the concept that surgical excision of a pancreatic cancer might be worthwhile even in the case of vascular involvement, in contrast to Crile's statement that resection and simple by-pass will achieve the same goal. Provided the surgeon has a low mortality rate, even palliative resection may be justified, since it will probably offer the patient a better quality of life when compared to non-resectional palliation. As a

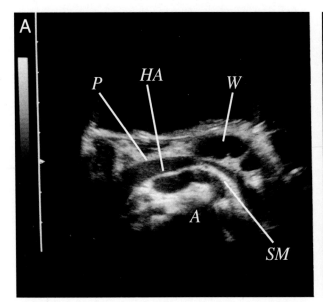
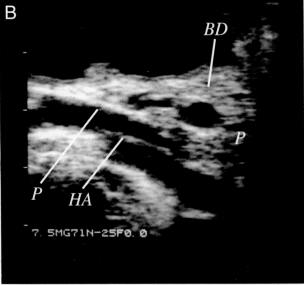

Fig 20.3 A Mechanical sector transverse scan in a case of pancreatic cancer, showing a dilated pancreatic duct (W), portal vein (P), aorta (A), and superior mesenteric artery (SM). Anomalous course of the common hepatic artery (HA). **B** Linear array scan in the same case, showing the anomalous retroportal course of the hepatic artery. BD: biliary duct; P: pancreatic head.

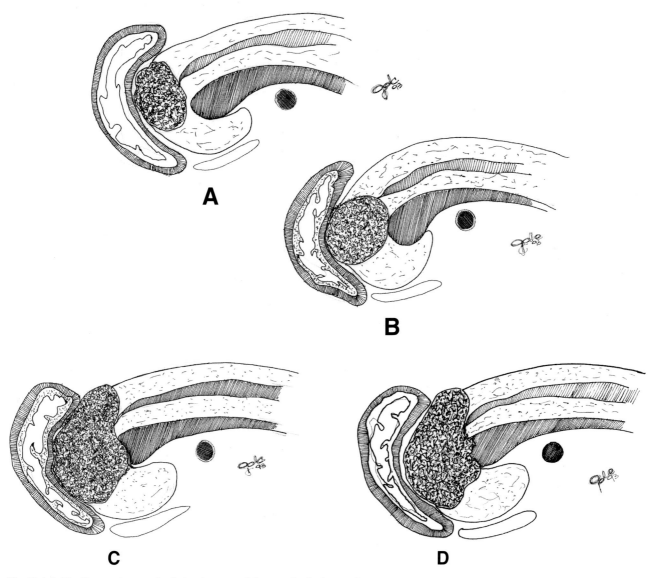

Fig 20.4 A–D   Progressive neoplastic involvement of the portal vein (see text).

consequence, fewer efforts are now made to identify pre-operative contraindications to surgery. Moreover, many surgeons believe that percutaneous or, preferably, endoscopic stent placement is not superior, in terms of prognosis, to biliary by-pass; in addition, many patients (up to 20–30%) will require gastroenteric by-pass to palliate duodenal obstruction.

US, CT and laparoscopy should represent the routine methods for preoperative staging of patients with pancreatic cancer, whilst IOUS provides the best assessment of tumor extension, particularly with respect to vascular infiltration. When IOUS suggests the tumor has involved the superior mesenteric artery or portal and mesenteric superior veins, a standard pancreatic head resection should be abandoned in favor of an 'en-bloc' resection which reduces intraoperative cancer dissemination and hemorrhagic complications.

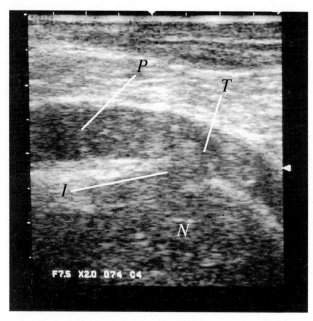

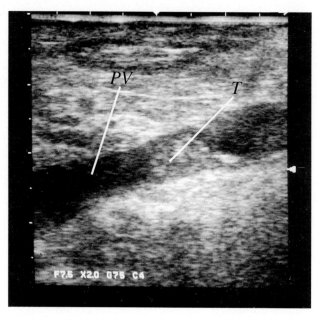

Fig 20.5 Oblique linear scan along the superior mesenteric vein and portal vein (P), showing neoplastic infiltration of the wall (I) and a neoplastic thrombus (T). N: neoplasm.

Fig 20.6 Oblique scan along the portal vein (PV) showing a neoplastic thrombus (T).

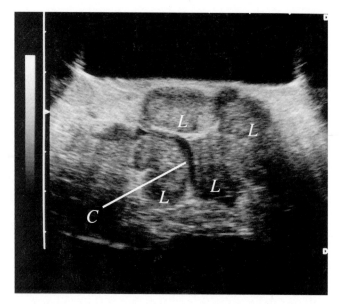

Fig 20.7 Celiac axis (C) infiltration by multiple involved lymph nodes (L) in a patient with cancer of the pancreatic body and tail.

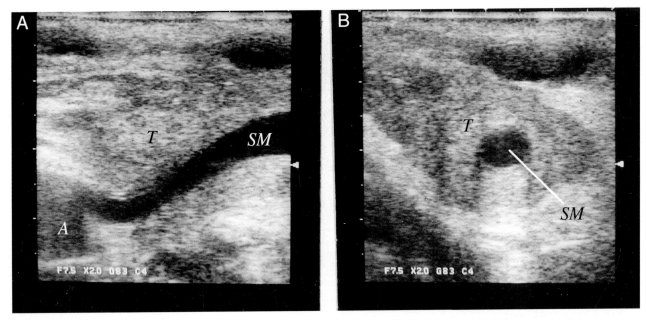

Fig 20.8   Neoplastic lymph node infiltration (T) around the superior mesenteric artery (SM), on oblique scan along the artery in (**A**) and on transverse scan in (**B**). A: aorta.

REFERENCES

1. Warshaw A L, Gu Z, Wittenberg J, Waltman A C 1990 Preoperative staging and assessment of resectability of pancreatic cancer. Arch Surg 125: 230–233
2. Warshaw A L 1991 Implications of peritoneal cytology for staging of early pancreatic cancer. Am J Surg 161: 26–30
3. Weiss S M, Skibber J M, Mohiuddin M, Rosato F E 1985 Rapid intra-abdominal spread of pancreatic cancer. Arch Surg 120: 415–416
4. Ferrucci J T, Wittenberg J, Margolies M N et al 1979 Malignant seeding of the tract after thin-needle aspiration biopsy. Radiology 130: 345–346
5. Printz H, Klotter H J, Nies C et al 1992 Intraoperative ultrasonography in surgery for chronic pancreatitis. Int J Pancreatol 12: 233–237
6. Machi J, Sigel B, Zaren H A, Kurohiji T, Yamashita Y 1993 Operative ultrasonography during hepatobiliary and pancreatic surgery. World J Surg 17: 640–646
7. Sigel B, Coelho J C U, Machi J et al 1983 The application of real-time ultrasound imaging during surgical procedures. Surg Gynecol Obstet 157: 33–37
8. Machi J, Sigel B 1989 Overview of benefits of operative ultrasonography during a ten-year period. J Ultrasound Med 8: 647–652
9. Jakimowicz J J, Rutten H, Jurgens P J, Carol E J 1987 Comparison of operative ultrasonography and radiography in screening of common bile duct for calculi. World J Surg 11: 628–634
10. Sigel B, Coelho J C, Spigos D G, Donahue P E, Wood D K, Nyhus L M 1981 Ultrasonic imaging during biliary and pancreatic surgery. Am J. Surg 141: 84–89
11. Rindsberg S, Radecki P D, Friedman A C, Au F, Mayer D 1986 Intraoperative localization of a small pancreatic pseudocyst. Gastrointestinal Radiol 11: 339–341
12. Kurohiji T, Sigel B, Machi J et al 1991 Detection of preoperatively unrecognized multiple pancreatic pseudocysts by intraoperative ultrasonography. Report of two cases. Am Surg 57: 668–672
13. Lewandrosky K B, Southern J F, Pins M R, Compton C C, Warshaw A L 1993 Cyst fluid analysis in the differential diagnosis of pancreatic cysts. Ann Surg 217: 41–47
14. Sigel B, Machi J, Kikuchi T, Anderson K W, Horrow M, Zaren H A 1987 The use of ultrasound during surgery for complications of pancreatitis. World J Surg 11: 659–663

15. van Heerden J A, Grant C S, Czako P F, Service F J, Charboneau J W 1992 Occult functioning insulinomas: which localizing studies are indicated? Surgery 112: 1010–1015
16. Brightbill T C, Templeton E O, Sperling D, Mooney L P 1992 Insulinoma: detection by intraoperative ultrasonography. JCU 20: 615–617
17. Doherty G M, Doppman J L, Shawker T H, Miller D L, Eastman R C, Gorden P 1991 Results of a prospective strategy to diagnose, localize and resect insulinomas. Surgery 110: 989–997
18. Bottger T C, Junginger T 1993 Is preoperative radiographic localization of islet cell tumors in patients with insulinoma necessary? World J Surg 17: 427–432
19. Angelini L, Bezzi M, Tucci G et al 1987 The ultrasonic detection of insulinomas during surgical exploration of the pancreas. World J Surg 11: 642–647
20. Cromack D T, Norton J A, Sigel B et al 1987 The use of high-resolution intraoperative ultrasound to localize gastrinomas: an initial report of a prospective study. World J Surg 11: 648–653
21. Norton J A, Cromack D T, Shawker T H et al 1988 Intraoperative ultrasonographic localization of islet cell tumors. A prospective comparison to palpation. Ann Surg 207: 160–168
22. Hirayama T 1989 Epidemiology of pancreatic cancer in Japan. J Clin Oncol 19: 208–215
23. Gordis L, Gold E B 1984 Epidemiology of pancreatic cancer. World J Surg 8: 808–821
24. Watanapa P, Williamson R C N 1992 Surgical palliation for pancreatic cancer: developments during the past two decades. Br J Surg 79: 8–20
25. Crist D W, Sitzmann J V, Cameron J L 1987 Improved hospital morbidity, mortality, and survival after the Whipple procedure. Ann Surg 206: 358–365
26. Braasch J W, Deziel D J, Rossi R L et al 1986 Pyloric and gastric preserving pancreatic resection: experience with 87 patients. Ann Surg 204: 411–418
27. Trede M, Schwall G, Saeger H 1990 Survival after pancreatoduodenectomy. Ann Surg 211: 447–458
28. Tsuchiya R, Tomioka T, Kunihide I et al 1986 Collective review of small carcinomas of the pancreas. Ann Surg 203: 77–81
29. Roder J D, Stein H J, Huttland W, Siewert J R 1992 Pylorus-preserving versus standard pancreatico-duodenectomy: an analysis of 110 pancreatic and periampullary carcinomas. Br J Surg 79: 152–155

30. Trede M, Schwall G, Saeger H 1990 Survival after pancreatoduodenectomy: 118 consecutive resections without an operative mortality. Ann Surg 211: 447–458
31. Trede M 1985 The surgical treatment of pancreatic carcinoma. Surgery 97: 28–35
32. Cameron J L, Crist D, Sitzmann J V et al 1991 Factors influencing survival after pancreaticoduodenectomy for pancreatic cancer. Am J Surg 161: 120–125
33. White M, Wittenberg J 1984 Pancreatic neoplasia. Semin US CT MR 5: 401–415
34. Sigel B, Machi J, Ramos J R, Duarte B, Donahue P E 1984 The role of imaging ultrasound during pancreatic surgery. Ann Surg 200: 486–493
35. Plainfosse M C, Bouillot J L, Rivaton F, Vaucamps P, Hernigou A, Alexandre J H 1987 The use of operative sonography in carcinoma of the pancreas. World J Surg 11: 654–658
36. Cane R J, Glazer G 1980 Intraoperative B-mode ultrasound scanning of the extrahepatic biliary system and pancreas. Lancet 2: 343–347

37. Smith S J, Vogelzang R L, Donovan J, Atlas S W, Gore R M, Neiman H L 1985 Intraoperative sonography of the pancreas. AJR 144: 557–562
38. Serio G, Fugazzola C, Iacono C et al 1992 Intraoperative ultrasonography in pancreatic cancer. Int J Pancreatol 11: 31–41
39. Moosa A R, Altorki N 1983 Pancreatic biopsy. Surg Clin North Am 63: 1205–1214
40. Kadir S, Lundell C, Saeed M 1991 Celiac, superior and inferior mesenteric arteries. In: Kadir S (ed) Atlas of normal and variant angiographic anatomy. Saunders, Philadelphia, pp 297–308
41. vanDamme J P, Bonte J 1990 Vascular anatomy in abdominal surgery. Thieme Medical, New York, pp 4–26
42. Bihel T, Traverso W, Hauptmann E, Ryan J 1993 Preoperative visceral angiography alters intraoperative strategy during the Whipple procedure. Am J Surg 165: 607–612
43. Dooley W C, Cameron J L, Pitt H A, Lillemoe K D, Yue N C, Venbrux A C 1990 Is preoperative angiography useful in patients with periampullary tumors? Ann Surg 211: 649–655

21

Liver intraoperative ultrasound

S. Miyagawa   M. Makuuchi

INTRODUCTION

As the liver surface has no landmarks which reflect intrahepatic structures, hepatic resection involved some risk before the introduction of intraoperative ultrasonography. While a tumor on the liver surface can be removed without ultrasonic guidance, safe and accurate resection of a tumor existing in deep portions of the liver is impossible without a device to visualize its location. Systematic hepatic resection based on hepatic anatomy can be carried out with intrahepatic vascular structure visualization, which can be achieved only using intraoperative ultrasonic guidance. Furthermore, intraoperative ultrasonography can detect small tumors which are overlooked by other preoperative imaging modalities and can predict the histologic nature of some tumors. The uses and merits of intraoperative ultrasonic examination for hepatic resection procedures are described below. In this chapter, Couinaud's terminology is used.

IDENTIFICATION OF INTRAHEPATIC ANATOMY

As the intrahepatic vascular structures can not be seen from outside, surgeons must reconstruct three-dimensional images of the spatial relationships between a tumor and the liver architecture on the basis of the two-dimensional information provided by intraoperative ultrasonography. In order to do this accurately when carrying out hepatectomy, surgeons need to understand the approximate spatial relationships represented by the preoperative image. When an unknown vessel is encountered during ultrasonic scanning, its site of origin must be established by tracing its course proximally; usually it will be identified as a tributary of a known main branch, providing the surgeon has a good understanding of intrahepatic vascular anatomy. The basic intrahepatic vascular anatomy should therefore be imprinted on the minds of hepatic surgeons as a three-dimensional image. Our intrahepatic portal map[1] is shown in Figure 21.1.

The right hepatic vein runs along the intersectoral plane between the right paramedian and lateral sectors, and drains mainly the latter and a small part of the former, particularly segment 8.[2] In almost all cases, the right hepatic vein is divided and transected extrahepatically following mobilization of the right liver from its diaphragmatic attachments and division of the inferior vena cava (IVC) ligament. This maneuver can reduce operative blood loss during hepatic parenchymal transection.[3] In patients with a small right hepatic vein, segment 6 is drained by the thick tributary of the middle hepatic vein or the thick short hepatic vein (the inferior right hepatic vein),[4] with which segment 6 can be preserved when the right hepatic vein must be resected. In the majority of patients, the middle hepatic vein runs along Rex-Cantlie's line and forms a common trunk with the left hepatic vein. It drains the right paramedian sector and part of segment 4 and only rarely drains

segment 6. One or two innominate hepatic veins sometimes drain the superior part of segment 4, and join the trunk (Fig. 21.2). The left hepatic vein usually has a superficial branch, and its trunk is also divided extrahepatically. Dissection is carried out around the junction of the right hepatic vein and trunk with the IVC until an index finger can be inserted between the right hepatic vein and trunk. The Arantius duct is severed at its confluence with the venous trunk, then the dorsal surface of the trunk and ventral surface of the IVC are exposed after dissecting and dividing the cranial portion of the caudate lobe between the trunk and the IVC. The portal vein divides into the right and left portal venous branches at the hepatic hilum in the majority of cases. Alternatively, it trifurcates into the right paramedian, right lateral and left branches, or the right lateral portal vein branches off from the main portal vein. The right paramedian portal venous branch runs in a craniodorsal direction from the hepatic hilum and divides into the dorsal branch of segment 8 and the paramedian portal venous trunk,[5] which divides further into the ventral branch of segment 8 and the branches of segment 5 (Figs 21.3, 21.4). The anterior inferior branch is usually thin and comprises 3–5 branches. The right lateral branch of the right portal vein runs vertically in a dorsal direction from the hepatic hilum and then bifurcates into the segment 6 and 7 branches. The left portal venous branch runs toward the left lateral side of the hepatic hilum (the transverse portion), then vertically in a ventral direction and ends at the cul de sac. The segment 2 branch originates at the corner of the transverse and umbilical portions. The segment 3 and 4 branches arise from the cul de sac. A few portal venous branches to the caudate lobe arise from the craniodorsal side of the right and left portal veins at the hepatic hilum.

DIFFERENTIAL DIAGNOSIS USING INTRAOPERATIVE ULTRASONOGRAPHY

Compared with other imaging modalities, including computed tomography, magnetic resonance imaging and angiography, intraoperative ultrasonography can detect small hepatocellular carcinomas which have been missed preoperatively.[6,7] Hepatic tumors larger than 2 cm can be diagnosed easily using intraoperative ultrasonography alone, as their ultrasonic features are characteristic and reflect their histologic nature. The ultrasonic diagnosis is made on the basis of the following six features: shape of margins, halo, internal echogenicity, anechoic areas, lateral shadows, and posterior echoes. Table 21.1 summarizes the ultrasonic characteristics of hepatocellular carcinomas, hemangiomas, and cholangiocellular carcinomas or secondary liver tumors.[8] Recently, Takayama et al reported malignant transformation of adenomatous hyperplasia to hepatocellular carcinoma[9] and classified the ultrasonic appearances of small hepatic tumors (about 1 cm or less in

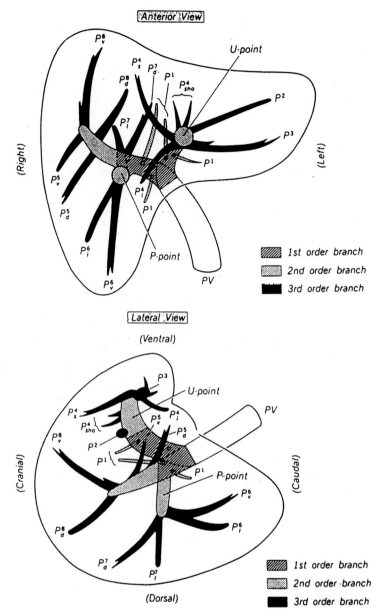

Fig. 21.1   Map of intrahepatic portal venous branches from reference 1).
Anterior and lateral views of the liver. The superscripts refer to the eight hepatic
subsegments and the subscripts to the subsegmental branches named after their
major subsegmental feeding areas – v: ventral; d: dorsal; l: lateral; s: superior;
i: inferior; PV: portal vein; U/P point: umbilical/posterior point; sho: short
branches.

diameter) on the basis of their pathologic diagnoses.
Although adenomatous hyperplasia showed as simple
hypoechoic or hyperechoic nodules, the ultrasonic patterns
of early hepatocellular carcinoma presented as simple hypo-
or hyperechoic, two-layered, or mosaic-like nodules (Fig.
21.5), which suggests that two-layered or mosaic-like
nodules indicate early hepatocellular carcinoma.[10]
However, intraoperative histologic examination of needle
core biopsy of tumor specimens is indispensable for differential diagnosis.

INTERVENTIONAL ASPECTS

Guidance for needle puncture for staining and biopsy procedures

At present, two techniques are available for intraoperative
needle puncture under ultrasonic guidance: one involves
using an adapter for puncture and the other is a free-
hand technique (Fig. 21.6). The free-hand technique is
preferable for needle biopsy in a narrow space or when a
skilful surgeon carries out ultrasound-guided puncture, as

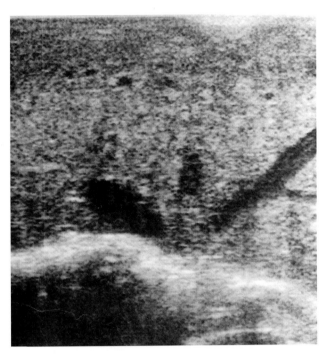

Fig. 21.2 A few innominate veins enter the left, middle, or the confluence of the left and middle hepatic veins.

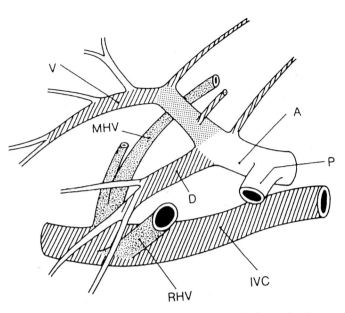

Fig. 21.3 Schema of right anterior segmental standard portal and hepatic venous architecture – RHV: right hepatic vein; MHV: middle hepatic vein; P: posterior portal vein; A: anterior portal vein; D: dorsal branch of the segment 8; V: ventral branch of the segment 8; IVC: inferior vena cava (from reference 14).

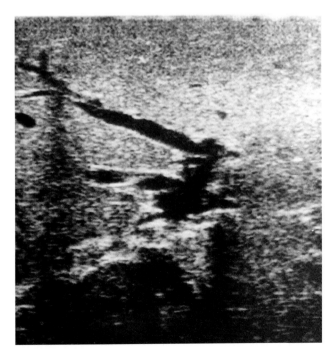

Fig. 21.4 Echogram of the ventral and dorsal portal venous branches of segment 8.

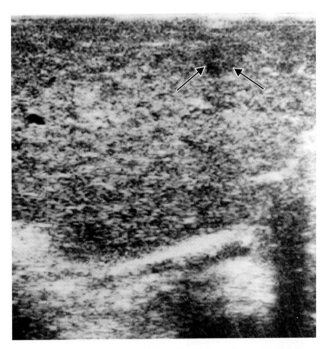

Fig. 21.5 Hypoechoic nodule 13 mm in diameter (arrows), which was confirmed histologically to be a very well differentiated adenocarcinoma (Edmondson's grade I).

Table 21.1 Ultrasononographic characteristics of liver tumors (from reference 8)

Observation feature	Hepatocellular carcinoma	Hemangioma	Cholangiocarcinoma or metastatic liver tumor
Shape of margins	Round and smooth	Fine saw-toothed	Cauliflower-like
Halo	Thin	Absent (echogenic ring is sometimes present)	Thick
Internal echogenicity	Mosaic-like	Hyperechoic (round anechoic area is often seen)	Target appearance
Anechoic area due to liquefactive necrosis	Small, star-shaped, scattered, not central	Absent	Large, round, central
Lateral shadows	Present	Absent	Absent
Posterior echoes	Enhanced	Slight enhancement	Attenuated

fine adjustment of the angle and direction of the needle is limited by using an adapter. A target with a diameter greater than 5 mm can be punctured easily, but when the target size is only a few millimeters, it can be hit and punctured only by the most skillful use of the ultrasound-guided technique. If the ultrasonic image of the needle is lost during insertion, the probe should be tilted to and fro without shifting the position of the scanner, and the needle should be moved 1–2 mm to and fro. Filling the needle's lumen with air facilitates ultrasonic identification of its tip because air is strongly reflective. When a small target is punctured in the longitudinal direction of the probe (Fig. 21.6), the probe should be placed where the clearest ultrasonic image of the target is obtained on the screen, as the highest ultrasonic intensity occurs at the center of the ultrasonic beam. The needle should then be inserted and advanced along this ultrasonic beam plane and its angle and direction adjusted finely (Fig. 21.7). If very clear ultrasonic images of both the target and needle are not obtained, the possibility that the needle has not hit the target, even if the sonogram suggests it has, should be considered.

Staining of the portal area for anatomic hepatectomy

The liver surface has no landmarks reflecting the internal portal area. So, when sectoriectomy of the right liver is carried out, the hepatic arterial and portal venous branches are ligated at the hepatic hilum; ischemic color changes can then be demonstrated on the corresponding liver surfaces, enabling anatomic resection of the required portion of the liver to be carried out. Left liver segments can be discolored by dissecting and ligating the segmental vessels in the

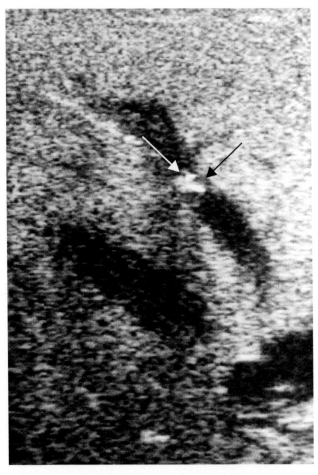

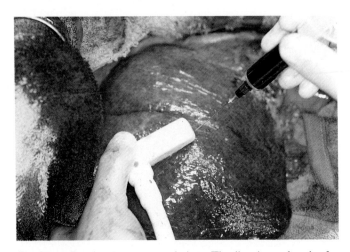

Fig. 21.6 Free-hand puncture technique. The direction and angle of the needle are finely adjusted according to the image on the screen.

Fig. 21.7 The portal venous branch is punctured for portal area staining. The echogenic line (arrow) is a reflection from the needle.

umbilical fossa. It is very difficult to ligate the segmental arterial and portal venous branches at the hepatic hilum in the right liver, and anatomic resection of areas smaller than this sector using the conventional methods described for the right lobe is difficult. Furthermore, accurate identification of the segmental area is particularly difficult in the moderately or severely cirrhotic liver due to its characteristic right lobar atrophy and left lateral sector hypertrophy.

Small portal areas less than the whole sector can be identified using the following staining method.[11] A portal venous branch which feeds the tumor is identified and then punctured 1–2 cm distal from the point to be ligated under ultrasonic guidance; a dye (3–5 ml of indigo-carmine) is then injected at a suitable speed to prevent regurgitation into other portal venous branches that are to be preserved. This stains the liver surface corresponding to the required portal area (Fig. 21.8) and the stained area is marked using electrocautery. Patent-blue is not a suitable stain, as it remains in the body for several days and the patient looks cyanotic after the operation. Indigo-carmine is excreted rapidly from the body and stains as effectively as patent-blue. When the portal area has an arterioportal shunt, the injected dye is regurgitated into the other portal branch, which results in no staining of the required portal area and staining of the other segmental area supplied by the shunt. In such instances, clear staining of the required liver surface is obtained by occluding the relevant hepatic artery at the hepatic hilum or puncturing the arterial branch that feeds the tumor and then injecting the dye. When staining cannot be achieved using these methods, a counterstaining technique can be tried.[12] Other instances of blurred staining or non-staining of the portal area occur when the liver is compressed as a result of high lifting after extensive mobilization, packing with towels or gauze around the liver, or by the ultrasonic probe itself. In such circumstances, puncture is performed using a bent needle to avoid com-

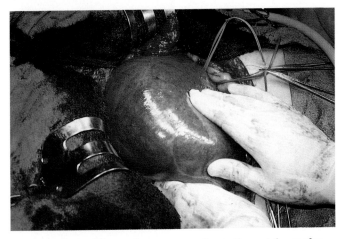

Fig. 21.8 Stained liver surface corresponding to the portal area after dye injection.

pressing the liver after it has been replaced in its natural position. Fibrosis of the liver surface due to previous surgery or peritonitis also results in blurred staining. When multiple portal venous branches are punctured, the dorsal branch should be punctured first, then the ventral one, because small air bubbles entering the ventral branch disturb sound penetration into the deeper hepatic structures. As the hepatic resection volume is restricted in patients with cirrhosis, the appropriate volume to be resected is decided using our hepatic resection criteria published in previous reports.[13] We will describe the resection procedure for segment 8, which is a typical segmentectomy, and caudate lobectomy below.

Resection of segment 8

The standard three-dimensional structure[14] of the hepatic veins and portal venous branches in segment 8 is shown in Figure 21.3. The portal venous branches supplying this segment comprise two main branches (dorsal and ventral branches) (Fig. 21.4), between which, in most cases, a large tributary of the middle hepatic vein runs. In a few cases, the right hepatic vein branch runs there. After identifying the portal area of segment 8 by staining, as described above, the liver parenchyma is resected about 1 cm to the left of Cantlie's line under hemihepatic vascular occlusion of the left liver[15] or using the Pringle maneuver.[16] After about two thirds of the right side of the middle hepatic vein has been exposed, the parenchyma between segments 8 and 5 and between 8 and 7 is transected. The ventral branch of segment 8 is exposed, ligated, and divided, after which parenchymal transection is continued further proximally and the dorsal branch is exposed and divided. When these procedures have been completed, an ischemic color change corresponding to segment 8 is seen on the liver surface. During parenchymal division along the proximal one third of the middle hepatic vein, care should be taken near its confluence with the IVC, where there is usually a large branch of the middle hepatic vein draining segment 8. Next, the parenchymal transection proceeds along the right hepatic vein, which is located 1–2 cm dorsolateral to the ligated point of the dorsal branch.

Intraoperative ultrasound is particularly useful for orientation of the right hepatic vein. For precise anatomic subsegmentectomy, division of the hepatic vein tributaries along the main hepatic vein is required and no Glissonian triads, except their feeding portal pedicles, should be encountered during parenchymal transection. When bleeding from the right hepatic vein near its confluence with the IVC starts, the bleeding point should be compressed by an index finger inserted from behind while lifting the liver ventrally. Bleeding can be minimized using this procedure and safe suture ligations achieved. When segment 8 has been resected completely, the main trunk of the middle and right hepatic veins and two stumps of the segment 8

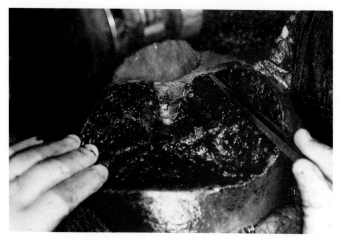

Fig. 21.9 The raw surface of the liver following resection of segment 8. The main trunk of the middle and right hepatic veins and ventral and dorsal branches of the segment 8 portal pedicles can be seen on the raw surface of the liver.

portal pedicles are exposed on the raw surface of the liver (Fig. 21.9).

Caudate lobectomy

Segmental resection of the caudate lobe is a difficult surgical procedure.[17] The caudate lobe comprises three parts: the Spigelian lobe, the caudate process, and the paracaval portion.[18] The cranial portion of the caudate lobe borders the three main hepatic veins, but there is no landmark for its right-hand side margin. The right-hand side border can

be visualized by staining the posterior segment using the counterstaining method. After full mobilization of both the right and left liver from the diaphragmatic attachments and retroperitoneum, both sides of the IVC ligament are divided and the short hepatic veins are dissected and divided from the retrohepatic vena cava right up to the three main hepatic veins. The caudate branches of the hepatic artery and portal vein are dissected, ligated, and divided at the hepatic hilum, and parenchymal transection is performed from both the left- and right-hand sides. Another segmental caudate lobectomy technique (isolated caudate lobectomy using the transhepatic approach) is also available[19] and caudate lobectomy can be combined with other types of hepatic resection in patients with good liver function (Fig. 21.10).

Orientation of the plane to be transected during hepatic parenchymal division

Intraoperative ultrasonic examination is indicated for confirming the distance between the transected point and a tumor, identifying unknown vessels encountered during parenchymal division, and deciding at which point the vessels should be transected. In order to obtain an accurate orientation for parenchymal division, the liver is scanned after replacing the divided surfaces in their natural positions, and the transected plane appears as a glittering line on the sonogram (Fig. 21.11), which is due to a tiny amount of air between the divided surfaces; alternatively, a sonolucent layer due to blood between the raw surfaces of the liver is apparent. When neither a glittering line

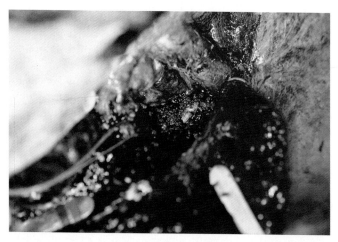

Fig. 21.10 The raw surface of the liver following caudate lobectomy with resection of the right lateral sector. The right hepatic vein is exposed and the retrohepatic vena cava can be seen.

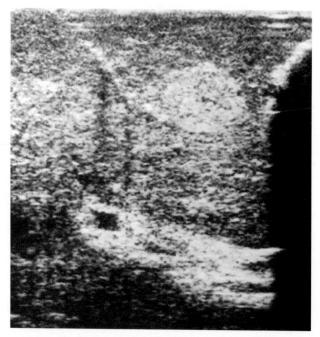

Fig. 21.11 The transected plane of the liver appears as a glittering line when the divided planes are apposed in their natural position.

nor a sonolucent layer is present on the sonogram, the orientation can be confirmed by inserting an index finger between the transected planes and moving it to and fro. In order to avoid the risk of failing to resect a tumor, it is vital to confirm the spatial relationships between the transection point and the tumor repeatedly using ultrasound until the echogenic line of the transected plane has passed over the tumor and reached its other side. When multiple tumors are removed en bloc, repeated visualization of the spatial relationships with ultrasound is particularly important to avoid failing to resect them all. Care should be taken to resect the tumor at its proximal margin, to preserve the hepatic parenchyma, and to prevent tumor exposure and rupture at the resected surface of the specimen.

Examination of the resected specimens to determine whether a tumor has been properly resected

Ultrasonic examination of the resected specimen immersed in saline is important to avoid the risk of failing to resect a tumor and is useful for counting the number of tumors. Furthermore, the distance between the raw surface of the specimen and the tumor can be measured without cutting it (Fig. 21.12).

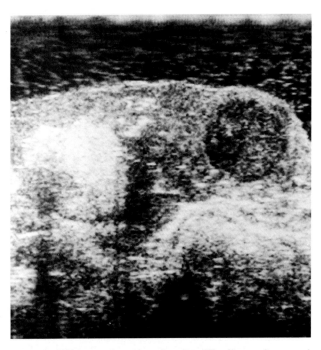

Fig. 21.12 The resected specimen in saline. The distance between the tumor and raw surface and the number of tumors included in the resected specimen can be confirmed using ultrasound.

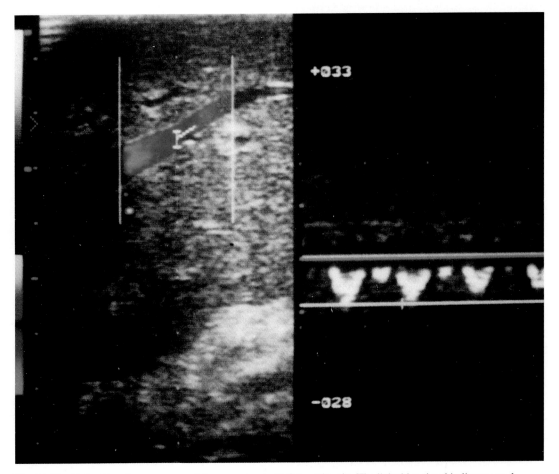

Fig. 21.13 Color Doppler sonogram of the reconstructed left hepatic vein. The light-blue signal indicates good hepatic blood flow and vessel patency.

Intraoperative biliary drainage for jaundiced patients in whom percutaneous transhepatic biliary drainage is difficult

Intraoperative biliary drainage under ultrasonic guidance is a safe procedure for patients with slightly dilated intrahepatic biliary ducts or ascites, in whom percutaneous transhepatic biliary drainage is difficult and dangerous. The technique used for intraoperative biliary drainage is the same as that for needle biopsy, with subsequent insertion of a guide wire through the puncture needle, which is replaced by a polyethylene catheter.

Evaluation of arterial and venous patency and blood flow after reconstruction of the resected vessels

Intraoperative color Doppler ultrasonography has been reported to be useful for identifying thromboses in the hepatic artery, portal venous branch, and hepatic vein during living-related partial-liver transplantation.[20] Extended surgery combined with vascular resection has been indicated for improving the resectability of hepato-pancreatobiliary malignancies which had been thought to be non-resectable. After reconstruction of the resected vessel, its patency can be assessed using color Doppler ultrasonography, which is non-invasive and enables repeated postoperative assessment of blood flow to be carried out easily (Fig. 21.13).

REFERENCES

1. Takayasu K, Moriyama N, Muramatsu Y, Shima Y, Yamada T 1985 Intrahepatic portal vein branches studied by percutaneous transhepatic portography. Radiology 154: 31–36
2. Nakamura S, Tsuzuki T 1981 Surgical anatomy of the hepatic veins. Surg Gynecol Obstet 152: 43–50
3. Makuuchi M, Yamamoto J, Takayama T et al 1991 Extrahepatic division of the right hepatic vein in hepatectomy. Hepatogastroenterology 38: 176–179
4. Makuuchi M, Hasegawa H, Yamazaki S, Bandai Y, Watanabe G, Ito T 1983 The inferior right hepatic vein: ultrasound demonstration. Radiology 148: 213–217
5. Makuuchi M, Hasegawa H, Yamazaki S, Takayasu K 1987 Four new hepatectomy procedures for resection of the right hepatic vein and preservation of the inferior right hepatic vein. Surg Gynecol Obstet 164: 68–72
6. Makuuchi M, Hasegawa H, Yamazaki S, Takayasu K, Moriyama N 1987 The use of operative ultrasound as an aid to liver resection in patients with hepatocellular carcinoma. World J Surg 11: 615–621
7. Sheu J C, Lee C S, Sung J L, Chen D S, Yang P M, Lin T Y 1991 Intraoperative sonography – An indispensable procedure in resection of small hepatocellular carcinoma. Surgery 109: 91–103
8. Makuuchi M 1987 Abdominal intraoperative ultrasonography. Igaku-shoin, Tokyo
9. Takayama T, Makuuchi M, Hirohashi S et al 1990 Malignant transformation of adenomatous hyperplasia to hepatocellular carcinoma. Lancet 336: 1150–1153
10. Takayama T, Makuuchi M, Kosuge T, Yamazaki S, Hasegawa H 1990 Ultrasonographic diagnosis of early hepatocellular carcinoma and borderline lesions. Jpn J Med Ultrason 17 (suppl 1): 109–110 (in Japanese)
11. Makuuchi M, Hasegawa H, Yamazaki S 1985 Ultrasonically guided subsegmentectomy. Surg Gynecol Obstet 161: 346–350
12. Takayama T, Makuuchi M, Watanabe K et al 1991 A new method for mapping hepatic subsegment: counterstaining identification technique. Surgery 109: 226–229
13. Makuuchi M, Takayama T, Yamazaki S, Hasegawa H 1987 Strategy of surgical treatment for hepatocellular carcinoma with liver cirrhosis. Gekasinryo 29: 1530–1536 (in Japanese)
14. Makuuchi M 1986 Standard running of the vessels in the right anterior segment based on ultrasonography. Acta Hepatol Jpn 27: 391 (in Japanese)
15. Makuuchi M, Mori T, Gunven P, Yamazaki S, Hasegawa H 1987 Safety of hemihepatic vascular occlusion during resection of the liver. Surg Gynecol Obstet 164: 155–158
16. Pringle J H 1908 Notes on the arrest of hepatic hemorrhage due to trauma. Ann Surg 48: 541–549
17. Lerut J, Gruwez J A, Blumgart L H 1990 Resection of the caudate lobe of the liver. Surg Gynecol Obstet 171: 160–162
18. Kumon M 1985 Anatomy of the caudate lobe with special reference to portal vein and bile duct. Acta Hepatol Jpn 26: 1193–1199 (in Japanese)
19. Yamamoto J, Takayama T, Kosuge T et al 1992 An isolated caudate lobectomy by the transhepatic approach for hepatocellular carcinoma in cirrhotic liver. Surgery 111: 699–702
20. Kasai H, Makuuchi M, Kawasaki S et al 1992 Intraoperative color Doppler ultrasonography for partial-liver transplantation from the living donor in pediatric patients. Transplantation 54: 173–175

22

Laparoscopic ultrasound

A. Pietrabissa   G. Di Candio   F. Mosca

INTRODUCTION

Over the last few years laparoscopic techniques have become an integral part of general surgical practice throughout the world. As with the laparoscopic approach to gallstone disease, the use of diagnostic laparoscopy to stage and manage abdominal neoplasms is a new and rapidly changing field. The development of these techniques was made possible also by the progress of endo-surgical technology which is still evolving so quickly that no textbook on the topic can be up to date.

A major problem with laparoscopy is the almost complete absence of tactile sensation and a lack of depth perception due to the two-dimensional video representation of three-dimensional anatomy. This may limit the surgeon's ability to define the nature of visualized structures and detect deep lesions. The combination of laparoscopy and ultrasound allows the surgeon to overcome some of these problems, resulting in a diagnostic potential which is stronger than that of either modality alone. It can therefore be speculated that laparoscopic ultrasound will be more valuable than traditional intraoperative ultrasound.

GENERAL ASPECTS OF LAPAROSCOPIC ULTRASOUND

Specially designed ultrasound probes are introduced into the abdominal cavity through 10 mm cannulae. The position of the access cannula is crucial because it will determine the orientation of the rigid probe in relation to the structure to be examined. To obtain the best angle of view with a rigid probe, in fact, it is often necessary to change the direction of the probe by using more than one access cannula. Flexible probes with directable tips have been designed to overcome this problem,[1] but they are in general less handy and more expensive. Before being used the ultrasound probe should be either gas-sterilized or soaked in a disinfecting solution.[2] Disposable sterile covers are not used because they have a high friction coefficient with the inside of the cannula which limits the movement of the probe. Linear array probes with a side viewing capability are better than sector ones as they outline the anatomy in greater detail. Real-time B-mode ultrasound systems are generally used, employing 7.5 MHz transducers which are preferred over ones with lower resolution. Color Doppler imaging systems have also been employed. This adds considerably in the interpretation of the anatomy, particularly when the surgeon is not familiar with ultrasound images. Complete decompression of the stomach and duodenum with a nasogastric tube is recommended during the examination since endoluminal air will impair the formation of ultrasound images. To provide a good acoustic coupling, saline solution is poured into the abdominal cavity. When needed, tilting of the table will move the saline by gravity in the area to be examined. Finally, the availability of a video-editor allows both the video-camera images of the ultrasound probe during the scanning and the ultrasound images that this produces to be displayed simultaneously on the same monitor, thus lowering the degree of hand–eye coordination which is required. Studies of the various application of laparoscopic ultrasound are still in progress.[3–8] In the following paragraphs the current role of this technique and its potential benefits in biliary tract, liver, and pancreatic surgery are discussed.

LAPAROSCOPIC ULTRASOUND IN BILIARY TRACT SURGERY

Laparoscopic cholecystectomy is the new standard treatment for uncomplicated cholelithiasis.[9] The use of diagnostic imaging during biliary tract surgery has always been a controversial issue. Contrast trans-cystic cholangiography is currently advocated as a routine measure in many centers.[10] Others believe that preoperative ultrasound or i.v. cholangiogram may be used instead of intraoperative cholangiography to exclude stones in the common bile duct and define the ductal anatomy.[11,12] Several benefits can be postulated for intraoperative ultrasound routine examination of the bile ducts over trans-cystic cholangiography. These include no need for previous tissue dissection, avoidance of contrast injection, reduced cost, and increased safety. Ultrasound examination avoids radiation exposure to both patient and surgical team, and the possibility of adverse reactions to the contrast medium is obviated. It can be performed more rapidly than radiologic examination, requires fewer consumables, and employs equipment that is usually less expensive than image intensifiers. In addition, useful information on the vascular anatomy of the hepato-duodenal ligament and its frequent anomalies can be obtained.

Longitudinal scanning of the extrahepatic ductal anatomy is first performed, when using a rigid probe, by advancing it through the operative cannula. This is usually located to the left of the midline, below the right costal margin (Fig. 22.1). The ultrasound probe can also be introduced through the infraumbilical cannula, giving sections almost parallel to the common bile duct. Examination of the extrahepatic biliary tree is best achieved with a probe stand-off technique in which the probe is placed one centimeter away from the hepatoduodenal ligament with the interposition of saline solution, thereby avoiding compression and visual distortion of underlying hollow structures (Fig. 22.2).

The potential advantages of laparoscopic ultrasound have to be weighed against its limitations, which include a long learning curve for what is clearly an operator-related test. The infraduodenal common bile duct is not always seen and the intrahepatic ducts are visualized only when dilated. For these reasons it is unlikely that it will replace cholangiography except in those cases in which the contrast

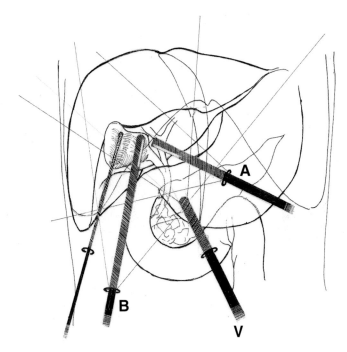

Fig. 22.1   Laparoscopic ultrasound of the hepatoduodenal ligament during biliary surgery. The access cannula acts as a fixed point and the range of movement of the rigid probe is described by a cone. A and B: sites of entrance of the laparoscopic ultrasound probe; V: site of entrance of the telescope.

LAPAROSCOPIC ULTRASOUND IN LIVER SURGERY

The technique of laparoscopic ultrasound of the liver does not differ from what has already been described for traditional intraoperative contact ultrasonography.[14] Its major limitation is again the reduced ability to move the long rigid probe on the surface of the liver as a result of the fixed position of the access cannula.

Ultrasound examination of the liver is very effective in staging primary hepatic tumors and detecting secondary deposits, with a reported accuracy superior to any other imaging technique.[8] However, with the continuous refinement of modern preoperative imaging techniques, the percentage of liver nodules detected only with intraoperative ultrasound has fallen to less than 10% in most institutions. Moreover, since a number of these lesions will require surgical excision and/or palliative management of the primary tumor, the place of laparoscopy to stage these conditions is dependent on the feasibility of a laparoscopic approach for the surgical treatment required. Although isolated cases of laparoscopic hepatectomies have been reported by few institutions, these procedures still have limited application. Similarly, laparoscopic bowel resection is being performed but is not yet clearly safe or advantageous.[9]

A possible future application of laparoscopic ultrasound of the liver will be in the field of cryotherapy of unresectable hepatic lesions. A laparoscopic cryoprobe will be ultrasound guided to the center of the target lesion; the growth of the freeze front, which forms as the tissue around the cryoprobe freezes, will also be monitored with ultrasound.

examination is technically difficult to perform or, at the opposite end of the spectrum, in easy cholecystectomies as a quicker method to exclude unsuspected stones.[13]

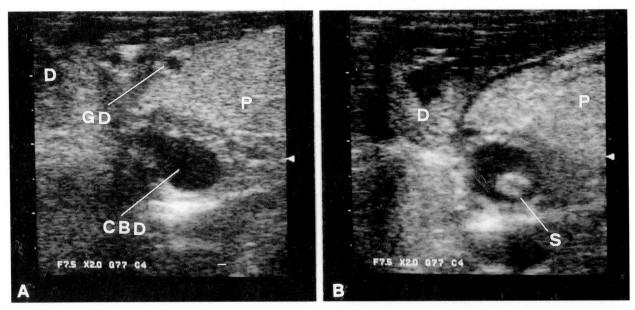

Fig. 22.2   Ultrasound detection of a stone in the distal common bile duct during laparoscopic cholecystectomy. A: dilated CBD above the stone; B: gallstone within the lumen of the distal CBD; D: duodenum; GD: gastroduodenal artery; P: pancreas; S: gallstone.

LAPAROSCOPIC ULTRASOUND IN PANCREATIC SURGERY

Despite modern imaging techniques, accurate preoperative staging of pancreatic cancer remains a common problem. Whilst in colo-rectal and, to some extent, gastric cancer palliative resection plays an important role in preventing and relieving symptoms, in patients with pancreatic cancer the laparoscopic finding of metastatic or locally advanced disease can result in avoidance of major surgery, particularly if endoscopic or percutaneous palliation is available. Local extension of the primary pancreatic tumor and secondary vascular involvement are best assessed with the help of laparoscopic ultrasound. Laparoscopic access to the pancreas can be gained either by a supragastric approach, through the pars flaccida of the lesser omentum,[15] or by an infragastric route.[16–18] The latter entails division of the omentum close to the greater curvature of the stomach and surgical dissection of the anterior surface of the pancreas from the gastric body and antrum. Contact laparoscopic ultrasound scanning of the body and tail of the gland can then be performed by advancing the probe through a 10 mm cannula positioned to the right of the umbilicus (Fig. 22.3). Transverse plane images of the pancreas can be obtained from the neck of the gland to the splenic hilum. Laparoscopic ultrasound assessment of the head of the pancreas should follow a Kocher dissection of the duo-

denum. The probe is then placed face up between the vena cava and the gland. Invasion of the portal vein and superior mesenteric vessels are best assessed through this approach, which requires an umbilical access cannula for the ultrasound probe (Fig. 22.4). Accurate localization of occult insulinoma by laparoscopic ultrasound has also been reported.[19] With new and effective technological innovations, laparoscopic localization of islet cell tumors of the body and tail, followed by laparoscopic excision, will constitute a considerable advance in the management of these patients.

CONCLUSIONS

As the benefits of diagnostic laparoscopy are becoming increasingly clear, the addition of laparoscopic ultrasound examination can offer the best assessment of patients, particularly in the staging of cancer.[20] However, at present, laparoscopic ultrasonography is of value if it can demonstrate unsuspected progression of a tumor, resulting in a decision not to operate. When the surgeon is committed to resection, the role of laparoscopic staging is dependent on the feasibility of proceeding via the laparoscopic approach. Further technological developments will be needed before laparoscopic US can be extensively and permanently employed.

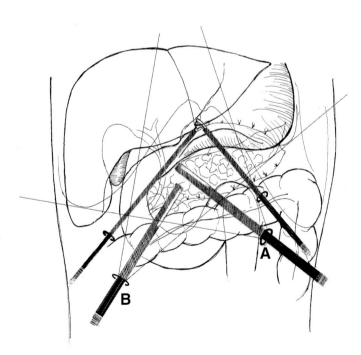

Fig. 22.3 Laparoscopic visual and ultrasound inspection of the pancreatic body and tail through the infragastric approach. A and B: sites of entrance of the laparoscopic ultrasound probe.

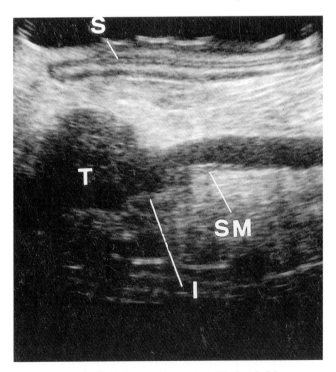

Fig. 22.4 Longitudinal ultrasound scanning of the head of the pancreas. The tumor involves the superior mesenteric vein. S: stomach; T: tumor; I: area of invasion; SM: superior mesenteric vein.

REFERENCES

1. Yamashita Y, Kurohiji T, Hayashi J, Kimitsuki H, Hiraki M, Kagegawa T 1993 Intraoperative ultrasonography during laparoscopic cholecystectomy. Surg Laparosc Endosc 3: 167–171
2. Melzer A, Buess G, Cuschieri A 1992 Instruments for endoscopic surgery. In: Operative manual of endoscopic surgery. Springer-Verlag, Berlin, p 14
3. Yamakawa K, Wagai T 1963 Diagnosis of intra-abdominal lesions by laparoscope. Ultrasonography through laparoscope. Jap J Gastroenterol 55: 741–745
4. Okita K, Kodama T, Oda M et al 1984 Laparoscopic ultrasonography. Diagnosis of liver and pancreatic cancer. Scand J Gastroenterol 19 (suppl 94): 91–100
5. Frank K, Bliesze J A, Bonhof J A et al 1985 Laparoscopic sonography: a new approach to intra-abdominal diseases. JCU 13: 60–65
6. Fornari F, Civardi G, Cavanna L et al 1989 Laparoscopic ultrasonography in the study of liver diseases. Preliminary results. Surg Endosc 3: 33–37
7. Miles W F A, Paterson-Brown S, Garden O J 1992 Laparoscopic contact hepatic ultrasonography. Br J Surg 79: 419–420
8. Cuesta M A, Meijer S, Borgstein P J, Sibinga Mulder L, Sikkenk A C 1993 Laparoscopic ultrasonography for hepatobiliary and pancreatic malignancy. Br J Surg 80: 1571–1574
9. Warshaw A L 1993 Reflections on laparoscopic surgery. Editorial. Surgery 114: 629–630
10. Sackier M J, Berci G, Phillips E, Carrol B, Shapiro S, Paz-Partlow M 1991 The role of cholangiography in laparoscopic cholecystectomy. Arch Surg 126: 1021–1026
11. Metcalf A M, Ephgrave K S, Dean T R, Maher J W 1992 Preoperative screening with ultrasonography for laparoscopic cholecystectomy: an alternative to routine intraoperative cholangiography. Surgery 112: 813–817
12. Barkun J S, Fried G M, Barkun A N et al 1993 Cholecystectomy without operative cholangiography. Implications for common bile duct injury and retained common bile duct stones. Ann Surg 218: 371–379
13. Cuschieri A, Berci G 1992 Laparoscopic biliary surgery. Blackwell Scientific, Oxford, pp 189–190
14. Machi J, Sigel B, Zaren H A, Kurohiji T, Yamashita Y 1993 Operative ultrasonography during hepatobiliary and pancreatic surgery. World J Surg 17: 640–646
15. Meyer-Burg J, Ziegler U, Palma C 1969 Zur supragastralen pancreaskopie. Ergebnisse aus 125 laparoscopien. Dtsch Med Wochenschr 97: 1969
16. Strauch M, Lux G, Ottenjann R 1973 Infragastric pancreascopy. Endoscopy 5: 30
17. Cuschieri A, Hall A W, Clark J 1978 Value of laparoscopy in the diagnosis and management of pancreatic carcinoma. Gut 19: 672–677
18. Cuschieri A 1988 Laparoscopy for pancreatic cancer: does it benefit the patient? Eur J Surg Oncol 14: 41–44
19. Pietrabissa A, Shimi S M, Vander Velpen G, Cuschieri A 1993 Localization of insulinoma by laparoscopic infragastric inspection of the pancreas and contact ultrasonography. Surg Oncol 2: 83–86
20. Easter D W, Cuschieri A, Nathanson L K et al 1992 The utility of diagnostic laparoscopy for abdominal disorders. Audit of 120 patients. Arch Surg 127: 379

INDEX

Numbers in bold print refer to illustrations and their captions.